Lee's
Synopsis of
Anaesthesia

Twelfth edition

To our wives:
Gill Rushman, Juliet Davies and Kate Cashman

Among the experiments that may be tried on man, those that can only harm are forbidden; those that are innocent are permissible; those that are beneficial are obligatory. – Claude Bernard (1813–1878)

A new scientific truth does not triumph because it convinces its opponents making them see the light, but rather because its opponents eventually die and a new generation grows up that is familiar with it. – Max Plank (1858–1947)

Eternal vigilance is the price of safety.

Primum non nocere – First of all, do no harm.

The proper dose of any drug is enough.

Knowledge is of two kinds; we know a subject ourselves or we know where we can get information about it. – Samuel Johnson (1709–1784)

Worry enough, but not too much. – C. L. Hewer

I esteem it the office of the physician not only to restore health but to mitigate pain and dolors. – Francis Bacon

The relief of pain is purchased always at a price. – Ralph Waters

Lee's
Synopsis of
Anaesthesia

G. B. Rushman MB BS FRCA
Consultant Anaesthetist, Southend Hospital, UK

N. J. H. Davies MA DM MRCP FRCA
Consultant Anaesthetist, Southampton General Hospital, UK

J. N. Cashman BSc MD FRCA
Consultant Anaesthetist, St George's Hospital, London, UK

Twelfth edition

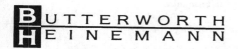
BUTTERWORTH
HEINEMANN

OXFORD AUCKLAND BOSTON JOHANNESBURG MELBOURNE NEW DELHI

Butterworth-Heinemann
Linacre House, Jordan Hill, Oxford OX2 8DP
225 Wildwood Avenue, Woburn, MA 01801-2041
A division of Reed Educational and Professional Publishing Ltd

 A member of the Reed Elsevier plc group

By J. Alfred Lee
First edition 1947
Second edition 1950
Third edition 1953
Reprinted with
minor amendments 1955

Reprinted 1956
Reprinted 1957
Fourth edition 1959
Reprinted 1960
Italian first edition 1963

By J. Alfred Lee and
R. S. Atkinson
Fifth edition 1964
Spanish edition 1966
Sixth edition 1968
Seventh edition 1973
French edition 1975
Portuguese edition 1976
German edition 1977

By R. S. Atkinson, G. B. Rushman and J. Alfred Lee
Eighth edition 1977
Reprinted 1979
Ninth edition 1982
Tenth edition 1987

Greek edition 1979
Polish edition 1981
Spanish second edition 1981
Italian second edition 1986
German second edition 1986

By R. S. Atkinson, G. B. Rushman
  and N. J. H. Davies
Eleventh edition 1993
Reprinted 1993, 1994

By G. B. Rushman, N. J. H. Davies
  and J. N. Cashman
Twelfth edition 1999
Reprinted 2000

© Reed Educational and Professional Publishing Ltd 1999

British Library Cataloguing in Publication Data
A catalogue record for this book is available from the British Library

Library of Congress Cataloguing in Publication Data
A catalogue record for this book is available from the Library of Congress

ISBN 0 7506 3247 X
ISBN 0 7506 3248 8 (Butterworth-Heinemann International Edition)

Typeset by BC Typesetting, Bristol
Printed and bound in Great Britain by MPG Books Ltd, Bodmin, Cornwall

Contents

SECTION 4   ANAESTHESIA FOR VARIOUS SURGICAL OPERATIONS AND SITUATIONS

SECTION 5   REGIONAL TECHNIQUES

SECTION 6   CHRONIC PAIN

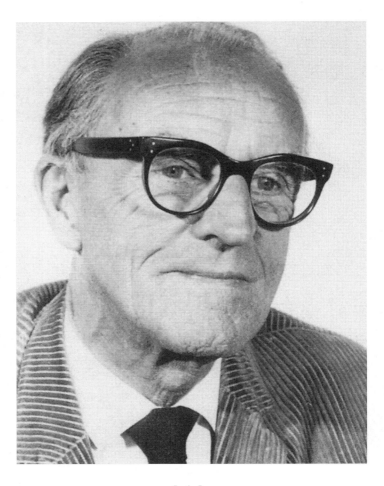

J. A. Lee

John Alfred Lee
(1906–1989)

Alfred Lee was born near Liverpool in 1906 and qualified from Newcastle upon Tyne, in 1927. His early experience of anaesthesia was that expected of the House Surgeon of that time, usually an open-drop method and occasionally a primitive Boyles machine or a Clovers inhaler. After moving to Southend-on-Sea as a general practitioner, he continued to maintain an interest in anaesthesia and took up anaesthetic sessions at the hospital. In 1939, on the outbreak of hostilities, Alfred Lee became a wholetime specialist in the Emergency Medical Service, working at Runwell Hospital, near Southend. In 1948, the inauguration of the National Health Service enabled him to become a Consultant Anaesthetist, a post he held up to his retirement in 1971, when he became Honorary Consulting Anaesthetist. He continued his interest in anaesthesia and travelled extensively, attending many regional, national and international meetings right up to the month of his death in April 1989.

After the war years, there was a return of anaesthetists from the Services to civilian life. There were few texts on anaesthesia for them and Alfred Lee approached John Wright and Sons Ltd of Bristol who asked him to submit some specimen chapters. The result was the publication of '*A Synopsis of Anaesthesia*' in 1947. Alfred Lee was to participate in 11 editions over the next 40 years, some being translated into Italian, Spanish, French, Portuguese, German, Greek and Polish. He was also the author of many papers, wrote and edited a number of other texts and was for a time Assistant Editor and later Chairman of the Editorial Board of '*Anaesthesia*'. His special interests included pre-operative care (he started an outpatient clinic for the pre-operative assessment of patients), postoperative care (Southend was the first non-specialist hospital to have a Postoperative Observation Ward adjacent to the theatres), regional analgesia (he advocated and taught extradural block long before it became common practice) and history (he was the first President of the History of Anaesthesia Society).

He examined for the Final Fellowship Examination, was a member of the Board of Faculty of Anaesthetists, and President of the Association of Anaesthetists of Great Britain and Ireland. He served as President of the Section of Anaesthetics of the Royal Society of Medicine and in 1975 received the Hickman Medal. He was an Honorary Fellow of the Faculty of Anaesthetists of the Royal College of Surgeons in Ireland (1970), Gaston Labat

Lecturer to the American Society of Regional Anesthesia (1985), Thomas Seldon Lecturer to the International Research Society (1985), and Koller Gold Medallist and Lecturer in Vienna (1984) to commemorate the centenary of local analgesia.

Preface to the twelfth edition

In this 12th Edition of *Lee's Synopsis of Anaesthesia*, there has been total revision of the structure and text. The history of anaesthesia has been removed and published as a separate volume, *Short History of Anaesthesia*. Intensive Care has been removed now that there are clear and authoritative texts in this subject. In recent years there has been a revolution in the area of references to published articles; the Internet and Search systems such as Medline now provide a source of recent references on every subject in Medicine, anywhere in the world. However, there is as yet no vetting system on the accuracy or validity of the mountain of information available by this route. The Synopsis continues to provide the orthodoxy, the breadth of experience and the wisdom which are the springboard for exploration on the information superhighway.

This book is about practical anaesthesia, where the art as well as the science is essential to success. We have tried to indicate these professional skills throughout the book, while being very conscious that authors too, are lifelong students. It has been forged on the floors of the theatre and the ward, where the yawning gaps between the ideal world of the textbook or the courtroom, and the real world are only too apparent.

The 'Synopsis' has become smaller and more vigorous in the area of practical anaesthesia and pain management, and continues to provide ready access of the relevant information and advice. The reduced bulk of the book makes it more portable and easier to place in the pocket, on the anaesthetic machine, and on the office table.

In this edition we bid farewell to Dr R. S. Atkinson, who has co-authored the Synopsis, with distinction, for 30 years with generosity, charm, humour and the wisdom born of long experience. We wish him a very long and happy retirement. We welcome Dr Jeremy Cashman of St. George's Hospital, London, as co-author, who brings a wealth of editorial and teaching experience.

GBR
NJHD
JNC

From the preface to the first edition

This book is not designed to take the place of larger textbooks of anaesthesia and analgesia. It is a summary of current teaching and practice, and it is hoped that it will serve the student, the resident anaesthetist, the practitioner and the candidate studying for the Diploma in Anaesthetics as a ready source of reference and a quick means of revision.

January 1947   JAL

Acknowledgements

Dr Thomas Boulton, whose long association with the authors of this book has been a help and encouragement; Dr David Zideman for much helpful advice on resuscitation, Dr Frank Walters, for stimulation, inspiration and new ideas; Dr S. Yentis, for advice about management of obstetrics; Dr Simon Dolin for the chronic pain section; Wendy Robson, Head nurse, Recovery room, Wellesley Hospital, Melanie Tait and Myriam Brearley, of Butterworth-Heinemann for much help with the practical aspects of publishing.

Section 1
WARD CARE

Preoperative assessment and premedication

Assessment of a patient about to undergo an operation is the foundation of an anaesthetist's good clinical practice. This should include development of a professional relationship, a medical history, relevant physical examination, checking the results of tests or investigations, and prescribing any drugs for premedication (if needed). It also allows the patient to ask questions, and express any anxieties. The anaesthetist will wish to explain to the patient what will happen before and after the operation.

We should also plan the anaesthetic technique, and include any special techniques (e.g. controlled hypotension, regional blockade, etc.). The anaesthetist should also consider whether to discuss any risks and complications that may result from the proposed anaesthetic technique, so as to enable informed consent.

There are several ways of organizing preoperative assessment. It may take place in a special anaesthetic out-patient clinic, which can be helpful in preventing late cancellations.[1] Assessment may also be part of a surgical out-patient clinic, or done when an in-patient. The patient should be asked to complete a medical questionnaire, or have been taken through one by a suitably trained nurse[2] (Fig. 1.1.1).

Patients have a full responsibility to tell doctors and nurses about all their diseases and conditions. The incidence of medical disease in surgical patients is high. A **preoperative consultation** in the ward or in an anaesthetic out-patient clinic allows special investigations to be ordered, autologous blood donation organized, and treatment started to render the patient as fit as possible by the time he or she is admitted to hospital. When necessary, the patient can be followed up by repeated attendances at the clinic. In-patient stay may thus be reduced. Optimization of the condition of sick patients may usefully be done in the intensive care unit.

The admission of patients on the morning of even major surgery is common, and tends to trap the unwary anaesthetist into rushing the assessment. Enough time must be allowed to ensure the assessment is adequate and up-to-date, even when the operating schedule is produced late or a patient is added. The anaesthetist is often the final safeguard that prevents dangerous surgical practice. Beware the 'I'll see them in the anaesthetic room' trap!

Date:

Name:

Age, weight, height:

Surgeon, proposed operation:

Have you had an anaesthetic before?

Have you or your relatives had a complication from an anaesthetic?

Have you got any crowns, caps or bridges on your teeth?

Have you got any loose teeth?

Are you allergic to any medicines? If so, give details

Do you, or did you smoke? If so, how much?

Do you get short of breath after climbing stairs? If so, how many stairs, how fast?

Have you ever had:
   High blood pressure   Hepatitis
   Pain in the chest   Diabetes
   Heart disease   Asthma
   Epilepsy   Bronchitis
   Bleeding problems   Tuberculosis
   Other medical condition?

Do any medical conditions run in your family? If so, give details

Are you on the pill?

Are you taking any medicines? If so, give details

Do you take aspirin? If so, when was the last dose?

Is there anything else the anaesthetist might need to know about you?

If the answer to any of these questions is yes, please give a few details.

Figure 1.1.1 Preoperative assessment questionnaire

There is, however, a yawning gap between the ideal situation and the real, practical world of the busy hospital the relevant risks of anaesthesia are explained.

HISTORY (Fig. 1.1.2)

Check the medical notes, and with the patient for the following.

1 General medical and surgical history. Ask especially for respiratory symptoms (such as shortness of breath, cough, sputum, wheezing), and those relating to the cardiovascular system (such as angina, orthopnoea, ankle swelling, previous myocardial infarction).
2 Previous anaesthetics, and any ill-effects. Nausea and vomiting after anaesthesia will affect the choice of anaesthetic and analgesic drugs.
3 Drug therapy, including oral contraceptives. Aspirin is often a component of non-prescription medicines.
4 Does the patient take aspirin, bruise easily, or bleed for a long time when cut?
5 Excessive alcohol intake. The alcoholic patient may suffer from cirrhosis of the liver, cardiomyopathy, diminished adrenocortical response to stress, electrolyte imbalance, hypoglycaemia, bone marrow depression, neuropathy and psychosis.
6 Allergies.
7 Pregnancy. Non-urgent surgery may need to be postponed if pregnancy is suspected.
8 Smoking history.
9 Loose teeth, crowns, bridge-work and dentures.
10 Time of last intake of food and drink.
11 A consent form, signed by patient and surgeon.
12 Appropriate laboratory findings, results of special tests, e.g. echocardiography, and availability of cross-matched blood, if required.

Note that patients may not always tell doctors about their disabilities, particularly if they are afraid of having their operation cancelled.

PHYSICAL EXAMINATION

This will be guided by the surgery to be performed and, most importantly, by the patient's medical history. The following are of particular interest to the anaesthetist.

1 Respiratory system: cyanosis, finger clubbing, pattern of breathing, mediastinal shift, localizing signs, presence of added sounds on auscultation.
2 Cardiovascular system: pulse (rate, rhythm and character), venous pressure and character, peripheral dependent oedema, blood pressure, apex beat, thrills, extra heart sounds and murmurs.

Patients with serious heart disease may have no symptoms whatsoever! In particular, this is true of severe aortic stenosis (which may be detected by the slow-rising pulse and small pulse pressure), myocardial ischaemia and hypertension. The first reading of blood pressure taken on admission is often high in an anxious patient, but this does necessarily mean an increased risk to the patient.[3] If lability of blood pressure persists in subsequent readings, the morbidity is similar to that in the known hypertensive patient. The risks of surgery and anaesthesia in patients with congestive cardiac failure are very high. Patients with cardiac prostheses on anticoagulant therapy should be changed from warfarin to the relatively short-acting heparin, so that their anticoagulation can be stopped for a minimum time.

3 State of nutrition, malnutrition or obesity.
4 Skin colour, especially pallor, cyanosis, jaundice or pigmentation.
5 Psychological state of the patient, degree of anxiety.
6 The airway. Assess the difficulty of airway maintenance and laryngoscopy, even if intubation is not planned (*see* Chapter 2.6). Assess the dentition, e.g. prominent or loose teeth, caps, crowns, veneers, bridge-work, especially at the front. Their presence should be recorded, and the patient usually warned of possible damage.
7 Ease of venous cannulation.

INVESTIGATIONS

The anaesthetist is advised against accepting patients for elective surgery unless the appropriate investigations are available. The simpler tests that are often indicated include the following.

1 Urine tests, especially for sugar, ketones and protein.
2 Haemoglobin and blood count, including Sickledex tests for patients at risk of carrying the sickle cell gene.
3 Blood urea (or creatinine) and electrolytes, especially if the patient may have renal impairment, is taking drugs that affect electrolyte balance (such as diuretics), or before surgery that will interrupt oral feeding post-operatively.
4 Other biochemical screening tests are sometimes justified, e.g. blood glucose.
5 Electrocardiogram, in patients with suspected cardiovascular disease. Some authorities recommend routine electrocardiograms (ECGs) on all patients over a certain age, since abnormalities are picked up increasingly as patients get older.
6 Chest radiograph. Seldom indicated purely for the purposes of anaesthetic assessment of a patient who is undergoing non-thoracic surgery. It is more likely to be useful in the elderly. The history, physical examination and, if indicated, echocardiography are probably better at detecting and quantifying abnormalities that will influence anaesthetic technique. A chest radiograph will be useful if lung bullae are suspected.

7 Simple lung function tests, such as forced expiratory volume in 1 second, vital capacity and peak expiratory flow rate can be readily performed at the bedside using pocket-sized spirometers and a Wright peak flowmeter.
8 Bedside pulse oximetry. The measurement of arterial O_2 saturation breathing air and a high O_2 concentration gives a useful and rapid index of pulmonary gas exchange.
9 Echocardiogram. This is a useful non-invasive test that shows anatomical abnormalities in the heart, assesses ventricular function and pressure gradients across stenosed valves, and detects valvular regurgitation. It can be done at the bedside, but needs expensive equipment and a skilled operator.
10 Other special investigations may be ordered where indicated.

Medical conditions?	Medication?
Previous anaesthetics?	Fasting?
State of teeth	Blood tests?
Pre-surgical complications?	Airway problems?

Figure 1.1.2 Simple questions for the preoperative assessment

ASSESSMENT OF 'PHYSICAL STATUS'

The American Society of Anesthesiologists (ASA) classified patients into a number of grades according to their general condition.[4]

ASA 1: The patient has no organic, physiological, biochemical or psychiatric disturbance. The pathological process for which operation is to be performed is localized and does not entail a systemic disturbance.

ASA 2: Mild to moderate systemic disturbance caused either by the condition to be treated surgically or by other pathophysiological processes, e.g. mild organic heart disease, diabetes, mild hypertension, anaemia, old age, obesity, mild chronic bronchitis.

ASA 3: Limitation of lifestyle. Severe systemic disturbance or disease from whatever cause, even though it may not be possible to define the degree of disability with any finality, e.g. angina, severe diabetes, and cardiac failure.

ASA 4: Severe systemic disorders that are already life-threatening, not always correctable by operation, e.g. marked cardiac insufficiency, persistent angina, severe respiratory, renal or hepatic insufficiency.

ASA 5: Moribund. Little chance of survival, but submitted to operation in desperation. Little if any anaesthesia is required.

If the operation is an emergency, the letter E is placed beside the numerical classification, and the patient is considered to be in poorer physical condition.

The ASA scheme is the most commonly used system for describing the physical condition of a patient, although different anaesthetists do not always agree about the classification of a particular patient. The ASA grading does not cope with an asymptomatic patient who, for example, may have severe coronary artery disease. It also ignores the added insults and risks of the proposed operation. It is therefore not synonymous with the risk of perioperative morbidity and mortality.

Many other schemes of assessment have been invented and are useful.

The special needs of patients who have suffered trauma, or who are due for other emergency surgery are considered in Chapters 4.1 and 4.4.

SOME COMMON PREOPERATIVE PROBLEMS

Some common problems may need attention before elective surgery.

Poor dentition is likely to be less at risk of damage if the patient seeks the opinion of a dentist.

Smoking needs to be stopped 6 weeks before operation to minimize pulmonary complications of surgery, which include infection, laryngospasm and bronchospasm. Stopping for just 12 h prevents the adverse effects of carbon monoxide and nicotine on myocardial oxygen supply and demand.[5] Stopping for a few days will improve ciliary activity. Smoking may also interfere with wound healing. If children are passively exposed to the smoking habits of others, it increases the incidence of airway complications if they have a general anaesthetic.[6]

Malnutrition may need correction with an appropriate diet, vitamins, etc. Intravenous feeding may be useful preoperatively in, for example, carcinoma of the oesophagus.

Obesity is a common enemy of both surgeon and anaesthetist. Treated properly by a 1000-kcal diet, excellent results may be obtained, even in the few weeks at the anaesthetist's disposal. The patient should be referred to a dietician. 'Whatever the quantity that a man eats, it is plain that if he is too fat, he has eaten more than he should have done' (Samuel Johnson, 1709–1784). One definition is a body mass index (weight in kilograms divided by the square of the height in metres) exceeding 30. The morbidly obese are over twice their ideal weight.

Oxygen consumption is increased, chest (and even lung) compliance reduced, increasing the work of breathing. The diaphragm is displaced headwards, and functional residual capacity is reduced below closing volume. Hypoxaemia develops, exacerbated by anaesthesia, the supine or Trendelenburg positions. Postoperative chest complications are common. Hypoxic pulmonary arterial constriction with right ventricular strain. A few obese patients develop the Pickwickian syndrome – somnolence due to chronic hypercapnia and hypoxia.[7] Total blood volume, blood pressure and cardiac output and work are increased. Coronary disease, stroke, postoperative thrombosis and varicose veins are common.

There may be a hiatus hernia, a higher volume of resting gastric juice which has a lower pH than normal (antacid and H_2-antagonist prophylaxis may be useful). There is an increased incidence of burst abdomen and the possibility of diabetes, cholelithiasis, gout, hepatic and renal dysfunction.

Obese patients are difficult to nurse, move, lift and position on the table. There is less tolerance of Trendelenburg and lithotomy positions. Venesection and placement of needles for regional analgesia are awkward. Intended intramuscular injections may be placed subcutaneously. It is difficult to maintain patent airway. The need for tracheal intubation is increased and because of short thick neck this may be troublesome; awake intubation under local anaesthesia may even be needed. Access by the surgeon to the abdomen, chest and mouth is difficult. If the blood pressure cuff is too small for an obese arm, inaccuracies will result. Intra-arterial monitoring may be preferred. There are similar problems with tourniquets. The volume of the epidural space is decreased, reducing requirements for local analgesics.

Psychological factors. Occasionally patients are terrified of anaesthesia, or of a particular anaesthetic technique (face mask, spinal anaesthesia). A little time spent in discussion with these patients is invaluable and may even help some patients to agree to a necessary operation.

Preoperative preparation of specific medical diseases is discussed in Section 3.

SHOULD OPERATIONS BE POSTPONED OR EVEN REFUSED?

The anaesthetist frequently has to make a decision about whether a patient is fit for surgery, or whether they should be postponed or even denied possible anaesthesia. This calls for skilful judgement, and the safety of the patient must be the overriding concern. Although considerable risks may have to be taken, they should not be taken unless the perceived benefits clearly exceed these risks. There should be full discussion with the patient and perhaps the relatives. Patients may want to take serious risks because they believe that they personally will not die as a result.

An elective operation should always be postponed if there has been insufficient time for adequate preparation. The anaesthetist must be firm with his or her surgical colleagues in this regard! Postponement may also be needed when postoperative facilities, such as an intensive care bed, are temporarily inadequate. As a last resort, consider transfer to another hospital.

Decisions about postponement or cancellation of surgery call for great tact with all those affected, and must be tightly argued. Subsequently, the patient may be accepted by another (often less experienced) anaesthetist without being informed about the previous cancellation! It may be humbling to discover that your colleague 'got away with' the risks you thought were unjustified.

THE EFFECTS OF PRE-EXISTING DRUG THERAPY

Antihypertensive drugs are normally continued up to the time of surgery. Adequate therapy restores a normal blood volume, and minimizes the risk of a dangerous fall of arterial pressure at induction of anaesthesia. Preinduction volume loading goes some way to preventing such a fall, and the avoidance of hypovolaemia during surgery is important. Bradycardia is common in those taking beta-blocking drugs.

Alternative parenteral medication may be needed for those antihypertensives which are oral-only drugs, e.g. angiotensin-converting enzyme (ACE) inhibitors.

Antianginal drugs such as calcium-channel blockers or nitrates (GTN) should not be stopped before surgery without a very specific reason, or angina may recur. If the oral route is impossible, transdermal glyceryl trinitrate patch dressings placed on the lateral chest wall last about 24 h. Reapplication should be at a fresh site. Sublingual GTN spray may be used for fast onset of action.

Lithium should be stopped 2 days before major surgery as it potentiates the non-depolarizing group of relaxants, and in emergency cases suxamethonium and regional blocks should be considered as alternatives. Lithium toxicity may occur when the patient is dehydrated. It is generally safe to continue lithium therapy before minor surgery, provided that due attention is paid to fluid and electrolyte balance.

Monoamine oxidase (MAO) inhibitors type A such as phenelzine, isocarboxazid, and especially tranylcypramine, should be discontinued 2 weeks before elective surgery. The mode of action of this group of drugs is imperfectly understood and cannot be explained solely in terms of MAO inhibition. Reactions to pethidine, and to a lesser extent to fentanyl and morphine, have been reported in patients taking these drugs and deaths have occurred. They include coma, muscle twitching, hypotension, ataxia, ocular palsies and cerebral excitement. Relief has been obtained following administration of 25 mg of chlorpromazine. Not all patients show adverse reactions, and small test doses of pethidine have been given, with monitoring of pulse and blood pressure. Severe hypertensive effects and even death may occur when pressor drugs (e.g. the adrenaline in local analgesic solutions) are given to patients on MAO-A inhibitors, but may be counteracted by phentolamine.

For postoperative analgesia in patients receiving MAO-A inhibitors, a combination of chlorpromazine and codeine has been used without ill effect. Regional blocks and non-steroidal anti-inflammatory drugs (NSAIDs) are also suitable.

Reversible MAO-A inhibitors (moclobemide) and *MAO-B inhibitors* (selegiline) are considered very much less dangerous during anaesthesia, although caution is still needed. The reversible inhibitors may be continued up to the day before surgery.

Selective serotonin uptake inhibitors are used commonly in depression and obsessive–compulsive disorders, e.g. fluoxetine (Prozac), sertraline, fluvoxamine. They have half-lives of several days, and can inhibit the metabolism of benzodiazepines. There are few other implications for the anaesthetist (unless taken in overdose), although the syndrome of inappropriate antidiuretic hormone (ADH) secretion has been described in the elderly, and rarely, platelet function is impaired.[8]

Disulphiram (Antabuse) blocks the normal metabolism of alcohol causing an accumulation of acetaldehyde. There may be a synergistic depressant effect with thiopentone.

Levodopa should be continued up to the time of surgery to prevent the recurrence of severe Parkinsonism, dysphagia and the risk of aspiration pneumonia. Butyrophenones antagonize the action of levodopa on dopaminergic receptors in the brain and should be used with caution.

Steroid therapy. Normal secretion of hydrocortisone from the adrenal cortex is 20 mg/day, but can rise to 300–500 mg/day in response to the stress of trauma or surgery. Steroid therapy suppresses adrenocorticotrophic hormone (ACTH) production by the anterior pituitary. In time the adrenal cortex atrophies and is thus unable to increase its secretion in response to this stress. This can result in profound hypotension during and after anaesthesia, with a decreased sensitivity to catecholamines. The first death from this cause was reported in 1952 following therapeutic doses of cortisone.[9] As short a course as 1 week may produce this depression of the cortex. Depression usually recovers by 2 months after stopping steroids, but may last over 1 year, and in some cases of prolonged therapy may never recover. There are no satisfactory simple tests for adrenocortical reserve.

Thus, it is generally safer to assume some diminution of adrenal reserve, and to give extra hydrocortisone over the period of surgery, e.g. hydrocortisone 100 mg i.m. just before surgery, and continued 6- to 8-hourly for 24 h after minor surgery such as hernia repair, or for 3 days in the case of major surgery. Intramuscular injections give more sustained plasma level than the intravenous route. Corticosteroids are often contraindicate patients with active infections, tuberculosis, peptic ulcer. They can aggra diabetes mellitus.

Insulin: see Chapter 3.1.

Oestrogen-containing ('combined') oral contraceptives increase the risk of deep venous thrombosis. Surgery and the combined pill both reduce the activity of antithrombin III. The risk is greatest following major pelvic, orthopaedic and cancer operations, and in those patients with Factor V Leiden mutation etc.

Combined pills should, if possible, be discontinued 4 weeks before major elective surgery or leg surgery such as varicose veins, and started again at the first period following an interval of 2 weeks after the operation providing that the patient is fully mobile. Should this not be possible, e.g. because of urgent surgery, prophylactic low-dose heparin should be considered. Additional risk factors are older age groups, obesity and cigarette smoking.

Progesterone-only pills or hormone replacement therapy need no special precautions to be taken.

THE DAY OF OPERATION

Food should be withheld for 6 h and clear fluids for 3 h before an operation in adults.[10] Excessive starvation and dehydration are to be avoided, especially in infants, who may suffer dangerous hypoglycaemia. Children are often given a clear drink 2 h before anaesthesia if there are no complicating factors. In all cases, trauma, labour, anxiety or prior administration of morphine are likely to greatly delay gastric emptying, and it should be assumed that the patient has a full stomach.

Lipstick, nail varnish and other cosmetics should be removed before the patient comes to theatre so that the anaesthetist can readily appreciate cyanosis etc. Dentures, artificial limbs, artificial eyes, contact lenses, etc. should be removed before the journey to the theatre, although some dentures can be useful to protect a solitary vulnerable tooth. Hearing aids may often be retained by the patient to help communication in the recovery area. The patient (and anaesthetist!) should not come to theatre with a full bladder.

Two identification labels are tied around the wrist or ankle, stating the name and hospital number. The site of operation should be marked on the patient's skin with ink by the surgeon. The availability of blood must be checked.

On arrival in theatre, the completed consent form and ID labels are inspected, and the patient asked to state their name and operation. More detailed consent forms may be required, e.g. for research procedures, sterilization, termination of pregnancy, and Jehovah's Witnesses. This is the responsibility of the surgical team.

PREMEDICATION

> Empirical procedures, firmly entrenched in the habits of good doctors, seem to have a vigour and life, not to say immortality of their own.
>
> (H. K. Beecher)

Reasons for administration of premedicants

1 To reduce fear and anxiety.
2 To reduce saliva secretion.
3 To prevent vagal reflexes, due to surgical stimulation, (e.g. squint operations, stretching of anal sphincter), or associated with medication (e.g. beta-blockers).
4 For specific therapeutic effects, e.g. steroids, H_2 blockers, transdermal glyceryl trinitrate patch dressings (Transiderm-Nitro), and potentially many other drugs.[11]

Sedative premedication does not lessen the need for kind, sympathetic care for patients at a time of great stress.

Drugs used for premedication

Sedatives

Benzodiazepines or phenothiazines are most commonly used. Patients in hot climates are more sensitive to sedative premedication than those living in temperate zones, due to their reduced basal metabolic rate. Sedative action is helped by the oral administration of a suitable benzodiazepine hypnotic the night before operation. Zopiclone 7.5 mg is a safe non-benzodiazepine alternative. Clonidine has been used to decrease requirements of volatile anaesthetics.[12]

BENZODIAZEPINES

These are all good premedicants, and can be given orally producing sedation, amnesia and freedom from anxiety. The chief difference between them is their duration of action, and they can be used singly or in combination. They can be combined with oral analgesics to add background analgesia for the operation. They have only a minor effect on the cardiovascular system and respiration, but do potentiate propofol and thiopentone. Patients who are already regular takers of benzodiazepines will be resistant to the action of these drugs.

Benzodiazepines have been given by other routes (such as intramuscularly or rectally). They all inhibit γ-aminobutyric acid (GABA) receptors, and have anticonvulsant properties. The amnesia produced is anterograde, and lasts some 10 min if given intravenously, but much longer after oral doses.

Temazepam: short-acting (4 h); adult dose 10–30 mg; useful for night sedation or for premedication in all types of surgery, including day-stay, and suitable for elderly patients. Syrup is available for children, 2 mg/ml. Dose 0.5 mg/kg.

Midazolam (Hypnovel): has been used for night sedation before surgery (15 mg) or as premedication. Can be given intramuscularly 70–100 mcg/kg 30–60 min before surgery. Most used as a sedative during endoscopy or regional analgesia (2–7.5 mg iv), often combined with a short-acting opioid such as fentanyl. This is useful in patients with severe learning disabilities.[13] It is also useful as an induction agent in a dose of up to 0.1 mg/kg in the elderly, or as a co-induction agent with propofol (*see* Chapter 2.4).

Lorazepam (Ativan): 1–4 mg (30–50 mcg/kg) orally, sublingually or intramuscularly given 2 h preoperatively. It is long-lasting (4–24 h) with appreciable anterograde amnesia. It abolishes the vasoconstriction that accompanies fear and attenuates the psychic sequelae of ketamine.

Diazepam (Valium, Diazemuls): 10–20 mg, orally or intramuscularly, duration 4–8 h. Combination with metoprolol greatly enhances its anxiolytic activity.[14]

Reversal of benzodiazepines – flumazenil (Anexate): this is a specific benzodiazepine antagonist, useful for reversing therapeutic doses and overdoses. Dose 100–200 mcg i.v. up to total of 1 mg. This only lasts about 30 min, and so further infusion may be needed (100–400 mcg/h). It can transiently increase pulse and blood pressure, or sometimes allow fits to recur.

PHENOTHIAZINES

Promethazine is sedative, anxiolytic, antihypertensive, antihistaminic and antiemetic, and is useful in combination with pethidine as a premedicant. Dose 25–50 mg i.m. Patients with alcoholic liver disease are very sensitive to phenothiazines.

Trimeprazine tartrate (Vallergan) is available as a syrup for oral administration to children. Dose 2 mg/kg 2 h preoperatively, although higher doses have been used with success. Many anaesthetists now use benzodiazepines in preference.

Analgesics

Narcotics usually produce euphoria, but at the price of some nausea in many patients (*see* Chapter 1.6). Hyoscine has been commonly used as an antiemetic, especially in children, as it also has useful antisialogogue and sedative properties. Preoperative analgesia is important in painful conditions, e.g. ischaemic limbs for amputation.

Long-acting NSAIDs give a useful background analgesia, upon which intraoperative and postoperative opiates develop an enhanced analgesic effect, with fewer side-effects. Ketoprofen (100–200 mg oral or rectal, 30 mg i.m., i.v.), piroxicam (20–40 mg oral), diclofenac (50–100 mg oral or rectal) will all give useful analgesia.

Anticholinergic agents (Table 1.1.1)

ATROPINE

The name is from Atropos, the oldest of the Three Fates who severed the threads of life, which were spun by Clotho and mixed, with those of good and evil fortune, by Lachesis. It is the alkaloid of the *Atropa belladonna* or deadly nightshade. Atropine was first suggested by E.A. Sharpey-Schaffer (1850–1935), an Edinburgh physiologist, in 1880 to prevent vagal cardiac arrest during chloroform anaesthesia, and advocated by Dudley Buxton (1855–1935), a London anaesthetist, 35 years later to inhibit secretions during ether anaesthesia. (*See also* Kessel J. *Anaesth. Intensive Care* 1974, **2**, 77.) Not used in premedication before 1890, although it was given, as the extract, per rectum, in 1861 to control patients resistant to chloroform.[15] The atropine group of alkaloids are esters of tropic acid with organic bases – tropine (atropine) and scopine (hyoscine). Atropine is the racemic mixture, but the laevo isomer is the more active.

Action on the nervous system
Competitive blocking action on muscarinic receptors supplied by postganglionic cholinergic nerves, e.g. smooth muscles and secretory glands. It has no effect on either production or destruction of acetylcholine, nor on its nicotinic effects. Complete vagal block requires a dose of 3 mg. It also stimulates the medulla and higher centres, the respiratory centre, and causes auditory hyperacusis. It inhibits sweating and so may be best avoided in pyrexial children. Occasionally, restlessness and delirium are seen (central anticholinergic syndrome).

Effects on the eye
Topical atropine paralyses the sphincter of the iris resulting in dilated pupils and loss of accommodation for up to a week. Parenteral atropine has little effect on the eye, and is not contraindicated in a patient with glaucoma, even of the narrow-angle type, since significant dilatation of the pupil does not occur. Down's syndrome patients may show resistance to parenteral atropine (and to sedatives).

Effects on the respiratory system
Sweat, bronchial and salivary glands are inhibited. Bronchial muscle is relaxed, causing bronchodilation and a slight increase in anatomical dead space. If given intramuscularly 1 h before anaesthesia, salivation is suppressed more efficiently than if given intravenously immediately before induction.

Action on the circulatory system
Tachycardia occurs due to the inhibition of vagal influence on the sinoatrial node. Heart rate can slow initially due to the Bezold–Jarisch coronary chemoreceptor reflex. The tachycardia decreases coronary filling time and increases myocardial oxygen consumption, and so it should be used with care in patients with coronary disease. Cardiac output and arterial pressure

is usually increased, with a fall in CVP. Atropine tachycardia is less marked in the elderly.

Reflex bradycardia and neostigmine-induced bradycardia are prevented. Atropine may cause nodal rhythm. It sometimes causes marked dilatation of the vessels of the face. Atropine can be considered for asystole, although it is no longer recommended as first-line treatment.[16]

Action on the alimentary canal
The tone and peristalsis of the gut and urinary tract are decreased. Like hyoscine and glycopyrronium, it lowers the opening pressure of the cardiac sphincter of the stomach and hence increases the chances of regurgitation.

Effect on the fetus
Atropine crosses the placenta rapidly (as a tertiary amine), and may protect the fetus and newborn from vagal reflexes occurring during birth and resuscitation.

Pharmacokinetics
Plasma half-life is 2–3 h, 50% protein bound. Elimination is slow in children under 2 years old and in the elderly. Excretion is partly by the kidneys, partly being destroyed in the tissues and the liver, with the formation of tropine and tropic acid.

Dose
Usual adult dose, 0.6 mg i.m. (in children 0.015 mg/kg) 1 h before operation. With neostigmine, 1–2 mg. Oral adult dose 2 mg (0.03 mg/kg in children), 90 min before operation. Black people may require larger doses than white people.

Overdose of atropine
'Mad as a hatter' (central stimulation).
'Hot as a hen' (inhibition of sweating and raising of metabolic rate).
'Blind as a bat' (paralysis of accommodation).
'Red as a beetroot' (facial vasodilatation).
'Dry as a bone' (salivary inhibition).

The central anticholinergic syndrome
Excitement, drowsiness or even coma may be seen especially in the elderly after treatment with atropine or hyoscine. There may also be thought impairment, memory disturbances, hallucinations, ataxia or behavioural abnormalities. They may be 'slow to wake up' in the recovery area. Treated with physostigmine salicylate, an anticholinesterase derived from the Calabar bean which has a tertiary amine, allowing it to cross the blood–brain barrier (neostigmine has a quaternary amine which prevents this).

Physostigmine 2 mg i.v. is given cautiously, and repeated if necessary. The drug has also been used in the treatment of depressant effects on the central nervous system of tricyclics and phenothiazines. It also modifies the psychotic side-effects of ketamine.

HYOSCINE HYDROBROMIDE (SCOPOLAMINE)

Similar actions to atropine, and also a Belladonna alkaloid. It is also a tertiary amine, so crosses the blood–brain barrier and causes sedation, with drowsiness, sleep, and amnesia in some patients. Occasionally it produces central anticholinergic syndrome. It is a mild respiratory stimulant, while its actions on the iris, the salivary, sweat and bronchial glands are stronger than that of atropine. It is a moderately powerful antiemetic. Action on heart, intestine and bronchiolar muscle is weaker than that of atropine.

The adult dose is 0.3–0.6 mg i.m. Combination of hyoscine 0.4 mg with pethidine 100 mg or papaveretum 20 mg has been widely used before surgery.

Hyoscine butylbromide (Buscopan) is used (like propantheline) as a gastrointestinal antispasmodic. It can be absorbed from skin, e.g. posterior to the pinna. Dose 10–30 mg.

GLYCOPYRRONIUM BROMIDE (ROBINUL, GLYCOPYRROLATE)

A quaternary ammonium compound with anticholinergic properties, which does not readily cross the placental or blood–brain barriers, and so does not cause central anticholinergic effects. Like atropine and hyoscine it reduces the tone of the lower oesophageal sphincter (the opposite effect to metoclopramide). It suppresses gastric secretion better than atropine or hyoscine, and results in less tachycardia and dysrhythmia. Effective at preventing bradycardia after suxamethonium. It efficiently dries up salivary secretions, being more potent than atropine and longer lasting. Faster emergence from anaesthesia than when atropine has been used. In clinical doses it does not affect the pupil size. It is not antiemetic. It is commonly used with neostigmine to reverse neuromuscular block.

Dose: premedication 0.2–0.4 mg (adult); 4–8 mcg/kg (child). Intravenous use to protect against bradycardia (adult) 0.2 mg, 4 mcg/kg (child).

Table 1.1.1 Comparison of anticholinergic drugs

	Atropine	*Hyoscine*	*Glycopyrronium*
i.v. dose (mcg/kg)	5–20	5–10	4–8
Onset time (i.v.)	1 min	1 min	1 min
Length of action	3 h	2 h	6 h
Effect on heart rate	+ + + +	+ + +	+ +
Inhibition of salivation	+ +	+ +	+ + +
CNS side effects	Yes	Yes	No

Antacids

These are commonly prescribed for patients thought to be at risk of regurgitation and aspiration. Ranitidine, 150 mg orally or 50 mg i.m. or slow i.v. injection, or nizatidine, 150 mg orally, block H2 receptors and decrease gastric acidity.

Drugs for specific effects

These include all drugs used to ensure optimal treatment of specific conditions right up to the time of surgery, e.g. salbutamol inhalation for asthmatics.

REFERENCES

1 Fischer S. P. *Anesthesiology* 1996, **85,** 196.
2 Badner N. H. et al. *Can. J. Anaesth.* 1998, **45,** 87.
3 Howell S. J. et al. *Anaesthesia* 1996, **51,** 1000.
4 *Anesthesiology* 1963, **24,** 111; Owens W. D. et al. *Anesthesiology* 1978, **49,** 239; Editorial, *Anesthesiology* 1978, **49,** 233; Keats A. S. *Anesthesiology* 1979, **51,** 179.
5 Nel M. R. and Morgan M. *Anaesthesia* 1996, **56,** 309–311.
6 Skolnick E. T. et al. *Anesthesiology* 1998, **88,** 1144.
7 Named for Mr Wardle's fat boy in Charles Dickens's (1812–1870) *The Pickwick Papers*, 1837; *see* Burwell C. S. et al. *Am. J. Med.* 1956, **21,** 811 (reprinted in 'Classical File', *Surv. Anesthesiol.* 1977, **21,** 477).
8 Kam P. C. A. and Chang G. W. M. *Anaesthesia* 1997, **52,** 982.
9 Fraser C. G. et al. *JAMA* 1952, **149,** 1542.
10 Strunin L. *Br. J. Anaesth.* 1993, **70,** 1–3 and 702–3.
11 Nimmo W. S. *Br. J. Anaesth.* 1990, **64,** 7.
12 Richards M. J. et al. *Br. J. Anaesth.* 1990, **65,** 157–163.
13 Tuel D. C. and Weis F. R. *Anesthesiology* 1990, **72,** 216.
14 Jakobsen C. J. et al. *Anaesthesia* 1990, **45,** 40.
15 Pithra J. *Medical Times* 1861, **2,** 121.
16 Vincent R. *Br. J. Anaesth.* 1997, **79,** 188.

Intravascular techniques, infusion and blood transfusion[1]

INTRAVENOUS CANNULATION

When inserting a cannula in a frightened patient, a benzodiazepine premedication is helpful to reduce anxiety, adrenaline levels and venous spasm. Suitable veins include the veins in the forearm, veins on the dorsum of the hand and veins above the wrist. In the shocked patient, the antecubital fossa or subclavian vein puncture are used.

In infants the internal or external jugular or scalp veins can be used or the umbilical vein. *In children*, the dorsum of the foot and ankle in addition to the upper limb.

Topical lignocaine–prilocaine cream (EMLA), amethocaine gel 4% or GTN may be useful, especially in children.[2]

Infusion flow rate is influenced by bag height, cannula size and viscosity of fluid. For blood, the latter is 2.5 times as great at 0°C as at 37°C. Blood at body temperature runs twice as fast as blood at 10°C. Fluids must be given cautiously to patients with impaired ventricular function. Self-adhesive skin patches of glyceryl trinitrate have decreased the rate of infusion failure three-fold, whether due to thrombosis or extravasation.[3] Any solution run continuously into a vein will eventually lead to thrombosis. Thrombophlebitis is early warning of infection to come. Cutaneous nerves may also be damaged, resulting in chronic neuropathic pain. Extravasation of intravenous fluids into the subcutaneous tissues occurs in about one-fifth of those receiving infusions. Usually no harm results but occasionally there is loss of skin, muscle and tendon, with permanent disability.[4]

NEEDLESTICK INJURIES

A written 'sharps drill' is required. Gloves, avoiding resheathing needles and the use of new cannulae designed for greater safety may lessen the risks.

Zidovudine prophylaxis may be indicated after an injury involving human immunodeficiency virus (HIV)-positive blood.[5]

THROMBOPHLEBITIS FROM INTRAVENOUS DRIPS[6]

Prevention

1 Re-site cannula every 24 h. Avoid leg veins if possible.
2 Use a larger vein, e.g. central venous catheter rather than a peripheral cannula. (A cannula is usually 7 cm in length or less; a catheter, more.)
3 Add hydrocortisone 10 mg/l or heparin 1 unit/ml to the infused fluid. Heparin-bonded, antibiotic-bonded and teflon cannulae are available.
4 Avoid hypertonic solutions.
5 Use a microfilter.

The pH of intravenous fluids may be a factor in causing thrombophlebitis, as may particulate matter. Some patients develop thrombophlebitis more easily than others, e.g. those with carcinoma.

Treatment

Heparinoid ointment may be applied but is of uncertain value. Venous thrombosis is more serious and calls for anticoagulation.

CENTRAL VENOUS CATHETERS

A catheter is inserted under full asepsis, from a more peripheral vein as far as the vena cava or right atrium. Risk factors for infection include prolonged duration of catheterization and immunocompromised patients.
   Prevention of infection:

1 full asepsis and sterilization of insertion site;
2 flushing catheters with antimicrobial/antithrombotic agents;
3 use of subclavian site rather than femoral;
4 heparin-bonded, antibiotic-bonded and teflon cannulae;
5 use of antiseptic catheter hubs;
6 maximal sterile barriers and use of transparent occlusive dressings;
7 tunnelling of catheters;
8 use of antibiotics and microfilters;
9 employment of a skilled infusion therapy team;
10 avoiding cut-downs for insertion;
11 avoiding frequent manipulations of catheter (e.g. PA catheter).

The veins which have been used include the following.

1 *Internal jugular vein.* The right side gives the best results. Cannulation is aided by a head-down tilt and head rotated to the other side.
   (a) The skin is punctured midway between the mastoid process and sterno-clavicular joint and the needle advanced under sternomastoid towards the sternoclavicular joint or ipsilateral nipple. On vein puncture, a guide wire is advanced into the lumen, over which the catheter is threaded.
   (b) In the relaxed, anaesthetized patient it may be possible to palpate the vein through the muscle and advance from the medial side.
   (c) Another approach is from the apex of a triangle formed by the sternal and clavicular heads of the sternomastoid to enter the vein beneath the clavicular head. This carries the risk of pneumothorax.
2 *External jugular vein.* Threading the cannula is more difficult.
3 *Subclavian vein.* Via skin puncture 1 cm below the middle of the clavicle, and directed under the clavicle towards the suprasternal notch until it pierces the vein (first described in 1952), but carries risk of pneumothorax.
4 *Axillary vein.*[7]
5 *Femoral vein,* medial to the artery below the inguinal ligament. Sometimes used in child.
6 *Basilic vein from antecubital fossa.* The catheter is connected to a pressure transducer. Respiratory fluctuations confirms that the tip lies within the thorax (larger fluctuations also indicate hypovolaemia). Sudden increases in pressure during systole indicate that the tip has entered the right ventricle. Catheter positions should be checked by X-ray (also to exclude pneumothorax), or by using the catheter as an electrocardiogram (ECG) electrode.

Complications of central venous catheters

1 Air embolus.[8]
2 Pneumothorax.
3 Migration of the tip.
4 Heart perforation.
5 Damage to thoracic lymph duct (on left side).
6 Thromboembolism.
7 Infection by bacteria and fungi migrating from the hub, skin, or blood; with septicaemia. Catheter sepsis is reduced by scrupulous asepsis; use of anti-biotic-coated catheters.[9] Salvage of infected haemodialysis catheters by antibiotics has been attempted with limited success.[10]
8 Local damage at point of insertion, e.g. to carotid artery.

INFUSION CONTROLLERS AND PUMPS

These can control flow given intravenously, intramuscularly, subcutaneously, intra-arterially, extradurally or by nasogastric tube. Their accuracy is useful in infants, or for infusion of drugs. Battery back-up is important.

PROBLEMS FROM INFUSION FLUID CONTAINERS

1 *Sepsis*. Growth of organisms in intravenous fluids can reach 10^6 or 10^7 organisms/ml without turbidity being detected and can cause severe septicaemia. Regular blood cultures are needed (including yeasts). A record of the batch number of containers used may help to trace the origin of infection. Giving sets should be changed every 24–48 h and always after blood has been used. Infusion teams to supervise intravenous drips have been helpful.
2 *Embolism*. May be of plastic, rubber, bacterial, air or dust. Added drugs may also cause precipitates.

In-line filtration is available, which removes particles during infusion without seriously impeding flow. The mesh size within a filter diminishes progressively in the direction of flow from about 10 μm down to around 0.1–0.5 μm. These filters cannot be used with blood transfusion. Ordinary filters on giving sets are 200 μm.

INTRAVENOUS FLUIDS

pH of some fluids

pH may vary by 1–2 pH units between batches. Typical values: normal saline, 5.0; compound sodium lactate solution (Hartmann), 6.5; 5% dextrose in water and 4% dextrose in 0.18% saline, 4.0; dextran in 5% dextrose, 4.5–5.0; dextran in 0.9% saline, 5.0–6.0; Haemaccel 7.3; Gelofusine 7.4; sodium bicarbonate 8.4%, 7.8; Hetastarch 5.5; Pentastarch 5.0.

Glucose (dextrose)

Five per cent solution is isotonic and may be used for fluid replacement and to keep an intravenous route open for medication. The preferred saline/glucose isotonic combination is 1/5 normal saline with 4.3% glucose. When stored blood is followed by glucose, rouleaux formation with clumping occurs in the drip set. Glucose of 10% or more readily produces thrombophlebitis.

Normal saline (0.9%)

First used in the treatment of shock in 1891. About one-third of its volume is retained in the circulation. Can cause sodium overload, especially in infants. Na, 154; Cl, 154 mmol/l.

Hartmann's solution (compound sodium lactate solution, BP)

One-sixth molar concentration of sodium lactate in Ringer's solution. The lactate is metabolized in the liver to form bicarbonate, to counteract acidosis. Large volumes have been used in the treatment of hypovolaemia instead of colloid. Na, 131; Cl, 111; K, 5; Ca, 2; Lactate, 29 mmol/l.

Human albumin

See below under 'Blood transfusion'.

Colloids

Colloids maintain or increase plasma oncotic pressure and so help draw fluid into the intravascular space. However, in disease they may leak into the extravascular space. They include the dextrans, gelatins, starches and albumin. Reactions occur to colloids, mainly mild pyrexia, especially in atopic patients, but anaphylaxis may occur rarely. No risks of transmitted viral diseases. Pre-emptive colloid fluid challenge may reduce perioperative morbidity in vascular cases.[11]

Dextran 70

Molecular weight (MW) 70 000 Da; 6% solution in saline, or 5% dextrose. Active for many hours. It is hyperoncotic; 500 ml will usually increase the circulating plasma volume by 750 ml. Has proved useful as a plasma volume expander, and in the prevention of venous thromboembolism. If more than 1.5 litres are infused in any 24-h period there is interference with blood grouping and cross-matching, owing to rouleaux formation (recipient cells must be washed before testing). Large infused volumes can increase bleeding by interfering with platelet stickiness, enhancing fibrinolysis.

Gelatins

Produced by hydrolysis of collagens. Haemaccel is 3.5% urea-linked gelatin, MW 35 000, in electrolyte solution which includes calcium 6.25 mmol/l and potassium 5.1 mmol/l. pH 7.2–7.3. Gelofusine is 4% succinylated (modified fluid) gelatin in normal saline, MW 30 000. pH 7.4. Short biological half-life, less than 12 h; no effect on blood cross-matching, and only a dilutional effect on clotting factors; 85% excreted by the kidney. Duration of useful plasma expansion is about 2 h. Gelatins have an incidence of adverse reactions, most of which occur after the first few millilitres infused. Haemaccel contains calcium and should not be given through the same infusion set as citrated blood or fresh frozen plasma. Can help promote a postoperative diuresis.

Hydroxyethyl starches (HES)

Hetastarch (Hespan) is a 6% solution in normal saline. Average MW 450 000. ph 5.5. Degree of substitution 0.7, i.e. 70 hydroxyethyl groups for every 100 glucose units. Pentastarch (Pentaspan) is a 10% solution in normal saline. Average MW 250 000. pH 5.0. Degree of substitution 0.45. Pentastarch results in the greater intravascular volume expansion. Both have long intravascular lives (but may pass into lung lymph[12]), and do not release histamine. Little effect on coagulation or cross-matching. Expand plasma volume for about 14 h. Serious anaphylactoid reactions are probably less common (1 in 16 000 for hetastarch) than with other plasma substitutes (except albumin) and are therefore safe.[13]

Blood substitutes

There is a strong clinical need for a non-toxic blood substitute with a good flow profile in narrowed vessels.

Perfluorocarbons

Various perfluorochemicals have been emulsified with phospholipid or synthetic surfactants and can carry enough O_2 to completely replace blood in animals. They have also been used as respirable liquids in humans.[14] Fluosol-DA has been used in man as a blood substitute. It is an inert emulsion of perfluorinated decalin and tripropylamine which dissolves over three times as much O_2 as plasma, obeying Henry's law. It provides useful O_2 transport, but only with a high inspired O_2 concentration. Newer emulsions may carry considerably more O_2.

Haemoglobin solutions

Solutions of polymerized haemoglobin with a 2,3-DPG analogue added can provide O_2 transport with a better carriage profile than perflurocarbons. Renal toxicity of the red cell stroma remnants is a problem.

Haemosomes

Synthetic red cells with stroma-free haemoglobin in lecithin capsules in synthetic plasma solution.

OTHER METHODS OF FLUID ADMINISTRATION

Intramedullary or intraosseous infusion

For transfusion of blood or fluid in the complete absence of a suitable vein, e.g. into the marrow of the manubrium sterni or long bones in children,[15] usually upper tibia. The cannula is sometimes locked in position by a screw thread.

Rectal administration

In the remote situation, tap water or dilute tea can be life-saving.

Hypodermoclysis

Subcutaneous administration of saline can be used, when the intravenous route is not available, retromammary or into outer side of thigh using *hyaluronidase*.

ARTERIAL PUNCTURE AND CANNULATION

Performed to measure the PaO_2, $PaCO_2$, SaO_2 and pH to clarify the acid–base and electrolyte status.

Any artery that can be compressed after puncture may be used (but not end-arteries), usually the radial (preferred), brachial, or femoral. Cannulation is more difficult in hypotension. Blood should pulsate into the attached syringe under its own power as colour is not a certain sign of arterial puncture. The adhesive tape and attached infusion pipes and taps are clearly marked to indicate **'ARTERY'** to avoid injections into them. Extreme care is taken to avoid air embolism from any system attached to an arterial line.

Radial artery: some workers perform Allen's test (pressure on radial artery while blanching skin of hand; an alternative arterial supply will cause rapid re-flushing of the skin) the wrist is extended. After palpation, the line of the artery may be marked on the skin. The needle or cannula is inserted at the level of the wrist skin crease (proximal to this the artery lies much deeper), at about 45 degrees to the surface, with local analgesia. Circulation of the fingers is checked.

Brachial artery: palpated medial to the biceps tendon. Circulation of the forearm and fingers is checked.

Femoral artery: palpated halfway between the pubic symphysis and the anterior superior iliac spine. The needle is advanced between the fingertips of the other hand which straddle the artery.

Dorsalis pedis artery: the line of the artery may be marked on the skin after palpation. The vessel presents a convex curve over the navicular and metatarsal heads, which makes entry easier, and is very superficial. In a modified version of Allen's test, the foot may be squeezed during pressure occlusion of this artery. If there is no satisfactory alternative blood supply, the blanched skin remains white until the occluding finger is taken off the dorsalis pedis.

MANAGEMENT OF BLOOD LOSS

In the acute situation

1 Stop the haemorrhage.
2 Replace blood volume: Adult: 10% of blood volume lost – replace with crystalloid/colloid infusion. Adult: 20% of blood volume lost replace with blood transfusion, monitored by central venous pressure (CVP). Child: 5% of blood volume lost – replace with crystalloid/colloid infusion. Child: 10% of blood volume lost – replaced with blood transfusion, monitored by CVP.
3 Replace clotting factors after transfusion of 50% of blood volume.

Note: the first infusion is given to replace blood *already lost*, as well as replace continuing blood loss.

Correction of preoperative anaemia

A new, simple, cheap haemoglobin test has been developed.[16] A haematocrit of 30–35% (Hb 10 g/dl) or more is the usual target. Lower levels may be accepted, especially in renal failure, those who refuse transfusions, where cross-infection risk is high and where temporary reduction of immuno-competence is to be avoided.

1 Preoperative iron therapy.
2 Recombinant human erythropoietin therapy 20–50 U/kg/day, i.v., s.c. Erythropoietin, a glycoprotein of total MW 34 000 Da, originating in the kidney renal cortical peritubular cells. Used in renal failure, chemotherapy and tumour anaemia with iron supplements.
3 Transfusion when the haemoglobin is low. Messmer Hb/cardiac output graph with O_2 flux.

Transfusion of one 540 ml unit of blood will raise the haemoglobin about 1 g/dl in the adult. If the haemoglobin is less than 6 g/dl, transfusion is desirable. If a major operation is to be performed and the haemoglobin is less than 10 g/dl, a blood transfusion is often indicated. Below 9 g/dl tissue oxygenation can be maintained only by increasing cardiac output.

At operation

1 Reduce blood loss if possible. (The surgeon must develop more effective haemostasis, especially in patients with a bleeding tendency.)
2 Use synthetic colloids in volume replacement, e.g. Haemaccel, Hetastarch, dextran 70, and Gelofusine.
3 Transfuse as above.
4 If haemorrhage is unexpected ('bleeding from everywhere'), check if the patient has taken aspirin recently. If so, give a platelet transfusion.
5 Autotransfusion:
   (a) preoperative harvesting;
   (b) intraoperative salvage of shed blood.
6 Need for postoperative O_2 therapy in the severely anaemic.
7 Accept lower haemoglobin limits where transfusion is not an option, with warning about morbidity for the patient.
8 Intravenous fluorocarbon therapy: see above.

BLOOD TRANSFUSION

Storage

Red cells last well in refrigerated (4–6°C) stored blood. More than 70% survive 24 h after transfusion. Clotting factors deteriorate progressively after 24 h storage. Citrate–phosphate–dextrose (CPD) blood contains no functioning platelets after 48 h. Factor V has decreased to 50% after 14 days, and factor VIII to 50% after 24 h and 6% after 21 days. Factor XI is only stable for 7 days. Citrate–phosphate–dextrose blood plus adenine preserves its adenosine triphosphate (ATP) and 2,3-DPG levels for up to 2 weeks with a slow fall thereafter and is stored for up to 35 days. Each unit contains 450 ml of blood and 60 ml of CPD solution. The pH may be 6.7 and the potassium content about 20 mmol/l after 3 weeks, with reabsorbtion into the erythrocytes after warming and infusion. Saline adenine glucose mannitol (SAG-M) also preserves red cells for 35 days.

Red cells can be washed, suspended in glycerol and stored frozen in liquid nitrogen for many years. Two hours are needed for thawing and washing to remove glycerol. They then should be used within 6 h. Main application is military.

Use of uncross-matched red blood cells

O-negative is the universal donor blood. Techniques are being developed to convert A, B and AB blood to group O, improving the usefulness of donated blood.

The chance of a reaction with group-compatible uncross-matched blood is 1 : 300 transfusions.[17]

Rhesus-negative blood should whenever possible be given to Rh-negative patients, who form about 15% of the population in the UK. This is important in:

1 Rh-negative patients of either sex who have either had a previous trans-fusion or may require a subsequent one;
2 Rh-negative girls and women of child-bearing age;
3 Mothers of infants who have haemolytic disease;
4 Infants with haemolytic disease.

Various blood products

1 *Packed cells* (erythrocytes). The commonest product. Most of the plasma is removed and stored as fresh frozen plasma (FFP).
2 Saline adenine glucose mannitol blood.
3 *Microaggregate-free (MAF) blood* is CPD blood from which the 'buffy coat' (containing leucocyte and platelet debris) has been removed.
4 *Whole blood* – uncommon except when specifically collected fresh for coagulopathies.
5 *Frozen blood.* See above.
6 *Plasma.* Available as FFP, 150 or 300 ml, used for its clotting factors. It contains citrate.
7 *Human albumin.* Available as albumin, salt-poor albumin, or 'plasma pro-tein fraction' (PPF), prepared by pasteurization of plasma with resulting precipitation of globulins and any viruses.
8 *Human fibrinogen*, for use in disseminated intravascular coagulation (DIC).
9 *Cryoprecipitate* (particularly rich in clotting factors).
10 *Platelets* may be transfused in severe thrombocytopenia ($< 80\,000/\mu l$). Platelet concentrates are slightly contaminated with donor red cells and so should be given to patients of the same ABO group; in the case of Rh-negative women anti-D immunoglobulin should be given. Ordinary filters on transfusion sets remove 5% of platelets, but microfilters remove over 30% and so should not be used.

The concentrate from each unit of whole blood contains about 50×10^9 platelets suspended in 50 ml plasma. The pooled concentrate from four O positive units is used in adults (1 unit per 10 kg in children) and raises the count by about 60 000 per microlitre. They last 7–10 days in the circulation.

Platelets from plateletapheresis are from one donor and are used on a group-specific basis.

11 *Factor VIII concentrate.*
12 *Factor IX concentrate.*
13 *Washed red cells.* Washed in saline. Used rarely for non-haemolytic transfusion reactions to plasma proteins.

Homologous blood transfusion

Each blood transfusion carries a certain risk and, in adults, single-unit transfusions are seldom necessary.

Acute haemolytic reaction

This is serious and may be fatal. An increased rate of destruction usually of the donor's red cells by antibodies in the recipient's plasma. May be immediate or delayed. ABO incompatibility usually causes a more immediate and severe reaction than one due to Rhesus or other factors. General anaesthesia and sedation mask the signs. The blood pressure and pulse rate should be taken every 5 min for the first 15 min with each new unit of blood. If there is a red rash, hypotension, tachycardia or cyanosis for which no other cause can be found, the transfusion should be stopped.

PATHOPHYSIOLOGY

Largely mediated by histamine released from mast cells in response to the activation of C3a and C5a cleavage products of complement by the antigen–antibody reaction. In addition, the action of anti-A or anti-B or both (IgM alloantibodies) causes erythrocyte disruption with release of aphospholipid procoagulant (e.g. erythrocytin) and DIC. The combination of intravascular fibrin deposition and vasospasm leads to acute tubular necrosis of the kidney.

SIGNS OF INCOMPATIBLE TRANSFUSION

In the conscious
 1 Headache.
 2 Precordial or lumbar pain.
 3 Urticaria or pruritus.
 4 Burning in limbs.
 5 Bronchospasm, dyspnoea, tachycardia and restlessness.
 6 Suffused face.
 7 Nausea and vomiting.
 8 Pyrexia and rigors.
 9 Circulatory collapse.
10 Later, haemoglobinaemia, haemoglobinuria and oliguria.

Under anaesthesia

Sometimes not easy to distinguish from the effects of haemmorrhage itself, especially during rapid transfusion > 100 ml/min.

1 *Immediate* rapid severe and progressive hypotension.
2 Tachycardia.
3 General oozing from wound.
4 Urticarial rash.
5 Bronchospasm, raising airway pressures on intermittent positive-pressure ventilation (IPPV).
6 *Later*, jaundice and oliguria in 5–10% of these patients. It strongly resembles anaphylactic reaction and the treatment is similar.

The incidence has been variously reported to be between 1–3000 and 1–15 000 transfused units.
The factors affecting the severity of the reaction are:

1 quality and quantity of recipient's antibody;
2 dose of antigen, i.e. volume of blood given, and antigen concentration per donor red cell;
3 the general fitness of the recipient.

DIFFERENTIAL DIAGNOSIS

1 Anaphylactic reaction to some other substance (e.g. a drug).
2 Acute septicaemia.
3 Transfusion of thermally damaged, infected or outdated blood.

MANAGEMENT OF SEVERE TRANSFUSION REACTION

1 Stop the transfusion.
2 Support blood pressure with intravenous colloids or crystalloids, and inotropes or vasoconstrictors if needed.
3 One hundred per cent O_2.
4 Induce a diuresis with mannitol 50 g or frusemide 10–20 mg.
5 Check acid–base balance and electrolytes.
6 Exchange transfusion in the desperate case.
7 High dose of steroids may be useful.
8 Antihistamines may be indicated in the early stages but may increase hypotension.
9 Where DIC is occurring, coagulation factors and platelets need to be replaced.
10 Transfer to high-dependency unit (HDU) or intensive therapy unit (ITU).

INVESTIGATION OF TRANSFUSION REACTIONS

The following are needed:

Immunological consequences of transfusion

Immediate
Minor febrile reactions (1%).
Urticaria.
Major reactions (see above).

Delayed
Modulation of immune system, e.g. improved transplant survival.
Possible increased postoperative tumour recurrence.
Increased postoperative infection rates; active suppression of cellular immunity.
Reduction in recurrence of Crohn's disease.
HIV cross-infection.

---

1 the blood samples used for the original compatibility test;
2 the remains of the blood used for the transfusion;
3 10 ml of the patient's blood taken 3 h after the transfusion reaction, collected into a plain sterile bottle, and 2 ml in an oxalated bottle,
4 a sample of urine.

Delayed reaction

Four to ten days after transfusion, there may be anaemia, jaundice and renal failure.

Other immune reactions

Can occur to leucocyte, platelet and plasma protein antigens. Mild urticaria or fever is common, but rarely acute anaphylaxis results. Immunosuppression occurs.

Post-transfusion immunosuppression in trauma has been blamed for early neutrophil priming and activation leading to the second-hit model of early multisystem organ failure (MOF).[18]

Graft-versus-host reactions may be seen in postmediastinal radiation cases and DiGeorge syndrome. In these cases, blood is irradiated before transfusion.

Coagulopathy

This is common in component transfusion, usually treated by infusion of FFP, after a transfusion of two or three units of plasma reduced blood. Desmopressin (DDAVP) 4 μg may also be helpful.

Transmission of infectious disease

VIRUSES

1 Hepatitis B,[19] 2–6 months incubation period. Jaundice may not be evident.
2 Hepatitis C[20] carried by up to 1% of the population; an antibody assay is now available.
3 HIV-I (or HIV-II in West Africa); donor screening for acquired immune deficiency syndrome (AIDS) started in 1985 in the UK. Prevalence less than 1 per million in the UK.
4 Cytomegalovirus.
5 Epstein–Barr virus.

BACTERIA[21]

1 Contaminants during collection or storage. Blood left out of the refrigerator or transfer box for more than 30 min should not be used; sudden and severe septicaemia with collapse from toxic shock may result.
2 Syphilis.
3 Brucellosis.
4 Yaws.

PARASITES[21]

1 Malaria. In areas where malaria is not endemic serology can exclude donors who may transmit the disease. Transfer of malaria can be prevented by giving chloroquine 600 mg to the recipient before transfusion.
2 Trypanosomiasis.
3 Leishmaniasis (Kala-azar).

Circulatory overloading

Those with heart disease, incipient left ventricular fibrillation (LVF), severe anaemia and old age are especially vulnerable. The jugular venous pressure should be watched, and the CVP or pulmonary wedge pressure monitored if needed. To make overload less likely, frusemide 20–40 mg i.v. can be given during the transfusion.

Hypothermia

Prevented by using a thermostatically controlled blood warmer. The temperature should never exceed 40°C (thermally damaged blood transfusion resembles acute haemolytic reaction).

Embolism

Blood filters (20–40 μm pore size) remove microaggregates of more than 20 μm diameter during transfusion. Three structures are in common use:

1 surface filters;
2 depth filters;
3 combination filters (pore size 40–100 μm depending on type of filter).

Various materials have been used in their construction, such as woven polyester screen, nylon screen, Dacron wool and polyester sponge. Must be fully primed with blood before use. They may prevent lung damage caused by microaggregates, but a consensus about this has not been reached. Problems and dangers of these filters include: slowing of rate of transfusion, complete blockage after 4–10 units of blood, embolism of particles from the filter, haemolysis and massive activation of the clotting process if FFP is infused through a filter. The ordinary infusion set filter pore size is about 170 μm.

Hyperkalaemia

Stored blood may contain up to 30 mmol/l of potassium by its expiry date. Children and patients with acidosis, hypothermia or renal failure are particularly at risk. Blood warmers reduce the risk of arrythmias.

Signs of hyperkalaemia include elevation of the T wave on the ECG and widening of the QRS complex. In emergency, slow intravenous injection of 5–10 ml of calcium chloride 10% (adult) will temporarily counteract the effects of potassium on the heart.

Citrate intoxication with hypocalcaemia

A warm oxygenated adult can metabolize the citrate content of 1 unit of CPD blood in 5 min. If the transfusion is faster than this, citrate intoxication may cause tremors, arrhythmias, acidosis and hypocalcaemia. Calcium gluconate 10% 10 ml (2.3 mmol Ca^{2+}) may be required. This is most likely in cold or cyanosed patients, or those with severe hepatic disease, e.g. in the anhepatic phase of liver transplantation.

During open-heart surgery and renal dialysis, heparinized blood may be preferred (5 u/ml). Heparinization does not interfere with calcium stores in the body and citrate intoxication does not arise, but its shelf-life is less than 2 days.

Acidosis

The pH of stored blood varies between 6.6 and 7.2 due to lactic acid, pyruvic acid, citric acid and raised $P\text{CO}_2$. This is only important in massive transfusion, as citrate is metabolized to bicarbonate in the liver.

Hypomagnesaemia

During massive transfusion, with particular loss from the myocardium.

Transfusion-related acute lung injury

Due to transfusion of the donor's leukocyte agglutinating antibodies. Rare, but causes damage to the lung microvasculature resulting in ARDS. Washed red cells only should be used from donors who cause this problem.

Massive blood transfusion

Defined as total blood volume replacement by stored blood in under 24 h or more than 1 ml/kg/min – this is common in major haemorrhage. It can be regarded as an organ transplant. Coagulation screening is important and can be done at the bedside or in theatre. A coagulopathy is common, due to lack of platelets, fibrinogen, factors V and VIII. Platelets and FFP should be given as indicated by measurements of platelet count, fibrinogen levels and INR.

Autologous blood transfusion (autotransfusion)

A *pre-deposit programme* can be used to collect 6 or more units of blood during the 5–6 weeks before an operation. The main drawback to this approach is the logistical support needed. The marrow of a patient on iron supplements replaces the cells in a unit of blood in 3–4 weeks. Erythropoietin therapy speeds this further (*see above*).

Blood is stored in CPD–adenine for up to 35 days. Oral iron is given to the patient during the pre-donation phase. Up to 450 ml of blood can be donated every 4–5 days up to 72 h prior to surgery, with 'piggybacking' or 'leap-frogging' (reinfusing the oldest unit at a donation) giving up to 5 units of blood up to 3 weeks old, from 6 weeks pre-donation. Careful documentation (sometimes done and signed by the patient) is essential. Written consent is often obtained. Blood is stored separately from the homologous supply. Unused blood may be given to the transfusion service.

Blood salvage

The Solcotrans system collects spilt blood in a containers primed with ACD and is infused directly through a filter. Useful for recovery of postoperative drainage. The Cell Saver collects from suckers which introduce heparin at their tips, and then centrifuges, washes and packs the red cells ready for retransfusion. Reinfusion of up to 10 litres has been performed,[22] although haemolysis limits the rate at which blood can be collected. Autotransfusion first described in 1874,[23] and first used in 1886![24] The need for homologous blood is not always eliminated, as salvage is incomplete and there is a delay before it is ready for transfusion.

CENTRIFUGAL SYSTEMS

1 Benefits to patient.
  (a) Elimination of cross-infection.
  (b) Serological compatibility is ensured.
  (c) Avoidance of alloimunization, and no rhesus immunization affecting any future pregnancy.
  (d) Minor transfusion reactions reduced.
  (e) Operative benefits of haemodilution, e.g. improved blood flow, reduced risk of venous thrombosis.
  (f) Psychological advantage to the patient in being more closely involved with the preoperative preparation for surgery.
  (g) May be acceptable to religious sects who might otherwise refuse transfusion.
2 Benefits to medical staff.
  (a) Obligatory pre-donation tests minimize risk of cross-infection.
  (b) Cross-matching unnecessary.
  (c) Stores of homologous blood are conserved, especially those of rare blood groups.
  (d) Reduced overall costs.

Preoperative haemodilution[25]

One litre of blood is drawn off into anticoagulated packs and replaced with an equal volume of colloid. This means that haemodiluted blood is spilt at surgery, which is replaced by the saved blood after haemostasis is secured. Although a haematocrit of 30% is widely used, there is disagreement about the degree of haemodilution that is safe, especially in patients with vascular disease.

Drugs to minimize blood loss and transfusion

Aprotinin, tranexamic acid are antifibrinolytic agents.[26]

REFERENCES

1 Park G. R. and Roe P. G. *Fluid Balance and Volume Resuscitation Made Easy*. Oxford University Press, Oxford, 1998.
2 Gunawardene R. D. and Davenport H. T. *Anaesthesia* 1990, **45,** 52.
3 Wright A. et al. *Lancet* 1985, **2,** 1148.
4 Burd D. et al. *Br. Med. J.* 1985, **290,** 1579.
5 Henderson D. K. and Gerberding J. L. *J. Infect. Dis.* 1989, **160,** 321.
6 Congo A. and Lensing A. W. A. et al. *Br. Med. J.* 1998, **316,** 17–20.
7 Taylor B. L. and Yellowlees I. *Anesthesiology* 1990, **72,** 55.
8 Fitchet A. and Fitzpatric A. P. *Br. Med. J.* 1998, **316,** 604–605.

9   Maki D. G., Stolz S. M., Wheeler S. and Mermel L. A. *Ann. Intern. Med.* 1997, **127,** 257–266; Raad I. et al. *ibid.* 267–274.
10 Marr K. A. et al. *Ann. Intern. Med.* 1997, **127,** 275–280.
11 Mythen M. *Arch. Surg.* 1995, **130,** 423.
12 Korent V. A. et al. *Am. J. Respir. Crit. Care Med.* 1997, **155,** 1302–1308.
13 Warren B. B. and Duriex M. E. *Anesth. Analg.* 1997, **84,** 206–212.
14 Fuhrman B. P. *J. Pediatr.* 1990, **117,** 73.
15 Fiser D. H. *N. Engl. J. Med.* 1990, **322,** 1579.
16 *J. Clin. Pathol.* 1998, **51,** 21–24.
17 McClelland R. and Phillips P. *Br. Med. J.* 1994, **308,** 1205–1206.
18 Moore F. A., Moore E. E. and Sauaia A. *Arch. Surg.* 1997, **132,** 620–625.
19 Hoofinagle J. H. *Transfusion* 1990, **30,** 384.
20 Choo Q-L. et al. *Br. Med. Bull.* 1990, **46,** 423; Wright R. *J. R. Coll. Physicians* 1990, **24,** 78.
21 Barbara J. A. J. and Contreras M. *Br. Med. J.* 1990, **300,** 386.
22 Lee D. and Napier J. A. F. *Br. Med. J.* 1990, **300,** 737.
23 Highmore W. *Lancet* 1874, **2,** 89; Blundell J. *Med. Chir. Trans.* 1878, **9,** 56.
24 Duncan J. *Br. Med. J.* 1886, **1,** 192.
25 Meikle M. *Anesth. Analg.* 1997, **84,** 26–30.
26 Lanpacis A. and Fergusson D. *Anesth. Analg.* 1997, **85,** 1258–1267.

Acid–base and electrolyte balance

HYDROGEN ION CONCENTRATION AND pH

The pH notation was described by S.P.L. Sorensen (1868–1939), Copenhagen physiologist.[1] pH is the negative logarithm (to the base 10) of the hydrogen ion concentration. The normal range for arterial blood is 7.36–7.44, which is a hydrogen ion concentration of 36–44 (nmol)/l. The pH range compatible with life is about 6.8–7.7 (20–160 nmol H^+)/l. Hydrogen ions actually exist in water as $(H_3O)^+$. The pH of blood rises by 0.0147 for each °C that its temperature falls, due to changes in the ionization of proteins.[2]

Hydrogen ions in:

pH units	nmol/litre	
6.8	160	This is the H^+ concentration of water at 37°C
7.0	100	This is the H^+ concentration of water at 20°C
7.2	63	
7.4	40	
7.6	25	
7.8	16	

ACIDOSIS AND ALKALOSIS

Acidosis is a condition which would tend to cause acidaemia (i.e. a higher than normal H^+ concentration) if uncorrected. Alkalosis tends to cause alkalaemia if uncorrected.

BUFFER SYSTEMS

Buffers act to minimize the change in pH of blood and body fluids that would otherwise occur when acid or alkali is added to them. The most important buffer is the bicarbonate system.

The bicarbonate buffer system and the Henderson–Hasselbalch equation

Carbonic acid is formed by the hydration of CO_2 (catalysed by carbonic anhydrase) and exists in a state of equilibrium with hydrogen ions and bicarbonate ions:

$$CO_2 + H_2O \longleftrightarrow H_2CO_3 \longleftrightarrow H^+ + HCO_3^-$$

By the law of mass action (i.e. when such a reaction has reached equilibrium, the product of the concentrations of the reagents on one side of the equation is proportional to the product of the concentrations of reagents on the other side):

$$[H^+] \cdot [HCO_3^-] = \text{constant} \times [H_2CO_3]$$

Furthermore, $[H_2CO_3]$ is taken to be proportional to PCO_2 so that:

$$[H^+] = 180 \times PCO_2/[HCO_3^-]$$

(if $[H^+]$ is expressed in nmol/l, PCO_2 in kPa, and $[HCO_3^-]$ in mmol/l)

Henderson (1878–1942, Boston physiologist) derived this, and Hasselbalch (1874–1962, Copenhagen biochemist) expressed it in logarithmic form:

$$pH = pK + \log \frac{[HCO_3^-]}{0.225 \times PCO_2}$$

pK varies with temperature and pH, but can normally be taken to be 6.1. This equation can also be expressed graphically as in the Davenport or Siggaard–Andersen diagrams.

The body tries to compensate for any acid–base disturbance by preserving the ratio of $[HCO_3^-]$ to PCO_2, and hence to keep the pH normal. PCO_2 is altered by changing ventilation, and $[HCO_3^-]$ by changing renal bicarbonate excretion. Because protein buffers also exist in blood, the change in bicarbonate resulting from a metabolic acidosis or alkalosis is less than expected, and so underestimates the true disturbance.

Other buffer systems

Haemoglobin is the most important buffer after the bicarbonate system. Reduced haemoglobin is a more effective buffer the oxyhaemoglobin.

Plasma proteins also act as buffers, but their concentration is only one-third that of haemoglobin. Phosphate buffers are present in low concentrations.

Standard bicarbonate and base excess

Standard bicarbonate is the bicarbonate concentration in the plasma of blood at 37°C, with a PCO_2 of 5.3 kPa and fully oxygenated haemoglobin. Normally 24 mmol/l. As with base excess, any abnormality indicates a metabolic disturbance. *Buffer base* is the sum of all the buffer anions in blood (including the proteins) in mmol/l. *Base excess* is the surplus or deficit of acid or base in mmol/l of blood, i.e. the amount of acid or base in mmol/l required for titration back to pH 7.40 at PCO_2 of 5.3 kPa at 37°C. This is the most useful clinical estimate of the metabolic component of any acid–base disturbance, and (like standard bicarbonate) takes account of non-bicarbonate buffers in blood, but not the buffers outside blood. By convention an acid surplus (base deficit) is referred to as a negative base excess.

METABOLIC (NON-RESPIRATORY) ACID–BASE DISTURBANCES

Acid–base disturbances due to any substance other than carbon dioxide. Metabolic acidosis results in a negative base excess (i.e. a base deficit) and a low standard bicarbonate, and the converse with alkalosis.

Metabolic acidosis

This may occur due to an excess acid production or ingestion:

1 ketoacidosis from diabetes or starvation;
2 uraemic renal acidosis;
3 salicylate poisoning;
4 lactic acidosis after, for example, severe exercise, tissue ischaemia and hypoxia, cardiopulmonary bypass, during rewarming after hypothermia, severe liver disease.

These all result in the measured cations (Na and K) greatly exceeding the measured anions (bicarbonate and chloride), or a high *anion gap*. The normal anion gap is 10–18 mmol/l and is mainly due to negatively charged proteins in blood.

Metabolic acidosis may also be associated with a normal anion gap. This occurs when there is a loss of bicarbonate:

1 diarrhoea;
2 hyperkalaemia;
3 renal tubular acidosis;
4 to compensate for a respiratory alkalosis.

Clinical effects

1 Increased, gasping respiration, which is stimulated via the peripheral chemoreceptors.
2 Tachycardia, vasoconstriction, increased catecholamines, positive inotropy, ventricular arrhythmias.
3 Nausea and vomiting.
4 Hyperkalaemia.

The hyperventilation reduces the PCO_2 and this partially compensates for the acidosis.

Treatment

Treatment is mainly of the primary cause. This will often render treatment with intravenous sodium bicarbonate unnecessary. If indicated, it is normally given as 8.4% solution which contains 1 mmol/ml. Dose may be calculated by:

dose of bicarbonate (mmol) = $1/3 \times$ base deficit $\times$ body weight (kg)

The disadvantages of giving bicarbonate are that it is hyperosmolar, includes a high sodium load, and that CO_2 is formed which diffuses into the cells and worsens any intracellular acidosis. This latter hypothesis has in the past led to it being avoided if possible.

Metabolic alkalosis

This may occur following:

1 ingestion of large amounts of bicarbonate or other alkalis;
2 loss of acid, as in pyloric stenosis, vomiting, nasogastric drainage, hypokalaemia;
3 retention of bicarbonate as in respiratory acidosis.

The body compensates by underventilation and increased renal bicarbonate excretion. Renal potassium loss causes hypokalaemia.

Treatment

Treatment is again mainly of the primary cause. The alkalosis itself is more difficult to treat than acidosis. High doses of potassium chloride are needed (up to 150 mmol daily). Ammonium chloride can be given orally or intravenously, with the dose calculated as above.

RESPIRATORY ACID–BASE DISTURBANCES

This is caused by changes in respiration and hence in arterial PCO_2. Normal range is 4.8–5.9 kPa. High values mean a respiratory acidosis, and low values a respiratory alkalosis.

Respiratory acidosis

Hypercapnia (hyper, over + kapnos, smoke) is the ill effects of CO_2 excess, and was first emphasized in anaesthesia by Waters.[3]

Causes in anaesthetic practice

1 Impairment of ventilation due to respiratory obstruction, depression, or paralysis.
2 Severe chronic obstructive lung disease.
3 Accidental administration of carbon dioxide.
4 Faulty CO_2 absorption.
5 During apnoea.
6 Overproduction of CO_2, as in hyperpyrexia.

Mild hypercapnia is probably not as serious as was once thought, although PCO_2 up to 10.5 kPa commonly causes arrhythmias during anaesthesia. As the PCO_2 rises towards 25 kPa, narcosis deepens into coma. This can occur during respiratory depression in the recovery ward with apparent delayed awakening. Over 25 kPa and profound narcosis and respiratory failure resembling curarization occur. Supercarbia, PCO_2 over 50 kPa, is associated with tolerance in animals, when respiration becomes possible again.

Effects of hypercapnia

CENTRAL NERVOUS SYSTEM

1 Cerebral vasodilatation and increased intracranial pressure. If the hypercapnia is chronic, as in emphysema, the cerebrospinal fluid (CSF) bicarbonate rises, restores the CSF pH, and so sets a new baseline for cerebral vascular resistance.
2 Progressive narcosis.

AUTONOMIC NERVOUS SYSTEM

1 Sympathetic activation with a rise of circulating catecholamines, although reduced sensitivity of the end organs to these catecholamines, and sweating.
2 Parasympathetic activation (though overshadowed by the sympathetic effect).

RESPIRATORY SYSTEM

1 Carbon dioxide stimulates the respiratory centre.
2 Right shift of the haemoglobin dissociation curve, the Bohr effect, facilitating oxygen release in the tissues.

CARDIOVASCULAR SYSTEM

1 Inotropy, tachycardia and increased cardiac output due to direct effect of CO_2 on the heart, reflex sympathetic stimulation, and increased circulating catecholamines.
2 Arrhythmias, particularly during halothane anaesthesia.
3 Peripheral resistance: central effect leads to sympathetically mediated vasoconstriction, abolished by spinal anaesthesia; peripheral effect leads to dilatation.
4 Blood pressure often rises.

BIOCHEMICAL

1 Compensatory metabolic alkalosis, by renal retention of bicarbonate.
2 Rise of serum potassium.

EFFECTS ON ACTION OF DRUGS

1 Acidosis affects the ionization and protein-binding of many drugs.
2 Conflicting reported effects on the action of muscle relaxants. Usually antagonized, with difficult reversal.

Reduction of carbon dioxide

Recovery from severe respiratory acidosis may be associated with hypophosphataemia, so the serum phosphate needs to be carefully monitored.[4]

If the PCO_2 is reduced too rapidly after a long period of hypercapnia, there may be:

1 sudden hypotension;[5]
2 a sudden release of potassium from heart muscle and liver causing hyperkalaemia and arrhythmias;
3 a left shift of the haemoglobin dissociation curve which impedes oxygen release in the tissues;
4 a rapid rise in CSF pH leading to cerebral vasoconstriction and convulsions.

Respiratory alkalosis

This is caused by hyperventilation, producing hypocapnia and a rise of pH. Intermittent positive pressure ventilation (IPPV) under clinical conditions may readily reduce the $PaCO_2$ from a normal of 5.3 kPa to half of this value. Other causes of hyperventilation are in response to hypoxia, high altitude, acidaemia or due to localized neurological disease, e.g. hyperventilation syndrome.

If a relaxant is adequately reversed, respiration will usually start again even in the presence of a lower PCO_2 than existed preoperatively, provided that there is not undue depression by opiates. It is not normally necessary to administer CO_2 at the end of an anaesthetic.

Effects

NERVOUS SYSTEM

1 Cerebral vasoconstriction and reduced cerebral blood flow.
2 Clouding of consciousness and analgesia.[6] Voluntary hyperventilation to lessen the pain of surgery was described by Bonwill in 1876.[7]
3 Tetany due to fall in ionized calcium.

CARDIOVASCULAR SYSTEM

Fall of blood pressure and cardiac output, despite vasoconstriction.

CHANGES IN THE BLOOD

1 Fall of plasma potassium.
2 Left shift of the haemoglobin dissociation curve.

FETUS

Hyperventilation causes a reduction in uteroplacental blood flow which, with the left-shifted haemoglobin dissociation curve, causes a fall in fetal oxygen and acidosis.

ELECTROLYTE BALANCE

Sodium

Total amount of sodium in the adult body is about 105 g; about one-third of this is in bone. Basic need of body is 1–2 g/day, but as much as 15 g may be taken with food, the excess being excreted in the urine (normal, 5 g/l). Normal serum levels are 132–145 mmol/l of sodium and 98–106 mmol/l of chloride.

Hyponatraemia[8]

CAUSES

1 Salt loss, such as vomiting, diarrhoea, intestinal fistulae or drainage, intestinal obstruction, diuretic therapy in the elderly.[9]
2 Water retention which dilutes the serum sodium, such as inappropriate antidiuretic hormone (ADH) secretion (part of the endocrine stress response to surgery or trauma), administration of excessive 5% dextrose, glycine absorption during resection of the prostate.
3 The 'sick-cell syndrome' with sodium moving into the intracellular space.

SYMPTOMS

Lassitude, apathy, weakness, anorexia, vomiting, peripheral circulatory failure.

EFFECTS

1 Lowered osmotic pressure of extracellular fluid, excretion of water by the kidneys, and decreased extracellular fluid volume. There may be a rise in blood urea.
2 The disturbance of acid–base balance depends on the relative loss of sodium and chloride ions. Loss of gastric juice leads to hypochloraemia and alkalosis. Loss of other intestinal fluid results in more sodium loss and acidosis.

TREATMENT

1 Treatement of the primary cause.
2 Twice normal saline intravenously (1.8%).
3 Stronger solutions of saline.

Hypernatraemia

This may occur if sodium is retained with water, as in oedema, or by itself. Usually accompanied by hyperchloraemia. May be due to:

1 *Excessive intake* as in overinfusion, excessive oral intake, or use of sodium-containing medicines in babies;
2 *Inability to excrete* as in primary hyperaldosteronism, Cushing's syndrome, excessive steroid therapy.

Hypernatraemia also results from excess water loss, as in pituitary diabetes insipidus. Effects are: mild oedema, thirst, confusion, apathy, leading to coma. Treated by withholding sodium and giving frusemide or thiazides.

Potassium

Most of the body potassium is found within the cells and only about 2% is in the extracellular compartment. Total average values may be taken as 3200 mmol for a 70-kg man. The average dietary intake of a normal healthy adult is 40–120 mmol (3–9 g) per day. Normal serum levels are 3.5–5.0 mmol/l. Normal intracellular concentration is 135–150 mmol/l. Daily urine loss is about 50–75 mmol.

Potassium depletion – hypokalaemia

CAUSES

1 Excessive loss from the gastrointestinal tract, vomiting, diarrhoea (contains 50–100 mmol/l), biliary fistula, etc.
2 Excessive loss in the urine if diuresis is marked.
3 Absence of normal potassium intake especially in the presence of excessive loss, and when the patient is reliant on intravenous fluids.
4 In congestive heart failure with diuretic therapy.
5 May occur when patients are receiving intravenous glucose and saline for long periods.
6 Hyperadrenal states or intensive steroid therapy.
7 Insulinoma (drives potassium into cells).
8 Familial periodic paralysis.
9 Diabetic ketosis.
10 Renal tubular disease.

Alkalosis is a common cause of hypokalaemia as the ion moves into the cells.

EFFECTS

A clinical picture of lethargy, apathy, anorexia and nausea related to disordered function of the three types of muscle:

1 smooth muscle – constipation, distension and ileus;
2 skeletal muscle – hypotonia, weakness and paralysis;
3 cardiac muscle – hypotension, arrhythmias and arrest.

DIAGNOSIS

Suspicion should arise when there is excessive fluid loss from urinary or gastrointestinal tracts, particularly when potassium intake is low or absent. It may be a factor in prolonged paralytic ileus or metabolic alkalosis not responding to normal treatment. Diagnosis is confirmed by:

1 serum potassium estimation, although this can sometimes be normal in the presence of intracellular depletion;
2 Electrocardiogram (ECG) changes – depression of ST segment, lowering, widening or inversion of T waves, prolongation of PR and QT interval, appearance of U waves; these are a reflection of intracellular potassium deficiency;
3 response to treatment.

MANAGEMENT

Complications are likely when the serum potassium is below 3.0 mmol/l. In the previously fit adult patient, this may represent a deficit of 200 mmol which in anaesthesia and intensive care may be replaced intravenously using up to 200 mmol of potassium chloride diluted in 500–1000 ml of 5% dextrose over 4–8 h, although slower rates of replacement may be safer. Clinical judgement should be exercised before active treatment. The correction of hypokalaemia contributes to the correction of concurrent metabolic alkalosis and vice versa.

Proposed surgery may have to be delayed if the serum potassium is below 3.0 mmol/l, because of the risk of cardiac dysrhythmias, potentiation of digitalis, muscle weakness, inability to reverse relaxants, myopathy and renal failure.

Hyperkalaemia

This is dangerous, chiefly because of its effects on the heart.

CAUSES

1 Overzealous intravenous replacement therapy.
2 Renal failure.
3 Administration of suxamethonium causes an acute rise in serum potassium, although less after pretreatment with non-depolarizing relaxant. This occurs within 1–7 min of injection and is of the order of 0.5 mmol/l in normal patients or 1.8 mmol/l in patients with trauma and burns, muscle injury (may be late), muscle diseases such as myopathies, motor neuron disease, muscular dystrophy, denervation and spinal cord transection and tetanus.
4 Metabolic acidosis.
5 Potassium-sparing diuretics.
6 Adrenal insufficiency.

Toxic manifestations may occur at concentrations above 7 mmol/l, when the ECG shows a tall peaked T wave with a narrow base, diminished amplitude of R wave, absence of P wave, widening of QRS and finally a biphasic QRST. Ventricular fibrillation may supervene. Stored blood may contain 25 mmol/l (*see* Chapter 1.2).

TREATMENT

1 Glucose and insulin, which causes a shift of potassium into cells.
2 Bicarbonate infusion 150 mmol has a similar effect.
3 Calcium salts can be given because calcium ions oppose the action of potassium ions on the heart.
4 Long-term treatment includes diet, resonium cation exchange, peritoneal and haemodialysis.

Calcium

The normal range is 2.1–2.6 mmol/l. Half is ionized, and this is of clinical importance in certain patients.

Hypocalcaemia

The level may be lowered as a result of the following.

1 Changes in ventilation affecting PCO_2 (hyperventilation lowers serum ionized calcium).
2 Transfusion with citrated blood. This is seldom important in the healthy individual as the small changes, 0.1–0.2 mmol/l, last only for minutes. When there is a disorder of citrate metabolism (eg. in hypothermia and hepatic transplantation), administration of calcium may be indicated.
3 In some patients with prolonged electrolyte losses through fistulae, etc. Hypocalcaemia results in a long QT interval.
4 After removal of the parathyroids.

Hypercalcaemia

This may be caused by hyperparathyroidism, pseudohyperparathyroidism or chronic renal failure. The ECG shows a short QT interval. Emergency treatment of dangerously high levels (coma and cardiac arrythmias) is with potassium infusion. Elective treatment is by removal of cause, high water intake to prevent renal calculi, phosphate administration (but carries risk of calcification), propranolol (in primary hyperparathyroidism).

Magnesium

Serum magnesium levels may fall after prolonged intravenous therapy in ill patients with electrolyte losses, diuretic therapy, in chronic alcoholics, and major burns. Magnesium is a cofactor in various cellular enzymes. Clinical signs associated with low magnesium include tremors, twitching, tetany, muscular weakness, confusion and hallucinations. It may be given as magnesium chloride, 2 mmol/kg in 4 h. Normal values, 0.9–1.1 mmol/l.

Zinc

It is suspected that lack of zinc may be a factor in delayed wound healing after prolonged severe illness with electrolyte imbalance. It is given with enteral and parenteral nutrition.

Phosphate

Hypophosphataemia exists when the serum phosphate is below 1 mmol/l. Signs are confusion, disorientation, dysarthria, paraesthesia, coma. The oxygen-dissociation curve shifts to the left, and this results in lactic acidosis and pulmonary oedema. There is also poor leucocyte function. The condition is seen mainly during intravenous feeding when fats and phosphate are not provided. The maintenance requirement is at least 10 mmol/day in the adult, given as sodium phosphate, orally or intravenously.

REFERENCES

1 p = Potenz or power; pH (Sorensen SPL C. R. *Trav. Lat. Carlsberg* 1909, **8,** 1).
2 Rosenthal T. B. *J. Biol. Chem.* 1948, **173,** 25; Severinghaus J. W. *J. Appl. Physiol.* 1966, **21,** 1108.
3 Waters R. M. *N. Orl. Med. Surg. J.* 1937, **90,** 219; *Can. Med. Assoc. J.* 1938, **38,** 240.
4 Storm T. L. *Br. Med. J.* 1984, **289,** 456.
5 Brown E. B. and Miller F. *Am. J. Physiol.* 1952, **169,** 56.
6 Robinson J. S. and Gray T. C. *Br. J. Anaesth.* 1961, **33,** 62.
7 Bonwill W. G. A. Penna *J. Dent. Science* 1876, **3,** 57 (reprinted in 'Classical File', *Surv. Anesthesiol.* 1964, **8,** 377).
8 Foote J. *Hospital Update* 1990, **16,** 248–258.
9 Hornick P. and Allen P. *Hospital Update* 1990, **16,** 554.

Nutrition

BACKGROUND

Nutritional requirements

The daily basal requirements are shown in Table 1.4.1.

The calorie requirement of an acutely ill patient is highly variable. Indirect calorimetry (measuring O_2 consumption), may help, but such a patient will need about 30–35 kcal/kg/day. Calorific needs can be increased in various situations as follows: 6% per °C temperature rise; 10% for elective operative stress; 25% for a long-bone fracture; 30% for peritonitis; 50% for multiple

Table 1.4.1 Typical daily nutritional requirements

	Requirement per kg/day body weight	Requirement for 70-kg man per day
Water	25–35 ml	1500–2500 ml
Protein	1 g	70 g (4 kcal or 17 kJ/g)
Nitrogen	0.15–0.2 g	10.5–14.0 g
Carbohydrate	2 g	140 g (4 kcal or 17 kJ/g)
Fat	1–2 g	140 g (9 kcal or 38 kJ/g)
Calories	30 kcal (125 kJ)	2100 kcal (8750 kJ)
Sodium	1.5 mmol	100 mmol
Potassium	6 mmol/g Nitrogen	60–80 mmol
Calcium	0.11 mmol	8 mmol
Magnesium	1 mmol/g Nitrogen	10 mmol
Phosphate	0.5–0.75 mmol	35–50 mmol

The proportion of fat and carbohydrate is very variable. Minerals, vitamins and some trace elements are also necessary. Alcohol provides 7 kcal (29 kJ) per g.

injuries or major sepsis; The area of any burns (25% if <20%, 75% if 20–40%, 100% if >40%).

Indications for artificial feeding include:

1 any cause of gastrointestinal failure such as prolonged paralytic ileus, multiple fistulae or blind loops;
2 major surgery, trauma, burns, sepsis;
3 preoperative malnutrition;
4 some patients with kidney or liver failure (where the usual dietary restrictions apply with equal force to enteral and parenteral nutrition);
5 chemotherapy resulting in intractable nausea and vomiting;
6 coma;
7 severe anorexia nervosa.

Assessment of nutritional status

1 *Simple measurements:* body weight; mid-triceps skinfold thickness (indicates fat stores) should be more than 10 mm in men and 13 mm in women; mid-arm muscle circumference (indicates muscle mass), which is mid-arm circumference minus (π × triceps skinfold thickness), and should be more than 23 cm in men and 22 cm in women. These are subject to errors if oedema is present.
2 *Biochemical estimates of protein lack:* serum albumin; transport proteins with a rapid turnover, e.g. transferrin, thyroxine-binding prealbumin, retinol-binding protein; ratio of urinary creatinine to patient's height. Note that there is normally a turnover of some 100 g of protein per day.
3 *Tests of immunity:* lymphocyte count, suppression of cell-mediated delayed hypersensitivity, e.g. skin reactions to mumps, streptokinase, Candida. Of limited value.

ENTERAL NUTRITION

Enteral feeding

When the patient cannot take oral food, but has a functioning gut, enteral feeding with a liquid diet is more effective and less hazardous than intravenous nutrition. Although a normal gastric tube can be used, a 1-mm internal diameter (ID) plastic tube, with a stylet to stiffen it for insertion, is more comfortable, causes less trauma to the oesophagus and stomach, and may be left in place for up to a month. It can be placed in the stomach or duodenum, but may be misplaced into the lungs. The position is checked by X-ray or endoscopy. The feed is given intermittently from a reservoir, controlled by a clamp or pump. Some regimens give the feed over 12–18 h and rest the gut overnight. Gastrostomy and jejunostomy are important alternative routes, especially for longer term feeding.

The protein sources used are casein, milk or soya. The degree of protein hydrolysis varies. Vegetable oils are used as sources of fat, and starch or corn syrup for carbohydrate. The latter usually provides over half the calories. Most feeds have about 1 kcal (4.2 kJ)/ml. Clinifeed, Isocal and Ensure are widely used. Clinifeed ISO has 260 g of carbohydrate, 56 g of protein, 82 g of fat and 2000 kcal (8400 kJ) per 2000 ml. It provides the recommended 200 kcal (840 kJ) of non-protein calories per gram of nitrogen (1 g nitrogen is equivalent to 6.25 g protein). Vitamins, minerals and trace elements are included, it is low in sodium and the osmolality is 270 mosmol/kg. Vivonex and Flexical have a high proportion of elemental, predigested nutrients. Such feeds have a higher osmolality which can cause diarrhoea, and the indications for them are uncertain.

Some nutrients such as glutamine, short-chain fatty acids and poly-unsaturated fatty acids may be trophic to the gut and be of particular benefit to septic patients.

Complications

1 *Of the tube:* trauma and ulceration of nose, pharynx and gut mucosa; sinusitis (if nasal); misplacement in the lungs; regurgitation and aspiration, reflux can be reduced by nursing the patient at 10 degrees head up.
2 *Gastrointestinal:* change of gut flora, vomiting, regurgitation, large residue on aspiration of the nasogastric (NG) tube, and diarrhoea. The latter is common and may be due to infection of the feed, antibiotics, lactose intolerance or high osmotic pressure of feed. The feed should be slowed, diluted with water or changed. Loperamide 2 mg, up to 16 mg daily, or codeine phosphate 30 mg, up to 180 mg daily, are useful.
3 *Metabolic:* fluid balance and electrolyte abnormalities, hyperglycaemia, folate deficiency.

PARENTERAL NUTRITION

Parenteral feeding

Intravenous nutrition is used when feeding via the gut is not possible. May be total (TPN) or supplement partial oral or tube feeds. Maintains the patient until the gut failure is corrected, and is usually started after a few days' starvation, or when prolonged feeding difficulties are expected, e.g. major abdominal surgery. Total parenteral nutrition aims to provide:

1 nitrogen in the form of amino acids in order to reduce muscle breakdown;
2 calories;
3 essential amino acids;
4 electrolytes, phosphate, trace elements, folate and vitamins.

Nitrogen loss in a moderately catabolic patient will exceed 15 g/day, and can be easily measured as urinary urea, adding any proteinuria or rise in total body urea:

Nitrogen loss (g/day) =

daily urinary urea $\dfrac{\text{grams}}{2}$ or $\dfrac{\text{mmol}}{30}$

+ daily urinary protein excretion $\dfrac{\text{grams}}{6.25}$

+ body wt (kg) × daily rise in blood urea $\dfrac{\text{mg/dl}}{360}$ or $\dfrac{\text{mmol/l}}{60}$

(1 g urea = 17 mmol urea = 0.47 g nitrogen)

The loss of 15 g of nitrogen represents the breakdown of 94 g of protein, or 450g of muscle. It is usually recommended that 200 kcal (840 kJ) of non-protein calories per gram of nitrogen should be given, although this may have to be reduced to 150 kcal (630 kJ) per gram nitrogen in the sickest patient. If glucose is the only non-protein energy source, protein anabolism is not optimal, and CO_2 production is higher, putting a strain on patients with poor respiratory reserve. Non-protein energy is best provided equally from glucose and fat.

Carbohydrate

Body stores of carbohydrate are limited, the average adult having only 5 g of blood glucose and 100 g of liver glycogen. Adequate carbohydrate is needed to allow fat utilization without ketosis, the minimum for this being 400 kcal (1.7 MJ) of carbohydrate energy per day, although normally at least 50% of the administered calories are from glucose. Fructose, sorbitol, ethanol, xylitol have all been used as alternative carbohydrate energy sources in the past but offer no advantage over glucose, and indeed can cause metabolic problems, such as lactic acidosis or an osmotic diuresis.

Glucose provides 4.0 kcal (17 kJ) per gram. One litre of isotonic (5%) solution provides only 200 kcal (840 kJ), so concentrated solutions are needed to give enough calories without overhydration. Twenty-five per cent glucose supplies 250 g glucose and 1000 kcal (4 MJ) per litre. Twenty-five per cent or 50% are commonly used, and these solutions need a central vein. The metabolic response to surgery or trauma includes impaired glucose tolerance, but insulin does not often need to be given if less than 500 g glucose is given per day. If needed it may be given intravenously by infusion, normally about 1 unit per 4 g glucose infused, keeping the blood glucose below 12 mmol/l.

Fat

Fat provides 9.0 kcal (38 kJ) per gram. Advantages include iso-osmolarity and neutral pH (can be given into a peripheral vein). No losses occur in faeces or urine. Fat is provided as a 10% or 20% soya oil emulsion, with particle diameters 0.2–1.0 μm, much the same as a chylomicron. The surfactant is egg phospholipid and glycerol is added to make the solution isotonic. Five hundred millilitres of 20% emulsion provides 1000 kcal (4.2 MJ). this provides the essential fatty acids. It is well utilized in all patients. The fasting patient's spun plasma may be examined each day for excessive milkiness (which calls for a reduction in fat intake). This is more likely in liver insufficiency, acute pancreatitis, uraemia and septicaemia. Occasional side-effects are shivering, flushing and fever.

Patients on infusions of propofol for sedation may receive a considerable proportion of their daily fat requirements by this route and this should be taken into consideration when planning a TPN regimen.

Protein

Given as a mixture of essential and non-essential crystalline amino acids in the physiological laevo-rotatory form. Solutions with higher proportions of branched-chain amino acids (valine, leucine, isoleucine) have no advantage in most patients, except those suffering from hepatic failure. Most solutions have nitrogen contents ranging from 9 to 18 g/l, are hyperosmolar and have a pH around 5.6. Some, however, have 5 g nitrogen per litre, an osmolality of only 370 mosmol/kg and so can be given peripherally. There is no point in giving more than 24 g of amino acid nitrogen per day, as it then cannot be handled by the liver. A typical dose in most clinical situations would be 0.2–0.25 g nitrogen/kg/day. The electrolyte composition varies, some are nearly electrolyte-free. Extra electrolytes may be added by the pharmacy.

Additives

These are conveniently provided by commercial additive preparations.

ELECTROLYTES

Daily requirements very variable with the clinical situation, but approximately: sodium 100 mmol and potassium 60 mmol or 6 mmol/g nitrogen, more if febrile; phosphate 40 mmol, less if in renal failure and more if very catabolic – should not be mixed with calcium or magnesium for injection; calcium 5–15 mmol; magnesium 10 mmol or 1 mmol/g nitrogen. Chloride is also present in most additives.

VITAMINS

Daily requirements: thiamine (B_1) 3 mg: riboflavine (B_2) 3.6 mg; pyridoxine (B_6) 4 mg; nicotinamide 40 mg; vitamin B_{12} 5 μg; biotin 60 μg; pantothenic acid 15 mg; folic acid 0.4 mg; vitamin A 1 mg; vitamin C (ascorbic acid) 100 mg; vitamin D 200 IU; vitamin E 10 mg; vitamin K 150 μg. The B vitamins degrade when exposed to light.

TRACE ELEMENTS

Daily requirements: iron 20 μmol; zinc 100 μmol (more if very catabolic); copper 20 μmol; manganese 5 μmol; chromium 0.2 μmol; selenium 0.4 μmol; molybdenum 0.2 μmol; fluorine 50 μmol; iodine 1 μmol.

Management

A central venous catheter is needed for most TPN solutions, inserted under aseptic conditions, and used for nothing else. There is disagreement as to the necessity for subcutaneous tunneling of the catheter (for insertion, *see* Chapter 1.2). If a multilumen catheter is used, one lumen should be reserved exclusively for TPN. Some lower osmolality solutions (lipids, and low nitrogen amino acid solutions) may be given through a peripheral vein using a fine-bore silicone catheter. Total parenteral nutrition is generally managed by a multidisciplinary team and can be carried out at home for patients with, for example, Crohn's disease. The desired mixture is made up in pharmacy, presented in a 3-litre bag and infused over 24 h with a controlled volumetric pump. Albumin or red cells should be given to patients with hypoproteinaemia or anaemia although albumin may be ineffective at correcting the plasma level.

Complications

These can largely be prevented by adequate biochemical monitoring.

1 *Glucose metabolism:* hyperglycaemia, due to excess hypertonic glucose or insufficient insulin. Ketoacidosis may occur. May progress to hyperosmolar syndrome (facial flushing, lethargy, coma) with a poor prognosis. Hypercapnia may occur with too much glucose.
2 *Amino acid metabolism:* patients in acute renal failure will have to be dialysed or have haemofiltration more frequently due to prerenal uraemia. Patients with hepatic encephalopathy may benefit from a higher proportion of branched chain amino acids. Metabolic acidosis may be due to excessive chloride in some amino acid solutions.
3 *Fats:* the sicker patients may be less able to metabolize fat. Essential fatty acid deficiency.
4 *Water and electrolytes:* circulatory overload, excess water and hyponatraemia relatively common. Electrolyte deficiencies include potassium, calcium (tetany and muscle spasm), phosphate (weakness, metabolic bone disease resembling osteomalacia, left-shift oxygen dissociation curve), magnesium (tetany, weakness, tremor, dysrhythmias).
5 *Vitamin and trace element deficiencies:* thiamine deficiency for even 1 month may produce cardiac failure from acute beri-beri. Lack of vitamin B_{12} or folate causes anaemia, and lack of vitamin K causes clotting defects. Zinc deficiency causes acrodermatitis enteropathica (crusty skin lesions around the mouth, nostrils and sites of trauma), chronic infections and diarrhoea.

Copper deficiency causes anaemia, osteoporosis, leucopenia and reduced red cell superoxide dismutase.

6 *Catheter sites:* infection, thrombophlebitis, complications of central venous cannulation (pneumothorax, damage to arteries and nerves, etc.).

7 *Miscellaneous:* cholestasis may occur, possibly due to overgrowth of intestinal bacteria. It has been prevented by metronidazole, suggesting anaerobic infection.

FURTHER READING

Philips G. D. and Odgers C. L. *Parenteral and Enteral Nutrition: A Practical Guide*, 3rd edn. Edinburgh: Churchill Livingstone 1986.

Immediate postoperative care (recovery)[1]

The anaesthetist is directly responsible for anaesthetic aspects of the patient until the patient is conscious (patients unconscious prior to surgery are, of course, exceptions), or until function has returned after regional block; and vital functions are stable and can be preserved without assistance. This normally takes place in a recovery ward,[2] where respiratory and circulatory care and analgesia are managed to an agreed standard.[3] The patient is transferred to the surgical ward when conscious, comfortable and with an adequate ventilation and a stable circulation. (In the UK, the primary medical responsibility for patient care after return to the general ward lies with the surgical team.) There is no consensus on the degree to which anaesthetists and pain teams are involved in ongoing patient care – this is a matter of healthy topical debate.

A possible scheme of shared perioperative management	
Item of care	->->Time (pre- & postoperative days) ->->
Oxygenation	Anaesthetist/physiotherapist/surgeon
Pain control	Anaesthetist/pain team ->-> surgical team
Nutrition	Surgical team/nutrition team/nurses
Wound care	Surgical team
Mobilization	Surgical team

The anaesthetist must hand over carefully to the recovery nurse drawing attention to any unusual features of the patient, surgery or anaesthesia, institute monitoring and leave clear instructions for the patient's care (*see* protocol below). It may be helpful to write these in the notes. Failure of immediate postoperative care is an important contributing factor to mortality and morbidity associated with anaesthesia.

Management of haemorrhage is the responsibility of the surgeon.

THE POSTOPERATIVE RECOVERY WARD

Transfer from theatre to recovery ward should be as short as possible. The patient should receive oxygen.

Location

The postoperative recovery ward should be as close as possible to the operating theatre, and the intensive therapy unit (ITU)/high-dependency unit (HDU) (with which it is continuous), and part of the 'clean' area. Curtains for privacy should be available. Different areas are designated for different types of case, and for different ages and sexes. Requirements vary with the type of surgery performed. Three beds per theatre will be needed for busy specialities. A floor space of 9.3 m^2 (100 ft^2) per bed has been recommended.[4]

Equipment

This should include oxygen therapy equipment, ventilators, self-inflating resuscitation bags and monitors, intravenous drip apparatus, beds and trolleys which can be easily tipped, proper lighting and suction apparatus. There is equipment for resuscitation, intubation, chest drainage and bronchoscopy, with piped oxygen and suction at each bed-head. Entonox may be valuable.

Staffing is likely to be needed through 24 hours except in daycase recovery.

Functions

In the postoperative room the nursing and medical staff observe, record and, if necessary, remedy:

1 the comfort of the patient, including consciousness and sedation, relief of pain,[5] restlessness, nausea, vomiting and shivering;
2 the airway, respiratory activity (rate/depth), oxygenation, capnography;
3 cardiovascular stability – the pulse rate, blood pressure, various other vascular pressures, peripheral perfusion, arrythmias;
4 body temperature;
5 the intravenous infusions (including nutrition);
6 neuromuscular function, where relaxants have been used;
7 surgical drains, catheter, etc.;
8 urine output, if appropriate;
9 other specialized care, e.g. spinal blocks, intracranial pressure;
10 haemorrhage/ wound site.

Staffing

The postoperative ward should be staffed to allow for a nurse for each high-dependency case, a nurse for each three 'medium-dependency' cases, and a nurse for each four 'low-dependency' cases; three beds being sufficient for each operating room, on average.

The handover procedure

A simple verbal protocol may include the following information:

1 The patient's name.
2 The operation and surgeon.
3 The anaesthetic used, e.g. general, local.
4 Drugs given, e.g. which opiates and how and when they were given.
5 Regional blocks, and which drug(s) were used.
6 The state of the teeth, e.g. crowns, bridges and loose teeth.
7 Blood loss (and whether it has been stopped) and the intravenous regimen.
8 Any complications, e.g. difficulty in reversal of relaxants.
9 Arterial pressure and respiration – adequate? Stable?
10 Details of the analgesia given and prescribed.
11 Other medical conditions, even social information if relevant.
12 (In oral surgery), whether the throat pack has been removed.

PROBLEMS OF THE IMMEDIATE POSTOPERATIVE PERIOD

Inadequate respiration[6]

Pulse monitors, capnography and apnoea alarms help the visual monitoring of nurses here. To prevent obstruction, the head is extended, the mandible

---

Causes of postoperative hypoventilation

1 obstructed airway

2 anaesthetic drugs – especially volatiles and opioids

3 incomplete reversal of relaxants

4 pain

5 shock

6 CO_2 narcosis (caused by, and a cause of, hypoventilation)

7 obesity and medical problems of the patient, e.g. myasthenia, pulmonary disease, raised intracranial pressure

displaced anteriorly, an airway inserted, the patient turned on the side, head down and 100% oxygen given, with intermittent positive-pressure ventilation (IPPV) if necessary, and pharyngeal suction if appropriate. Hypoxia causes cyanosis, restlessness, and tachycardia, followed by bradycardia, circulatory arrest and brain damage.

Action plan for low postoperative SpO$_2$

1 quickly check the monitor, probe and patient colour for accuracy of reading. Seek help

2 diagnose the cause
   (a) obstruction of airway (tongue, vomit, mucus) and/or tube (kink, cuff herniation)
   (b) inadequate respiration (is the patient breathing, e.g. apnoea, breath-holding, bronchospasm, pulmonary oedema)
   (c) failure of oxygen supply
   (d) a cardiac/circulatory problem, e.g. hypotension
   (e) other rare problems: pneumothorax etc.

3 quickly listen to the chest

4 increase FiO$_2$ and ventilation

5 check circulatory status – is the heart beating, what is the blood pressure? Is there anaphylaxis?

6 consider other rare problems

Hypercarbia causes tachycardia, sweating, hypertension, cutaneous vaso-dilatation, arrythmias, and clouding of consciousness. **The cause is then found and corrected.** At particular risk are the obese, elderly, snoring 'sleep apnoea' patients, even during the first few postoperative nights, when continuous oxygen is prescribed and respiration is monitored by the nurses.

Paediatric recovery[7]

Small children are particularly at risk, from narrower airways, operations around the upper airway, hypothermia, longer duration of drug action and faster onset of hypoxia.

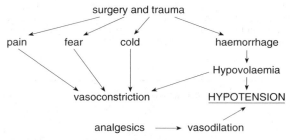

Figure 1.5.1 Cardiovascular instability

After major cases, especially vascular and cardiac surgery, the peripheral circulation may remain 'shut down' for 3–5 h. During this time some body water goes into 'the third space'. Then, often with warming, over a matter of $\frac{1}{2}$ h, the peripheral circulation 'opens up' with falls of peripheral resistance, venous and arterial pressure. Lactate, washed in from the peripheral tissues causes acidosis. Generous colloid infusion and dilating inotropic support is prophylactic. Intraoperative active warming, analgesia and adequate hydration are important preventive measures. The base deficit is a good guide to therapy.

Position of patient

The lateral position (perhaps with slight head-down tilt) is safest for the airway, with one or other knee drawn up to prevent rolling. After some orthopaedic and other procedures, it may be impossible to place the patient on the side, and there is greater risk of airway obstruction or aspiration. Head-down tilt is of little value in a patient lying on the back, owing to the angle the trachea makes with the horizontal.

Monitoring

Hypoxaemic episodes are especially common, both in the postoperative room[8] and during transfer to it from the operating theatre. They are often not recognized by simple clinical observation, and not certain to be prevented by the routine administration of oxygen (although this is recommended).[9] Monitoring of the circulation and respiration should continue for as long as needed. Pulse oximetry is especially useful.

Some classic signs of haemorrhage, i.e. tachycardia and restlessness, are often absent in the postoperative ward. Measurement of the actual loss (or the CVP) assumes greater importance. Increasing girth is of little help in the diagnosis of intra-abdominal haemorrhage. Non-invasive arterial pressure monitoring remains a routine.

Postoperative restlessness

This can be dangerous, leading, for example, to dislocation of hip prostheses, and removal of drains and drips. After hypoxaemia, pain, haemorrhage and full bladder have been corrected, this usually responds to a small intravenous dose of benzodiazepine. The sudden return of pain after remifentanil infusion may cause restlessness.

PAIN ASSESSMENT

Pain assessment: verbal scale

'Which word best describes the pain you have when you move or breathe deeply?'

0 = no pain

1–2 = mild pain

3–5 = moderate pain

6–7 = severe pain

8–10 = unbearable pain

POSTOPERATIVE PAIN MANAGEMENT

See Chapter 1.6.

POSTOPERATIVE NAUSEA AND VOMITING (PONV)

Antiemetics

These are required after about 15% of general anaesthetics, and after nearly half of postoperative opioid administrations and gynaecological operations.

Ondansetron 4 mg i.m., iv., works well in combination with other antiemetics.

Prochlorperazine (Stemetil) 6.25–12.5 mg i.m. only.

Cyclizine 25–50 mg, i.m., i.v., may cause mild tachycardia. It is very effective to prescribe this on a regular routine basis, e.g. 8- or 12-hourly. for the first 1–2 days after inpatient surgery.

Perphenazine 5 mg i.m. only.

Metoclopramide 10 mg. – very few side-effects except in high dosage. It acts centrally and also increases gastrointestinal motility. It also increases the tone of the gastro-oesophageal sphincter, reducing chance of regurgitation.

Droperidol 1–5 mg, powerful, but with more side-effects, even within the usual therapeutic range, e.g. dysphoria, dyskinesia, bad dreams and hallucinations.

SCORING SYSTEMS FOR RECOVERY FROM ANAESTHESIA

Salim ABC recovery score based on physical signs			
	3	2	1	0
Airways	can cough or cry	maintains airway without holding jaw	holding of jaw needed	holding of jaw and other measures taken to maintain airway
Behaviour	can lift the head	can open eyes and show tongue	some non-purposeful movements	no movement at all
Consciousness	fully awake, can talk, well orientated	awake but needs support	responds to stimuli only	no response

A score of **8 is the minimum for discharge** from the recovery room

OTHER TESTS OF RECOVERY (none has proved to be reliable)

1 Critical flicker fusion threshold – visual and auditory, a measure of sensory impairment.
2 Picture recall: nine or so objects from a memory card are memorized for a minute.

(a) after the test event, the subject is asked to recall them;
(b) for the forgotten ones, the verbal cued recall score is made using simple clues to help the subject;
(c) a further card of 20 or so pictures, containing the nine original pictures is shown, and the subject asked to pick out the originals (visual recognition score).

3 Backward spelling of common 4-letter words!
4 Serial 7s – time for backward counting in 7s from 100 to 44.
5 P letter deletion: usually crossing out 'b's or 'p's from a page full of letters.
6 Forward and backward digit span.
7 Time for reverse counting from 1000 to 976.

(Fitness to drive a car or operate machinery still awaits exact definition despite these tests, so the old 24-h rule is usually applied. The greatest danger is when the patient subjectively feels wonderful but objectively has slow reaction times.)

THE POSTANAESTHETIC CONSULTATION

Day-case patients are reviewed later on in the day prior to discharge. In-patients are reviewed at an appropriate time, usually 24–48 h after anaesthesia. The following items are noted and the visit recorded in the patient's notes (very important):

1 How the patient feels. Are there any residual side-effects from anaesthesia?
2 Whether the patient's pain is being adequately controlled. Does the patient need further advice about the PCA? (Note that the outcome of surgery is not related to the route by which opioids are given, and side-effects are related only to the total dose of opioid.[10]) Responsibility for pain control will return to the surgical team, (with the advice and help of the acute pain team). Oral long-acting opioids are useful at this hand-over.[11]
3 Does the patient have any nausea or vomiting? Are the antiemetics being given as prescribed?
4 If there is an intravenous infusion, is the drip site satisfactory? Is the patient receiving adequate nutrition? (equally important in day-cases!) Note that the management responsibility for fluid balance and nutrition will return to the surgical team about this time.
5 Are the patient's vital signs still stable? This is an area for discussion with the nurses and surgical team.
6 Have the patient's regular medications been resumed? (An example is steroid therapy.)
7 Is the patient's oxygenation satisfactory? Is respiration adequate? Can the patient cough properly?
8 Has there been a return of usual cognitive function?
9 Is the patient sleeping well at night? (Both surgery and morphine reduce rapid eye movement sleep.)[12]

10 Has the patient any other morbidity? Seventy per cent of these are non-cardiac,[13] about half are gastrointestinal and about a quarter related to ambulation.

The anaesthetist is sometimes referred to as the perioperative physician, optimizing the patient, organizing pre- and postoperative referrals, with graded hand-over of various aspects of the patient's care postoperatively. A postoperative care team has a role in directing patients to HDU or ITU.[14]

PROGRESSIVE POSTOPERATIVE CARE AND HIGH DEPENDENCY UNITS (HDUs)[15]

The trend towards more major surgery on older and sicker patients, and the need to make best use of scarce resources, has led to the development of HDUs, usually as an extension of the recovery ward. The nursing staff here are more numerous than on a general ward, and are trained in specialized monitoring techniques. The patients for such a unit are chosen by their need for a particular level of care. Patients are transferred to the ITU for organ support and life support. Patients likely to benefit are: after major surgery, significant trauma, major acute medical conditions, and specialized drug administration (e.g. epidural infusions). Invasive monitoring is routine. When the period of higher risk is judged to have passed, the patient may be returned (or 'progress') back to the original ward.

Location

It may be a single designated place within a hospital (in this case, defining the responsibility for patient care is often a problem) or high-dependency areas within wards in multiple sites in a hospital. In the latter arrangement, the responsibility for patient care is more obviously with the admitting team. The bed area may be similar to that in a general ward, but with piped oxygen, suction and a dozen power points.

Equipment

Multiple racks and shelves hold monitoring equipment:– ECG, invasive and non-invasive arterial pressure, CVP, pulse oximetry, capnography, temperature, urine flow. Additional monitors include ICP, cardiac output (invasive and non-invasive), and simple haematology and biochemistry. A defibrillator is always near.

Staffing

In a centralized unit, a clinical coordinator ensures interpretation of established guidelines and communication between staff groups. There must be clear written guidelines as to which group of medical staff are responsible for which aspects of the patient's care. An operating theatre manager often holds the budget.

Nursing levels: opinions vary between three and five whole-time equivalents per bed.

Advantages: improvement in the care of the severely ill patients with high nursing dependency.[16]

Disadvantages: in a centralized unit, physicians and surgeons may feel some loss of control of their patients; reduced sense of continuity of patient care for the nurses in the unit; nursing interest on the ordinary wards may decline.

REFERENCES

1 Hatfield A. and Tronson M. *The Complete Recovery Room Book*. Oxford University Press, Oxford, 1996.
2 Jolly C. and Lee J. A. *Anaesthesia* 1957, **12,** 49; Discussion, *Proc. R. Soc. Med.* 1958, **51,** 151.
3 *Standards for Postanesthesia Care*. American Society of Anesthesiologists, 1988.
4 Department of Health and Social Security, *Operating Department*. Health Building Note 26. HMSO, London,1975.
5 McQuay H. J., Moore R. A. and Justins D. *Br. Med. J.* 1997, **314,** 1531–1535.
6 Zelcer J. and Wells D. G. *Anaesth. Intensive Care* 1987, **15,** 168.
7 Mather S. J.and Hughes D. G. *A Handbook of Paediatric Anaesthesia.* Oxford University Press, Oxford, 1996.
8 Jones J. G. et al. *Anaesthesia* 1990, **45,** 563.
9 Moller J. T. et al. *Anesthesiology* 1990, **73,** 890.
10 Kehlet H. et al. *J. Clin. Anesth.* 1996, **8,** 441–445.
11 Smith G. and Power I. *Anaesthesia* 1998, **53,** 521–522.
12 Rosenberg A. et al. *Br. J. Anaesth.* 1994, **72,** 145; Cronin B. *Br. J. Anaesth.* 1995, **74,** 188.
13 *Crit. Care Med.* 1997, **1,** 103.
14 Lee A., Lum M. E., O'Regan W.J. and Hillman K.M. *Anaesthesia* 1998, **53,** 529–535.
15 *The High Dependency Unit*. Association of Anaesthetists, London, 1991.
16 *See* Brampton W.J. and Rowan K.M. *Anaesthesia* 1998, **53,** 612, for audit.

Acute pain management

The relief of pain is purchased always at a price.

(Ralph Waters)

There are many causes of acute pain other than postsurgery; including trauma, infection, cancer and medical conditions (such as sickle-cell crisis and rheumatic disease). Rarely postsurgical pain may become persistent (chronic). In theory, pain should be controllable. In practice there is often a gap between the ideal and the achievable. Perfect analgesia cannot be guaranteed and patients should not expect that it can.

PATHOPHYSIOLOGY OF ACUTE PAIN

Tissue damage and inflammation

Noxious stimuli sufficient to cause tissue damage are associated with release of numerous inflammatory mediators.[1,2]

Inflammatory mediators may be directly algogenic or enhance the algogenic effects of other stimuli. Chemical mediators of inflammation exert their effect on membrane ion channels of nociceptive neurones either by direct coupling to membrane receptors for specific substances (hydrogen ion, adenosine triphosphate, serotonin 5-HT_3), or more commonly by an indirect action mediated by intracellular second messengers (bradykinin, cytokines, prostanoids, histamine H_1, serotonin 5-HT_1). Some mediators act on other parts of the neurone to control the expression of receptor proteins and ion channels or to control the release of mediators by other cells. In addition, many inflammatory cells express receptors for neuropeptides that are released from peripheral nerve terminals (substance P, calcitonin gene-related peptide (CGRP)).[2,3]

Yet other mediators such as platelet-activating factor (PAF) enhance the process by acting on blood vessels and inflammatory cells to evoke long-lasting arteriolar vasodilatation.[4] Important mediators involved in inflammatory hyperalgesia include bradykinin, cytokines (interleukin IL-1, IL-6, IL-8, tumour necrosis factor (TNF-α)), and eicosanoids (prostaglandins and leukotrienes LTB4, LTD4).

Inflammatory mediators

Bradykinin: The autocoid bradykinin is cleaved from inactive precursors in response to tissue damage. Bradykinin is a potent algogenic agent which also sensitizes nociceptors to the action of other algogens, increases vascular permeability and enhances leucocyte chemotaxis. Bradykinin receptor activation releases prostaglandins from sympathetic fibres as well as from other tissues.[2] Binding sites for bradykinin are found on sensory nerve fibres and in the dorsal horn. Two subtypes of the bradykinin receptor have been characterized. Both are members of the G-protein superfamily. BK-2 is a constitutive member whilst BK-1 exhibits low expression but is upregulated by cytokine-driven inflammatory processes.[2,5]

Catecholamines have been implicated in nociception at the spinal cord level, the effect being mediated by the α_2-adrenoceptor.

Cytokines are regulatory peptides produced in all cells. They have pleiotropic actions; anti-inflammatory cytokines and growth factors contribute to inflammatory hyperalgesia. Thus, TNF-α release is stimulated by bradykinin. This stimulates the production of IL-1 and IL-6, which induce hyperalgesia via the production of cyclo-oxygenase products. The effect of IL-8 is mediated via sympathetic nerve fibres.[2]

Histamine released from damaged cells and mast cells in response to substance P and nerve growth factor (NGF) causes activation of nociceptors, vasodilatation and oedema.

Serotonin released by platelets in response to PAF is directly algogenic and enhances the nociceptive effect of bradykinin on sensory nerves. Both 5-HT$_1$ and 5-HT$_3$ receptors are involved.[2]

Protons: inflammatory exudates tend to be acidic and there is evidence that protons at the site of tissue damage enhances the action of algogenic substances as well as exciting neurones directly.

Prostaglandins: tissue damage releases phospholipids from cell membranes which are broken down by phospholipase to form arachidonic acid. Cyclo-oxygenase-catalysed oxidation of arachidonic acid results in the production of cyclic prostaglandins. The cyclo-oxygenase enzyme is encoded by two genes and two forms of the enzyme (COX-1 and COX-2) have been characterized.[2] COX-1 is produced in quiescent conditions and is a constitutive member of normal cells; important in circumstances where prostaglandins have a protective function, such as gastric mucus production and renal blood flow maintenance. COX-2, the inducible form of the enzyme, is the major isozyme associated with inflammation. COX-2 is induced in endothelial cells, macrophages and synovial fibroblasts, mast cells chondrocytes and osteoblasts after tissue trauma by inflammatory agents.[2,6,7] Prostaglandins sensitize nociceptors to the action of other algogenic substances and to mechanical stimuli.

Leukotrienes, the lipoxygenase products of arachidonic acid metabolism, may also have algogenic properties.

Pain signalling and modulation

Information signalling acute injury is transmitted along fast conduction velocity (20 m/sec) myelinated A-δ fibres (sharp first pain) and slow conduction velocity (0.5–2.0 m/sec) unmyelinated C fibres (dull second pain).

These first-order neurones synapse with second-order neurones in the dorsal horn of the spinal cord. A-δ fibres terminate mainly in lamina I, while C fibres terminate in lamina II. There is increased release of neuropeptides such as substance P, and excitatory amino acids such as glutamate, in the dorsal horn. Projection of nociceptive information to the thalamus is conducted up the spinothalamic tracts. Synapse of second-order with third-order neurones in the ventral portion of the thalamus results in onward transmission of the nociceptive impulse to the sensory cortex, where it is ultimately perceived as pain.

Endogenous opioid modulation

Considerable modulation of pain sensation, both facilitatory and inhibitory, occurs within the central nervous system (CNS) and at peripheral afferent nerve endings. Endogenous opioid peptides are found in high density in areas of the CNS involved in nociception. Three groups of endogenous opioids (enkephalins, β-endorphins and dynorphins) have been identified. Endogenous opioids modulate nociception by binding to specific receptors. There are several types of opioid receptor (μ_1 and μ_2, κ, δ, ε, σ) each mediating a spectrum of pharmacological effects. Activation of the μ-receptor is largely responsible for supraspinal analgesia whereas activation of the κ- and δ-receptors results in spinal analgesia. The ε- and σ-receptors have been less clearly characterized although it seems that the σ-receptor is responsible for the production of psychotomimetic effects. β-endorphin is the prototypic endogenous opioid ligand at the μ-receptor, enkephalin is the prototypic ligand at the δ-receptor and dynorphin is the prototypic ligand at the κ- receptor. Recently opioid receptors have been reclassified as OP$_1$ (δ), OP$_2$ (κ) and OP$_3$ (μ).[8]

Opioids also act peripherally to block the release of inflammatory mediators, but this action is only manifest in injury and inflammation.

Endogenous non-opioid modulation

Inhibition by a descending monoaminergic pathway may modulate pain traffic at the spinal level. Peripheral chemical sensitization of the receptor transduction mechanism is, however, independent of central connections.[9]

Hyperalgesia

Tissue damage induces a state of hyperalgesia (increased response to a given stimulus intensity).

Primary hyperalgesia occurs within the area of injury and is due to sensitization of primary afferent neurones by inflammatory mediators.[5]

Secondary (mechanical) hyperalgesia develops in the surrounding uninjured tissue and is thought to be due to activation of the *N*-methyl-D-aspartate (NMDA) receptor (a subtype of the glutamate receptor) in the dorsal horn of the spinal cord; the phenomenon of 'wind-up'.[5,9,10]

In addition to producing immediate electrophysiological wind-up, noxious stimuli can cause long-lasting modification of cell phenotype by altering the expression of immediate early onset genes (IEG). Activation of the NMDA receptor may induce transcriptional activity of the IEG *c-fos*. Expression of *c-fos* is associated with increased production of dynorphin and other neurotrophic factors such as NGF, which affect the growth and survival of neurones.[1] Nerve growth factor regulates the synthesis of substance P and CGRP and has a prohyperalgesic action by increasing nociceptor excitability.

ACUTE POSTOPERATIVE PAIN

Pain measurement

Knowledge of the incidence and severity of postoperative pain is essential for the establishment of effective pain treatment programmes. Acute pain is commonly assessed using single-dimension pain scales (behavioural, verbal and numerical rating scales; visual analogue scale) as opposed to multidimensional pain scales (McGill pain questionnaire). Clinically verbal rating scales (VRS) tend to be preferred to visual analogue scale (VAS) for the measurement of acute postoperative pain because of their perceived greater ease of use.

Pain scoring

The simplest subjective measure of pain is to ask the patient whether or not he or she feels any pain. Greater sensitivity is obtained if ordered categories are used to grade the pain but the maximum number of grades of pain that a patient can define is no more than 21.

A simple VRS with which a patient is asked to describe the amount of pain that he or she feels according to an arbitrary scale is:

None
Mild /Slight pain
Moderate pain
Severe pain
Very severe/Intolerable

As many opioids are also sedatives, 'sedation scores' may also be recorded.

Incidence of postoperative pain

Between one-third and a half of all surgical patients experience significant postoperative pain. The incidence and severity of acute surgical pain depends on:

1 the site of operation (in one large series of operations, postoperative analgesia was required in 74% of thoracic cases; 63% of upper abdominal cases; 51% of lower abdominal cases and 23% of body-wall operations);[11]
2 age;
3 sex;
4 premedication;
5 anaesthetic agents;
6 Psychological factors;
7 Diurnal factors.

Adverse effects of uncontrolled postoperative pain

Adverse sequelae of uncontrolled postoperative pain include delayed postoperative recovery, increased postoperative morbidity, delayed return of normal physiological functions, restriction of mobility with risk of thromboembolism and heightened catecholamine response leading to increased oxygen consumption. Uncontrolled pain is recognized as the primary cause of pulmonary dysfunction after surgery with reduced sputum clearance, atelectasis, regional underventilation, perfusion inequality, shunting of venous blood and reduced Functional Residual Capacity (FRC), all contributing to hypoxia.

The problem of postoperative pain

Pain has a physiological protective function and is not necessarily bad. It is essential to consider both the management of pain on return of consciousness and the continuing management of pain when the first postoperative dose of analgesic has worn off (the 'pain gap'). Opioid analgesics are the mainstay for relief of postoperative pain but have tended to be underused because of excessive concern about creating drug dependency and fear of inducing respiratory depression. These risks are overstated; the incidence of addiction among patients who receive opioids for pain relief is less than 0.1% and the incidence of respiratory depression is no more than 1%.[12]

Several approaches have been made to solve this problem.

1 Use of non-opioid analgesics on their own or in combination with opioid analgesics.
2 Use of regular injections of opioids rather than injections at the discretion of the nurse.
3 Use of continuous intravenous or subcutaneous infusion of opioids.

4 Use of 'patient-controlled analgesia' (PCA).
5 Use of extradural route of opioid administration.
6 Use of the very long-acting oral opioids.
7 Use of long-acting regional blocks where appropriate. The quality of this analgesia is usually better than that provided by opioids and non-steroidal anti-inflammatory drugs (NSAIDs), but regional analgesia is limited by time constraints and by side-effects.

An enormous amount of concern and effort is made by doctors and nurses to relieve pain. In the perioperative setting, the acute pain team is very important (*see below*).

Drugs used in acute postoperative pain management

Non-steroidal anti-inflammatory drugs[13]

Non-steroidal anti-inflammatory drugs may be sufficiently effective as sole analgesics after minor to intermediate surgery. They are also useful after major surgery when their opioid-sparing effect ($\sim 30\%$) will help contribute towards a reduction in overall side-effects. They may usefully be combined with paracetamol.

Table 1.6.1 Chemical classification of non-steroidal anti-inflammatory drugs.

Carboxylic acids	
Salicylic acids	
Acetylated	Aspirin
Nonacetylated	Diflunisal, Salicyl, Salicylate
Acetic acids	
Indoleacetic acids	Acemetacin, Indomethacin, Sulindac
Phenylacetic acids	Aceclofenac, Diclofenac
Pyrolleacetic acids	Ketorolac, Tolmetin
Naphthylacetic acid	Nabumetone
2-Aryl propionic acids	
Phenyl propionic acids	Ibuprofen, Fenbufen, Fenoprofen, Flurbiprofen, Ketoprofen, Tiaprofenic acid
Naphthyl proprionic acids	Naproxen
Fenamates	
n-Phenylanthranilic acid	Mefenamic acid
Enolic acids	
Pyrazolones	Azapropazone, Phenylbutazone
Oxicams	Piroxicam, Tenoxicam, Meloxicam

SUMMARY OF ACTIONS

Prostaglandins are involved in regulating a wide variety of cell processes. Hence, NSAIDs will have widespread actions. They:

1 inhibit synthesis of prostaglandin E;
2 exert a direct analgesic effect on higher centres;
3 modify the nociceptive responses caused by bradykinin;
4 reduce stickiness of blood platelets;
5 cause hypothrombinaemia in large doses;
6 lower body temperature in pyrexia, in low dosage;
7 lower blood sugar in low dosage; reverse effect in high dosage;
8 cause acid–base imbalance and acidosis (rarely).

Inhibition of prostaglandin biosynthesis is considered to be the main mechanism of analgesic action of NSAIDs. However, there is evidence that some NSAIDs also exhibit significant prostaglandin-independent mechanism(s) of action, which augments the analgesia.[14]

COX-selective non-steroidal anti-inflammatory drugs
Theoretically the 'ideal' NSAID would inhibit COX-2 without influencing COX-1. It is possible that COX-2-selective inhibitors might produce analgesia with fewer adverse effects.

COX-2-specific inhibitors have a number of characteristics in common:

1 absence of a -COOH group;
2 lipid soluble rather than water soluble;
3 do not uncouple oxidative phosphorylation.

Currently there are only three COX-selective NSAIDs (Etodolac COX 1:2 ratio between 1.24 and 10; Meloxicam COX 1:2 ratio 100; Nabumetone COX 1:2 ratio approximately 7).

Table 1.6.2 COX selectivity of current NSAIDs.

COX-1 : COX-2 ratio > 1	Intermediate COX-1 : COX-2 ratio = 1	COX-1 : COX-2 ratio < 1
Etodolac	Diclofenac	Aspirin
Meloxicam	Ketoprofen	Indomethacin
Nabumetone	Naproxen	Ibuprofen
		Piroxicam

Enantioselective non-steroidal anti-inflammatory drugs
Ketorolac and all of the profen group of NSAIDs are formulated as racemic mixtures. There may be benefits to using the S-enantiomer as opposed to racemic mixtures as stereoselectivity is exhibited in pharmacokinetics, COX inhibition is also enantioselective.

Naproxen is the only profen marketed as the S(+) enantiomer. S(+) ibuprofen and S(+) ketoprofen exhibit greater peak and faster time to peak plasma concentration compared with racemic preparations.[14]

ROUTES OF ADMINISTRATION

Many NSAIDs are available in a range of formulations including oral, sublingual, rectal, and topical. Parenteral preparations of aspirin, diclofenac, indomethacin, ketoprofen, ketorolac, piroxicam and tenoxicam are available.

PHARMACOKINETICS

Non-steroidal anti-inflammatory drugs are rapidly absorbed from the gastrointestinal tract, the speed of absorption is increased using arginine salts. They are highly protein bound (> 90%), and are metabolized in the liver. Some are given as inactive 'prodrugs', which are converted to active drugs in the liver, e.g. sulindac, fenbufen. Glucuronic acid conjugation is followed by excretion of inactive metabolites in the urine. The rate of elimination is reduced in the elderly and in those with renal impairment.

ADVERSE EFFECTS

Non-steroidal anti-inflammatory drugs can damage gastrointestinal mucosa, impair renal function and may be associated with an increased risk of postoperative haemorrhage. They can also provoke asthma in susceptible patients.[13,15] Clinical guidelines for their safe use in the perioperative period have been produced. (See *Guidelines for use of Non-Steroidal Anti-Inflammatory Drugs in the Perioperative Period*, Royal College of Anaesthetists, London, 1998.)

They should be avoided in patients with a history of gastrointestinal ulceration or bleeding, when there is evidence of fluid retention or renal impairment, in patients with hepatic impairment or who are hypovolaemic or in circulatory arrest. They may worsen ulcerative colitis. They should be used with caution in the elderly. Blood dyscrasias are rare (except with phenylbutazone).

Strategies for reducing the gastrointestinal injury
The risk of NSAID-induced gastropathy can be reduced by co-prescription of cytoprotective drugs such as the synthetic prostaglandin E_1 analogue, misoprostal or an histamine H_2-receptor antagonist (less effective).

An alternative approach is to use NSAIDs devoid of gastroduodenal toxicity such as selective inhibitors of the COX enzyme or enantioselective NSAIDs.[15]

NON-STEROIDAL ANTI-INFLAMMATORY DRUGS FOR POSTOPERATIVE PAIN MANAGEMENT

In the UK, acemetacin (a glycolic acid ester of indomethacin), ibuprofen, flurbiprofen, mefenamic acid and tiaprofenic acid are licensed for use for postoperative analgesia. Diclofenac, indomethacin, ketoprofen and naproxen (250 mg) may also be used for postoperative pain relief after certain, specified types of operation, viz. orthopaedic, dental and minor surgery. Only ketorolac is specifically (and solely) indicated for the relief of pain associated with surgical procedures including major abdominal surgery. However, as a result of reports to the Committee on Safety of Medicines of serious and fatal adverse reactions associated with the use of ketorolac the recommended dose and duration of parenteral administration for ketorolac has been reduced.[16]

Diclofenac is versatile and can be given orally, i.m., i.v. or p.r. during or after the operation.[17] Intramuscular diclofenac should be avoided as it may be very painful for a long time. A combination oral preparation of diclofenac with misoprostal is available. Dose: 150 mg/day by any route.

Indomethacin can be given orally as well as intravenously and per rectum. Dose: 150–200 mg/day.

Ketorolac is structurally related to zomepirac and tolmetin. Provides analgesia equivalent to opioids in single-dose studies. May adversely affect renal function. Peak plasma concentrations achieved within 30–60 min after oral and parenteral administration. In excess of 99% is plasma protein bound. It is metabolized in the liver, conjugated and excreted by the kidneys. Dose and duration should be reduced in the elderly. Can be used as continuous intravenous infusion and in PCA. Dose: 10–30 mg i.v. or i.m. (*See also* Gillis J. C. and Brogden R. N. *Drugs* 1997, **53**, 138.)

Piroxicam has a very long half-life hence dosing is 'once daily'. Dispersible (sublingual) tablets are available.

Meloxicam: a new COX-2-selective NSAID. However, *see* Anon., *Drug. Ther. Bull.* 1998, **36**, 62, which suggests that equi-effective doses may be no better than other NSAIDs with respect to adverse gastrointestinal events. (*See also* Distel M. et al. *Br. J. Rheumatol.* 1996, **35** (suppl. 1), 68.) Dose: 7.5–15 mg/day.

Other non-opioid analgesic drugs

Paracetamol: this is an active metabolite of phenacetin. It works centrally; it is analgesic and antipyretic, although not anti-inflammatory. It inhibits prostaglandin synthesis within the CNS. It does not cause gastric irritation and is relatively non-toxic in therapeutic doses, but 5 g may be enough to cause centrilobular hepatic necrosis. Aspirin and paracetamol form an effective mixture. Dose: 10–15 mg/kg orally and per rectum. Max 60 mg/kg/day.

Opioid analgesic drugs

Opiates are very effective as postoperative analgesics. Opiates influence the emotional aspects of pain, such as anxiety and fear, as well as reducing the actual pain threshold, so making intolerable pain, tolerable. They act on specific opioid receptors in the brain and spinal cord. The piperidine ring structure is essential for opioid activity.

Table 1.6.3 Opioid drugs.

Agonists	*Mixed agonist/ antagonist*	*Antagonist*
Phenanthrene alkaloids of opium		
Codeine		Methylnaltrexolone
Morphine		
Papaveretum		
Thebaine	Buprenorphine	
Semisynthetic alkaloids		
Diamorphine		
Dihydrocodeine		
Dihydromorphinone		
Oxycodone		
Oxymorphone	Nalbuphine	Naloxone
Synthetic agents		
Morphinans		
Levorphanol	Butorphanol	
	Dezocine	
Benzomorphinans		
	Meptazinol	
	Pentazocine	
Phenylpiperidine derivatives		
Alfentanil		
Fentanyl		
Pethidine		
Phenoperidine		
Remifentanil		
Sufentanil		
Tramadol		
Diphenylheptane derivatives		
Dipipanone		
Dextromoramide		
Methadone		
Piritramide		
Propoxyphene		

Opiates can be arranged depending on their affinities for endorphin receptors, ranging from pure agonists, through partial agonists and partial antagonists to pure antagonists. Some, e.g. morphine, are more active at the supraspinal μ receptor, while others, e.g. nalbuphine, are more active at spinal δ and κ receptors. (*See also* Bovill J. G. *Curr. Opin. Anaesthesiol.* 1990, **3**, 581.)

Opiate analgesia can be potentiated by pretreatment with oral clonidine, a partial α_2-adrenoceptor agonist, 50–150 μg, orally, i.v., i.m. or epidurally. Clonidine acts at the spinal level.

Naloxone antagonizes opioid analgesia as well as most side-effects.

SUMMARY OF ACTIONS OF OPIOIDS

Central nervous system
Depress: awareness, anxiety, pain sensation and respiration.
Stimulate: vomiting centre, secretion of antidiuretic hormone, Edinger–Westphal nucleus (causing small pupils), hallucinations (rarely).

Smooth muscle
Depress: vascular tone and peristalsis
Stimulate: bronchoconstriction, bowel sphincters, biliary sphincter, fallopian spasm, erectores pilorum

Note the relative lack of effects on the vascular system, even in large doses.

Addiction
Psychological and physical: patients may develop both tolerance (and tachyphylaxis) and dependence (or addiction). In addicts, withdrawal results in agitation, severe abdominal cramps, diarrhoea and lacrimation ('cold turkey'). Relieved by further doses of morphine or methadone.

Other
Stimulate: secretion of catecholamines.
Depress: metabolism.
Release: histamine.
Induce: vagally mediated bradycardia (especially short-acting opioids).

ROUTES OF ADMINISTRATION OF OPIOIDS

Oral[18]
Oral opiates can give good analgesia. There are several oral formulations of oral morphine; morphine in solution, immediate release and controlled-release tablets. Peak plasma concentrations occur within 1 h of morphine in solution and immediate-release tablets, analgesia lasting 4 h. Oral diamorphine analgesia comes on quicker but is of shorter duration. Controlled-release morphine tablets produce delayed peak plasma concentrations and long-lasting analgesia (12 h MST; 24 h MXL). The potency ratio of oral to parenteral morphine is 1:6 for acute pain but 1:2 to 1:3 for non-acute pain. An antiemetic may be needed.[19]

Rectal
Morphine suppositories have similar bioavailability and duration to oral morphine. The potency ratio to oral morphine is $1:1$.[19]

Parenteral
Traditionally opioids have been given intramuscularly. Neonates, infants, the elderly and the unfit are more susceptible to respiratory depression. Children and young adults are often quite resistant.

Continuous intravenous infusions of opioid analgesic can be given until pain is relieved, and then the dose titrated against the pain. Infusions of fentanyl efficiently relieve postoperative pain.[20] Opioid infusions need not be followed by either psychological dependence or physical sequelae[21] (*see also* PCA). This gives good pain relief at a lower dosage than intramuscular injection.

Postoperative pain relief can be provided by a continuous subcutaneous infusion. A simple infusion regimen for subcutaneous morphine is 0.8 mg/kg/24 h. Continuous subcutaneous pethidine infusion (2 mg/h) has also proved successful and free of side-effects.[22] A bolus facility for extra pain (dressings, turning) or to regain pain control is useful.

Opioid requirements of patients receiving high doses of corticosteroids is less than normal in the control of postoperative pain.[23]

Transdermal
The high lipophilicity of fentanyl makes it ideal for transdermal delivery (TTS). Fentanyl patches provide sustained delivery of 25–100 μg/h. It is not recommended for acute pain management in view of the high incidence of sedation. It may also be possible to deliver morphine transdermally.

Extradural
Lipophilic opioids are no more potent by this route than when given systemically, unless they are mixed with local analgesics. *See* Chapter 5.3. (*See* Eisenach J.C. et al. *Anesthesiology* 1989, **71**, 640; Motsch J. et al. *Anesthesiology* 1990, **73**, 1067; Vercauteren M. et al. *Anaesthesia* 1990, **45**, 531.)

ADVERSE EFFECTS

1 Nausea and vomiting in up to 50% of cases.
2 Respiratory depression.
3 Considerable variation of individual response, (up to 10-fold) making it difficult to predict the correct dose.
4 Bradycardia with short-acting opiates.
5 Relatively slow onset of analgesia. Intravenous alfentanil and pethidine are fastest (1–2 min); papaveretum, and fentanyl may take 15–20 min to produce analgesia; but respiratory depression has a faster onset.
6 Addiction in susceptible individuals. Tachyphylaxis in the more chronic situation, and occasional hallucinations with prolonged administration.
7 Antagonism of their analgesia by other drugs acting at the spinal level, e.g. reversal of neuromuscular relaxation.

OPIOID AGONISTS

Naturally occurring alkaloids of opium

Morphine: (Morpheus, Greek, god of dreams, son of Somnos, god of sleep). Morphine has been in use for over 2000 years and is still the best available analgesic (first used by Theophrastus in the third century BC). Opium comes from the dried latex of unripe capsules of the poppy head (Papaver somniferum). Morphine is one of over 25 alkaloids (alkaloid = like alkali) contained in opium but only morphine, codeine and papaverine have wide clinical use. The concentration of morphine in opium is 9–17%. Morphine was isolated from opium by F.W.A. Seturner in 1803, its chemical structure determined in 1925 and was synthesized in 1952. Morphine salts are not destroyed by boiling.

Pharmacodynamics:
1 Central nervous system: morphine is analgesic, sedative, anxiolytic, euphoric, addictive, a respiratory depressant, and causes nausea and vomiting. More effective against dull, continuous, visceral, than against sharp, intermittent pain. Very rarely, restlessness and delirium follow its injection and dysphoria follows. The intracranial pressure is increased because of the raised $PaCO_2$.
2 Effect on the eye: miosis by central action, via the oculomotor nerve, stimulating the Edinger–Westphal nucleus. Atropine can counteract this miosis. Intraocular tension reduced in both normal and glaucomatous eyes.
3 Cardiovascular system: mild vasodilatation in clinical doses, sometimes bradycardia. Patients in shock should be given morphine intravenously, so that it does not accumulate unabsorbed in the ischaemic tissues, only to produce a massive effect when absorption occurs with improvement in the circulation. Only small doses needed.
4 Respiratory system: the response of the respiratory centre to $PaCO_2$ is

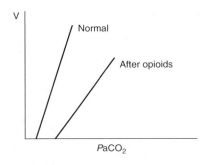

Figure 1.6.1 Respiratory depression caused by opioids

diminished, with 50% depression of the $PaCO_2$ response curve at plasma levels of 100 μg/l (postoperative analgesia occurs at 12–25 μg/l).[24]

Respiratory rate, rather than tidal volume, is decreased. Arterial and alveolar $PaCO_2$ are not usually much raised. Respiratory depression is difficult to define or measure clinically, and the respiratory rate is often used, by default. Breathing may become periodic (Cheyne–Stokes) or irregular. Bronchoconstriction occurs, worse in asthmatic patients. Maximal respiratory depression comes on 30 min after intramuscular injection, sooner after intravenous injection. Depresses the cough reflex.

5 Gastrointestinal tract: morphine constricts the sphincters of the gut and reduces peristalsis, more so when given intramuscularly than when given orally.[25] Nausea and vomiting are due to central stimulation. This is seen most strongly with the allied drug, apomorphine. Vomiting after morphine depends partly on the movements of the body and the position of the patient; it sensitizes the vomiting centre to vestibular movements. Early ambulation after morphine will cause more nausea than quiet bedrest. Antiemetics can control this nausea, some more effectively than others. About one-third of postoperative patients feel sick after opioids, females much more so than males. Morphine contracts the sphincter of Oddi, raising the pressure in the bile ducts, which rarely causes severe pain. Atropine does not fully antagonize this action, but nitroglycerin, nalorphine, levallorphan, adrenaline, aminophylline and amyl nitrite do.

6 Genitourinary tract: the tone and peristalsis of the ureters and other smooth muscle, e.g. of the hollow viscera, bladder sphincter, fallopian tubes, etc., are increased, an action antagonized by atropine. The tone of the vesical sphincter is increased and may hinder micturition, a common postoperative problem. Urinary output decreased due to stimulation of secretion of antidiuretic hormone. There is little relaxation of uterus during labour. Morphine crosses placental barrier and depresses fetal respiration.

7 Endocrine system: posterior pituitary and adrenal medulla are stimulated, therefore antidiuretic hormone and blood catecholamine levels increased. Morphine may cause rise in blood sugar.

8 Other: morphine sometimes causes itching, especially of the nose. It may occasionally cause anaphylactoid and allergic reactions, ranging from slight syncope, due to histamine release, to anaphylactic shock. It is useful in the management of paroxysmal nocturnal dyspnoea (cardiac asthma). Sweating may be stimulated.

Pharmacokinetics:

1 Routes: oral, buccal, intramuscular, intravenous, subcutaneous, rectal, transcutaneous, intra-articular.

2 Morphine has a pKa 7.9, is poorly lipid-soluble, 40% bound to plasma albumin (30% in neonates), exhibits triexponential elimination kinetics. The elimination half-life varies with age – neonate 629 min; infant 233 min; child 120 min; adult 180 min.[26]

3 Oral morphine undergoes significant first-pass metabolism. Biotransformation is by conjugation with glucuronic acid in the liver, followed by excretion in the bile and by the kidneys. There are both active

(morphine-6-glucuronide; M6G) and inactive (morphine-3-glucuronide; M3G) metabolites. Deficient renal excretion may cause accumulation and respiratory depression.[27]

4 It appears in breast milk, saliva and sweat.
5 Special care is necessary in infants under 6 months, aged or debilitated patients and in patients with a raised $PaCO_2$, suprarenal insufficiency, myasthenia, myotonia, hypothyroidism, asthma, raised intracranial pressure, respiratory depression, hepatic failure, renal failure, acute alcoholism, diverticulitis and labour.
6 Dose: 0.15 mg/kg. i. m., 0.03 mg/kg i.v. (very roughly 0.1–1 mg/kg i.v. prevent the 'stress response'); infusion rate 0.03 mg/kg/h, (5–15 μg/kg/h in neonates).
7 Onset of analgesia: 3–10 min (i.v.); and 10–20 min (i.m.).
8 Duration: 3–4 h.

Papaveretum: originally a mixture of purified opium alkaloids in the proportion found in nature; reformulated in 1993 following concerns regarding toxicity of noscapine. Now contains only three alkaloids – morphine, papaverine and codeine – in same ratio as before; thus, overall concentration of morphine has decreased. Papaveretum 15.4 mg is equivalent to 10 mg of morphine sulphate. There is no evidence that papaveretum causes fewer unpleasant side-effects than morphine.

1 Dose: 10–20 mg i.m.
2 Onset: 20 min.
3 Duration: 2–4 h.

Papaverine: isolated from opium in 1848. Does not suppress intestinal peristalsis. Relieves spasm in arteries. Has almost no central effects. Dose: up to 30 mg i.v. or i.a.(very slowly); 120–250 mg orally.

Codeine phosphate: from the Greek name for 'poppy head'. Methyl morphine; together with morphine and papaverine forms the chief alkaloidal derivative of opium. Isolated in 1832. A superb cough suppressant, useful in ophthalmic and neuroanaesthesia. It depresses respiration less, causes less constipation and vomiting than morphine. Analgesic effect is one-tenth that of morphine. Non-sedating, non-addictive, excreted unchanged by the kidneys; widely used as a paediatric analgesic (1 mg/kg oral or i.m.), but may release histamine.[28] Undergoes very little first-pass metabolism hence oral route is effective. Should not be given intravenously as by this route it depresses cardiac output. Adult dose: 15–50 mg i.m., oral, as analgesic, antitussive and antidiarrhoeal agent. Duration 4–12 h. May be combined with paracetamol in oral preparation.

Semi-synthetic alkaloids of opium

Diamorphine hydrochloride (heroin): the diacetyl ester of morphine. A prodrug which is hydrolysed to 6-monoacetyl morphine and morphine. It is a drug of addiction, because of the euphoria it creates. Introduced into medicine in 1898. In the US and in Australia its use is proscribed. Should be freshly prepared from powder. Depresses the respiratory centre and the cough reflex more than morphine and is twice as efficient as an analgesic. Diamorphine 5 mg has a quicker onset of activity and fewer emetic sequelae than morphine 10 mg. An excellent postoperative analgesic although its effect does not last as long as that of morphine. In coronary occlusion, 5 mg i.v. cause little cardiovascular depression or vomiting, if given slowly. Useful by mouth in the treatment of chronic pain in doses up to 30 mg[19,29] and as an epidural opioid. Excretion is chiefly by the kidneys after conversion to morphine in the body. Dose: 2.5–5 mg, i.v. or i.m. Onset: 5 min (i.v.); 10 min (i.m.).

Dihydrocodeine tartrate: analgesic, constipator, and antitussive. May cause nausea, dysphoria and vertigo. Releases histamine. Dose: 0.5 mg/kg, oral, i.m. or i.v.

Synthetic alkaloids of opium

Pethidine hydrochloride (meperidine hydrochloride): the hydrochloride of the ethyl ester of 1-methyl-4-phenyl-piperidine-4-carboxylic acid.

Pharmacodynamics:
1 Analgesic: relieves most types of pain, especially those associated with plain muscle spasm. Depresses respiratory centre and cough reflex. Is also a local analgesic. No effect on ciliary body or iris. Raises the cerebrospinal fluid (CSF) pressure. Can cause addiction.
2 Has a direct papaverine-like effect on the smooth muscle of the bronchioles, intestine, ureters and arteries. Will often relieve bronchospasm. Vasodilatation may be unwelcome in trauma cases and uncontrolled hypertensives.
3 Has an atropine-like effect on cholinergic nerve endings.
4 May release histamine from tissues.
5 Side-effects include sweating, hypotension, vertigo and limb tingling. Postoperative nausea is similar to that following morphine, but comes on earlier. Worse after intravenous than after intramuscular injection. Like morphine, pethidine may cause hypotension if the head of the patient is raised, or with sudden movement. Because of its circulatory depressant effects it is probably not the ideal drug for the relief of pain in myocardial infarction. Phenobarbitone enhances the production of toxic metabolites of pethidine. These two drugs should not be given together.[30]
6 Pethidine in labour. *See* Chapter 4.3.
7 Precautions: the administration of pethidine to patients receiving monoamine oxidase inhibitors may cause severe reactions and even death. There is restlessness, hypertension, convulsions and coma with absent tendon jerks and an extensor plantar response; hypotension may also be seen. The reaction is said to be due to interference with the microsomes in liver cells which detoxicate pethidine. Treatment is supportive, and with 25 mg prednisolone or chlorpromazine.

Pharmacokinetics:
Routes of administration same as morphine. Oral bioavailability 45–75%; 64% bound to plasma protein. Pethidine is metabolized at the rate of 17%/h. The biological half-life is 3–4 h in humans.[31] Eighty per cent is hydrolysed in the liver. About 5–10% is excreted unchanged by the kidneys. One metabolite, norpethidine, may cause convulsions or hallucinations if pethidine is given in large doses, for prolonged period or with monoamine oxidase inhibitors. Dose: 0.5 mg/kg i.v. , 1.5 mg/kg i. m. Onset: 2–5 min (i.e. rapid). Duration: 2–4 h.

Phenoperidine; Fentanyl; Alfentanil; Sufentanil; Lofentanil; Remifentanil: See Chapter 2.4.

Tramadol: a synthetic 4-phenyl-piperidine analogue of codeine. Weak central action on opioid receptors, also acts on descending monoaminergic pathways. The M1 metabolite shows higher affinity for opioid receptors than the parent drug. Half-life 5 h after oral dosing. Potency comparable to pethidine. Can be given orally, rectally, intravenously and intramuscularly. Less likely to depress respiration than morphine. Dose: 100 mg p.o. or i.v. to maximum of 250 mg. Duration: 3–6 h after 100 mg p.o. (*See also* Besson J.-M. and Vickers M. D. *Drugs* 1994, **47** (suppl. 1.)

Methadone hydrochloride: a powerful analgesic. Causes less sedation and has a more prolonged action than morphine (half-life 40–90 h, increasing with subsequent doses). Exhibits high oral bioavailability. Absorption from fatty sites (e.g. subcutaneous and epidural) is very slow. Has been used to wean addicts from morphine and for chronic pain. (*See also* Bullingham R. E. S. *Br. J. Hosp. Med.* 1981, **5**, 59; Gourlay G. K. et al. *Anaesth. Intensive Care* 1981, **9**, 183.) Dose: 0.1 mg/kg i.m. or 0.05 mg/kg i.v. Onset: 1 min i.v.; 5 min i.m.

Dextropropoxyphene: the only one of the four isomers of propoxyphene to have analgesic activity. Undergoes extensive first pass metabolism. May cause dependence and, if taken with alcohol, respiratory depression. Commonly combined with paracetamol; co-proxamol contains dextropropoxyphene 32.5 mg and paracetamol 325 mg. Overdose will result in liver toxicity and respiratory depression.

Dextromoramide acid tartrate: a morphine-like analgesic but twice as potent. Relatively non-soporific. Can be given by mouth. Dose: 5-mg tablet or 5–10 mg by intramuscular injection.

MIXED AGONIST/ANTAGONISTS AND PARTIAL ANTAGONISTS OF OPIUM

Buprenorphine: a powerful, long-acting synthetic thebaine derivative, with agonist/antagonist properties. Duration of action up to 10 h. A single dose may therefore last throughout the night, important in postoperative analgesia. Buprenorphine may accentuate urinary obstruction.[32] A dose of 0.3 mg relieves the pain of ureteric colic.[33] It has different disposition in patients with renal impairment.[34] Only partly reversed by naloxone but because of its agonist/antagonist properties, respiratory depression shows a 'ceiling effect' and apnoea, or even a respiratory rate below 4/min, is very unlikely to occur. It is associated with a particularly high incidence of emesis, especially in mobilizing patients. Routes: sublingual, intramuscular, intravenous, epidural. Dose: 0.2–1 mg.

Butorphanol: A synthetic morphinan derivative and potent opioid agonist/ antagonist. Undergoes significant hepatic first-pass metabolism after oral dosing with only 5–17% bioavailability. Extensively metabolized in the liver by hydroxylation, only 5–10% excreted unchanged by the kidney after a single intravenous dose. Respiratory depression is dose related, ceiling reached with 2 mg dose. Can be given transnasally. Dose: 1–2 mg i.m.

Pentazocine: an opioid agonist/antagonist analgesic derived from benzmorphinan. Agonist at κ/σ-receptors and very weak opioid antagonist, one-fiftieth the activity of nalorphine. Respiratory depression is dose related but has a ceiling effect. Non-addictive and not euphoric. Raises rather than lowers blood pressure and the dextro-isomer has a positive inotropic effect on the myocardium (α-receptor stimulation).[35] Does not influence pupil size or intraocular tension. Crosses the placental barrier less easily than pethidine. Hallucinations may follow its use but may be controlled by diazepam. Routes oral and intramuscular. Dose: 30 mg, i.v. Onset: 20 min.

Nalbuphine hydrochloride: partial κ-receptor agonist and μ-receptor antagonist. Undergoes extensive first-pass metabolism with oral bioavailability of only 10%. Has been used for perioperative analgesia. Has less effect on delay of coordinated bowel motility than morphine.[36] Not likely to cause bronchoconstriction in asthmatics. Dose: 10–20 mg.

Meptazinol: An opioid agonist/antagonist with partial agonist activity at the μ_1 receptor and some cholinergic activity. Shorter duration of action than morphine. Used for perioperative analgesia. Dose: 200 mg, orally repeated; 75–100 mg i.m.

OPIATE ANTAGONISTS

Specific antagonism to opioids were first described in 1915. Antagonists are usually the *n*-allyl derivatives of opiate analgesics. The more potent the narcotic, the smaller the dose of its allyl derivative necessary to antagonize opioid-induced respiratory depression. They have high receptor affinity and low receptor activity. They do not lead to addiction. They may cause signs of withdrawal in narcotic addicts. Probable mode of action is competition at receptor sites on cell surfaces. Antagonists counteract the analgesia produced by morphine, pethidine and oxymorphone (although less so than morphine).

Naloxone: n-allyl noroxymorphone, derived from oxymorphone. First synthesized in 1972. It also antagonizes the respiratory depression caused by pentazocine and dextropropoxyphene. Short duration of effect (1 h) may be less than the opiate it is designed to antagonize, so that repeat dosage or an infusion may be necessary. Relaxes spasm of the sphincter of Oddi induced by opiate analgesics. With careful titration of dosage, analgesia is not reversed. Can be used in the treatment of opiate-induced respiratory depression and in midwifery to reverse fetal respiratory depression due to opiates. Naloxone reverses respiratory depression but not the analgesia of intrathecal morphine.[37] May raise blood pressure in septic shock, suggesting that endorphins may contribute to this hypotension.[38] Can cause acute pulmonary oedema in previously fit patients.[39] Has caused dysrhythmia and even sudden death.[40] Can be given intramuscularly for a more prolonged effect.

Pharmacokinetics: half-life 20 min. Metabolized in the liver.

Dose: 0.1–0.4 mg i.v. repeated. (0.01 mg/kg in neonates).

Methylnaltrexolone: epoxymorphinan. Has a very long half-life. Main use is as an aid in maintaining abstinence in opioid withdrawal. Has been suggested that with careful titration of dosage, analgesia is not reversed.

OPIOID OVERDOSE[41]

Coma, respiratory depression, hypoxia, acidosis, muscle compression (from deep sedation) all leading to rhabdomyolysis and acute renal failure. Pulmonary oedema (non-cardiogenic), cerebral oedema, convulsions, aspiration pneumonia also occur. Treatment is by immediate reversal with naloxone and by organ support, e.g. oxygenation/intermittent positive-pressure ventilation (IPPV).

Controlled drugs and drug dependence

There are legal requirements relating to the prescription of controlled drugs (CDs). The Misuse of Drugs Regulations 1985 divides drugs into five schedules, whilst the Misuse of Drugs Act 1971 divides drugs into three classes according to their harmfulness when misused.

Most opiates are CDs and as such subject to full controlled drug requirements relating to prescription, safe custody and need to keep a register. There are a few notable exceptions such as pentazocine and oral (but not parenteral) codeine which are subject to special prescription but not safe custody requirements.

MANAGING ACUTE PAIN

Methods of pain relief

Identify and if possible remove cause of pain (e.g. distended bladder). Thereafter treatment may be by pharmacological (viz. analgesics and regional blocks) or non-pharmacological (e.g. hypnosis, acupuncture methods). (*See also* Commission on the Provision of Surgical Services, Royal College of Surgeons and College of Anaesthetists. London, 1990.)

Pharmacological

SIMPLE ANALGESICS

Non-steroidal anti-inflammatory drugs: see above.

COMBINATION PREPARATIONS

Aspirin–papaveretum, aspirin–paracetamol, codeine–paracetamol, ibuprofen–codeine, paracetamol–dextropropyxphene.

Caffeine: caffeine has been shown to have adjuvant analgesic activity when combined with simple oral analgesics. A dose of > 65 mg is needed. In a large meta-analysis of > 10 000 patients analgesia from paracetamol or paracetamol and aspirin with caffeine 65 mg added was approximately 1.4 times more potent than without added caffeine.[42]

OPIOID ANALGESICS

See above.

PATIENT-CONTROLLED ANALGESIA[43]

This refers to the on-demand, intermittent, self-administration of analgesic drugs by a patient. Predominantly used to deliver opioid analgesics but other classes of drugs can be administered in this way. Any opiate can be used. The traditional route of drug delivery has been intravenous (IV-PCA) but subcutaneous (SC-PCA) and epidural (PCEA) routes can also be used. The quality of analgesia is normally good, and allows for wide inter-patient variation. The basic variables of PCA are: demand (bolus) dose, lock-out interval (length of the time between patient demands), background infusion rate (if used), and hourly or 4-hourly limit.

The use of background infusion in adults is controversial, tending to increase sedation and other side-effects without improving analgesia. In children, use of a background infusion (4–10 μg/kg/h) is standard.

The majority of PCA infusors incorporate sophisticated pump technology with a lockable syringe compartment to prevent tampering (non-disposable). Compact ambulatory devices are a further refinement. Alternatively light-weight disposable infusors which combine an elastomeric pressure mechanism (a cylinder containing the analgesic drug within an elastic balloon) with a non-electronic non-programmable 'wristwatch' control device are available.

A one-way Y-connector enables use with intravenous infusions. Antireflux valves are recommended to prevent reflux delivery of drug into gravity-fed infusion tubing in the event of an occlusion. However, these valves may store a large bolus of drug, or impede the intravenous infusion.[44]

Preoperative counselling in the use of PCA is helpful.

Opiates administered by PCA are associated with less severe falls in oxygen saturation compared with when given as intermittent intramuscular boluses.[45]

Pain control, respiration and sedation should be monitored.

Epidural PCA with lipophilic opioids may be improved by addition of local analgesics.

Patients express high satisfaction with PCA. The advantages welcomed by patients include not having to bother nurses; rapid pain relief; self-control of their own pain; exact titration of dose; lack of intramuscular injections.[46]

Some patients worry about overdose, addiction, lack of personal contact with nurses and machine dysfunction.

Patient-controlled analgesia is also useful in children over 5 years,[47] in obstetrics, in acute medical diseases, e.g. sickle-cell crisis and malignant pain. Parent-controlled analgesia, nurse-controlled and spouse-controlled analgesia have all been described.[48]

Drawbacks of PCA include: problems with patient selection/education. Opioid side-effects especially respiratory depression (rare 0.019%) and excessive sedation. Also nausea, vomiting, itching, ileus and hallucinations. Complex equipment leading to programming errors. Equipment malfunction occurs in 5% of cases; underutilization, overutilization and syphoning.

REGIONAL LOCAL ANALGESIC BLOCKADE, INCLUDING EPIDURAL INFUSION ANALGESIA[49]

Avoid the side-effects of the opioids etc, can be applied to an area of the body no larger than the source of pain, and can give supremely good analgesia. Prolonged action is possible with insertion of micocatheters to the site of the block, and top-ups or infusion of local analgesic. Particular postoperative care is needed when epidural opioids have been given.[50]

Blockade of pain afferents by regional techniques, e.g. postoperative high extradural analgesia, intercostal and paravertebral nerve block, axillary and femoral sheath catheters and subcutaneous bupivacaine after herniorrhaphy. A continuous intravenous lignocaine drip (2 mg/min) has been used with success and absence of signs of toxicity.[51]

KETAMINE INFUSION

Low-dose (5–15 mg/h) continuous intramuscular infusion of ketamine has been successfully used.

INHALATION OF ANALGESIC GASES AND VAPOURS

Entonox can be used for dressing changes.

Non-pharmacological

TRANSCUTANEOUS ELECTROSTIMUTATION[52]

CRYOANALGESIA

Cryoanalgesia of intercostal nerves is no longer used because of the high incidence of dysaesthesia.

ACUPUNCTURE

HYPNOSIS

Where the skills are available.

The acute pain team

An *acute pain service* can teach, encourage and oversee the delivery of analgesia. It involves surgeons, physicians, pharmacists, anaesthetists and nurses.

The relief of postoperative pain can be badly managed, simply by neglect. Failure can occur at the point of writing prescriptions and at the point of delivery of analgesia by nurses. Experience with 'pain teams' has heightened awareness of this, but the risk is that the whole of the pain (and fluid and other) management of the hospital may be transferred by default to the team by those surgeons and nurses who previously looked after it. Thus, pain-team activity may need to be mainly advisory in continuing effective analgesia and developing even more efficient methods by nurses, surgeons etc. Perfect pain relief is often not attainable in practice, and sometimes not even desirable, since pain is a protective mechanism and the experience of pain on excessive movement may persuade the patient to take proper rest after surgery or trauma. 'Pain-free at rest' is a reasonable aim.

FURTHER READING

Breivik H. Post-operative pain management *Baillière's Clinical Anaesthesiology, Volume 9/Number 3.* Baillière Tindall, London, 1995.
Ferrante F. M. and VadeBoncouer T. R. (eds.) *Postoperative Pain Management.* Churchill Livingstone, New York, 1993.

REFERENCES

1 Dray A. *Br. J. Anaesth.* 1995, **75,** 125.
2 Dray A. and Bevan S. *Trends Pharmacol. Sci.* 1993, **14,** 287.
3 Rang H.P. et al. *Br. Med. Bull.* 1991, **47,** 534.
4 Watanabe M. et al. *Br. J. Pharmacol.* 1995, **116,** 2141.
5 Rice A. S. C. *Acute Pain* 1998, **1,** 27.

6 Vane J. R. et al. *Proc. Natl. Acad. Sci. USA* 1994, **91,** 2046.

7 Seibert K. et al. *Proc. Natl. Acad. Sci. USA* 1994, **91,** 12013.

8 Lambert D. G. *Br. J. Anaesth.* 1998, **81,** 1.

9 Woolf C. J. *Br. Med. Bull.* 1991, **47,** 523.

10 Coderre T. J. and Melzack R. *J. Neurosci.* 1992, **12,** 3665.

11 Loan W. B. and Dundee J. W. *Practitioner* 1967, **198,** 759.

12 Angell M. *N. Engl. J. Med.* 1982, **306,** 98; Commission on the Provision of Surgical Services Royal College of Surgeons and College of Anaesthetists, London, 1990.

13 Orme M. *Prescribers J.* 1990, **30,** 95.

14 Cashman J. N. *Drugs* 1996, **52** (suppl. 5), 13.

15 Cashman J. and McAnulty G. *Drugs* 1995, **49,** 51

16 Committee on Safety of Medicines and Medicines Control Agency. *Curr. Prob. Pharmacovigil.* 1993, **19,** 5.

17 Hodsman N. B. A. et al. *Anaesthesia* 1987, **42,** 1005.

18 Gordon A. *The Physician*, 1988, **7,** 33; Hillier E. H. *Br. Med. J.* 1983, **287,** 701.

19 Hanks G. W. et al. *Br. Med. J.* 1996, **312,** 823.

20 Nimmo W. S. and Todd J. G. *Br. J. Anaesth.* 1985, **57,** 250.

21 Morgan R. J. M. *Anaesthesia* 1983, **38,** 492.

22 Davenport H. T. et al. *Ann. R. Coll. Surg.* 1985, **67,** 379.

23 Korman B. and McKay R. J. *Anesth. Intensive Care* 1985, **13,** 395.

24 Lynn A. M. and Slattery J. T. *Anesthesiology* 1987, **66,** 136.

25 Park G. R. *Anaesthesia* 1984, **39,** 645.

26 Aitkenhead A. R. et al. *Br. J. Anaesth.* 1984, **56,** 813.

27 McQuay H. and Moore A. *Lancet* 1984, **2,** 284.

28 Shanahan E. C. et al. *Anaesthesia* 1983, **38,** 40.

29 Twycross R. G. *Br. Med. J.* 1975, **4,** 212.

30 Stambough J. E. et al. *Lancet* 1977, **1,** 398.

31 Mather L. E. et al. *Clin. Pharmacol. Ther.* 1975, **17,** 21.

32 Murray K. *Br. Med. J.* 1983, **286,** 761.

33 Finlay I. G. et al. *Br. Med. J.* 1982, **284,** 1830.

34 Hand C. W. et al. *Br. J. Anaesth.* 1990, **64,** 276 ; Bullingham, R. E. S. et al. *Anaesthesia* 1984, **39,** 329; Derbyshire D. R. et al. *Anaesthesia* 1984, **39,** 324.

35 Appleyard T. N. *Proc. R. Soc. Med.* 1975, **68,** 770.

36 Shah M. et al. *Br. J. Anaesth.* 1984, **56,** 1235.

37 Jones R. D. M. and Jones J. A. *Br. Med. J.* 1980, **2,** 646.

38 Peters W. P. et al. *Lancet* 1981, **1,** 529; Annotation, *Lancet* 198l, **1,** 538.

39 Taff R. H. *Anesthesiology* 1983, **59,** 576.

40 Dhamce M. S. and Ghandi S. K. *Anaesthesia* 1982, **37,** 342.

41 Conti G. et al. In *Update in Intensive Care and Emergency Medicine 10*, Vincent J.-L. (ed.), Springer-Verlag, London, 1990.

42 Laska E. M. et al. *J. Am. Med. Assoc.* 1984, **251,** 1711.

43 Ferrante F. M. et al. (eds) *Patient Controlled Analgesia.* Blackwell Scientific Publications, Oxford, 1990.

44 Kluger M .T. and Owen H. *Anaesthesia* 1991, **45,** 1059.

45 Wheatley R.G. et al. *Br. J. Anaesth.* 1990, **64,** 267.

46 Kluger M. T. and Owen H. *Anaesthesia* 1991, **45,** 1072.
47 Lawrie S.C. et al. *Anaesthesia* 1991, **45,** 1074.
48 Wakerlin G. and Larson C.P. Jnr. *Anesth. Analg.* 1990, **70,** 119.
49 Wildsmith J. A. W. and McClure J. H. (eds). *Conduction blockade for post-operative analgesia.* Edward Arnold, London, 1991.
50 Ross N. L. *Anesthesiology* 1990, **72,** 212 ; Ready B. L. and Edwards W. T. *Anesthesiology* 1990, **72,** 213.
51 Cassuto J. et al. *Anesth. Analg. (Cleve.)* 1985, **64,** 971.
52 Baker S. B. C. et al. *Can. Anaesth. Soc. J.* 1980, **27,** 150.

Safety in anaesthetic practice and audit

PATIENT SAFETY

Concerns about the safety of anaesthesia have been expressed since the first reported deaths under ether and chloroform in 1847 and 1848 respectively. Death due to anaesthesia was criticised far more than death due to surgery! In 1896 Hewitt[1] stressed the need for education and training, but anaesthesia was not included in the undergraduate medical curriculum by the General Medical Council until 1912. Today, an increasing public awareness and often unrealistic expectation of surgery and anaesthesia without morbidity and mortality have led to increased litigation and a related interest in patient safety.

The International Committee on Prevention of Anesthesia Mortality and Morbidity[2] and the Anesthesia Patient Safety Foundation[3] were started in the 1980s in the US. The Australian Patient Safety Foundation first reported in 1988.[4] In the UK, the *Report of the Confidential Enquiry into Perioperative Deaths (CEPOD)* was first published in 1987, and nationwide audits of deaths during or after sugery published regularly since.[5] The large literature details the multifactorial nature of most anaesthetic accidents: Murphy's Law is one of the foundation principles of medical practice 'If it can happen, it will happen'.

The anaesthetist

Even after the period of training, knowledge and skills must be maintained by continuing education, including regular practice audit, and discussions of any morbidity and mortality. Assessment, treatment or resuscitation of the patient before surgery may be inadequate. Delegation to a junior colleague may be inappropriate. Special techniques of training, such as computer-based simulators,[6] are useful for infrequent but particularly hazardous situations, e.g. failed intubation, cardiac arrest, anaphylaxis, malignant hyperpyrexia. Objective structured clinical examinations (OSCE) have been introduced to aid the assessment of practical skills. Anaesthesia examinations objectively test both knowledge and skills.

The anaesthetist needs to prepare for the unexpected and be alert. Commonsense says we should be allowed a reasonable amount of sleep and rest before taking a patient's life into our hands. This is a legal requirement in New York State.[7] All anaesthetists should have skilled assistance throughout an operation.

Anaesthetic errors can be categorized as of technique, judgement or failure of vigilance. No anaesthetist (particularly a trainee) should be persuaded to treat a patient beyond his or her capabilities. The General Medical Council have introduced a procedure designed to protect patients from serious deficiencies in the performance of doctors.[8] It is recognized that anaesthesia is a stressful speciality, and wise counsel from colleagues can be especially valued.[9]

Equipment and drugs

The anaesthetist must understand the working of all the equipment, and be satisfied that it has been properly maintained and checked before use.[10] Accidental disconnection of parts of the breathing circuit is an ever-present hazard. Ill-fitting tapers should be discarded. Modern anaesthetic machines are unable to deliver hypoxic gas mixtures, limit CO_2 flow, and have built-in monitors. Further features such as digital control of gas flows and vaporizers, and servo control of vapour concentration may provide additional safety.

The safety of electrical equipment is governed by BS 5724 and by International Electrotechnical Commission (IEC) 601. The Department of Health (UK) publish their evaluations as *Health Equipment Information* and issue cautionary notes (*Safety Action Bulletins*) and urgent warnings (*Hazard Notices*) to relevant parties. The last two are published in *Anaesthesia*. Electronic bulletin boards are becoming widely used. In the US the Food and Drug Administration regulates medical devices. It divides them into Classes I, II and III in increasing order of patient risk. In the European Community (EC) the 'CE' mark allows the sale of medical devices throughout the EC.

Adverse drug reactions should be reported to the Committee on Safety of Medicines on the special yellow card for anaesthetic drugs. New drugs require special vigilance and are marked by an inverted black triangle in the *British National Formulary*.

Monitoring

Few doubt the contribution that monitoring has made to safe anaesthesia, and many countries have introduced minimum standards[11] (*see* Chapter 2.2) These usually include the continuous presence of an anaesthetist and monitors of the anaesthetic machine (oxygen failure alarm; inspired oxygen concentration; ventilator disconnect alarm), and of the patient (circulation – electrocardiogram (ECG), pulse, blood pressure; respiration – bag movement, capnography; pulse oximetry; temperature; neuromuscular transmission). Such standards are legally enforced in certain states and have led to some reductions in malpractice insurance premiums in the US. An analysis of closed insurance claims in the US over 15 years concluded that additional monitors, especially capnography and pulse oximetry, would have prevented 31.5% of the accidents.[12] Critical incident studies have yielded similar conclusions.

Time and motion studies of anaesthetists in the operating theatre[13] reveal much time *not* spent observing the patient, and an implicit reliance on monitors and their alarms. The anaesthetist must know the limitations of the monitors, set appropriate alarm limits, know how to check that they are working correctly and be able to interpret the data. An excessive number of monitors may lead to distractions, complacency and a blind adherence to 'standards'.

The patient is exposed to nearly as much danger in the postoperative recovery room as in theatre. Hypoxaemic episodes there are common.[14] Monitoring of the circulation and respiration should continue as needed. There should be a safe hand-over of the patient to recovery staff. *See* Chapter 1.5.

The patient

Patients have a responsibility to fully disclose details of all factors relevant to their medical and nursing care, analogous to full disclosure of details for insurance purposes. The development of a national NHS number in the UK enables checks on patients' veracity. Patients are also fully responsible for obeying instructions given by doctors and nurses.

The surgeon

Dangers (and problems for the anaesthetist), are caused by failure of communication, e.g. last-minute changes to operating lists, unannounced entry into the thoracic cavity, and unannounced haemorrhage; failure of technique, e.g. uncontrolled haemorrhage, air embolism; and unreasonable demands, e.g. for severe hypotension, darkness in the theatre, or excessively long operating lists.

ANAESTHESIA RECORDS

Pioneers in anaesthetic record-keeping include Harvey Cushing in 1895[15] and Ralph Waters in 1936.[16] E.I. McKesson's (1881–1935) 'Nargraf' machine of 1930 could produce a semi-automated record of inspired oxygen, tidal volume and inspiratory gas pressure.[17] Nosworthy's cards[18] carried details of the patient, operation and anaesthesia, and had notches to allow rapid sorting with a knitting needle.

A record should be kept of all administrations of anaesthesia. Its value is as follows.

1 To contribute to patient care. Although about 11% of an anaesthetist's time may be consumed by keeping the record,[19] it probably stimulates vigilant anaesthesia, and helps any future anaesthetist caring for that patient.
2 As an aid for audit of an anaesthetist's work.
3 For teaching.
4 For medico-legal reasons. Much harm may be done to an anaesthetist's defence of a civil claim if his record is not full, accurate, contemporaneous and legible.

Although patient care should always take precedence over record-keeping, events should be recorded as soon as possible after they happen. Any corrections should be made in a way that will not arouse suspicion that the record has been falsified.

Even the simplest record should contain the patient details, date of operation, surgeons and anaesthetists involved, operation performed, a summary of the preoperative assessment, techniques and drugs used, record of vital signs such as pulse and blood pressure, complications, instructions to staff in the recovery room. Intravenous fluids given during operation should be recorded, including the serial numbers of any units of blood. Vital signs are traditionally recorded at 5-min intervals, although this may not be appropriate for all operations.

Anaesthetists have been noted to fail to record manually the extremes of blood pressure readings indicated (sometimes erroneously) by automatic recorders.[20] They also seldom record critical incidents,[21] and if they do, errors are common.[22] The use of computers to record both data from monitors and other aspects of anaesthetic technique is attractive, although the interface with the anaesthetist is often unsatisfactory in practice. A keyboard, touch-responsive screen, light pen, digitizing pad and voice recognition systems have all been tried.

MEDICO-LEGAL CONSIDERATIONS

In the UK, *criminal law* concerns offences prohibited by the state, has sanctions that punish and deter the offender, and does not compensate the victim (although the Criminal Injuries Compensation Board may do so). *Civil law* involves the private concerns of individuals and awards compensation to the victim that aims to restore him to the financial position he would otherwise have occupied. Criminal matters are rare in medical practice, although anaesthetists have been convicted of manslaughter, i.e. causing death by criminal neglect, but claims for civil offences ('torts'), usually negligence, are all too common. Criminal offences have to be proven 'beyond all reasonable doubt', but torts merely 'on the balance of probabilities'.

Negligence

To prove negligence, the plaintiff has to show that the doctor had a duty of care, that he or she breached that duty, and that the plaintiff has suffered damage as a result.

The Bolam case is widely quoted to establish whether the standard of care is negligent: 'the test (of negligence) is the test of the ordinary skilled man exercising and professing to have that special skill. A man need not possess the highest expert skill; it is well established law that it is sufficient if he exercises the ordinary skill of an ordinary competent man exercising that particular art'.[23]

A defence must be able to muster 'a body of competent professional opinion' in support, even if it is in a minority. The trial judge is helped in his decision on these matters by 'expert witnesses' called by both sides.[24] These experts often disagree.[25] The burden of proof is usually on the plaintiff unless the doctrine *res ipsa loquitur* (the thing speaks for itself) is invoked, in which case it is obvious, even to a layman, that negligence has occurred, and the burden of proof thus shifted to the doctor. The plaintiff still has to establish a causative link between the negligence and the harm done. This link is often disputed. Lord Woolf has proposed methods of streamlining the legal process in the United Kingdom.

Note that the standards expected are effectively determined by one's colleagues in the guise of expert witnesses, and *not* by the legal profession. Very often these colleagues will sense 'there but for the Grace of God . . .'

Consent[26]

Consent to treatment must be freely given after an opportunity for the patient to discuss the operation and anaesthetic. Anyone of 16 years or over and of sound mind may give valid consent. A patient who has been premedicated is unlikely to be able to do so. It is not considered necessary, or even always in the patient's best interest, to discuss all possible complications, however unlikely. Each case has to assessed on its own merits. There would be a duty to inform the patient of 'substantial risk of grave adverse consequences' unless there was 'some cogent clinical reason why the patient should not be informed'.[27] If this was the case it should be recorded in the notes. Consent forms are normally used, and are of value in subsequent litigation. *See Information and Consent for Anaesthesia*, Association of Anaesthetists, London, 1999.

In practice

The potential for litigation should never be underestimated, nor should the stressful effect it can have upon the doctor. Much trouble may be avoided by the following:

1 *Better communication* with the patient and relatives.
2 *Careful preoperative assessment.*
3 *Informing the patient of what to expect postoperatively*, e.g. temporary muscle weakness and numbness if a major regional block is to be given as well as general anaesthesia; the possibility of imperfect epidural blockade; presence of catheters etc.; the use of a suppository of analgesic drug; an oxygen mask over the face.
4 *Informing the patient of any special risks*, e.g. to fragile front teeth. He or she may wish to insure against damage to expensive dental work.
5 *Keeping full, legible, contemporaneous and signed records*, particularly of any unusual events.
6 *Compliance with the law on controlled drugs.*
7 *Dealing compassionately with any injury that the patient suffers.* An honest and full explanation should be given, with apologies and sympathy if appropriate.

The anaesthetist should not judge his or her own negligence and liability, and it is unwise to admit these. Expert help from a defence organization should be sought as soon as possible.

Jehovah's Witnesses[28] and members of some other sects may wish to restrict some aspects of treatment, e.g. blood transfusion. The consequences of this should be explained fully in the presence of a witness. The patient should sign a statement of the restriction which should be countersigned by the witness. Special consent forms are available. An entry should also be made in the notes. With a child, his own best interests normally take priority over the wishes of his parents. Special legal procedures may be undertaken for his protection.

Patient identification requires a clearly defined system, discipline and vigilance.[29] A patient may give the wrong name and agree to the wrong operation. The very old, the very young and the mentally ill may be unable to verify these details at all. Beware: (i) too much haste; (ii) too much work; (iii) too little rest for the anaesthetist; (iv) changes in the operating list.

Deaths associated with anaesthesia[30]

In England and Wales, deaths are normally reported to HM Coroner (in Scotland to the Procurator Fiscal) if the death: (i) occurs during an operation, or before recovery from an anaesthetic; (ii) was sudden or unexplained; (iii) may have been caused by neglect, violence, poisoning, abortion or industrial injury or disease.

The sick anaesthetist

Anaesthetists are at risk of drug and vapour abuse. In England, after a patient died in theatre while under the care of an anaesthetist who was an addict, a procedure was adopted in the NHS to try to protect patients from ill doctors. This is the 'Three Wise Men' approach, as detailed in HC(82)13 *'Prevention of harm to patients resulting from physical or mental disability of hospital or community medical or dental staff'*. Professional associations have set up voluntary schemes to help colleagues whose competence has been affected by sickness. Employers or the General Medical Council may act if a sick doctor refuses to take advice.

AUDIT

Medical audit is the process by which doctors review, evaluate and improve their practice in the context of prescribed targets and standards: a systematic, critical analysis of the quality of medical care. It also impinges on resource provision and financial audit. It is an important component of all medical practice, a professional obligation. The Audit Commission has audited the NHS since 1990. Health Circular (91)2 outlines the arrangements for audit mandatory in UK hospitals from 1991. The Professional Standards Review Organization in the US was legislated in 1972.

Historical development

Government has attempted to regulate medicine from time immemorial. Doctors have realized that it is more effective to do it themselves. 'The price of clinical freedom is eternal professional vigilance'. The 1518 charter of the Royal College of Physicians states that one of the College's functions is to uphold the standards of medicine 'both for their own honour and in the name of the public benefit'. Although outcome studies of particular operations had been published in the late 19th century,[31] the first systematic attempt to link outcome with the care in hospital was associated with the establishment of the American College of Surgeons in Illinois in 1912.[32] Some early results were so shocking that they were incinerated!

Anaesthetists have a strong record. The first large-scale survey was of 599 548 anaesthetics administered over 5 years in 10 teaching hospitals in the US, with annual feedback of results to participating hospitals.[33] It recognized that anaesthesia, surgical care and intercurrent disease were inextricably bound up with each other. Mortality related to anaesthesia was 1 in 1560. Another important large survey at that time was of 10 098 spinal anaesthetics with no long-term neurological sequelae.[34]

Methods of audit

Audit is a cyclical process: current practice is observed, standards of practice are set, the results of current practice are compared with these standards, change is implemented, practice is observed again, and so on.

There is a wide choice of outcomes of practice that may be observed, e.g. questionnaires of patient satisfaction, administrative data (e.g. hospital stay), morbidity from anaesthesia, mortality. Sometimes one unexpected death may trigger a comprehensive review of patient care. Audit of the anaesthetist's involvement in obstetrics, intensive therapy and the treatment of chronic pain presents particular problems. The reporting of 'critical incidents' (events which if uncorrected would lead to harm) avoid the malpractice implications raised by some morbidity or mortality studies.[35]

Results of recent audit

Although methods vary widely, mortality associated with anaesthesia has probably gradually fallen.[36] The first *Confidential Enquiry into Perioperative Deaths* in 1987 which looked at just three English regions attributed only 3 out of 4034 deaths solely to anaesthesia. This amounted to about 1 in 185 000 operations.

The deficiencies revealed have been repeated to a greater or lesser extent in the subsequent nationwide reports, e.g. inadequate supervision of trainees and communication with superiors, especially out of hours; poor results of surgeons operating in specialist areas outside their sphere of expertise; unjustified emergency operations; inadequate preparation of the patient for surgery.

NCEPOD has established four useful categories of surgical priority: *emergency* = immediate life-saving operation, should take place within 1 h; *urgent* = as soon as possible after resuscitation, within 24 h; *scheduled* = early, e.g. for cancer, within 1–3 weeks; *elective* = anytime.

The *Confidential Enquiry into Maternal Deaths* is run jointly between the Department of Health and the Royal College of Obstetricians and Gynaecologists and began in 1952. Anaesthetic assessors are involved in this enquiry.

Important results have come from studies of the legal consequences of anaesthetic complications, despite the uncontrolled method of patient selection. Data from death certificates and inquests were used to examine deaths in the *dental surgery*.[37] Although general anaesthesia in this situation is now used less, the risk of death was about four times greater with operator anaesthesia. The *closed insurance claims studies* in the US have been of particular importance.[38] Analysis of 1175 such claims showed that nearly a third might have been prevented by monitors of O_2 saturation and respired CO_2.[39] Closed claims relating to 14 cardiac arrests during *spinal analgesia*[40] showed how easy it is to give too much sedation and that α-agonists and postural change are the most effective treatment of sympathetic blockade. Six of these patients died and only one survivor could return to independent self-care.

REFERENCES

1 Hewitt F. W. *Practitioner* 1896, **57,** 347.
2 Cooper J. B. *Can. J. Anaesth.* 1988, **35,** 287.
3 Cooper J. B. and Pierce E. C. *Anesth. Patient Safety Foundation Newslett.* 1986, **1,** 1.
4 Runciman W. B. *Anaesth. Intensive Care* 1988, **16,** 114.
5 Buck N. et al. *Report of the Confidential Enquiry into Perioperative Deaths.* London: Nuffield Provincial Hospitals Trust and the Kings Fund for Hospitals, 1987; subsequent reports of the National Confidential Enquiry into Perioperative Deaths.
6 Spence A. A. *Br. J. Anaesth.* 1997, **78,** 633; Kapur P. A. and Steadman R. H. *Anesth. Analg.* 1998, **86,** 1157.
7 Dyer C. *Br. Med. J.* 1988, **297,** 938.
8 Hatch D. J. *Anaesthesia* 1997, **52,** 193.
9 Dickson D. E. *Anaesthesia* 1996, **51,** 523; Seeley H. F. *Anaesthesia* 1996, **51,** 571.
10 *Checklist for Anaesthetic Apparatus* – 2. London: Association of Anaesthetists, 1997.
11 *Recommendation for Standards of Monitoring during Anaesthesia and Recovery* 1994, London: Association of Anaesthetists.
12 Tinker J. H. et al. *Anesthesiology* 1989, **71,** 541.
13 McDonald J. S. et al. *Br. J. Anaesth.* 1990, **64,** 582.
14 Jones J. G. et al. *Anaesthesia* 1990, **45,** 563.
15 Beecher H. K. *Surg. Gynecol. Obstet.* 1940, **71,** 689.
16 Waters R. M. J. *Indiana St. Med. Assoc.* 1936, **29,** 110.
17 Westhorpe R. *Anaesth. Intensive Care* 1989, **17,** 250.
18 Nosworthy M. *Curr. Res. Anesth. Analg.* 1945, **24,** 221; *St. Thomas' Hosp. Rep. (London)* 1937, **2,** 54; Nosworthy M. D. *Anaesthesia* 1963, **18,** 209.
19 McDonald J. S. et al. *Br. J. Anaesth.* 1990, **64,** 582.
20 Cook R. I. et al. *Anesthesiology* 1989, **71,** 385.
21 Sanborn K. V. et al. *Anesthesiology* 1996, **85,** 977.
22 Byrne A. J. *Br. J. Anaesth.* 1998, **80,** 58.
23 Bolam v Friern Hospital Management Committee 1957, *2 All ER* 118.
24 *Medico-Legal Reports. Appearing in Court.* London: Medical Protection Society, 1989.
25 Posner K. L. et al. *Anesthesiology* 1996, **85,** 1049.
26 Palmer R. N. *Anaesthesia* 1987, **43,** 265; *Consent. Confidentiality. Disclosure of Medical Records.* London: Medical Protection Society, 1988.
27 Sidaway v Bethlem Royal Hospital Governors and others. *1 All ER* 643 HL.
28 *Management of Anaesthesia for Jehovah's Witnesses.* Association of Anaesthetists, London, 1999.
29 *Theatre Safeguards.* Medical Defence Societies and Royal College of Nursing, 1986.
30 Aitkenhead A. R. *Anaesthesia* 1997, **52,** 477.

31 Haidenthaller J. *Arch. Klinische Chir.* 1890, **40**, 493; Bassini E. *Arch. Klinische Chir.* 1894, **47**, 1.
32 Codman E. A. *Surg. Gynecol. Obstet.* 1914, **18**, 491.
33 Beecher H. K. and Todd D. P. *Ann. Surg.* 1954, **140**, 2.
34 Dripps R. D. and Vandam L. D. *J. Am. Med. Assoc.* 1954, **156**, 1486.
35 Cooper J. B. *Anesthesiology* 1996, **85**, 961.
36 Edwards G. et al. *Anaesthesia* 1956, **11**, 194; Dinnick O. P. *Anaesthesia* 1964, **19**, 536; Derrington M. C. and Smith G. *Br. J. Anaesth.* 1987, **59**, 815.
37 Coplans M. P. and Curson I. *Br. Dental J.* 1982, **153**, 357.
38 e.g. Morray J. P. et al. *Anesthesiology* 1993, **78**, 461.
39 Tinker J. H. et al. *Anesthesiology* 1989, **71**, 541.
40 Caplan R. A. et al. *Anesthesiology* 1988, **68**, 5.

Section 2

GENERAL ANAESTHESIA TECHNIQUES

Chapter 2.1

Anaesthetic equipment

'We shape our tools, and thereafter our tools shape us'.

There is value in standardization of equipment within a unit, but there is also a good argument for a variety of equipment to meet the varying requirements of individual patients and for training purposes.

Evaluation of medical anaesthetic equipment

British Standard 5724:
 Part 1 (1979 & 1989) – safety
 Part 2 – specifications
 Part 3 – performance
European equivalent is IEC 601.
The European Medical Device Directives
 Implantable Active Devices, e.g. pacemakers
 Medical Devices
  Class 1. Heart valves
  Class 2. Powered non-implantable devices, e.g. anaesthetic
    equipment
 In vitro diagnostics

The accredited mark is 'CE'. 'Horizontal standards' concern electrical safety, sterilization, biocompatibility. 'Vertical standards' concern clinical investigation protocols and standards specific to a given device.

ANAESTHETIC MACHINES

Apparatus for administration of inhalation anaesthesia

Anaesthetic machines provide either continuous or intermittent flow. Vaporizers may be plenum or 'draw-over'.

The 'Boyle machine'[1]

The modern Boyle's apparatus bears little resemblance to the original. Gases are delivered from pipelines (or cylinders) via a reducing valve, which reduces the pressure to the flowmeters where flow is controlled by a needle valve. Two or more vaporizers are usually provided. Gases then pass into an anaesthetic breathing system. Modern anaesthetic machines, with or without built-in monitoring, are complex items of equipment which are increasingly dependent on electronics. This provides a high level of sophistication but at the price of vulnerability to electronic device and mains failure.

Cylinders

UK colours and pressures when full at 15°C: O_2 (international colour is white: but only the shoulder is white in UK) – 137 bar; N_2O (blue in UK) – 54 bar; air (grey body/black and white quartered shoulders in UK) – 137 bar; entonox (blue body/white and blue quartered shoulders in UK) – 137 bar; CO_2 (grey in UK) – 50 bar. (Note cyclopropane (orange) – 5 bar is no longer available in the UK.)

Cylinders are made of molybdenum steel. They are checked at intervals by the manufacturer for defects by subjecting them to tests.

1 *Tensile test:* this is carried out on at least 1 out of every 100 cylinders manufactured. Strips are cut and stretched – the 'yield point' should not be less than 15 tons/in^2.
2 *Flattening, impact and bend tests:* also carried out on at least 1 out of every 100 cylinders made.
3 *Hydraulic or pressure test:* usually a water-jacket test.

The filling ratio of a cylinder is the ratio of weight of gas in the cylinder to weight of water the cylinder could hold. Nitrous oxide cylinders are filled to a filling ratio of 0.75. Great care is taken that the gas is free from water vapour, otherwise when the cylinder is opened, temperature falls and water vapour would freeze and block the exit valve. Cylinder outlet valves use the pin-index system (British Standard 1319, 1955) so arranged that it is impossible to connect cylinders to wrong yokes,[2] and the yokes connected to flowmeters via non-interchangeable screw-threaded connectors (NIST). Before connection to the yoke, the cylinder valve is turned on briefly to flush out inflammable dust. After connection, the cylinder valve is slowly opened 2.5 turns. Machine backflow check valves prevent transfilling of cylinders.

Calculation of cylinder contents: N_2O by weight (1.87 g/l of gas); critical temperature 36.5°C, critical pressure 72 bar. (Note that nitrogen impurity exists in N_2O cylinders, especially at first opening.)[3] Oxygen and air content calculated by pressure gauges.

Table 2.1.1 Cylinder sizes.[4]

OXYGEN (international colour is white; but still black body/white shoulder in UK)

Size	Capacity (l)	Weight (kg)	Valve type
C	170	2	pin index
D	340	3.4	pin index
E	680	5.4	pin index
F	1360	14.5	bullnose

NITROUS OXIDE (blue in UK)

Size	Capacity (l)	Weight (kg) Cylinder	Gas	Valve type
C	450	2	0.85	pin index
D	900	3.4	1.7	pin index
E	1800	5.4	3.4	pin index
F	3600	14.5	6.8	wheel

Piped gas supplies[5]

Oxygen (white, 4 bar), N_2O (blue, 4 bar), Entonox (O_2 and N_2O mixture in equal volumes), compressed air (black, 7 bar for instrument use, 4 bar – medical quality) and vacuum (yellow) may be supplied by pipelines (UK colours). Banks of supply cylinders are housed in a ventilated fireproof room and automatically switch (with warning lights) to the reserve bank when the running bank is near exhaustion. The machine to pipeline connections are 'tug-tested' to ensure security.

Liquid oxygen supply[6]

Oxygen is stored in a thermally insulated vessel at a pressure of about 1200 kPa and at a temperature lower than the critical temperature (minus 119°C). Evaporation requires heat. Fresh supplies of liquid O_2 are pumped from a tanker into a storage vessel which rests on a weighing balance so that a dial measures the mass of liquid. Reserve banks of O_2 cylinders are kept in case of failure of supply. Liquid O_2 stores are housed away from main buildings because of the fire hazard.

Accidents have occurred due to the wrong connection of pipelines to anaesthetic apparatus. The union between hoses and the anaesthetic machine should be permanent.[7] The routine preanaesthetic drill will detect any such fault. Hoses are colour coded and when repairs are necessary a complete hose assembly is provided. A 'permit to work' system[8] requires in the UK a certificate in six parts to be signed as appropriate and is used when the action of one group of workers could directly or indirectly expose others to hazard. Three levels of hazard are identified:

1 *high*, when work involves cutting an in-service pipeline, with danger of cross-connection or pollution;
2 *medium*, work on a terminal unit where more than one gas is supplied, with danger of cross-connection;
3 *low*, where only one gas is involved.

Hazards include mechanical, electrical failures, and failures of correct inter-action between anaesthetist and machine. There must be enough light shining on the machine (and the patient) to see everything clearly.

Pressure and contents gauges

These indicate the cylinder contents in the case of O_2 and CO_2. In the case of N_2O they read 'full' until the last liquid is vaporized, when the pressure declines with the last $\frac{1}{2}$ h use of the contents. The BS 4272 (1968) gives a scale marked '0; $\frac{1}{4}$; $\frac{1}{2}$; $\frac{3}{4}$; full'.

The preanaesthetic machine checklist

The following procedure has been recommended.[9] At the start the apparatus is disconnected from all piped medical gases and the O_2 and N_2O cylinders turned off.

1 Calibrate O_2 analyser and place it at common gas outlet.
2 Confirm correct insertion of pipelines by 'tug test'.
3 Check that the O_2 cylinder contains sufficient gas.
4 Check any other gas cylinders that are needed.
5 Turn off cylinders.
6 Check pipeline pressure gauges (400 kPa).
7 Open O_2 flowmeter to read about 5 l/min and check O_2 analyser approaches 100%.
8 Check operation of other flowmeters and turn them all off.
9 Check operation of O_2 emergency bypass control and that it does not cause pipeline pressure to fall significantly.

The contents, closure, backbar locking, and control knob function of vaporizers are checked and also any electrical devices, e.g. monitors. The circuit systems are checked for leaks and loose connections by occluding the outlet while gas flows. The bobbins dip slightly, and the pressure relief valve opens. This test should not be performed if there is no pressure relief valve.
    The whistle discriminator enables the nature of a gas issuing from a pipeline to be determined. With N_2O the note falls $1\frac{1}{2}$ tones from the oxygen note.

Pressure-reducing valves (pressure regulators)

Reducing valves are used: to give safe working pressures; to prevent equipment damage; maintain constant pressure within the machine; and to allow delicate control of gas flows. The classic reducing valve is the Adams valve in which a toggle mechanism occludes the orifice when pressure rises. The Medishield 5 valve reduces to 810 kPa and the M valve to 405 kPa. The McKesson valve to 465 kPa. In the US, regulating valves vary from these values.

Dust filters are incorporated.

Flow restrictors

Pipeline gas supplies at 405 kPa (about 4 atmospheres) are commonly transferred to the flowmeters without interposition of a reducing valve. Sudden pressure surges are prevented by the use of a flow restrictor which is a constriction in the low-pressure circuit upstream to the flowmeter. The fine-adjustment control would require recalibration if the pipeline pressure changed markedly. Flow restrictors are also used downstream of vaporizers to prevent back-pressure effects.

Flowmeters

Theory

Flow rate through a tube is proportional to the pressure difference. With a given pressure difference across an orifice, flow rate of gas is proportional to the square of the diameter of the orifice. Flow rate along a tube depends on the viscosity of a gas. Flow rate through an orifice depends on density and varies as the reciprocal of the square root of the density.

Types of flowmeter

These may be divided into variable orifice and fixed orifice types.

VARIABLE-ORIFICE METERS (FIXED-PRESSURE DIFFERENCE)

The rotameter

This is the type used today in most modern machines. Gas is led to the base of a finely wrought glass tube, slightly smaller on cross-section at bottom than at top. A light metal float (bobbin) rides the gas jet and notches in its edge cause it to rotate. As the bobbin rises with increased flow, the size of the annulus between it and the glass tube increases. Height of top of float gives rate of flow, the gas escaping between the rim of the metal float and the walls of the glass tube. The glass tubes must be vertical, and clean, and the float rotate freely. A wire stop keeps the float in sight at the top. The calibration of the glass tubes takes into account both the density and the viscosity of the gases passing through them. Viscosity is important at low flows as gas flow round the bobbin approximates to tubular flow (diameter of orifice less than length), but density is important at high flows (diameter of orifice greater than length). Hence, a rotameter calibrated for CO_2 will not read true for cyclopropane, because although their densities are similar (44 : 42) their viscosities are different (1 : 0.6). The needle valve control knob carries the name of the gas and is colour coded. The oxygen control knob commonly protrudes further out than the others to assist recognition.

The needle valve may be upstream of the rotameter (UK), or downstream (US), which maintains a more constant pressure in the rotameter tube. The rotameter bank may have the oxygen on the left (UK) or right (parts of US). In either case, oxygen is the last gas to enter the stream, which diminishes the risk from leaks at the top of the oxygen rotameter.

FIXED-ORIFICE METERS (VARIABLE-PRESSURE DIFFERENCE)

Pressure differences across an orifice vary with changes in flow. Pressure varies as the square of flow rate.

Pressure gauge meter
The pressure build-up proximal to the constriction is measured utilizing a Bourdon pressure gauge, which is then calibrated for flow (used on some air cylinders).

Water depression meter
Pressure on two sides of the fixed orifice is measured by means of a water manometer.

Inaccuracies and dangers of rotameters

1 Static electricity and dirt can cause as much as 35% inaccuracy. Can cause sticking of the bobbin, especially when low flows are used.
2 Cracked flowmeter tubes with consequent leaks may result in delivery of a hypoxic mixture. It is safer to place the oxygen flowmeter last in the flowmeter bank. An internal arrangement at the top of the rotameters allows this to be achieved even with the oxygen rotameter on the left, and the bank on the left side of the machine.
3 A defect in the top sealing washer of a rotameter can cause fatal deprivation of oxygen.[10]
4 The rotameter tube must be vertical.
5 Back-pressure (*see below*).

In the past the small bobbin of a cyclopropane or CO_2 flowmeter could become jammed at the top of the rotameter tube so that the anaesthetist was unaware that gas was flowing. On older anaesthetic machines a blanking plug is recommended for the CO_2 cylinder yoke.

Effect of barometric pressure

Flowmeters are calibrated for use at sea level. They become inaccurate at high altitudes or in hyperbaric chambers.

Flowmeters also become inaccurate when a restriction at the outlet causes a pressure build-up. This may occur when some humidifiers, nebulizers, etc. are in use. Flow is then greater than indicated with variable-orifice-type flowmeters. In the fixed-orifice type a large flow may be indicated even when there is complete occlusion of the outlet. These inaccuracies can be corrected by placing the control valve distal to the orifice. In this pressure-compensated flowmeter, pressure in the flowmeter itself is the same as that in the supply line. The flowmeter is calibrated in terms of litres the gas will occupy after discharge to atmospheric pressure.

Oxygen flush (bypass)

The control should not be able to be left on accidentally, or it will dilute anaesthetics and allow awareness. The flow rate is in excess of 35 l/min.

Vaporizers

These may be draw-over (e.g. EMO for ether) or machine gas driven ('plenum'; variable bypass and measured-flow).

Both variable-bypass (tec-type; 'tec' = 'temperature compensated') and measured-flow (kettle-type) vaporizers when fully turned off can leak anaesthetic vapours into the circuit.

Some machines inject liquid agent into the gas stream in exact amounts controlled by feedback from vapour analysers further down the stream, and the required percentage dialled in by the operator. This is analogous to fuel injection.

A wide variety of vaporizers are now available. In general they are designed for use with a particular agent (sometimes, e.g. 'Selectatec', with lock-outs preventing use of more than one at a time) or in a particular situation (e.g. 'Triservice' type). Some are designed to prevent spillage if not kept vertical (e.g. Mk 4 fluotec).

Hook-on mountings, e.g. 'Selectatec', can cause major leaks of anaesthetic gas if not locked on properly.

Concentration distal to vaporizer depends on the following:

1 Saturated vapour pressure (SVP) of the inhalation agent (sevoflurane 21.3 kPa; enflurane 22.9 kPa; isoflurane 31.9 kPa; halothane 32.5 kPa; desflurane 88.5 kPa). The higher the SVP, the greater the concentration delivered; the gas diverted through the vapour chamber becomes fully saturated with the volatile agent.

2 Temperature (by raising the SVP). The heat for vaporizing the agent comes from the liquid agent itself, which cools as a result. (*See* Compensation, below.)

3 The 'splitting ratio' i.e. the proportion of the total flow which is diverted to the vaporizing chamber.
4 The surface area of the vapour chamber, including wick.
5 Flow characteristics through the vapour chamber.
6 The amount of liquid in the vapour chamber (concentration falls when nearly empty).

Compensation devices to stabilize the delivered concentrations

Efforts are made to overcome change of concentration with ambient temperature, rate of evaporation and the degree of heat gain from the vaporizer jacket or the surroundings as follows.

1 Automatic variation of the outlet port of the vaporizing chamber with temperature. The use of bimetallic (zinc–copper or zinc–brass) bars or a thermosensitive capsule, or both.
2 By bubbling the gas through the agent as in the 'copper kettle' to provide a saturated vapour which can be diluted to obtain the desired concentration. (The vapour chamber of a 'tec' type also produces a saturated vapour, due to the large surface area.) Desflurane was initially administered by this method.[11]
3 To maintain the liquid at constant temperature. The use of a water bath or calcium chloride crystals to provide extra heat. (e.g. in EMO).

Many vaporizers have interlocks to prevent more than one being on at one time. Some have spill-proof devices to prevent liquid loss if placed in non-vertical positions. Keyed filling ports which only connect with specific filler tubes of specific bottles of specific agents are common. Vaporizers are serviced at regular intervals, e.g. yearly.

Desflurane poses a specific problem in that its boiling point is near to room temperature, it may have to be kept in cooled vaporizers or in warmed cylinders.[11,12]

Oxygen failure warning (alarm) devices

The properties of the ideal oxygen failure warning device are:

1 It should not depend on the pressure of any gas other than the oxygen itself.
2 The alarm system should not utilize battery or mains power.
3 The signal should be audible and of sufficient length, volume and character.
4 There should be a warning of impending failure, and a further warning that failure has occurred.

When it comes into operation; other gases should cease to flow; the breathing system should open to the atmosphere; inspired oxygen concentration should be at least equal to that of air, and build-up of CO_2 should not occur; It should be impossible to resume anaesthesia until the oxygen supply has been restored.

Pressure-relief valves

These prevent damage to the machine, should the outlet become obstructed (flow restrictors are satisfactory only as a means of smoothing surges of pressure). Pressure relief valves are combined non-return and pressure relief valves and are usually fitted at the end of the back bar, downstream from the vaporizers. They are set to operate at 30–40 kPa (BS 4272 Part 1 1968).

Pressure-limiting valves

These aim to prevent damage to the patient's airways. They have a much lower opening pressure (e.g. 4 kPa) than pressure-relief valves. Such valves may be built into breathing systems. In addition, the 2-litre rubber reservoir bag, when distended with pressure, seldom reaches pressures above 5 kPa before it splits[13] (but plastic disposable bags used in the US can develop high pressures[14]). A pressure-limiting reservoir bag used in conjunction with a pressure-limiting valve has been described.[15] Unfortunately, a steady pressure of 4 kPa (28 mmHg) at the alveoli will stop the pulmonary circulation (PA systolic pressure = 25 mmHg), so this hazard is not prevented by these valves.

Expiratory valves

These are one-way, spring-loaded, fully adjustable valves. When open, they should have minimal resistance to expiration (1–5 mmHg). During spontaneous breathing they should always be fully opened (when the 'opening pressure' is 1–5 mmHg), as their setting determines the mean pressure in the anaesthetic circuit and in the patient's respiratory tract. During manual intermittent positive-pressure ventilation (IPPV) they are usually nearly closed with a small leak. During ventilator IPPV, they are usually completely closed. Heidbrink-type expiratory valves should be sterilized by autoclaving as antiseptic solutions may produce corrosion, stickiness and consequent increased resistance to opening pressure. Partial closure of the valve during spontaneous respiration produces a crude form of positive end-expiratory pressure (PEEP).

Other apparatus for administration of inhalation anaesthesia

Intermittent flow machines

Now of historical interest only. The McKesson is one example. BS 4272 Part 1 (1968) defined their standards. Many could deliver continuous flow.

Portable anaesthetic machines

Triservice, Portablease, Fluoxair. Many of these use a low-resistance draw-over vaporizer and an inflating bellows with one way valves and facilities for O_2 enrichment.

Computerized machines

With direct injection of volatile agents.

Reservoir bags

These are usually made of antistatic rubber and should be large enough to supply the patient's inspiratory volume (e.g. 2 litres for an adult). They also act as an excellent visual monitor of spontaneous respiration. (*See* also Pressure-limiting valves, above.) In paediatric anaesthesia a smaller bag gives a better indication of tidal excursion.

Face masks

These should be easy to clean and sterilize after each patient, and be antistatic. They should provide a good fit with the patient's face and add minimal dead space. The dead space of an adult face mask may be considerable (up to 7–198 ml) and this may equal or exceed the anatomical dead space. In children and infants it is possible for the mask and attachments to double or treble the dead space. The Rendell–Baker–Souchek face mask greatly reduce this dead space. However, clear latex face masks are now available which mould to the contours of the child's face; these should be preferred to the Rendall–Baker mask. The face mask connectors also add to the dead space (Ruben valve: 9 ml; angle connection and expiratory valve: 28–30 ml). A disposable face mask is available. An airtight seal between a face mask and the edentulous patient can often be improved by retention of dentures.

'Brain' laryngeal mask[16]

(*See also* Chapter 2.6.) An easy alternative to a face mask. They are normally inserted blind to behind the larynx. In difficult cases this is facilitated by extension of the head, insertion with the aperture facing backwards, then rotation to the forwards position within the pharynx. May be lubricated with lignocaine jelly to reduce coughing. The depression of pharyngeal reflexes by propofol is particularly advantageous in assisting their insertion immediately after induction. Malposition may be due to the mask being: not far enough in; too far in – within the oesophagus; or having pushed the epiglottis down between it and the glottis.[17] Repositioning is straightforward. Several sizes are available: sizes 1, 2 and $2\frac{1}{2}$ suitable for children, and sizes $2\frac{1}{2}$, 3, 4 and 5 for adults. The cuff of size 3 takes about 20 ml, size 4 about 30 ml. Can be used when intubation is difficult or impossible.[18] Designed for spontaneous respiration, but have been used for IPPV,[19] in which case they do not protect the airway from aspiration of stomach contents.[20] Thus, they are not appropriate for caesarean section.[21]

The pilot balloon has been exploded off during sterilization, and entered the pipe of the laryngeal mask.[22]

Entonox apparatus

The premixed gases are supplied from the cylinder via a two-stage valve. The first stage is a simple reducing valve which decreases pressure to about 1350 kPa (200 lb/in^2). The second incorporates a tilting valve which opens to the negative pressure of inspiration but is closed when the positive pressure of expiration pushes down a sensing diaphragm. Little inspiratory effort is needed to produce a high flow rate. Gas cannot flow when pressure in the cylinder falls below 1350 kPa (200 lb/in^2) so that a proportion of gas is wasted. This is a safety factor should separation of the premixed gases have occurred since residual gas is likely then to be rich in N_2O. The apparatus is compact and portable, weighing 6.1 kg with a full 500-litre cylinder. BS 4272 Part 2 (1968) defines their standards.

Premixed gases can also be used with a calibrated flowmeter and the Magill circuit.

ANAESTHETIC GAS DELIVERY SYSTEMS

These use rubber or plastic pipe. Rubber pipe is made antistatic by addition of carbon, which is responsible for its black colour. Corrugations make the pipes kink-proof. Connections are made with 8.5 (paediatric), 15, 22, or 30 (exhaust) mm tapers, with or without locking rings. There is inevitably resistance to flow and dead space in such tubular systems.[23] Some rebreathing is almost inevitable, and the patient compensates for this by physical and perhaps physiological means. Attempts to reduce rebreathing usually employ either valves or large gas flows. It can be assessed by capnography.[24]

Factors affecting carbon dioxide elimination

1 Fresh gas flow rate.
2 Apparatus dead space, both static and dynamic.[25]

3 Leaks in the anaesthetic system (especially ventilators).
4 Waveform and settings of the ventilator.
5 Design of the systems.
6 Patient's alveolar ventilation (patient's respiratory drive and performance; patient's respiratory waveform).

Semi-closed methods

These methods may allow some degree of rebreathing and may or may not be used in conjunction with CO_2 absorption. If the Magill attachment (Mapleson System A) is used effective CO_2 elimination requires spontaneous respiration, an expiratory valve of minimal resistance and a total gas flow greater than the alveolar ventilation (roughly 70% of the respiratory minute volume of the patient). There is no rebreathing if the fresh gas supply is more than 5 l/min for a 70-kg patient. Studies of the effect of fresh gas flows lower than alveolar ventilation indicate that with mild rebreathing the system acts as simple added dead space, but with gross rebreathing the entire system acts as a mixing device. Variations in tidal volume can be significant.

Classification

The Mapleson classification of anaesthetic systems is shown in Fig. 2.1.1.

MAPLESON SYSTEM A

The most satisfactory with spontaneous respiration (e.g. Magill system). A flow of about 5 l/min is required (in young healthy patients) to flush CO_2 from the system. In *assisted* or *controlled respiration* the expiratory valve must be partly closed. The Magill system is efficient with regard to CO_2 disposal in spontaneous ventilation with gas flows of 5–6 l/min.

An advancing cone front of laminar flow may explain how some hypo-ventilating patients, breathing spontaneously under anaesthesia with small tidal volumes (e.g. 100 ml), may ventilate reasonably effectively. The gas in the centre of a tube may reach the end of the tube preferentially. This only occurs with laminar flow. Furthermore, the higher the patient's alveolar CO_2 the more CO_2 is excreted at each breath.

VARIATIONS OF THE MAPLESON A SYSTEM

The Lack system[26]
The patient breathes through concentric tubes; the outer tube is inspiratory, the large inner tube is expiratory; the valve is situated near the anaesthetic apparatus. The commercial version has an inspiratory limb capacity of 500 ml and resistance to respiration is acceptable. The Lack system, unlike

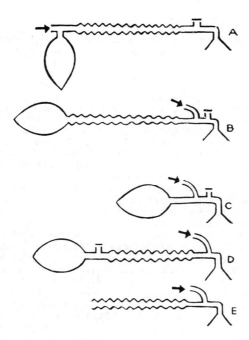

Figure 2.1.1 The Mapleson classification of anaesthetic systems

the Bain, does not readily permit the use of mechanical ventilators. It can be easily adapted for use with scavenging systems. The Lack Parallel system has two tubes side by side.

Miller preferential flow system
Similar to the Lack but has no valves.

Enclosed afferent reservoir[27]
The inspiratory reservoir bag is inside a rigid bottle (to which the expired gases pass via a one-way valve, before being vented). It is equally efficient during spontaneous respiration or IPPV.

MAPLESON B

Not in common clinical use.

MAPLESON C

The 'Waters' system used in many postoperative recovery wards is an example.

MAPLESON D

For example the Bain co-axial system.[28] The system is a modification of the Mapleson D system (*see* Fig. 2.1.1) in which the fresh gases enter the system by means of a narrow-bore inflow tube which lies within the lumen of the exhalation limb to terminate close to the patient end (Fig. 2.1.2).

Advantages: the system carries a single tube to the patient. It is light in weight and can be used in all age groups. It is adaptable to all types of anaesthetic procedures and can be used with spontaneous respiration and IPPV. (The Bain expiratory valve is normally closed for mechanical IPPV, the expired gases exiting via the ventilator.) It is controlled entirely from the machine end of the system. Scavenging of expired gases is facilitated. The Penlon co-axial system is a modification in which the inner tube is made of antistatic material while the outer tube is transparent to facilitate inspection. The Penlon co-axial valve is used to fit the system to the outlet of the anaesthetic apparatus. Hazard can occur if the inner tube becomes broken or dislodged as considerable dead space may then occur. This is tested for in the preanaesthetic checklist by occluding the exit port of the inner tube with the little finger while gas is flowing from the machine, and noting the drop in flowmeter bobbins (only if the machine has a pressure-release valve).

With IPPV a fresh gas flow of 70 ml/kg (5 l/min for a patient of 70 kg) produces normocapnia, and 100 ml/kg mild hypocapnia $PaCO_2$ is related to fresh gas flow in patients weighing more than 40 kg. Below this, more CO_2 is produced per unit of body weight and a minimal flow of 3.5 l/min has been recommended for patients weighing less than 50 kg. A flow of about 3 l/min is used with small children and infants.

With spontaneous respiration recommended fresh gas flow rates have varied from three times the minute volume to between 90 and 160 ml/kg. The differences probably reflect the respiratory depression caused by premedication, the depth of anaesthesia and the ratio of inspiration to expiration. In view of the higher gas flows required during spontaneous respiration, the Mapleson A (Magill) system is then more appropriate than the Bain.

Variations of the Bain include the Mera F-type with twin hoses.

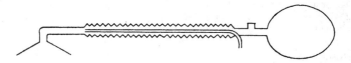

Figure 2.1.2 The Bain system

Recommended fresh gas flows for use with spontaneous respiration are: Lack, 58; Magill, 80; Bain, 100 ml/kg/min. These flows should be increased by about 10% for each C above 37°C.[29] Routine capnography enables fresh gas flows to be adjusted for individual patients. In particular, the elderly produce far less CO_2 and require much less fresh gas. (Note that capnograph sampling from the patient end of a Bain system may give false results because of the jet of fresh gas impinging on the sampling port.)

MAPLESON E

For example the Ayre's T-piece[30] (*see also* Chapter 4.2). Advocated primarily for use in infants and young children. In order to prevent dilution of inspired gases with air on the one hand, or rebreathing with CO_2 accumulation on the other hand, it is recommended that the total fresh gas flow should be about twice the minute volume of the patient, and the volume of the reservoir tube equal to about one-third of the tidal volume. Classically modified by Jackson Rees who added a bag for monitoring and IPPV.[31] Gases can be scavenged.

The main advantage of the T-piece technique is the absence of resistance to expiration, a factor of crucial importance in small children.

Efficiency of systems with spontaneous respiration:

$$A > D \& E > C > B$$

Efficiency of systems with IPPV:

$$D \& E > B > C > A$$

THE HAFNIA SYSTEMS

These are modifications of Mapleson A, B, C and D systems, using suction directly from the system to prevent atmospheric pollution. The expiratory valve is replaced by a suction port and an ejector flowmeter.

THE BURCHETT AND BENNETT CO-AXIAL BREATHING SYSTEM

This combines the benefits of the Mapleson A, D and E systems.

THE HUMPHREY (ADE) SYSTEM[23]

A single lever changes from one system to the other. This combines the Mapleson A, D and E principles.

REBREATHING AND DEAD SPACE[25]

The patient's dead space is increased by most anaesthetic apparatus, and efforts are made to reduce this to a minimum, by adequate fresh gas flows (70% of MV for Magill system; ranging to 200% of MV for T-piece). Rebreathing of some alveolar gas occurs with most anaesthetic breathing systems (especially the Bain), but in practice does not greatly raise the patient's $PaCO_2$, as a reasonably lightly anaesthetized person can compensate for this.

NON-REBREATHING VALVES

Advantages: no possibility of rebreathing provided the dead space of the valve itself is small; can be used for spontaneous or controlled respiration; and can be used to measure minute volume, if the flowmeters are accurate. Ideal for draw-over vaporizers, e.g. EMO.

Disadvantages: wasteful; variations of minute volume during spontaneous respiration require frequent adjustment of the flowmeters to prevent collapse or distension of the reservoir bag; valves may stick; and some valves are noisy.

Examples of non-rebreathing valves.

1 *The Ruben valve:* a bobbin moves against a spring to act as a unidirectional valve and an outlet valve prevents admission of atmospheric air. Dead space 9 ml. Low resistance. The resuscitation version has no outlet valve so that a patient breathing spontaneously will inhale air from the atmosphere.
2 *The Ambu valves:* uses one or two silicone rubber flaps. The valve can be dismantled easily for cleaning and sterilization. It is possible to reassemble the valve incorrectly with consequent risk of hypoxia. It can be used with a self-inflating bag. The valve with one flap is only suitable for IPPV. The valve with two rubber flaps is suitable for IPPV or spontaneous respiration. It has a very low dead space.

INSUFFLATION TECHNIQUES

Tracheal insufflation via a small catheter occasionally finds a use in upper airway manipulations.

Rebreathing with carbon dioxide absorption – closed systems, low-flow systems

The closed, circle, or low-flow system

Founded on principle that if sufficient oxygen is added to supply body's basal needs and CO_2 is absorbed, the same mixture of gases can be rebreathed repeatedly. Adult basal oxygen consumption varies between 200 and 400 ml/min. The system may be completely closed, or it may have a leak, when used with slightly larger flows. There is a rubber reservoir bag in the system. The system may be 'to-and-fro' or 'circle'.

ADMINISTRATION OF THE VOLATILE AGENT

1 *By vaporiser:* the vaporizer may be outside the breathing circuit (VOC) in the fresh gas supply line, or the vaporizer may be inside the breathing circuit (VIC) when the patient's inspirations or expirations go through the vaporizer, which must then be of 'low-resistance' type. (Plenum types are completely unsuitable for VIC use.) In this case the vaporizer increases the vapour tension with each breath and is potentially very dangerous.
2 *By direct injection of liquid agent into the system:* carefully calculated amounts of liquid volatile agent have been injected at 1-min intervals into

the expiratory limb of the circle system. Computer-controlled servo injection systems acting on feedback from in-circuit vapour analysers are used for the more expensive agents, e.g. desflurane.

Initially, larger flows are used to fill the system with the desired mixture of anaesthetics and oxygen, then, after 2 min, the gas flows are reduced.

Soda-lime

Used to absorb CO_2. A mixture of 90% calcium hydroxide with 5% sodium hydroxide and 1% potassium hydroxide, with silicates to prevent powdering. It is essential for effective absorption that moisture (14–19%) be incorporated within the granule. The hydroxides combine with CO_2 in the presence of water to form carbonates. It can absorb about 20% of its own weight of CO_2. Soda-lime granules are 3–6 mm in size to minimize resistance to breathing and to allow plenty of surface for absorption. Air space in the charged canister should equal the patient's tidal volume. Nearly half the volume in a properly packed canister consists of intergranular space. The chemical change involved in absorption results in water and the carbonate of the respective metals, and heat production, the heat of neutralization. All volatile anaesthetic agents (with the exception of desflurane) may be decomposed by the heat produced as a result of absorption of CO_2 by soda-lime. Thermal decomposition of trichloroethylene, and possibly also sevoflurane, results in toxic compounds; it has been suggested therefore that neither agent should be used with soda-lime. Storing soda-lime in its container does not interfere with its efficiency.

Durasorb is an improved soda-lime with a prolonged effective life which does not overheat. Its pink colour turns to white when it becomes inactive. Baralyme (barium hydroxide lime, USP) is 80% calcium hydroxide with 20% barium octohydrate. It is said to be less caustic, and to produce less heat than soda-lime. No silica is necessary to produce hardness. It contains mimoza Z and ethyl violet as indicator; the pink granules change to purple when exhausted. Used in spacecraft.

The soda-lime must be fresh and tidal exchange must be adequate for efficient CO_2 elimination. Vertical position of the canister prevents 'channelling' of gas flow down the edges, but even so, the centre of the canister tends to be used preferentially, resulting in loss of efficiency which is not evident to the naked eye because the visible soda-lime has not yet changed colour. In practice this is rarely a problem because most systems have a huge excess of efficiency.

The 1-lb canister will last about 6 h intermittently, 2 h continuously. In practice it is unwise to wait until the soda-lime is completely exhausted. Fresh absorbent should always be used if there is any doubt as to its efficiency.

Temperature during absorption

Nearly all from the heat of the chemical reaction of neutralization which is exothermic. The temperature within the canister may reach 60°C in that

---

Signs of exhaustion of soda-lime

1 Change of colour of granules.
2 Monitoring: rise in measured inspired CO_2 on the capnograph.
3 Clinically: rise in blood pressure followed eventually by a fall.
4 Rise in pulse rate.
5 Deepening of spontaneous respiration.
6 Increased oozing from wound and perhaps sweating.

---

part of the canister where active absorption is occurring, especially where much CO_2 is produced, as in malignant hyperthermia.

Monitoring the low-flow system

Inspired oxygen and end-tidal CO_2, anaesthetic agent, tidal volume, respiratory rate, airway pressure, basal oxygen consumption.

Applications

Economy in use of gases; less pollution of theatre atmosphere; and humidification and warming of inspired gas.

Disadvantages

1 Hypoxia may occur as the circuit gases have a different concentration to the added fresh gases. Circuit oxygen concentration is monitored. Added volatile agents are also diluted.
2 Hypercapnia may occur. Circuit CO_2 concentration should be monitored.
3 Even small leaks have a disastrous effect on circuit gas concentrations.
4 Greater risk of disconnections, due to greater complexity of pipework.
5 Alkaline dust may pass to patient;
6 Resistance to breathing and dead space may be high.
7 Increased CO_2 content of inspired gas, as absorption is far from perfect.
8 Dilution of gases in reservoir bag by nitrogen in the circuit in the early part of the administration.
9 Volatile agents may be adsorbed to soda-lime, lowering the initial concentration and 'hanging over' to subsequent patients.

Apparatus

1 The Waters 'to-and-fro' single-phase system (Fig. 2.1.3).[32] Gases pass through the canister during both inspiration and expiration. Fresh gases are led to the patient close to the mask.
2 The circle or two-phase system. An inspiratory and expiratory tube are used, with valves to ensure a one-way flow of gases; breathing and low dead space. The soda-lime can be by-passed and the canister can be easily removed for recharging. Fresh gases must not enter just before the

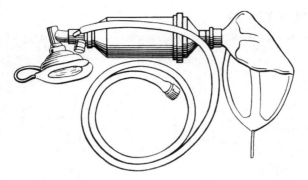

Figure 2.1.3 The Waters' 'to and fro' carbon dioxide absorber (British Oxygen Company Ltd)

expiratory valve, or they will be wasted and hypoxia may occur. A pop-off valve must not be placed between patient and inspiratory valve.

Circle absorption and fresh gas flow: at higher flows the system behaves like a semi-closed system and soda-lime is unnecessary. With basal flows, rebreathing is total and expired CO_2 is removed by soda-lime. At fresh gas flows of 1–2 l/min, the circuit concentration of volatile agents is about half the fresh gas concentration. At fresh gas flows of 3–4 l/min, circuit volatile concentrations are about equal to the fresh gas concentrations. Circuit gas concentrations are monitored. The fresh gas flow rates required for rebreathing systems have been studied using a mathematical model.[33] With a flow rate of 7 l/min, nitrogen elimination is complete in 5 min for practical purposes. With the flow reduced to 500 ml/min, the nitrogen concentration in the system is still 20% after 1 h. With an inflow of 500 ml/min Entonox, FIO_2, falls to dangerously low levels, but at 1000 ml/min FIO_2 remains at about 40% (assuming an oxygen consumption of 225 ml/min).

A low-flow regimen of 1000 ml/min N_2O and 600 ml/min O_2 will provide an FIO_2 between 35 and 25% over a range of oxygen consumption between 150 and 300 ml/min. Nitrous oxide uptake declines exponentially from 462 ml/min to 110 ml/min after 2 h.

Mechanical dead space

Mechanical dead space is the addition to dead space which is produced by the anaesthetic apparatus.[25] It increases the $PaCO_2$, but, provided FIO_2 is generous, may not affect PaO_2. It may be used deliberately to keep the $PaCO_2$ normal during hyperventilation intended to prevent alveolar collapse.

Mechanical dead space in a circle absorber is space between face and beginning of double corrugated tubing. Cope's modification of Waters' absorber is designed to minimize dead space when anaesthetizing children.

Scavenging systems

Collection of effluent gases from anaesthetic systems requires the use of a collecting valve and the use of tubing to duct the waste to atmosphere. Scavenging systems may be classified as:

Passive

The total flow resistance should not exceed 50 Pa (0.5 cmH$_2$O) at 30 l/min and copper pipes of 28–35 mm outer diameter are thought to be satisfactory. The discharge point should avoid wind pressures. A T-termination with a downward right-angle bend at each end is preferred, placed above a flat roof.

Assisted passive

The extract duct of a non-circulatory theatre ventilation system can be used instead of an exterior discharge point.

Active scavenging

The patient should be protected from negative pressures greater than 100 Pa (1 cmH$_2$O). There should be a reservoir which can take the form of an open T-piece to protect the patient from subatmospheric pressures. Piped suction has been used and this may be combined with the use of activated charcoal to remove anaesthetic vapours. A paediatric scavenging device has been described. (*See* Sik M.J. et al. *Br. J. Anaesth.* 1990, **64,** 117.)

The Papworth block incorporates a safety valve opening at 500 Pa (5 cmH$_2$O) and a reservoir bag to absorb peak pressures. The latter also acts as a monitor of the system.

The Cardiff Aldasorber contains activated charcoal which removes anaesthetic vapours but not N$_2$O. Its duration of active use is gauged by the gain in weight due to adsorbed agent.

Monitoring inhaled gases and vapours (*see also* Chapter 2.2)
Oxygen

Polarographic – reliable. The fuel cell analyser can be affected by water vapour and needs replacing every year or so. Paramagnetic – a common method.

Carbon dioxide

Infra-red absorption – most of these require removal of a gas sample from the system for analysis, but at least one has the infra-red cell in the anaesthetic system. Reliable and robust.

Volatile agents

Infra-red absorption – as for CO_2, but with gas-specific spectra; Drager Narkotest – silicone rubber lengthens in the presence of halothane, related to its concentration; and change in frequency of a quartz crystal oscillator (the Engstrom Emma) – affected by water vapour, which usually raises the reading by 0.3–0.5%.

MECHANICAL VENTILATORS

Some points to consider when acquiring a ventilator for theatre or intensive therapy unit (ITU).[34]

1 *Physical characteristics:* valve resistance important where spontaneous intermittent mandatory ventilation (SIMV), pressure support and continuous positive airway pressure (CPAP) are used.
2 *Triggering:* there is a tendency to place the trigger sensor nearer to the patient to get a faster response and higher sensitivity, especially where tachypnoea (commonly) exists.
3 *Safety and reliability:* automatic alarm for disconnection requires automatic oxygen flow if gas supply fails, automatic battery backup if mains fail, automatic ventilation if apnoea occurs. Partial ventilatory support features which are now added to the range of CPAP, IMV, SIMV and extended mandatory minute ventilation (EMMV), with extremely rapid response times for use in severe tachypnoea.
4 *Pressure support (PS):* with various rise times, and ability to combine with SIMV. Features desirable in CPAP include:
   (a) the inspiratory flow must always exceed that of the patient, e.g. 60 l/min;
   (b) minimal effort is needed to trigger the system;
   (c) minimal resistance in expiration;
   (d) the provision of full alarms and automatic override in CPAP;
   (e) gas usage is economical.
   (f) Built-in monitoring of airway resistance, calculation of auto-PEEP, peak inspiratory pressure are important for assessing the patient's progress.
6 *Built-in monitoring:* SpO_2 and end-tidal CO_2 may be included in the ventilator itself, but a higher number of monitoring functions included in one machine means more disruption when one of them fails and the machine is removed for service. DO_2 and VO_2 are valuable.

See also Hayes B. Ventilators: a current assessment. In Atkinson R. S. and Adams A. P. (eds) *Recent Advances in Anaesthesia and Analgesia – 18.* Churchill Livingstone, London, 1994.

ACCIDENTS ASSOCIATED WITH EQUIPMENT

Accidental disconnection

Constant vigilance is required. Ill-fitting tapers should be discarded. Minor leaks may have serious consequences and disconnection monitors (signalling if 10 cm H_2O is not reached at least every 20 s; and if airway pressure exceeds 50 cm H_2O during IPPV) are required. *See also* Chapter 1.7.

MAINTAINING THE AIRWAY

To maintain a patent airway in an anaesthetized patient it is usually necessary to displace the mandible anteriorly (holding up the jaw) by pressure just superior to the angle of the mandible. Some pressure may be required and both skill and experience are necessary for success. The patient's head is extended to 25 degrees beyond the horizontal, which tends to lift the epiglottis out of the way. If this method fails, a pharyngeal airway is inserted, but this may cause coughing in light anaesthesia. With the head extended, the tongue will sit over the curved shaft of the airway, leaving the end clear in the laryngopharynx. Airway obstruction is usually due to the tongue but the epiglottis may be responsible.

Many airways have been designed but today most anaesthetists use the Guedel pharyngeal airway.[35] Every attempt is made to avoid the use of these in patients with frontal crowns, caps, veneers, or very loose teeth, because a powerful bite will put great pressure (0.25 metric tonne) on these and may dislodge them (*see* Chapter 1.7). Then the use of a rubber or plastic nasopharyngeal airway is appropriate.

Alternative airways

1 Brain laryngeal mask (*see above*).
2 Postpalatal and postglossal variants (rather dissappointing).
3 Tracheal tube.

Laryngoscopes

See Chapter 2.6.

TRACHEAL TUBES AND CONNECTIONS

See Chapter 2.6. These tubes are of rubber or plastic. A red additive/preservative gives the rubber tubes their characteristic colour. The markings indicate: the maker; the inside diameter in millimetres; the outside diameter in millimetres; 'oral' or 'nasal' design (the pilot tube of a nasal tube enters the shaft of the tube much nearer to the connector); single or multiple use; code of the implantation test (IT); the markings of the number of centimetres from the tip.

Transducers: calibration and care

See Chapter 2.2.

Monitors

See Chapter 2.2.

Automated record-keeping

See Chapters 2.2.

Syringe pumps[36]

These are usually electrically driven by mains, battery or both with a motor turning a leadscrew. Alerts are frequently provided for power failure, empty syringe, occlusion of delivery pipe. Battery backup is particularly important in patient transfer situations.

Ideal properties include: reliability, electrical safety, accuracy, ease of use, robustness, ability to use a variety of syringe types and sizes, clear displays and instructions, RS232 or similar interface for computer control.[37]

Applications include control of diabetes, pain relief, total intravenous anaesthesia (TIVA) (*see* Chapter 2.4), cardiovascular support,[38] relaxants and sedation in intensive care.

Equipment for developing situations[39]

Low capital and revenue costs have high priority. Cylinders have relatively little place. Monitoring is primarily clinical, as instrumental monitoring is highly vulnerable, not least to frequent power failures. Syringe drivers have proved too complex.

1 Draw-over anaesthesia (*see* Chapter 2.3) with self-inflating manual ventilation bags. The Ambu E and Laerdal IVA valves play an important part in these systems.
2 Open ether with Schimmelbusch mask (*see* Chapter 2.3).
3 Intravenous techniques: ketamine, propofol, benzodiazepines, opioids.
4 Oxygen concentrators.[40]

5 Low-cost volatile agents: halothane, ether.
6 Simple electric ventilators with battery backup.

CARE AND STERILIZATION OF EQUIPMENT

Disinfection is the killing of non-sporing microorganisms. Sterilization is the killing of all microorganisms including viruses. fungi and their spores, if any.

Methods of sterilization

Heat sterilization

MOIST HEAT

Moisture increases cellular permeability and heat coagulates protein. Boiling (100°C) for 15 min kills bacteria, but spores may escape destruction. Increased pressure makes it possible to produce higher temperature. In the modern autoclave, air is exhausted and replaced by steam at 134°C and 32 psi pressure for $3\frac{1}{2}$ min. To remove moisture, the steam is evacuated and replaced by sterile air. The cycle takes about 10 min. Useful for metal objects and fabrics. This will kill all living organisms provided the material treated is properly wrapped to allow penetration. Deterioration of rubber and plastics is hastened by this method and exposure for 15 min to a temperature of 121°C may be substituted. Sharp instruments become dulled. Low-temperature (73°C) steam sterilization (290 mmHg pressure) takes just over 2 h; if formaldehyde is added spores are also killed: this is a method for materials harmed by steam at higher temperatures.

DRY HEAT

One hour at 160°C. Useful for powders, greases, oils and glass syringes.

Chemical sterilization

Useful for objects which will not withstand heat, e.g. endoscopes. Chemicals kill by coagulation or alkylation of proteins. Non-sporing bacteria, viruses, the tubercle bacillus and spores are resistant to destruction (in ascending order). Chemicals only act on exposed surfaces, some react with metals, some impregnate materials (e g. rubber) and remain as a source of irritation. Rubber and plastics are particularly subject to destruction by strong chemicals.

Formaldehyde
Can be used for endoscopic equipment, catheters, etc. Residual formaldehyde may persist after prolonged airing and may harm the skin or bring tears to the endoscopist's eye.

Ethylene oxide (C_2H_4O)

A colourless gas which is a good bactericidal agent, although very toxic to inhale. It has good penetrability and few materials are harmed. It is effective against all organisms, but is slow (8–12 h). The gas is explosive in excess of 3% in air, and it is necessary to use a 10% mixture with CO_2 at a relative humidity of 30–50%. This is a good method of sterilizing complicated and delicate apparatus (e.g. pump oxygenators, Ruben's valves, plastic tubing, Teflon prostheses, catheters, etc.), although the method is expensive and time-consuming. The accepted method of removing adsorbed ethylene oxide by allowing 7 days' shelf-life is inadequate, and the pulling of six poststerilization vacuums is advised. Even this, however, is not accepted by all authorities. It has also been used for sterilization of artificial ventilators after prolonged use in dirty cases and at least 4 h flushing with air is recommended on completion of the process. It is the preferred method of sterilization of respiratory equipment.

The cylinders containing the mixture are identified by aluminium paint; the shoulder is red and below it is a circular band of yellow paint.

LIQUIDS

Phenol (1–5%): used to clean surfaces of apparatus. Should not be used on equipment which comes into contact with the patient. Does not kill spores.

Iodine (0.5–2% in alcohol): may irritate or burn the skin. Povidone-iodine (Betadine) is less irritant.

Ethyl alcohol 70–80% is more efficient than absolute (100%) alcohol. Isopropyl alcohol, 50–70%, can be used.

Hexachlorophene (pHisoHex; 50–70%): one of the few antiseptics that does not lose its properties in the presence of soap.

Chlorhexidine (Hibitane): 0.1% aqueous solution for 20 min for sterilization of endotracheal tubes and other anaesthetic equipment; 0.5% in 50% ethyl alcohol for skin sterilization (30 s).

Glutaraldehyde (Cidex): Commonly used for endoscopes. Used in 2% solution made alkaline by the addition of 0.3% sodium carbonate. This will kill bacteria in 15 min and spores in 3 h. Users wear gloves, and if the room is not very well ventilated, gas masks.

Hypochlorites (e.g. Milton): used for human immunodeficiency virus (HIV).

Liquid disinfectants must make contact with all the inside area of the immersed tubing which must then be dried in a heated ultrafiltered drying chamber. Improper cold sterilization is potentially hazardous.

Gamma rays (ionizing radiation)

Lethal dose for bacteria is 2.5 Mrad. Usually obtained from a cobalt-60 source. Tubes, catheters, etc. can be sterilized in a transparent plastic envelope.

Ultraviolet light

Has been used to kill organisms by submitting the whole operation area to the light. Patients and staff must be protected from sunburn. All skin must be covered and plain spectacles worn with an eyeshade.

Filtration

Filters are used to prevent contamination by organisms. They will remove all particles down to a diameter of 0.5 μm with a 99.99% efficiency. The filters themselves can be autoclaved. The Millipore filter is commonly used for repeated injections via indwelling epidural catheters. Anaesthetic vapours in the concentrations generally produced in anaesthetic equipment cause a reduction in viability of such organisms as Esherichia coli. A particular concern is hepatitis C.

Tracheal tubes, suction catheters, airways, tubes

The use of presterilized disposable articles is now common. Where this is not possible they may be washed with soap and water and well rinsed. A suitable brush should be used to clear the inside of tubes and airways. They may then be sterilized by boiling, although this tends to soften the rubber tracheal tubes. Corrugated tubing, face masks and reservoir bags can be pasteurized (75°C for 10 min). Portex tubes should be boiled with a stylet in situ so that they retain their curvature. Armoured latex tubes should be handled with care since they may be compressed by Chealte's forceps, when hot. Alternatively, tubes may be soaked in a solution of 0.1% chlorhexidine (Hibitane). They should be stored in dust-free containers.

Another method is to place all suitable equipment in a domestic dishwater in which temperatures of 70°C are reached. A commercially supplied detergent, providing 33 ppm of available chlorine, is used. Although this does not guarantee absolute sterility, the method kills those pathogenic organisms with which anaesthetic equipment is likely to be contaminated, except spores and some viruses.

Laryngoscope blades

These may be boiled or autoclaved, provided they are detachable; stand in 5% phenol for 30 min; formalin oven; or simply wipe with 70% alcohol or 0.1% chlorhexidine in 70% alcohol.

Circle absorbers

These may be sterilized by γ radiation, formaldehyde vapour or ethylene oxide. Alternatively, they should be frequently dismantled, cleaned and disinfected with spirit. Another approach is to prevent entry of organisms by using a filter on the expiratory limb of the circuit.

Ventilators

Proper sterilization is essential. The methods available include: autoclaving; internal irrigation with antiseptics, provided the circuit is watertight; ultrasonic nebulization with alcohol, although this prevents a flammability hazard; ultrasonic nebulization with hydrogen peroxide; use of disposable patient-breathing circuits; use of a filter to prevent entrance of organisms.

Humidifiers

Water-bath humidifiers provide an ideal environment for bacterial growth. Prevented by use of 60°C running temperature for 'pasteurization'. Copper sponges have also been advocated as the metal has an antibacterial effect. Disposable heat and moisture exchangers are very widely used.

Contamination with tubercle bacilli

This may be expected after anaesthesia in the presence of open pulmonary tuberculosis. The tracheal tubes, suction catheters, rebreathing tubing, etc. should be disposable, but if not they may be placed immediately in an antiseptic solution (e.g. 0.1% chlorhexidine for 1 h). They can then be cleaned and scrubbed with soap and water with less danger to personnel. After this they can be sterilized by boiling or autoclaving. Boiling for 3 min will kill tubercle bacilli.

Hepatitis B and C

See Chapter 2.8. The virus is not destroyed by boiling but by pasteurization at 60°C for 10 h. It is killed by autoclaving and γ radiation. Of the chemical disinfectants the best results are obtained with hypochlorite.

Syringes and needles

Plastic, disposable, presterilized syringes and needles are now generally used.

Disposable syringes are made from polystyrene or polypropylene. Plunger grommets are attacked by paraldehyde and some X-ray contrast media. In remote and difficult situations, syringes can be sterilized by boiling for 5 min in distilled water.

Instruments for local blocks

Gamma-ray-sterililized disposable sets are widely used. In remote and difficult circumstances, special packs can be made up for each type of procedure, containing needles, syringes, cotton drapes, swabs and dishes. These, and ampoules of local analgesic solutions, such as lignocaine, amethocaine hydrochloride and bupivacaine (and adrenaline) can be autoclaved once at 160°C for 20 min at 20 psi. Some double-wrapped bupivacaine ampoules have been sterilized by ethylene oxide, others by steam autoclaving.

Tests for sterility

The inclusion of heat-sensitive tape or a Browne's tube in the set is a safeguard. If the appropriate temperature has been reached, there is a change in colour. Indicator tape is more commonly used.

Tests for sterility in mass-produced preparations (e.g. intravenous fluids) are not easy to perform. *Product control* presents problems due to cultural, technical and statistical difficulties. There is no single medium which will allow growth of every organism. Sampling can also result in contamination so that false-positive results are obtained. Samples tested may not subsequently be available for use. *Process control*, by examination of the effect on a challenge organism, offers an alternative approach though with its own problems.

FURTHER READING

Ward C.S. *Anaesthetic Equipment*, 3rd edn. Baillière, London, 1995.

REFERENCES

1 Boyle H. E.G. *Br. Med. J.* 1917, **2,** 653; Hadfield C. F. *Br. J.Anaesth.* 1950, **22,** 107; Hewer C. L. *Anaesthesia* 1967, **22,** 357; Obituary of Boyle *Anaesthesia* 1967, **22,** 710; Watt O.M. *Anaesthesia* 1968, **23,** 103; Bryn T. K. *The Development of Anaesthetic Apparatus.* Blackwell, Oxford, 1975: Hewer C. L. *Anaesthesia* 1977, **32,** 908.
2 Rawstron R. E. and McNiell T. D. *Br. J. Anaesth.* 1962, **34,** 591 & 670.
3 Snowdon S. L. and Head-Rapson H. G. *Anaesthesia* 1991, **45,** 1084.
4 Howell R. S. C. In *Anaesthesia Review – 7.* Kaufman L. (ed.). Churchill Livinstone, Edinburgh, 1990.

5 *Health Technical Memorandum No. 22* (and Supplement). DHSS, London, 1977.
6 Bancroft M. L. et al. *Anesthesiology* 1980, **52,** 504.
7 *Health Equipment Information* 1975, **61,** 38, 75.
8 *Hospital Technical Memorandum* No. 22 (HTM 22, DHSS, 1972); Elton V. *Health and Safety Executive* 1976, **29,** 4.
9 *Checklist for anaesthetic apparatus* – 2. Association of Anaesthetists of Great Britain and Ireland, London 1997.
10 Gupta B. L. and Varshneya A. K. *Br. J. Anaesth.* 1975, **47,** 805.
11 Jones R. M. et al. *Br. J. Anesth.* 1990, **64,** 11.
12 Miller E. D. and Greene N. M. *Anesth. Analg.* 1990, **70,** 1; Jones R.M. et al. *Anesth. Analg.* 1990, **70,** 3.
13 Johnstone R. E. and Smith T. C. *Anesthesiology* 1973, **38,** 192.
14 Parmley J. B. et al. *Anesth. Analg.* 1972, **51,** 888.
15 Newton N. I. and Adams A. P. *Anaesthesia* 1978, **33,** 689.
16 Brain A. I. J. *Br. J. Anaesth.* 1983, **55,** 801.
17 Payne J. *Anaesthesia* 1989, **44,** 865.
18 Calder I. et al. *Anaesthesia* 1990, **45,** 137.
19 Hammond J. E. *Anaesthesia* 1989, **44,** 616.
20 Griffin R. and Hatcher I. S. *Anaesthesia* 1990, **45,** 1039.
21 Freeman R. and Baxendale B. *Anaesthesia* 1990, **45,** 1094.
22 Conacher I. D. *Anaesthesia* 1991, **46,** 164; *see also* Cyna A. M. et al. *Anaesthesia* 1990, **45,** 167.
23 Criswell J. et al. *Anaesthesia* 1990, **45,** 113.
24 Miller D. M. *Br. J. Anaesth.* 1990, **64,** 251.
25 Macfie A. G. *Anaesthesia* 1990, **45,** 145.
26 Lack J. A. *Anaesthesia* 1976, **31,** 259; Lack J. A. *Anaesthesia* 1976, **31,** 576; Lack J. A. and Davies R. J. *Anaesthesia* 1976, **31,** 951, and addendum, 1253.
27 Voss T. J. V. *Anaesth. Intensive Care* 1985, **1,** 98.
28 Bain J. A. and Spoerel W. E. *Can. Anaesth. Soc. J.* 1972, **19,** 426.
29 Radford E. P. *J. Appl. Physiol.* 1955, **7,** 451.
30 Ayre T. P. *Lancet* 1937, **1,** 561; *Curr. Res. Anesth. Analg.* 1937, **16,** 330; *Br. J. Surg.* 1937, **35,** 131 (reprinted in 'Classical File', *Surv. Anesthesiol.* 1967, **11,** 400); *Br. J. Anaesth.* 1956, **28,** 520; *Anaesthesia* 1967, **22,** 359.
31 Rees G. J. *Br. J. Anaesth.* 1960, **32,** 132.
32 Waters R. M. *Curr. Res. Anesth. Analg.* 1926, **5,** 160; *Ann. Surg.* 1936, **38,** 103; *Proc. R. Soc. Med.* 1936, **30,** 11.
33 Holmes C. McK. and Spears G. F. S. *Anaesthesia* 1977, **32,** 846.
34 Fernandez R. et al. *Intensive Care World* 1990, **7,** 32.
35 Guedel A. E. *J. Am Med. Assoc.* 1933, **100,** 1862 (reprinted in 'Classical File', *Surv. Anesthesiol.* 1966, **10,** 515).
36 Stokes D. N. et al. *Anaesthesia* 1991, **45,** 1062.
37 Tackley R.M. et al. *Br. J. Anaesth.* 1989, **62,** 46.
38 Colvin J. R. and Kenny G. N. C. *Anaesthesia* 1989, **44,** 37.
39 Nordberg E. M. *Br. Med. J.* 1984, **289,** 92.
40 Fenton P. M. *Anaesthesia* 1989, **44,** 498.

Monitoring[1]

It is a capital mistake to theorize before one has facts
(Memoirs of Sherlock Holmes)

There has been a little progress towards an international consensus in this field.[2] There are five phases to the monitoring process.

1 Collect the monitor readings (data).
2 Analyse the data.
3 Decide if action needs to be taken or not.
4 Decide on course of action.
5 Compare results with others.[3]

GENERAL PRINCIPLES

Clinical monitoring

The various senses of the attending doctor are the primary equipment for clinical measurement. The anaesthetist should also develop a sixth sense, a subconscious mental computation of observations, time and experience, which warns of impending events and prompts action to meet the needs of the patient.

Simple observations which can be made and their relevance include the following.

1 Colour of skin and blood – oxygenation.
2 Temperature of skin (especially of extremities) – body temperature, circulatory status, fluid balance, acid–base status.
3 Pulse character and rate – cardiac performance and arterial pressure.
4 State of peripheral circulation – circulatory status.
5 Degree of filling of jugular veins – circulating volume.
6 Urine flow (> 0.5 ml/kg/h) – circulatory status, fluid balance.
7 Respiratory movement – adequacy of lung ventilation.
8 Movement of anaesthetic 'bag' – adequacy of lung ventilation, and depth of anaesthesia.

9 Perspiration, lachrymation, movement of head with respiration – depth of anaesthesia.
10 Muscle tone and movement – relaxation; and depth of anaesthesia.
11 Pupils – depth of anaesthesia, (in crisis situations; the state of cerebral circulation).
12 Clotting time of blood (collected in glass test tube and kept warm in the hand while timing clotting).

It is also useful to listen to the surgeon's comments, which may (or may not) provide additional information on the state of relaxation, depth of anaesthesia.

Basic instrumental monitoring of patient

1 Circulation: non-invasive blood pressure (BP), electrocardiogram (ECG), pulse oximetry.
2 Respiration: with intermittent positive-pressure ventilation (IPPV), airway pressure, ventilatory volume, capnography, disconnection alarms, volatile agent monitoring, pulse oximetry.[4]
3 Metabolic status: capnography, blood glucose, acid–base balance.
4 Neuromuscular transmission: nerve stimulators when relaxants are used.

Basic instrumental monitoring of anaesthetic machine

1 Oxygen failure warning (alarms, gas analysers).
2 Airway pressure monitoring.
3 Ventilator failure alarms.

Additional instrumental monitoring

In many major surgical operations, central venous pressure (CVP), arterial lines and pulmonary arterial catheterization may be required.

1 Urine output and body temperature.
2 Transthoracic impedance apnoea alarms, intra-arterial blood pressure, intermittent or continuous blood gas analysis, transcutaneous and trans-conjunctival CO_2.[5]
3 Arterial blood gases and special blood tests, e.g. blood glucose, electrolytes, coagulation, hormone assays.
4 Non-invasive cardiac output, cerebral electrical and metabolic activity and oxygenation, bispectral index, state of awareness, etc.
5 In-theatre coagulation monitoring.

Noninvasive and minimally invasive monitoring are to be preferred if they give as accurate or as useful information as the invasive methods.

Accurate detailed recording is also fundamental. Pen and paper are the most reliable tools for anaesthetic records. Although automated recording is available (*see also* Chapter 1.7) automated records are not regarded as infallible. The anaesthetist should initialize all monitoring errors on any automated record sheet.

When monitors go wrong, and when monitors give inaccurate readings

A high index of suspicion should be directed to accuracy of monitors. This requires constant comparison with clinical observation – always being able to see and feel the patient, and facilities for checking the performance of each monitor. Monitors do get tired by the end of the day; calibration slips, zeroes drift. They do not always provide the unsleeping vigilance we would like. Many problems in instrumental monitoring are at the patient interface. For this reason, repeated clinical examination is still of primary importance. Pulse oximeter probes slip, cracks and blockages occur in gas sampling tubes etc.

Limitations of monitors

It is important to know the limitations of electronic surveillance monitoring, occasionally clinical signs and subjective feelings are better, e.g. visual observation of the movements of a 2 l. bag on a breathing system is a better guide to tidal volume than a capnograph trace. Electronic monitoring may not necessarily detect an abnormality until relatively late when the initial compensation by the body in the face of overwhelming physiological insult is eventually lost. Examples include: postoperative haemmorhage, where vascular parameters may be maintained up to the final collapse, but the feel of the peripheral pulse, the colour of the patient's skin and the nature of the patient's pain give much earlier warning; also post-thyroidectomy respiratory obstruction due to haemorrhage in the deep tissues of the neck in which respiratory monitoring may remain normal up to the point of collapse and cyanosis, but the patient's subjective sensation of being 'unable to breathe properly' gives much better advance warning.

Facial expression has been used as guide to respiratory failure and weaning from ventilators.

Like an aeroplane pilot, the anaesthetist must critically appraise the information from the monitors and act accordingly.

Safety in monitoring equipment

See Chapters 1.7 and 2.1.

CARDIOVASCULAR AND RESPIRATORY MONITORING

Pulse oximetry (SpO₂)

The measurement of oxygen saturation of the arterial blood.[7] The lobe of the ear, bridge of nose, or finger is placed between a two-wavelength light source and a detector. Only pulsating signals are analysed, so skin pigmentation or venous saturation is ignored.[8] Measurement of FIO_2/SpO_2 ratios is diagnostic of changes of status and of some medical conditions, e.g. pulmonary fibrosis, and is useful in the preoperative and postoperative phases.[9] Changes of cerebral blood flow have been predicted by use of the conjunctival oxygen tension/arterial oxygen tension index.[10]

Limitations of pulse oximetry[11]

The computed haemoglobin saturation can be confused by the following.

1 Presence of methaemoglobin, sulphaemoglobin or carboxyhaemoglobin in the blood.[12]
2 Methaemoglobin and sulphaemoglobin make the apparent saturation tend to 85%.
3 Carboxyhaemoglobin is seen as oxyhaemoglobin. (*see* Adams A. P. in *Recent Advances in Anaesthesia and Analgesia 17*. Atkinson R.S and Adams A. P. (eds), Churchill Livingstone, Edinburgh, 1991).
4 Bilirubin causes under-reading.
5 Haemoglobin F in neonates and preterm infants (SpO₂ of 92% at PaO₂ of 13 kPa).[13]
6 Time-lag of indicated SpO₂ on sudden desaturation due to hypoxic hypoxia.[14] Response time 5–20 s.
7 Polycythaemia of cyanotic congenital cardiac disease.[15]
8 Weak arterial pulsation and poor peripheral perfusion.[16]
9 Non-pulsatile arterial flow.
10 Excessive movement or diathermy.
11 Dyes in the blood, e.g. methylene blue.
12 Nail varnish (weak signal).
13 Digit too large for the sensor, causing constriction.
14 Nasal pulse oximetry reads nearly 5% higher than digital.[17]
15 Strong ambient light.[18]
16 Electronic failures.[19]

They are non-invasive, reliable and expensive. They may be inadequate in severe vasoconstriction. Readings are indicated as analogue or digital displays. Their detection of hypoxic events is not instantaneous.[20] Different models use different algorithms to calibrate the saturation.[16] There are problems of calibration at the lower end of the scale.

Arterial pressure[21]

In spite of the advent of more sophisticated physiological monitoring possibilities, this continues to hold pride of place in cardiovascular monitoring for anaesthesia and intensive care. The systolic pressure is the easiest to measure, and is necessary for calculation of the MAP. The mean arterial pressure (MAP) is important for estimating organ perfusion, especially renal. The diastolic pressure is useful for estimating coronary flow.

The compression cuff

Too narrow a cuff – low readings; too wide – high readings. The cuff should cover approximately two-thirds of the length of the upper arm or 20% greater than the diameter of the arm. It should not be too near the flexed elbow; it may move the forearm down into an abdominal operation site. The American Heart Association recommends a 12–14-cm rubber bag, long enough to encircle half the arm, centred over the brachial artery. The cloth cover should be made of non-extensible material so that pressure is exerted uniformly. Recommended cuff widths are: neonate 2.5 cm; 1–4 years 6.0 cm; 4–8 years 9.0 cm; adult 12–14 cm (15 cm for the adult leg). A conventional cuff overestimates arterial pressure on a fat or muscular arm, and underestimates it on a thin arm or on the arm of a child.

Automatic oscillotonometer

A cuff is inflated automatically at preset intervals, to above the previous systolic pressure. The time intervals may be set to 1 min at times of potential instability, e.g soon after induction of anaesthesia; or 2–5 min at more stable times. Oscillations of pressure due to emerging arterial pulsations beneath the cuff (or a second 'sensing' cuff) as the cuff pressure is steadily reduced below the systolic and then diastolic figures are detected by a transducer in the monitor, analysed, and presented as systolic, diastolic and a computed mean arterial pressure. The electronics include artefact rejection.

The automated oscillotonometer is accurate in children and adults.

Monitors using ultrasonic detectors (2–10 MHz) placed over the brachial artery to detect arterial pulsation in a similar way to the transducers above, require protection from movement artefact. Finger arterial pressure monitors (Finapres)[22] indicate non-invasive beat-to-beat pressure. This compares well with intra-arterial monitoring.[23]

Low alarm limits are often set at 2/3 of the baseline values to give warning for action before the pressure reaches the limit of half the baseline value. There are many situations where the limit will be set nearer to the baseline value, e.g. in cardiac and arterial disease. High limits are often set at 4/3 of the baseline values.

Direct intra-arterial methods *(see Chapter 1.2)*

Indications:

1 Expected large blood or fluid loss.
2 Expected highly unstable arterial pressure, e.g. operations on the arterial tree.
3 Non-pulsatile arterial flow (e.g. cardiopulmonary bypass).
4 Severe or prolonged induced hypotension.
5 Arterial blood sampling.

Radial artery cannulation is a low-risk, high-benefit method of patient monitoring. The risk of ischaemic complications (though not of partial or complete occlusion of the artery) is very slight.[24]

A 20–23 G Teflon cannula (parallel sided in preference to tapered) is inserted into an artery and connected via a column of fluid to a transducer. Radial arterial puncture can be painful.[25]

The dorsalis pedis artery is also a convenient site giving similar pressures to the aorta.[26]

Other arteries have been used. The transducer is usually a semi-conductor.

Arterial occlusion can be diagnosed by thermography.[27] Arterial occlusion does not often cause distal ischaemia, because of other collateral arteries, e.g. ulnar. Allen's test may be used to detect adequate ulnar artery collateral circulation. The hand is exsanguinated by the patient making a fist actively (or passively when unconscious) while the radial artery is occluded and the palmar flush of blood from the ulnar artery observed on opening the hand.

A continuous flush system delivers heparinized saline (1 unit/ml) at about 3 ml/h.[28]

The heart beat can also be monitored by the use of a precordial stethoscope, a method particularly suited to use in infants. In children and adults undergoing major surgery an oesophageal stethoscope is helpful. Also useful for diagnosis of air embolus during operation.

Cardiac output[29]

Swan–Ganz catheters (pulmonary artery catheters)[30]

These are balloon-tipped, flow-directed flexible pulmonary artery catheters, originally used for measuring pulmonary capillary wedge pressure. Swan and Ganz modified the design of the earlier Lategola balloon-tipped catheter[31] enabling pulmonary artery catheters to be used clinically. Special pulmonary artery catheters are used to measure SvO_2 fiberoptically.

For cardiac output, ice-cold saline is injected into the pulmonary artery proximal to the thermistor at the tip of the Swan–Ganz catheter. Its thermo-dilution is proportional to the pulmonary blood flow and, therefore, to the cardiac output.[32] A microprocessor calculates the actual readings and presents the data. Pulmonary artery (PA) wedge pressure (PAWP; a close index of left atrial pressure) is also recorded directly. Right ventricular ejection fraction can also be measured.

Computer-aided analysis of parameters and trends from a Swan–Ganz catheter is used for 'intelligent' diagnosis-making, and control of therapeutic interventions. Continuous cardiac output and mixed venous saturation monitoring is now also available. (*See* Munro H.M. et al. *Clin. Intensive Care* 1994, **5**, 52; Hogue C.W. Jnr. et al. *J. Cardiothor. Vasc. Anesth.* 1994, **8**, 631.)

INDICATIONS

Low cardiac output; pulmonary oedema; septic shock; and to sample mixed venous blood.

RELIABILITY

Certain criteria are used to ensure accuracy: The mean PAWP should be less than the mean PA pressure, and infusate should flow freely through the catheter, indicating that the catheter tip is free; the wedge tracing should have atrial waveform; the wedge PO_2 should be greater than the non-wedge PO_2. Room-temperature fluid can be as accurate as iced infusate. Three measurements per determination are better than one, and a minimum of 15% difference between successive measurements suggests a real change of cardiac output.[33]

PULMONARY ARTERIAL WEDGE PRESSURE

Normal pressure 5–10 mmHg. After cardiac surgery and severe myocardial infarction fluid loading up to wedge pressures of 10–30 mmHg may occasionally be required. *See* Cardiac output above.

ERRORS IN MEASUREMENTS

Errors are worst in spontaneously breathing patients where the instantaneous readings, especially those used in automated estimations, do not reflect accurately the waveforms throughout the respiratory cycle.[34] The wedge pressure is normally measured in end-expiration. Pulmonary artery catheters are inserted via standard central venous approaches (including arm veins). The supraclavicular route has the lowest incidence of misdirection. Progress of the catheter tip is monitored by X-ray control or by observation of the pressures being measured at the tip. Most pass into the right lower lobe artery. Measurements should be made in zone 3 for best accuracy.

COMPLICATIONS[35]

These include dysrhythmias, damage to the lung, infection, thromboembolism, obstruction of venous return during cardiopulmonary bypass, balloon rupture, catheter migration and knotting of the catheter.

Some of these may be prevented by deflating the balloon of the indwelling catheter while not being used for measurements. The balloon blocks 5–15% of the lung blood vessels.

Other methods of estimating cardiac output

An alternative to pulmonary artery catheterization is a system,[62] which uses a combination of central venous and arterial thermodilution measurement, estimating cardiac output, cardiac function index, intrathoracic blood volume[63] and extravascular lung water.

Doppler ultrasound cardiac output estimation records velocity flow and cross-sectional area of aorta for single beats, (multiplied by pulse rate for output) and is reasonably accurate,[36] but not always during acute blood loss.[37] Aortovelography gives reasonable sequential estimates of changes in output.[38] Thoracic impedance techniques have proved difficult in children.[39]

Combined ultrasound and Doppler probes give flow in other vessels, e.g. the umbilical artery in the fetus.[40]

Echocardiography gives an important measure of left ventricular ejection fraction, wall motion abnormalities and gradients across valves. Transoesophageal echocardiography is a clinically useful tool,[41] giving information on wall motion abnormalities and ventricular function, but can cause damage.[42]

Radio-imaging with a γ-camera after intravenous injection of 99m technetium[43] gives the left ventricular ejection fraction, either on a first-pass study or gated fraction studies. The computer multiplies this by the heart rate to give the cardiac output. This technique also gives information on the size, localization and reversibility of cardiac infarcts. Radio-thallium is also used.

The electrocardiogram

The ECG is an excellent non-invasive monitor of cardiac rhythm and especially of unexpected cardiac arrest or rate changes. For routine monitoring (not the 12-lead diagnostic trace), three electrodes are placed on the chest, as near to the heart as convenient. This increases the signal/noise ratio. Since 75% of ischaemic ECG patterns are best detected from the V5 position, the electrodes should be placed on the positions CM_5 if possible:

1 left clavicle;
2 manubrium;
3 fifth intercostal space, anterior axillary line.

It does not afford a measure of the efficiency of myocardial contraction or of cardiac output; in fact normal electrical activity may occur when there is no cardiac output. If the electrodes are placed on the patient's back ST depression may be seen in the normal heart.

The ECG signal can be processed to provide information on the beat-to-beat (R–R) interval. Variability in R–R intervals has been shown to be a good indicator of the balance between sympathetic and parasympathetic tone, and analysis of heart rate variability (HRV) shows promise as a measure of depth of anaesthesia. (*See* Pomfrett C. J. D. In *Recent Advances in Anaesthesia and Analgesia – 19*. Adams A. P. and Cashman J. N. (eds). Churchill Livingstone, Edinburgh, 1995.)

Artefacts

The ECG is liable to artefacts which may be caused by disconnection of an electrode, superimposition of potential from another person in contact with the patient, improper earthing of apparatus, etc. It is possible for interference to take the form of a sine wave giving rise to the appearance of ventricular tachycardia. Bizarre complexes occur, e.g. ST depression and widening of the QRS complex may be due to battery exhaustion.

Central venous pressure

Venous tone

More than half the total blood volume is accommodated in the systemic venous system, only about 15% in the arterial system. Alterations in venous tone play a large part in the regulation of the haemodynamics of the circulatory system.

The term central venous pressure refers to the pressure in the right atrium or the intrathoracic inferior or superior venae cavae. For technique of insertion *see* Intravascular techniques, Chapter 1.2.

Readings

The zero must be a chosen reference level, i.e. the mid-axillary line or the manubriosternal angle. Normal CVP may be taken as 3–10 cmH$_2$O (Table 2.2.1). High values may indicate right ventricular failure, pulmonary embolism, tamponade, or misplacement of the catheter tip into the right ventricle or pulmonary artery.

Complications

These include: thrombophlebitis, infection, septicaemia; pneumothorax; haemothorax; hydrothorax; brachial plexus injury; air embolus; pericardial effusion; lymph leakage; catheter breakage; arrythmias.

Table 2.2.1 Interpretation of CVP.

When the patient is	Usual CVP is: (cm H$_2$O)	When the patient has:	Usual CVP is: (cm H$_2$O)
Supine	+3 to +10	IPPV with PEEP	+5 to +15
Head down	+5 to +10	Congestive cardiac	
On IPPV	+5 to +10	failure	+5 to +10
Head up	−10 to −5	Pulmonary embolism	+5 to +20
Hypovolaemic	−5 to 0	Cardiac tamponade	+5 to +20
In ARDS	+5 to +20		

Central venous pressure measurements are not a good guide to daily fluid requirements and should not be used for this purpose. A patient can easily be waterlogged or dehydrated in the presence of a normal CVP. The reliability of right atrial pressure monitoring to assess left ventricular preload in critically ill septic patients has been questioned.[44]

Measurement of blood loss

Gravimetric method

The simplest and most commonly employed method. Blood loss is estimated by measurement of the gain in weight of swabs and towels, together with measurement of the contents of suction bottles; 1 ml of blood weighs 1 g. Weighing of swabs is said to underestimate blood loss by 25%.

Colorimetric method

Swabs and towels are mixed thoroughly with a large known volume of fluid, which is then estimated colorimetrically. Errors may occur due to incomplete extraction or contamination with bile. The patient's haemoglobin must be known. One common system uses the following formula:

$$\text{Blood loss (ml)} = \frac{\text{Colorimeter reading} \times \text{volume of solution (ml)}}{200 \times \text{patient's Hb (g\%)}}$$

In operations involving complex exchanges of blood (e.g. extracorporeal circulation), it may be useful to weigh the whole patient before and after operation.

Analysis of gas mixtures[45]

Oxygen

PARAMAGNETIC ANALYSERS

Gases are classed as paramagnetic or diamagnetic according to their behaviour in a magnetic field. The former seek the area of strongest, the latter of weakest flux. Of the gases of interest to the anaesthetist only O_2, NO and NO_2 are paramagnetic, others are weakly diamagnetic. This principle is used in commercial apparatus for analysis of oxygen concentrations in a gas mixture.

Theatre monitor O_2 analysers are commonly of the polarographic or the microfuel cell type. These cells last about a year and are easily replaced.

For evaluation of O_2 analysers *see* reference.[46]

Carbon dioxide (capnography or capnometry)[47]

THE INFRA-RED ANALYSER

This type is commonly found in theatre monitors. Gases whose molecules contain two dissimilar atoms or more than two atoms absorb radiation in the infra-red region of the spectrum.

CAPNOGRAPHY[48]

Continuous recording of CO_2 in anaesthetic systems and in intensive care. A continuous sample of respired gas is withdrawn from as near to the trachea as possible, and the CO_2 content displayed on a continuous recorder. Sensors placed directly in the breathing system are also available. The highest CO_2 content is found at the end of expiration, and is called the end-tidal CO_2 ($ETCO_2$). In spite of theoretical interference by anaesthetic agents, especially N_2O, and the fact that $ETCO_2$ is not exactly the same as $PaCO_2$, the measurement is extremely useful. A colorimetric device is available and has been used to identify succesful tracheal intubation.[49] (*See also* O'Flaherty D. In *Principles and Practice Series*. Hahn C. E. W and Adamc A. P. (eds). BMJ Publishing Group, London, 1994.)

Analysis of capnogram
There are three areas of particular interest:

1 The end-tidal value:
   (a) intubation of oesophagus, (or trachea);
   (b) adequacy of ventilation;
   (c) emboli (because the embolized area does not exchange CO_2 into alveolar gas);
   (d) sudden changes in cardiac output.
   (e) malignant hyperpyrexia.
2 The shape of the expired capnogram:
   (a) inspiratory effort;
   (b) V/Q maldistribution.
3 Inspired portion:
   (a) rebreathing, deliberate or accidental;
   (b) CO_2 rotameter on.

Capnography is useful because:

1 careful control of CO_2 levels is important in most types of surgery;
2 it warns of airway, intubation and ventilation errors;
3 it monitors special dangers such as air embolism, shock, etc.;
4 it warns of inspired CO_2 rising (e.g. rebreathing);
5 the shape of the capnogram may show diaphragmatic inspiratory effort (early relaxant failure) as a 'dip' at the end of expiration, or V/Q maldistribution as a rising expiratory plateau; and
6 the efficiency of the closed system can be continuously monitored.

It can be monitored during high frequency positive pressure ventilation (HFPPV).[50]

Volatile anaesthetic agents

METHODS

1 Absorption of infrared radiation (often found in theatre monitors).
2 Mass spectrometry.
3 Absorption of ultraviolet radiation.
4 Piezo-electric crystal.
5 Absorption into silicone rubber (e.g. halothane).
6 Raman spectrometry.

Simultaneous analysis

Simultaneous analysis of various gases from several theatres can be carried out using the following:

THE MASS SPECTROMETER

Molecules are ionized, accelerated by an electric field and deflected by a magnetic field. The angle of deflexion is related to molecular weight. Carbon dioxide and N_2O have the same molecular weight, as do CO and nitrogen, but special electronic circuits can differentiate these gases. Response time < 100 ms. One instrument can serve several operating rooms; it also has applications in intensive care.

GAS CHROMATOGRAPHY

Separation of components by means of a partition column. It accepts a discrete gas sample and takes several minutes to analyse it, but is extremely sensitive, e.g. for measurement of anaesthetic pollution.

The term is a contraction for gas/liquid chromatography and is not concerned with 'colour', the word 'chromatography' being handed down from an older technique of liquid–liquid separation in which the components were identified by colour.

Respiration

Tidal volume and minute volume

INFERENTIAL METERS

Volume is inferred from the number of revolutions of a vane rotated by the gas stream. Now commercially available as small and light apparatus, which may be connected directly to a face piece or catheter mount.

1 Wright anemometer: gas passes through 10 tangential slots in a cylindrical stator ring to turn a flat two-bladded rotor. A recent development displays gas volumes on a calibrated meter and is not affected by water condensation. The Wright anemometer is a simple, robust, lightweight, accurate and cheap device, ideally suited for use in the intensive care ward. Its accuracy is slightly dependent on the wave form of the gases passing through it. There are various similar instruments.

2 *The pneumotachograph:* continuously measures gas flow by measuring pressure drop across a resistor. It is compact and forms part of modern ventilator circuits.

3 *Thoracic impedance plethysmography:* the electrical impedance of the chest changes during respiration and can be used to compute volume changes.

4 *Infant apnoea mats.*

Blood-gas measurements[51]

Arterial oxygen tension

THE OXYGEN ELECTRODE

This consists of a platinum cathode and a silver anode in a potassium hydroxide solution. Platinum gives up electrons to O_2 and the resulting voltage change can be measured and expressed in terms of O_2 tension. Platinum receives a deposition of protein when used in biological fluids, so the electrode system must be isolated from the blood sample by a thin gas-permeable membrane. The Clark electrode[52] is the basis of the modern O_2 electrode, although modifications have been produced.

BLOOD SAMPLES

These must be drawn from an artery into a syringe whose dead space has been filled with heparin. The O_2 consumption of whole blood at sufficient to cause a fall in PO_2 of about 0.4 kPa/min. Samples should therefore be analysed at once, or kept cool to reduce O_2 consumption. Oxygen may also diffuse into the substance of the plastic syringe. The loss is greater when PaO_2 is high. Use of glass syringes obviates this source of error. Normal values may be as low as 10 kPa (70 mmHg) in the over-70 age group, compared with 13.5 kPa (100 mmHg) in younger age groups.

Venous samples show satisfactory correlation with arterial ones for pH, bicarbonate, and PCO_2 (1 kPa higher), but not for PO_2.

Transcutaneous oxygen electrodes[53]

In the Clark-type electrode, the O_2 diffuses through the skin and is measured by a polarographic technique. Information concerning the blood flow in a flap of skin or in the skin after reconstructive vascular surgery, can also be obtained. (*See also* Tremper K. K. Can. *Anaesth. Soc. J*. 1984, **31,** 664.)

These give accurate and continuous measurement provided that: the patient is not cold or vasoconstricted; the skin under the electrode is not degenerating as a result of prolonged electrode placement; and drift problems have been eliminated from the system.

The transcutaneous (tC) PO_2 is normally 1–3 kPa lower than PaO_2.

Transcutaneous carbon dioxide monitoring[54]

A glass electrode with special membrane is closely applied to the skin. Voltage output is logarithmically related to the PCO_2. Response time is slow. The electrode is heated to 44°C. Over time this may cause skin damage so regular moving of the probe is advisable. The $tCPCO_2$ reads 0.5 kPa higher than the $PaCO_2$.

Mixed venous oxygen content

This is an index of adequate cardiac output and tissue perfusion. Normal value is 14 ml/100 ml blood. Central venous oxygen content correlates well with mixed venous oxygen content.

Pulse oximetry

See above.

Arterial carbon dioxide measurement

1 The electrode consists of a pH electrode surrounded by a bicarbonate solution. The whole is contained in a membrane permeable to PCO_2, which diffuses in from the blood sample, altering the pH of the bicarbonate solution. Modern machines consist of PO_2, PCO_2 and pH electrodes and are fully automated in their handling of the blood sample and calibration, and only need 0.1 ml of blood.
2 End-expired gas analysis gives a useful non-invasive indication of $PaCO_2$, using the lung as a tonometer.

NEUROMUSCULAR AND NEUROLOGICAL MONITORING

Neuromuscular monitoring

(*See* also Ch. 2.5.)

Neuromuscular monitors should deliver a 50 Ma supramaximal stimulus. Stimulating and recording electrodes are positioned over the ulnar nerve at or above the wrist. The median nerve has been used. For analysis of the response, finger movement can be assessed manually, recording electrodes positioned over the small muscles of the hand, or a force-transducer applied to the thumb.

Neuronal monitoring

Sensory-evoked potentials (SEPs) are used for testing neurone integrity during spinal, cardiac and carotid surgery, and for unplanned awareness.[55] Transcutaneous SEPs require huge amplification of the signal and interference is always a problem.[56] *See also* Chapter 2.8.

Electromyography

See also Chapter 2.5.

The electroencephalogram[57]

The purpose of the electroencephalogram (EEG) in the intensive therapy unit (ITU) and during operations is as follows.

1 To assess sedation and awareness.[55] Sedation (e.g. propofol, opioids), slows the frequency progressively through the range 8 Hz (light) to 0.1 Hz (deep). Awareness is indicated by fast α activity. Pain may produce more β activity. Barbiturates in moderate doses give large slow waves, then burst suppression. Low-dose isoflurane shows 10–12 Hz, reduction to δ waves and finally burst suppression with increasing concentration.
2 To monitor epileptic activity, and to control antiepileptic drug infusions, especially in paralysed patients.
3 To monitor changes in conscious level.

Technique

The scalp electrodes should have low impedance, (5 Kohms) involving shaving, cleaning and abrasion. Positioning is on the 10–20 system, with a ground electrode on the forehead or mastoid process. A bandwidth of 0.5–30 Hz, eliminating mains interference, is reasonable for theatre and ITU

Types of wave

1 *Delta waves:* 0.3–3.5 Hz; amplitude 100 μV. Occur in infants and sleeping adults, and anaesthesia.

2 *Theta waves:* 4–7 Hz, 10 μV.

3 *Alpha waves:* 8–13 Hz, 20 μV in infants, 75 in children, 50 in adults. Augmented by closing eyes or mental repose. Reduced by visual and mental activity. A sign of awareness.

4 *Beta waves:* 14–25 Hz, 20 μV. May indicate pain.

5 *Gamma waves:* 26 Hz or more. 10 μV. Rare.

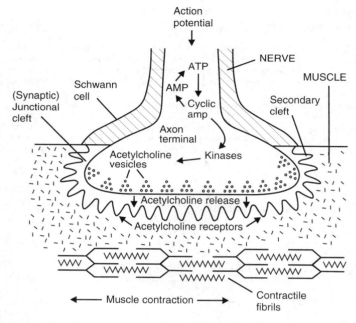

Figure 2.2.1 Diagram of neuromuscular junction

use, but cardiac and skeletal activity may still intrude. Artefacts may occur due to movement of the patient or to superimposition of an electrocardiogram if an electrode is placed directly over an artery.

Changes in the electroencephalogram

1 *Hypoxia.* Causes slowing of the frequency of the waves. After about 20 s of complete anoxia the recording becomes a straight line, e.g. after cardiac arrest. Lesser degrees of hypoxia may not affect the tracing until a level of 40% arterial O_2 saturation is reached.
2 *Hypotension.* A rapid fall of blood pressure is associated with slow high-amplitude waves or temporary cessation.
3 *Circulatory arrest.* Activity ceases. The recording can be used as a measure of cerebral circulation during cardiac massage. After cardiac arrest, the presence of α rhythm carries a good prognosis, while periods of wave suppression indicate a bad prognosis.
4 *Hypothermia.* Below 35–31°C some decrease in amplitude and frequency occurs. At 20°C there may be little activity.

The cerebral function monitor and cerebral function analysing monitor

The cerebral function monitor (CFM) and cerebral function analysing monitor (CFAM) have the advantage that the display is meaningful to non-neuroelectrophysiologists. They have been used to monitor depth of anaesthesia and sedation, cerebral ischaemia during cardiopulmonary bypass, coma levels in the ITU.

An amplitude value is computed from the integrated area under an assigned classical wave (α, β, δ, θ). The mean amplitude and the 10th and 90th centiles are displayed. The normal amplitude is between 5 and 15 μV. A fall below 5 μV can indicate a fall of cerebral perfusion, with corresponding fall of cerebral function. Epileptiform fits are also displayed as spikes of amplitude above 15 μV. The CFM can be used to titrate the dose of fentanyl for sedation, aiming for just above 5 μV.[58]

Magnetic resonance imaging[59, 60]

See Chapter 4.1.

OTHER MONITORING

Temperature[61]

1 *The standard mercury-in-glass clinical thermometer*. In a polythene sleeve to prevent cross-infection.
2 *Dial thermometers*. Simple instruments: a flat bimetallic spiral spring which winds or unwinds as temperature changes; the pressure gauge (Bourdon gauge) – a hollow ribbon of metal which winds or unwinds as temperature changes produce pressure changes within the coil.
3 *Thermocouple*. A circuit of two dissimilar metals produces an e.m.f. when the two junctions are at different temperatures. The e.m.f. is measured and calibrated according to temperature. The apparatus can be made small and it has a rapid response.
4 *Platinum resistance thermometry*. The resistance of a metal varies according to temperature, and the former is measured by means of a Wheatstone bridge. A platinum coil can be mounted within the lumen of a hypodermic needle for insertion in body tissues.
5 *Thermistor* (*thermally* sensitive *resistor*). A small bead of semi-conductor material can be sealed into hypodermic needles and PA catheters. Semi-conductors have negative coefficients of resistance, which can be measured using a Wheatstone bridge.
6 *Skin thermometers*. Difficulties may arise due to poor contact with the skin and because skin temperature itself falls as heat passes to the thermometer: (a) the magnetic thermometer – temperature affects its field strength; (b) the

radiometer. Infra-red rays, which are emitted by all substances at temperatures above absolute zero, are focused on a thermistor device.

The temperature can be taken from the mouth, rectum, skin, oesophagus or tympanic membrane. For evaluation of body temperature *see* Imrie M. M. and Hall G. M. *Br. J. Anaesth.* 1990, **64**, 346.

Monitoring during transfer of patients

Between hospitals and within hospital. This must reflect the severity of the patient's condition, and is as comprehensive as necessary. The patients are stabilized before transfer. Specially designed trolleys are available, and also framed units which fit on standard beds, to display parameters and prevent damage to expensive equipment. Battery power is necessary but batteries may fail after an hour. Special problems exist in helicopters due to vibration and noise, and even the most elementary measurements may be impossible. With rail and road transfers, a smooth trip is better than a fast trip.

FURTHER READING

Scurr C. S, Feldman S. A. and Soni N. (eds.) *Scientific Foundations of Anaesthesia*, 4th edn. Heinemann, Oxford, 1990.

REFERENCES

1 Atkinson R. S. and Adams A. P (eds). *Recent Advances in Anaesthesia and Analgesia* – 16. Churchill Livingstone, Edinburgh, 1989.
2 Winter A. and Spence A. A. *Br. J. Anaesth. 1990,* **64**, 263.
3 Shoemaker W. C. et al. *Crit. Care Med.* 1989, **17**, 1277.
4 Payne J. P. and Severinghaus J. W. (eds) *Pulse Oximetry*. Springer-Verlag, Berlin, 1986; Taylor M. B. and Whitman J. G. *Anaesthesia* 1986, **41**, 943.
5 Abraham E. et al. *Crit. Care Med.* 1986, **14**, 138.
6 Tremper K. K. and Barker S. J. *Anesthesiology* 1989, **70**, 98.
7 Adams A. P. In Atkinson R. S. and Adams A. P. (eds) *Recent Advances in Anaesthesia and Analgesia* – 16. Churchill Livingstone, Edinburgh, 1989; Yelderman N. and New W. *Anesthesiology* 1983, **59**, 349; Payne J. P. and Severinghaus J. W. (ed.) *Pulse Oximetry*. Springer-Verlag, Berlin, 1986; Taylor M. B. and Whitman J. G. *Anaesthesia* 1986, **41**, 943.
8 Striebel H. W. and Kretz F. J. *Anaesthesist* 1989, **38**, 649.
9 McKenzie A. J. *Anaesth. Intensive Care* 1989, **17**, 412.
10 Rutherford W. F, Panacek E. A. *Crit. Care Med.* 1989, **17**, 1328.
11 Kidd J. F. and Vickers M. D. *Br. J. Anaesth.* 1989, **62**, 355.
12 Bardoczky G. I. et al. *Acta Anaesth. Scand.* 1990, **34**,162.

13 Southall D. P. et al. *Arch. Dis. Child.* 1987, **62**, 882; Wasunna A. and Whitelaw A. G. L. *ibid*, p. 957.
14 Severinghaus J. W. and Naifeh K. H. *Anesthesiology* 1987, **67**, 551.
15 Ridley S. A. *Anaesthesia* 1988, **43**, 136.
16 Clayton D. G. et al. *Anaesthesia*, 1991, **46**, 3.
17 Rosenberg J. and Pederson M. H. *Anaesthesia* 1991, **45**, 1070.
18 Jobes D. R. and Nicolson S. C. *Anesth. Analg.* 1988, **67**, 186.
19 Duncan F. B. *Anaesthesia*, 1990, **45**, 1093.
20 Verhoeff F. and Sykes M. K. *Anaesthesia* 1990, **45**, 103.
21 O'Brien E. T. and O'Malley K. *Br. Med. J.* 1979, **2**, 851, 970, 1048, 1124.
22 Dorlas J. C. et al. *Anesthesiology* 1985, **62**, 342.
23 Kermode J.L. et al. *Anaesth. Intensive Care* 1989, **17**, 470.
24 Slogoff S. et al. *Anesthesiology* 1983, **59**, 42.
25 Clark G. S. et al. *Anaesthesia* 1982, **37**, 78.
26 Cole P., Rushman G. B. and Simpson P. *Anaesthesia* 1976, **31**, 69.
27 Evans P. J. D. et al. *Anaesth. Intensive Care* 1977, **5**, 231.
28 Morray J. and Todd S. *Anesthesiology* 1983, **58**, 187.
29 Crowther J. and Jenkins B. S. *Br. J. Clin. Equip.* 1980, **5**, 34.
30 Swan H. J. C. and Ganz W. et al. *N. Engl. J. Med.* 1970, **283**, 447; George R. J. D. and Banks R. A. *Br. J. Hosp. Med.* 1983, **29**, 286.
31 Lategola M. and Rahn H. *Proc. Soc. Exp. Biol. Med.* 1953, **84**, 667.
32 Landais A. et al. *Acta Anaesth. Scand.* 1990, **34**, 158.
33 Stetz C. W. et al. *Am. Rev. Respir. Dis.* 1982, **126**, 1001.
34 Cengiz M. et al. *Crit. Care Med.* 1983, **11**, 502.
35 Sprung C. L. et al. *Chest* 1981, **79**, 413.
36 Schuster A. H. and Nanda N.C. *Am. J. Cardiol.* 1984, **53**, 257.
37 Kamal G. D. et al. *Anesthesiology*, 1990, **72**, 95.
38 Haites N. E. et al. *Br. Heart J.* 1985, **53**, 123.
39 Donovan K. D. et al. *Crit. Care Med.* 1986, **14**, 1038.
40 Huntsman R. L. et al. *Circulation* 1983, **67**, 593.
41 Haggmark S et al. *Anesthesiology*, 1989, **70**, 19; Vandenberg B. F. and Kerber R. E. *Anesthesiology*, 1990, 73, 799; deBruijn A. and Clements J. *Intraoperative Use of Echocardiography*, Lippincott, Philadelphia, 1991.
42 Urbanowicz J. H. et al. *Anesthesiology*, 1990, **72**, 40.
43 Clements F. M. et al. *Br. J. Anaesth.* 1990, **64**, 331.
44 Knobel E. et al. *Crit. Care Med.* 1989, **17**, 1344.
45 Davies N. J. H. and Denison D. M. In Scurr C. S. Feldman S. A. Soni N. (eds) *Scientific Foundations of Anaesthesia*, 4th edn. Heinemann, Oxford, 1990.
46 Ilsley A. H. and Runciman W. B. *Anaesth. Intensive Care* 1986, **14**, 431.
47 Endler G. C. *Anesthesiology*, 1990, **72**, 214.
48 Kalenda Z. *Br. J. Clin. Equip.* 1980, **6**, 180; Kalenda Z. *Acta Anaesth. Belg.* 1978, **29**, 201; Hurter D. *Anaesthesia* 1979, **34**, 578; Smallhout B. and Kalenda Z. *An Atlas of Capnography*. Kerlebosch, Zeist Netherlands, 1980; Whitesell R. et al. *Anesth. Analg.* 1981, **60**, 508.
49 Goldberg J. S. et al. *Anesth. Analg.* 1990, **70**, 191.
50 Bourgan J.L. et al. *Br. J. Anaesth.* 1990, **64**, 327.

51 Parker D. *Br. J. Clin. Equip.* 1980, **5,** 31; Blackburn J. P. *Br. J. Anaesth.* 1978, **50,** 51.
52 Clark L. C. *Trans. Am. Soc. Artif. Intern. Organs* 1956, **2,** 41.
53 Rozkovec A. and Rithalia S. U. S. *Br. J. Clin. Equip.* 1980, **5,** 24; Goldman M. D. et al. *Anaesthesia* 1982, **37,** 944; Simpson R. M. and Bryan M. H. *Br. J. Hosp. Med.* 1982, **28,** 250.
54 Eberhard P. and Schafer R. *Br. J. Clin. Equip.* 1980, **5,** 224.
55 Klasing S. et al. *Anaesthesist* 1989, **38,** 664.
56 Lam H. S. *Can. J. Anaesth.* 1987, **34,** S232.
57 Spencer E. M. and Bolsin S. N. C. *Intensive Care World* 1990, **7,** 34; *Int. Anesthesiol. Clin.* 1990, **28(3)**.
58 *See also* Prior P. F. and Maynard D. E. Chapter 1, *Monitoring Cerebral Function*. Elsevier, Amsterdam, 1986.
59 Nixon C. et al. *Anaesthesia* 1986, **41,** 131.
60 Bydder G. M. and Steiner R. E. *Neuroradiology* 1982, **23,** 231; Bailes D. R. et al. *Clin. Radiol.* 1982, **33,** 395; Crooks L. E. et al. *Radiology* 1982, **144,** 843.
61 Imrie M. M. and Hall G. M. *B. J. Anaesthesia* 1990, **64,** 346.
62 Spiegel T. *Anaesthesist* 1998, **47,** 220–228; Priesman S. *Intensive Care Med.* 1997, **23,** 651–657.
63 Lichtwarck-Aschoff M. *Intensive Care Med.* 1992, **18,** 142–147.

The administration of volatile anaesthetics and gases

GENERAL PRINCIPLES OF INHALATIONAL ANAESTHESIA

The uptake of anaesthetic gases and vapours[1]

The word gas was invented by the Flemish chemist Johannes Baptiste van Helmont (1577–1644) from the Greek work Khos = chaos.

For this purpose, anaesthetic gases and vapours are assumed to be biologically inert. Their uptake is thus determined by physical principles. It can be separated into uptake in the lungs, diffusion into pulmonary blood, and then distribution by the blood and diffusion into the brain and other organs.

The alveolar concentration of any anaesthetic vapour during induction of anaesthesia is determined by the following:

1 *Inspired concentration*. If the body becomes fully saturated with vapour, uptake ceases and alveolar concentration will equal inspired concentration. This is never quite achieved in clinical practice, and alveolar concentration remains less than inspired concentration because of continuing uptake. Increasing the inspired concentration will speed induction provided that it does not cause breath-holding or laryngospasm. If the inspired concentration is high (e.g. N_2O), uptake into blood allows more fresh gas into the lungs. This accelerates induction (concentration effect). It also accelerates the rise of any volatile agent (second gas effect), so that gas induction with a volatile agent is more rapid if used with nitrous oxide as well as oxygen.
2 *Alveolar ventilation*. Alveolar concentration of anaesthetic agent will rise more quickly towards the inspired concentration if alveolar ventilation is increased, and will rise more slowly if there is respiratory depression or obstruction. This is a striking effect in clinical practice.
3 *Blood/gas partition coefficient*. The ratio (at equilibrium) of concentration in blood to that in gas. A high value denotes an agent very soluble in blood, and so large amounts diffuse from alveolar gas into the blood. This uptake means that a highly soluble agent will be one whose alveolar concentration

can only rise slowly. The rise of alveolar concentration of a highly soluble agent, and hence induction of anaesthesia, is speeded considerably by increasing the alveolar ventilation. The alveolar concentration of a poorly soluble agent will rise towards the inspired value more rapidly, and decay more rapidly when withdrawn at the end of surgery. In summary, agents with a low blood/gas partition coefficient mean that the alveolar, arterial, and hence brain partial pressures respond more quickly to a change in inspired concentration.

4 *Cardiac output or pulmonary blood flow.* The higher this is, the more agent will be taken away from the lungs, and hence the lower will be the alveolar concentration. This means that induction will be slower. This effect of cardiac output is more marked for the more soluble agents.

5 *Ventilation–perfusion relationships.* Gross disturbances delay the uptake of anaesthetic agents.

There is effectively no barrier to the diffusion of anaesthetic gases and vapours from alveolar gas into pulmonary capillary blood. They are then distributed in the arterial circulation.

The brain weighs only 2% of the body weight, but receives 14% of the cardiac output. Depth of anaesthesia depends on the partial pressure of agent in the brain. This rises more quickly if cerebral blood flow (CBF) is increased, e.g. by inhaling CO_2. In hypotension, CBF is maintained with a mean blood pressure down to about 40–50 mmHg, and CBF is a higher proportion of cardiac output, speeding equilibration between blood and brain. This is also true for intravenous anaesthetics.

Under basal conditions 75% of the cardiac output goes to the brain, heart, liver, kidney and endocrine glands, the *vessel-rich group*, which comprise only 7% of the body weight. *Muscles and skin* receive less than 20% of the cardiac output. The blood flow to fatty tissues is similar to muscle, but have a far greater capacity for anaesthetics, due to their higher solubility in fat. This slows induction and recovery in the obese. The *vessel-poor group* of tissues, bone, ligament, cartilage, etc. are 25% of body weight, but receive only a tiny blood flow.

In general, the speed with which an anaesthetic equilibrates with any tissue is faster if: (i) the blood flow is high, and (ii) the solubility in that tissue is low (as less agent needs to diffuse from the blood). The time constant for N_2O in brain is just over 1 min, but 100 min in fat. For halothane the respective figures are 3.3 and 2720 min.[1]

Minimal alveolar concentration

We assume that equilibration in the brain is rapid, and that brain concentration is equal to alveolar concentration. We can therefore speak of the *minimal alveolar concentration* (MAC) of an anaesthetic agent which will produce general anaesthesia.[2] The MAC produces a lack of reflex response to skin incision in 50% of subjects. Values are shown in Table 2.3.1. Strictly speaking, partial pressure rather than concentration is the important factor. Minimal alveolar concentration will vary with altitude, whereas minimal alveolar

Table 2.3.1 Physical properties of some inhalation anaesthetics

	MW	BP (°C)	Vapour pressure	Liquid density @ 20°C mmHg	Oil/water solubility	MAC	Blood/gas partition coefficient
Nitrous oxide N_2O	44	−89	5200	1.2	2.2	104	0.47
Halothane $CF_3.CHClBr$	197	50	243	1.87	220	0.75	2.3
Enflurane $CHF_2-O-CF_2.CHFCl$	184	56.5	174.5	1.52	120.1	1.68	1.9
Isoflurane $CHF_2-O-CHCl.CF_3$	184	48.5	238	1.50	120.1	1.15	1.4
Sevoflurane $CFH_2-O-CH(CF_3)CF_3$	200	58.5	160	–	53.0	2.0	0.69
Desflurane $CF_2H-O-CHF.CF_3$	168	23.5	673	–	19.0	6.0	0.42

pressure (MAP) would be reasonably constant.[3] The alveolar concentration needed to prevent reflex response in 95% of subjects is about 1.5 times the MAC value. When mixtures of agents are used their separate MAC fractions may be simply added to estimate total effect on the patient.

Recovery from anaesthesia

Recovery is the period from the cessation of the administration of anaesthesia until the patient is awake and with protective reflexes. It is a re-equilibration of the body with atmospheric air, and its speed depends on all the factors above. It is much more rapid after a short anaesthetic as there has not been time for the fatty tissues of the body to start to be saturated, and these tissues can act as very sizeable reservoirs for anaesthetic agents.

Clinical signs of anaesthesia

Since the early days of anaesthesia, it has been apparent that the anaesthetist must rely on a series of physical signs to indicate the onset of anaesthesia and to determine its depth. Arthur Eames Guedel's stages and planes of ether anaesthesia[4] were based on a progressive increase of muscular paralysis (ocular muscles, intercostals, diaphragm) and a progressive abolition of reflex response. These signs are less relevant now that muscle relaxants are so widely used. Some points, however, remain valid, e.g. excitement may occur in very light planes of anaesthesia, ocular movements occur in light anaesthesia as does lacrimation. Autonomic responses can still occur in the presence of full muscular relaxation, and neuroendocrine responses occur in response to surgery or trauma.

Anaesthesia may be regarded as having three basic components: (i) narcosis; (ii) analgesia (and associated suppression of reflexes and the neuroendocrine stress response); (iii) relaxation. With appropriate selection of drugs, these three components can be varied individually.

Is there an ideal inhalational anaesthetic agent?

The desirable properties for such an agent would include the following.

1 A stable molecule, not broken down by light, soda-lime, not requiring preservatives, and with a long shelf-life.
2 Non-flammable in air, O_2 or N_2O.
3 Potent enough to allow use with high concentrations of O_2.
4 Saturated vapour pressure high enough to allow easy vaporization, but not so high as to boil at room temperature.
5 Low solubility in blood to allow rapid induction and recovery, and rapid response to changes in inhaled concentration.
6 Pleasant and non-irritating to inhale.
7 Devoid of organ-specific toxicity.

8 Lack of toxic effect when inhaled in low doses by theatre staff.
9 Should not undergo metabolism in the body.
10 Minimal cardiovascular and respiratory side-effects.
11 Should provide some analgesia.
12 No stimulant effects on the nervous system.
13 No sensitization of the heart to catecholamines.
14 No interactions with other drugs.
15 Cheap to manufacture.

Environmental effects

There has been interest in the possible effects of gaseous and volatile anaesthetic agents on the environment. Chlorine-containing molecules are probably
more destructive than those with fluorine.[5] Anaesthesia contributes at most
0.01% to the total atmospheric burden of chlorine containing compounds
and will have a negligible impact on global warming.[6]

NITROUS OXIDE

Nitrous oxide was first prepared by Priestley in 1772, and its anaesthetic
properties suggested by Sir Humphry Davy in 1799. Horace Wells, a dentist
from Hartford, Connecticut, used it in dentistry in 1844, and had one of his
own teeth painlessly extracted that year. However, his demonstration of its
use at Massachusetts General Hospital was unsuccessful, and it became overshadowed by ether. Gardner Quincy Colton revived its use in dentistry in
1867/1868. It was introduced in dental practice in London in 1868 by
T.W. Evans. Later that year, the gas was supplied compressed into cylinders
and became available 2 years later as liquefied N_2O.
  Nitrous oxide is a weak anaesthetic agent, with a MAC value between 100
and 105%. It is a potent analgesic. Unplanned awareness may occur if it is
used as the sole anaesthetic. Tolerance has been demonstrated in volunteers
to the analgesic effects,[7] which can develop in 2 h, and may make awareness
more likely. It may cause the release of endorphins in the central nervous
system. There is evidence of reversal of its analgesia by naloxone.[8] Twenty-
five per cent N_2O has compared favourably with morphine for relief of
postoperative pain while having little general effect on consciousness. Psychomotor performance is not affected at concentrations of N_2O below 8–12%.
  This very useful agent has been in use for over 150 years. Some think that
its undesirable properties outweigh its benefits. The debate was argued in
Eger E. I. (ed.) *Nitrous Oxide*, Arnold, London, 1985.

Manufacture

By heating ammonium nitrate, as a solid or as an aqueous solution of 83%
ammonium nitrate to 240°C. At higher temperatures the percentage of

impurities increases. The issuing gas is collected, purified and compressed into metal cylinders at 50 kPa × 100 (750 psi). The cylinders are painted French blue (in the UK) and common sizes are D (200 gallons or 900 litres) and E (400 gallons or 1800 litres).

$$NH_4NO_3 \rightarrow 2H_2O + N_2O$$

Nitric oxide and nitrogen dioxide are produced as impurities so that the gases evolved must be washed with water and caustic soda, in turn, before being passed through activated alumina to remove water vapour. At various stages, monitors are used to detect the presence of higher oxides of nitrogen. As a further check, regular random sampling of cylinders is carried out.

The amount present in the cylinder can only be ascertained by weighing, as the gas is in liquid form and the gas pressure above the liquid level remains reasonably constant as long as any liquid remains. In fact, some fall in pressure occurs due to fall in temperature as the liquid N_2O evaporates using latent heat. Up to four-fifths of the contents of a full cylinder is in the liquid state, so, in use, cylinders must have their valves elevated above the horizontal. Just before exhaustion of the cylinder, when all the liquid is vaporized, the pressure quickly drops to zero. Cylinders are filled to a filling ratio (ratio of weight of N_2O to weight of water the cylinder could hold) of 0.75 in temperate and 0.67 in tropical climates. Cylinder weights, full and empty, are stamped on it; 100 gallons of N_2O weigh 850 g.

Physical properties

Sweet smelling, non-irritating, colourless gas. Boiling point −88.5°C. Molecular weight 44. Critical pressure 72.5 bar. Critical temperature 36.5°C. Density at 15°C is 1.875 g/l (1.5 times that of air). Velocity of sound in N_2O is 262 m/sec (compared with 317 for O_2) and a suitable whistle can be used to differentiate the two gases. Change from O_2 to N_2O causes the pitch to fall $1\frac{1}{2}$ tones.[9] Neither flammable nor explosive, but supports the combustion of other agents, even in the absence of oxygen, if a high temperature (above 450°C) is supplied to initiate decomposition into nitrogen and oxygen. For partition coefficients, *see* Table 2.3.1. It is eliminated unchanged from the body, mostly via the lungs, but partly through the skin. It is unaffected by soda-lime.

Impurities in nitrous oxide

Two cases of poisoning in the UK were reported in detail by Clutton-Brock,[10] in which there was contamination with NO and NO_2. Both are toxic, and one patient died. There was methaemoglobinaemia, and cardiorespiratory failure. Higher oxides of nitrogen can cause distress above 100 ppm, but clinical features may be delayed for several hours.

A crude test for contamination[11] is to put a piece of moistened starch-iodide paper into a large syringe and then fill this with the suspected N_2O mixed with

25% O_2 and wait for 10 min. If the gas is contaminated by over 300 parts per million, the starch iodide will turn blue.

Undesirable effects of nitrous oxide

Nitrous oxide is usually regarded as an extremely safe, non-toxic anaesthetic agent, provided that it is administered with a sufficient concentration of O_2. Undesirable effects may, however, sometimes occur.

Diffusion into gas-containing spaces

There is a 35-fold difference in the blood/gas partition coefficients of N_2O (0.47) and nitrogen (0.013), so for every molecule of nitrogen removed from gas-containing spaces, 35 molecules of N_2O will enter. The diffusion of N_2O between blood, tissue and gas is more rapid than nitrogen. There is thus an increase in the volume of the gas space when that space is compliant (pneumothorax, gut, air embolus) and an increase in pressure when the space cannot expand (sinuses, the middle ear).

In surgery for retinal detachment where sulphur hexafluoride is used, N_2O can diffuse in and considerably raise the intraocular pressure. It should be discontinued up to 15 min before the bubble is injected. The changes in middle ear pressure may cause postoperative hearing loss, and problems in otological surgery (e.g. myringoplasty) when tympanic grafts are used. It may be preferable to avoid N_2O.

Interaction with vitamin B_{12}

Nitrous oxide inactivates the cobalt in vitamin B_{12} and so irreversibly inactivates the enzyme methionine synthetase. The time course of this interaction is much slower in humans than in rodents, where it has been most extensively studied. Significant falls in plasma methionine concentrations during routine minor and intermediate surgery have not been demonstrated,[12] a period of at least 8 h of N_2O anaesthesia probably being needed to demonstrate a fall.[13] This interferes with the metabolism of folate and the synthesis of DNA and proteins. Megaloblastic anaemia has occurred after exposure of patients to N_2O for periods of 6–12 h.[14] Pretreatment with folinic acid prevents these megaloblastic changes.

In 1956 H.C.A. Lassen, Copenhagen physician, reported that very prolonged N_2O and O_2 anaesthesia, as in the treatment of poliomyelitis or tetanus, could cause bone marrow aplasia.[15]

Prolonged occupational exposure to N_2O may result in subacute combined degeneration of the cord. This emphasizes the need for the avoidance of pollution of the atmosphere of the operating room.

Teratogenicity

Although teratogenic changes have been observed in pregnant rats exposed to N_2O for prolonged periods, there is no evidence of harm to the fetus in humans.[16]

Cardiac effects

There is a minor depressant effect on the heart, but this is more than compensated for by an increase in catecholamines, which is more marked under hyperbaric conditions.[17]

Diffusion hypoxia[18]

Immediately after N_2O anaesthesia, hypoxia may occur, as N_2O diffuses out into alveolar gas faster than nitrogen (from room air) can diffuse in. The dilution of alveolar O_2 results in hypoxia. This may be prevented by giving 100% O_2 for a few minutes at the end of an anaesthetic, and the administration of O_2 in recovery.

Postoperative nausea and vomiting

This is now accepted to be more common when N_2O has been used, possibly associated with its diffusion into the middle ear.[19]

Advantages of nitrous oxide in anaesthesia

These include the analgesic properties, non-irritant properties, low blood solubility, and additive effects allowing lower doses of volatile agents. Nitrous oxide also speeds induction with volatile agents.

It is useful to supplement continuous or intermittent intravenous anaesthesia, in order to reduce the chances of awareness. When using a mainly inhalational technique, it is common practice to prevent awareness by adding a volatile agent to a mixture of O_2 and N_2O.

Premixed nitrous oxide/oxygen

Premixed N_2O /O_2 (80 : 20) at a maximum cylinder pressure of 47 kPa $\times$ 100 (700 psi) was used in the US in 1945.[20]

Certain mixtures of N_2O and O_2 will remain in the gaseous phase at pressures and temperatures at which N_2O by itself would normally be a liquid (Poynting effect).

Entonox

This is a 50 : 50 mixture of N_2O and O_2 and is readily available. The cylinder top is painted white and the body French blue. If such cylinders are exposed to cold temperatures ($-7°C$), some N_2O separates as a liquid and may lead to delivery of uneven mixtures, too much O_2 at the beginning and too much N_2O at the end of the cylinder life. Cooling due to expansion of gases while in use is not likely to cause this. Danger of separation can be avoided by immersing the cylinder in water at $52°C$ and inverting it three times, or by keeping it above a temperature of $10°C$ for 2 h before use. Uses of Entonox include analgesia for dressing wounds, chest physiotherapy, removal of chest drains, coronary infarction and dental surgery. It is often carried by ambulances. The English National Board for Midwifery permit its use by midwives on their own responsibility. For its use in obstetrics, *see* Chapter 4.3. Entonox may be supplied by pipeline.

ISOFLURANE

Isoflurane ($CHF_2–O–CHCl.CF_3$) is a fluorinated methyl ethyl ether synthesized by Ross Terrell in 1965, who had synthesized its isomer, enflurane, in 1963.[21] Used in clinical anaesthesia by Dobkin et al.[22] and Stevens et al. in 1971.[23]

Physical properties

A colourless volatile liquid, *see* Table 2.3.1. The saturated vapour pressure is similar to that of halothane, and so could theoretically be used in the same vaporizer as halothane though this is not recommended on safety grounds. Induction and recovery are rapid, partly because of the low blood/gas partition coefficient, but also because of a fairly low fat solubility. MAC is 1.15 in O_2 and 0.66 in 70% N_2O. Isoflurane is stable and no preservatives are necessary to prevent its decomposition. It does not react with metal in breathing systems.

Pharmacodynamics

Cardiovascular system

Isoflurane causes less myocardial depression than halothane or enflurane. Isoflurane lowers arterial blood pressure less than halothane or enflurane, principally as a result of vasodilatation. The cardiac rhythm is stable, and the myocardium is not sensitized to catecholamines. Heart rate often increases, especially in young patients.

Isoflurane is a powerful coronary vasodilator at normal concentrations. Therefore coronary steal may occur in patients with certain uncommon types of coronary artery disease, where healthy myocardium receives increased blood flow at the expense of myocardium supplied by the stenosed vessels. On the other hand, isoflurane with N_2O has improved the tolerance to pacing-induced myocardial ischaemia in patients with coronary artery disease.[24] Animal work on this subject has yielded conflicting results.

Respiration

Isoflurane causes a decrease in tidal volume and increase in respiratory rate. In terms of depression of normal breathing, it occupies a position intermediate between halothane and enflurane. The ventilatory response to hypercapnia is blunted. The response to hypoxia is abolished at just 0.1 MAC (as with all volatile agents). The incidence of coughing and laryngospasm during induction is greater than with halothane as the vapour is mildly irritant.[25]

Nervous system

Low concentrations up to 1 MAC do not cause any increase in CBF, provided that the PCO_2 is normal, and is preferred by many in neurosurgical anaesthesia. Larger concentrations do increase CBF. At 2 MAC the electroencephalogram (EEG) may be isoelectric, and so there may be some protection against the cerebral effect of hypoxia. It does not affect the development of cerebral oedema after trauma.

Muscle tone is reduced, as with other volatile agents. It potentiates nondepolarizing muscle relaxants.

The uterus

There is a dose-related relaxation of the pregnant uterus, but is suitable for Caesarean section in a concentration of 0.75%.

Liver

Repeated isoflurane administrations have failed to produce measurable changes in liver function.[26] However, isolated cases of fatal hepatic necrosis have occurred after the use of isoflurane.[27]

Pharmacokinetics

Only about 0.2% of inhaled isoflurane can be recovered as urinary metabolites.[28] Serum fluoride after 3 MAC-hours exposure amounts to only about 5% of the levels associated with renal toxicity.[29] The likelihood of renal or hepatic toxicity following isoflurane anaesthesia is considered to be minimal.

Indications

Of the various inhalation agents available, isoflurane has the advantage of providing stability of cardiac rhythm and lack of sensitization of the heart to exogenous and endogenous adrenaline. Rapid awakening is an advantage in the day-stay patient. Isoflurane is stable and is unlikely to be toxic. It produces hypotension with little cardiac depression. For maintenance with spontaneous breathing 1–2.5% is usually needed.

SEVOFLURANE[30]

Sevoflurane (CFH_2–O–$CH(CF_3)CF_3$) was first described in North America in 1971,[31] was first given to human volunteers in 1981, and has been used in clinical practice since 1990.

Physical properties

Molecular weight 200. Boiling point 58.5°C. Specific gravity 1.52. Saturated vapour pressure (SVP)162 mmHg at 20°C. The blood/gas partition coefficient is 0.63–0.69, and is the second-lowest of the volatile agents (desflurane is 0.4). Brain–blood partition coefficient 1.7. Minimum alveolar concentration 2%.

Clinical uses

Inhalation induction: Induction is rapid (1–2 min), non-irritant, and this method is well-tolerated in both children and adults.

It is poorly soluble in blood, pleasant smelling and fairly non-irritant to the upper airways. It therefore has a useful place as an induction agent. Various techniques have been used with success, either rapidly increasing the inspired concentration from 0.5% up to 4–8%, by taking a single vital capacity breath of 4.5% or higher, or by immediately breathing a high concentration (8%).[32] The incidence of coughing is acceptably low.

The trachea may be intubated under deep sevoflurane anaesthesia,[33] and a laryngeal mask airway inserted at about 1 MAC. Some workers recommend its use as an induction agent when the airway is likely to be difficult, although its superiority over halothane in this regard is not fully established.

Emergence from anaesthesia is more rapid than with isoflurane, and is comparable with that seen after continuous propofol anaesthesia. This makes it suitable for day-stay surgery.

Cardiovascular and respiratory effects

These are similar to isoflurane. However, sevoflurane's coronary vasodilator properties are less marked than isoflurane. It is also less likely than isoflurane to cause tachycardia.

Nervous system

Similar to isoflurane, with no increase in CBF or intracranial pressure (ICP) below 1 MAC. No excitatory phenomena. Reduces muscle tone, and potentiates non-depolarizing muscle relaxants.

Effects on the uterus

Similar to isoflurane, with a dose-related relaxation of the pregnant uterus. May be used in Caesarean section.

Toxicity

No known hepatic or renal toxicity, even after repeated administration. May trigger malignant hyperpyrexia in susceptible individuals. About 5% is metabolized by cytochrome P450 in the liver with the production of hexafluoroisopropanol and inorganic fluoride. Concentrations of inorganic fluoride are only likely to reach 50 μmol/l (the proposed threshold at which renal impairment may occur) after about 8 MAC-hours of sevoflurane anaesthesia. In clinical practice, sevoflurane does not cause renal damage. However, some workers caution against its use if renal function is significantly impaired.

Sevoflurane is absorbed into soda-lime and Baralyme, and degraded by them. Five breakdown compounds have been identified, compounds A to E. This degradation is more marked at higher temperatures. Compound A (PIFE, pentafluoroisopropenyl fluoromethyl ether) is the only one likely to be produced in clinical use, and is toxic to the liver, kidneys and central nervous system in rats. The concentrations of compound A found in patients have been generally less than 10 ppm, and are higher if Baralyme is used. Concentrations over 30 ppm have been recorded after very prolonged exposure using low fresh gas flows. These values are substantially less than the 200 ppm which seems the minimum dose needed to cause renal damage in rats. Compound A is almost certainly of no clinical significance, with the possible exception of when sevoflurane is used for a very long time with fresh gas flows under 2 l/min. For example, transient changes in renal function, attributed to compound A, have been noticed in volunteers after administration of 1.25 MAC of sevoflurane for 8 h with fresh gas flows of 2 l/min.[34]

DESFLURANE[35]

Desflurane ($CF_2H–O–CHF.CF_3$) was developed in the US.[36] First reports in the UK followed administration to volunteers at Guy's Hospital.[37] Like sevoflurane, it is halogenated only with fluorine.

Physical properties

Molecular weight 168. Boiling point 23°C. Saturated vapour pressure at 20°C 673 mmHg. Blood/gas partition coefficient 0.42. Minimum alveolar concentration in O_2 6.0%. No preservative required. Stable in soda-lime.

Vaporizer

Because of the boiling point close to room temperature, standard vaporizers are unsatisfactory and special heated vaporizers have been developed for clinical use.

Cardiorespiratory effects

These are similar to those of sevoflurane. However, some sympathetic hyper-activity has been reported when inspired concentration is increased rapidly, with rises in pulse rate and blood pressure.[38] Some depression of respiration is to be expected. The myocardium is not sensitized to catecholamines.

Although the vapour is not unpleasant to inhale, desflurane is more irritant to the airways than sevoflurane, with a higher incidence of coughing and laryngospasm at induction in both adults and children.[39]

Because of the extremely low blood/gas partition coefficient, induction, change of depth of anaesthesia and recovery will be rapid. It is therefore particularly suitable for day-stay surgery. Solubility in body tissues is low so that in a closed breathing system the concentration of vapour in the system will approach that in the basal flow more rapidly than in the case of other agents.

Biotransformation is negligible.[40]

No significant liver or kidney toxicity has been reported. May trigger malignant hyperpyrexia in susceptible individuals.[41]

ENFLURANE

The first clinical account of enflurane ($CHF_2-O-CF_2.CHFCl$) appeared in 1966.[42] Developed by Ross Terrell in the US in 1963.

Physical properties

Molecular weight 184. Boiling point 56.5°C. Saturated vapour pressure 175 mmHg. Minimum alveolar concentration 1.68% in O_2 and 1.28% in 70% N_2O. Blood/gas partition coefficient 1.9 (oil-gas 98.5). Concentrations above 4.25% are flammable in 20% O_2/80% N_2O. Stable with soda-lime and metals. Contains no preservative.

Clinical properties

Central nervous system

Electroencephalogram (EEG) changes of an epileptiform nature may occur which are more common during hypocapnia and may persist for several weeks.[43] Convulsions may occur at 2 MAC. Enflurane should be used with extreme caution in patients with epilepsy. Cerebral blood flow increased, doubled at 1 MAC.

Cardiovascular system

As depth of anaesthesia is increased, there is a reversible fall in arterial pressure mainly due to myocardial depression, but also with some vasodilatation. Serious dysrhythmias uncommon. Relatively safe when adrenaline infiltration used. Up to three times the adrenaline dose permitted with halothane is reported to be safe.[44]

Respiratory system

Pulmonary ventilation depressed; tidal volume decreased, perhaps with a rise in respiratory rate. Salivary and bronchial secretions not increased. May cause occasional sighing respiration.

Muscular relaxation

Produces moderate relaxation, and enhances the action of non-depolarizing relaxants.

Obstetrics

Satisfactory for Caesarean section using a concentration of 1%. Dose-related relaxation of the uterus is seen.

Toxicity

Enflurane is eliminated mostly via the lungs, although about 3% is metabolized in the body and the resultant fluoride ions excreted by the kidney. Peak fluoride concentrations are similar to those seen after sevoflurane anaesthesia, and are usually well below the possible toxic level of 50 μmol/l. Changes in renal function are not clinically significant, and enflurane seems to produce no further impairment of renal function even when this is impaired preoperatively.

Emergence is smooth and reasonably rapid, with shivering, nausea and vomiting infrequent.

HALOTHANE

Halothane ($CF_3.CHClBr$; 2, bromo-2-chloro-1, 1, 1, trifluoroethane) is a potent, non-flammable, relatively non-toxic anaesthetic agent. Its ease of use revolutionized practice in the 1950s.

Physical properties

A colourless liquid. The vapour is relatively non-irritant. Molecular weight 197, specific gravity of the liquid 1.87. Boiling point 50°C. Saturated vapour pressure at 20°C is 243 mmHg. Minimum alveolar concentration is 0.75%. Partition coefficients: blood/gas 2.3; oil/water 220; fat/blood 60.0; brain/blood 2.6. Decomposed by light (stabilized by 0.01% thymol), but is stable when stored in amber-coloured bottles. It can be used safely with soda-lime. The vapour is absorbed by rubber (rubber/gas partition coefficient at 20°C is 120). In the presence of moisture it attacks tin, brass and aluminium in vaporizers and circuits. Non-flammable and non-explosive when its vapour is mixed with O_2 in any concentration (or under hyperbaric conditions) used clinically. May be decomposed by an open flame liberating bromine.

Pharmacodynamics

Cardiovascular system

Arterial pressure falls, due mainly to myocardial depression, but with significant vasodilatation too. Dilates coronary arteries. Heart rate often slows, and this may be reversed by atropine. This is usually a sinus or nodal bradycardia.

There is increased myocardial excitability, with ventricular extrasystoles. These are more likely when there is CO_2 retention, sensory stimulation in light anaesthesia, and with the use of beta-stimulant drugs. Ventricular fibrillation has even occurred following adrenaline infiltration during halothane anaesthesia. Intravenous infusion of more than 10 μg/min of adrenaline is likely to provoke dysrhythmias.

Central nervous system

Halothane increases CBF threefold at 1 MAC and abolishes autoregulation. It should only be introduced in neurosurgery if the PCO_2 has previously been lowered to about 3.3 kPa (25 mmHg). Produces moderate muscle relaxation, and deep halothane anaesthesia allows relatively easy laryngoscopy. Potentiates non-depolarizing relaxants.

Respiratory system

Depresses respiration, by decreasing tidal volume and increasing respiratory rate. Causes bronchodilatation. Not irritant to airways, and depresses pharyngeal and laryngeal reflexes.

The uterus

One MAC causes significant relaxation of the uterus. This effect is dose related. A concentration as low as 0.5% may increase blood loss during therapeutic abortion even when oxytocin is administered.

Temperature

Induction of anaesthesia with halothane is soon followed by a drop of up to 1°C in oesophageal temperature, together with a rise of up to 4°C in skin temperature, due to redistribution between core and peripheral tissues. Later, skin temperature may fall as peripheral vasodilatation aids heat loss.

Shivering ('halothane shakes')

Shivering and tremor are common during the immediate postoperative period following halothane anaesthesia. It may be associated with a generalized increase in muscle tone, clonic or tonic. There may sometimes be an association between shivering and temperature falls during anaesthesia, and heat loss during surgery should be minimized. Pethidine has been recommended in management.

Liver toxicity

Massive hepatic necrosis following halothane anaesthesia was reported in 1958,[45] though widespread attention was not drawn to the problem until 1963. Subclinical 'halothane hepatitis' (lesser degree of liver impairment, with a hepatocellular pattern of elevated transferases) may also occur.[46] The most susceptible patients are middle-aged, female and obese.[47]

About 20% of the halothane taken up by the body is metabolized. Metabolites are slowly cleared from the body for as long as 3 weeks. The pathways are complex, but the products of the reductive pathways are more toxic than those arising from oxidative metabolism. There is also evidence, however, for an immune-mediated reaction, with the production of antibodies that react with liver cells sensitized to halothane.

Current advice from the Committee on Safety of Medicines is that:

1 a careful history should be taken relating to previous anaesthetics to see if halothane was given, and if so what effect it had;
2 halothane should not be used within 3 months of a previous halothane anaesthetic without 'overriding clinical circumstances';

3 unexplained jaundice or fever after a previous halothane anaesthetic is an absolute contraindication to halothane.

Many anaesthetists feel that (2) should not apply to children, in whom liver toxicity has been extremely rare. Pre-existing liver disease unrelated to halothane is not a specific contraindication to the use of halothane. Severe liver damage is unlikely to follow a single administration of halothane.

Other causes of postoperative jaundice include the effect of drugs (such as phenothiazines, monoamine oxidase inhibitors), blood transfusion, sepsis, hypotension, coincidental viral hepatitis. Stress and starvation may produce overt jaundice in subjects with Gilbert's syndrome (familial unconjugated hyperbilirubinaemia) but the serum transaminases remain normal.[48]

XENON

Isolated in 1898 by William Ramsey (1852–1916), Nobel prize winner in chemistry 1904. First used in 1951. Radioactive xenon is used in CBF studies. It has been suggested that xenon compares favourably with N_2O in terms of haemodynamic, neuroendocrine and analgesic properties.[49]

ETHER

Ether ($CH_3 . CH_2–O–CH_2 . CH_3$) is still a widely used anaesthetic agent in several continents. It was introduced to the profession by W.T.G. Morton of Boston on 16 October 1846.

Properties

Saturated vapour pressure at 20°C is 425 mmHg. Blood/gas partition coefficient 12.0. Slow induction and recovery. Minimum alveolar concentration 1.92. Flammable in air and explosive in O_2. Irritant vapour, which can readily induce laryngeal spasm, and make induction even slower.

Ether stimulates salivary and bronchial secretions, and so atropine premedication is given. Ether is commonly given from an EMO draw-over inhaler. Spontaneous respiration may be maintained, and the concentration of ether slowly increased, or the same apparatus may be used in conjunction with bellows for intermittent positive-pressure ventilation (IPPV) using air. Muscle relaxants need not be used as ether itself produces excellent relaxation. Their use would complicate an otherwise simple technique.

The use of concomitant regional block with local anaesthetic greatly reduces the concentration of ether needed, lessens the side-effects, and speeds recovery. Typical maintenance concentration is 5% without local block, and

2% with local block. The use of opiates will also reduce the necessary concentration of ether, but will make postoperative nausea and vomiting much worse. These will, however, respond to antiemetics.

Ether liberates catecholamines and tends to maintain blood pressure. There is little cardiac depression. Dysrhythmias are rare. Adrenaline is relatively safe with ether. Bronchial smooth muscle is relaxed. The products of its metabolism (alcohol, acetaldehyde and acetic acid) are relatively non-toxic. It should not be used when diathermy is needed in the airways, because of the risk of fire or explosion, although these have not occurred when air is used to carry the ether vapour.

GASES USED IN ASSOCIATION WITH ANAESTHESIA

Oxygen

Antoine Lavoisier and Pierre Laplace coined the term 'oxygène' (oxy = acid; gene = producer) in 1779. They were the first to compare the heat produced by respiration in animals and that from the combustion of carbon.

Medical O_2 is manufactured by the fractional distillation of liquid air (nitrogen comes off first). Boiling point of O_2 −183°C; of nitrogen −195°C. Oxygen cylinders are painted black with white shoulders in the UK, blue in some European countries and green in the US. The cylinders contain gaseous O_2 compressed to 137 bar. Also supplied as a liquid at about −183°C in insulated tanks at a pressure of around 10.5 bar. One millilitre of liquid O_2 gives 842 ml of gas at 15°C. Pipeline pressure is 4.1 bar.

The O_2 concentrator produces O_2 from ambient air by preferential absorption of nitrogen on zeolites (crystalline aluminosilicates). It behaves like a molecular sieve with a pore size of 0.5 nm. The resultant gas contains 6% of harmless impurities, mostly argon. It is suitable for use in hospitals, remote areas, developing countries and in the military. Small machines producing about 2 l/min are cheaper than cylinders for domestic use.

Properties

Molecular weight 32. Solubility in water 0.024 ml/ml at 37°C, 0.031 at 20°C, 0.049 at 0°C. Boiling point −183°C. Critical temperature −118.4°C. Critical pressure 50.8 bar. Specific gravity 1105 (air is 1000). Density 1.35 kg/m^3 at 15°C. Electric sparks convert it into ozone (O_3).

When compressed, O_2 may ignite grease or oil (as in a diesel engine). It encourages fires, although not itself flammable. Oxygen (and N_2O) cylinders should be turned on momentarily before being fitted to the machine to allow any dirt in the valve to escape. They should be turned on slowly after fitting to prevent sudden surges of pressure in the reducing valve and contents gauge.

Medical air

Atmospheric air contains 78.08% nitrogen, 20.95% O_2, 0.93% argon, 0.03% CO_2, plus traces of neon, helium, krypton, hydrogen and xenon in descending order of abundance. Medical air is supplied in the UK in grey cylinders with black and white shoulder quadrants, compressed to 137 bar. In many hospitals it is also supplied by pipeline at 4 bar. It is used as a respired gas and to drive ventilators. It also drives surgical drills, etc., but these need a pressure of 7 bar or above. Medical air has fewer impurities than industrial compressed air, no water and less than 0.5 mg/m^3 of oil mist.

Carbon dioxide

Discovered by Jean Baptiste von Helmont and isolated by Joseph Black in 1757 who showed that it was produced by respiration, combustion and fermentation. Used to produce 'suspended animation' and surgical anaesthesia in animals in 1824 by Henry Hill Hickman. Thirty per cent CO_2 was used by Ralph Waters to render humans unconscious in 1928.

Properties

Colourless gas, pungent odour in high concentration. Molecular weight 44. Boiling point $-78.5°C$. Solubility in water 0.88 ml/ml at 20°C. Critical temperature 31°C. Critical pressure 73.8 bar. Specific gravity 1520 (air is 1000). Density 1.87 kg/m^3 at 15°C.

Preparation and storage

In the UK it is obtained from four sources.

1 From fermentation in the brewing of beer.
2 By-product of manufacture of hydrogen in petroleum refining.
3 From the combustion of other fuels.
4 By heating magnesium and calcium carbonate in the presence of their oxides.

Only a small fraction of the CO_2 manufactured is used for medicinal purposes.

It is stored in grey cylinders at 50 bar (or for industrial use in refrigerated tanks). Solid CO_2 is stored and transported in insulated containers. The filling ratio in cylinders is 0.75 in temperate climates and 0.67 in the tropics. The liquid phase disappears when about 83% of the gas has been discharged.

Oxygen–CO_2-premixed cylinders are available in various combinations. Such cylinders are black with grey/white shoulder quadrants and filled to a pressure of 137 atmospheres.

Effects

Inspired air contains 0.03%, mixed expired gas 3.5–4% and alveolar gas 5.3%. Breathing 5% CO_2 in air or O_2 is tolerable, but higher amounts cause dyspnoea, headaches, etc. Above 10% the narcotic effect becomes more marked, while at 30% there is an isoelectric EEG and coma. Muscle twitching, a flap of the hands and fits may occur before coma supervenes. At 40% breathing is depressed. Carbon dioxide has been much used to anaesthetize small laboratory animals.

Hypercapnia by itself depresses the heart, but this is masked by a rise in plasma catecholamines. Multifocal ventricular extrasystoles may occur. Major physoiological factor influencing CBF.

Carbon dioxide has been used to hasten inhalational induction especially with agents of high solubility, to facilitate blind intubation, to facilitate the onset of respiration after passive hyperventilation, as a cerebral vasodilator in studies of CBF, to add to the oxygenator gas mixture during hypothermic cardiopulmonary bypass in order to maintain $PaCO_2$ and pH when these values are corrected to body temperature, and to insufflate the abdomen for laparoscopy.

Dangers

Carbon dioxide administration is a potential source of great danger.[50] It is normally recommended that a CO_2 cylinder should only be attached to an anaesthetic machine at the specific request of the anaesthetist, there should be a limit to the maximum flow, and bobbins on CO_2 rotameters should not rise above half-way to make them more visible. The routine use of capnography in all anaesthetics should help prevent the inadvertent administration of CO_2.

Water vapour

Water has a high specific heat (4.2 kJ/kg/°C, 10 times that of copper). Inspired air is warmed to body temperature and fully saturated with water vapour by the time it reaches the trachea. If the trachea is intubated this has to take place in the tracheobronchial tree. Air saturated with water vapour at 15, 20 and 37°C has partial pressures of water vapour of 12, 18 and 47 mmHg and water contents of 13, 19 and 50 mg/l respectively.

Helium

Isolated by Sir W. Ramsey (1852–1916) (British chemist and Nobel prize winner in 1904 for his work on the inert gases) in 1895.

Preparation

From natural gas, some gas wells in Poland, Texas and New Mexico contain about 1%. Natural gas from the North sea contains only 0.01–0.03%. Air contains 0.0005%. Helium cylinders are brown, helium–oxygen cylinders brown with brown/white shoulder quadrants. The pressure in a full cylinder is 137 bar.

Properties

Inert, colourless, odourless gas. Molecular weight 4. Boiling point −269°C. Solubility in water 0.0088 ml/ml at 20°C. Critical temperature −268°C. Specific gravity 178 (air is 1000). Critical pressure 2.3 bar. Density 0.17 kg/m^3 at 15°C. Second lightest gas (to hydrogen).

A mixture of 21% O_2 and 79% helium has a specific gravity of 341 (air is 1000). Its low density enables this gas mixture to flow through an orifice three times as fast as air, for the same pressure gradient. Thus, patients with upper airways obstruction will benefit. Since its viscosity is very similar to O_2 it will make no difference to the laminar flow in smaller airways, but the lower Reynolds number for helium mixtures will encourage laminar flow.

Helium's low solubility has led to its use in the measurement of lung volumes by gas dilution. Its diffusibility and low solubility make it less likely than nitrogen to be responsible for decompression sickness. It has a high thermal capacity which encourages loss of body heat.

REFERENCES

1 *See also* Kety S. S. *Anesthesiology* 1950, **11,** 517; Eger E. J. *Anesthetic Uptake and Action*. Baltimore: Williams & Wilkins, 1974.
2 Merkel G. and Eger E. I. *Anesthesiology* 1963, **24,** 346 (reprinted in 'Classical File', *Surv. Anesthesiol.* 1974, **18,** 594); Eger E. I. et al. *Anesthesiology* 1956, **26,** 271.
3 Fink B. R. *Anesthesiology* 1971, **34,** 403.
4 Guedel A. E. *Inhalation Anesthesia* 1937 and 2nd edn. Macmillan, London, 1951.
5 Logan M. and Farmer J. G. *Br. J. Anaesth.* 1990, **63,** 645.
6 Brown A. C. et al. *Nature* 1989, **341,** 635 and *Lancet* 1989, **ii,** 279.
7 Rupreht J. et al. *Acta Anaesth. Scand.* 1985, **29,** 635.
8 Yank J. C. et al. *Anesthesiology* 1980, **52,** 414.
9 Wright B. M. *Lancet* 1977, **2,** 1008.
10 Clutton-Brock J. *Br. J. Anaesth.* 1967, **39,** 388; *Br. J. Anaesth.* 1967, **39,** 343 et seq.; Editorial, *Lancet* 1967, **2,** 930.
11 Kain M. L. et al. *Br. J. Anaesth.* 1967, **39,** 425.
12 Nunn J. F. et al. *Br. J. Anaesth.* 1986, **58,** 1.
13 Amos R. J. et al. *Lancet* 1982, **2,** 835.
14 Nunn J. F. and Chanarin J. *Br. J. Anaesth.* 1978, **50,** 1089.

15 Lassen H. C. A. *Lancet* 1956, **1**, 525.
16 Konieczko K. et al. *Br. J. Anaesth.* 1987, **59**, 449.
17 Hornbein T. F. et al. *Anesth. Analg.* 1982, **61**, 553
18 Fink B. R. *Anesthesiology* 1955, **16**, 511; Fink B. R. et al. *Fed. Proc.* 1954, **13**, 354.
20 Barach A. L. and Rovenstine E. A. *Anesthesiology* 1945, **6**, 449.
19 Hartnung J. *Anesth. Analg.* 1996, **83**, 114.
21 Vircha J. F. *Anesthesiology* 1971, **21**, 4.
22 Dobkin A. B. et al. *Can. Anaesth. Soc. J.* 1971, **18**, 264.
23 Stevens D. J. et al. *Can. Anaesth. Soc. J.* 1971, **18**, 500.
24 Tarnow J., Markschies-Horning A., and Schulte-Sasse U., *Anesthesiology* 1986, **64**, 147–156.
25 Friesen R. H. and Lichter J. L. *Anesth. Analg. (Cleve.)* 1983, **62**, 411.
26 Brown A. C. et al. *Nature* 1989, **341**, 635 and *Lancet* 1989, **ii**, 279.
27 Weitz J. et al. *Anaesthesia* 1997, **52**, 884.
28 Holaday D. A. et al. *Anesthesiology* 1975, **43**, 325.
29 Mazze R. I. et al. *Anesthesiology* 1974, **40**, 536.
30 Smith I. et al. *Br. J. Anaesth.* 1996, **76**, 435.
31 Wallin R.F. and Napoli M.D. *Fed. Proc.* 1971, **30**, 442.
32 Sloan M. H. et al. *Anesth. Analg.* 1996, **82**, 528; Thwaites A. et al. *Br. J. Anaesth.* 1997, **78**, 356.
33 O'Brien K. et al. *Br. J. Anaesth.* 1998, **80**, 452.
34 Eger E. I. et al. *Anesth. Analg.* 1997, **84**, 160.
35 Eger E. I. *Anaesthesia* 1995, **50(S)**, 3.
36 Eger E.I., *Anesth. Analg.* 1987, **66**, 983.
37 Jones R.M. et al. *Br. J. Anaesth.* 1990, **64**, 11.
38 Ebert T. J. et al. *Anesthesiology* 1995, **83**, 88.
39 Taylor R. H. and Lerman J. *Can. J. Anaesth.* 1992, **39**, 6.
40 Wrigley S. R. et al. *Anaesthesia* 1991, **46**, 615.
41 Allen G. C. and Brubaker C. L. *Anesth. Analg.* 1998, **86**, 1328.
42 Virtue R. W. et al. *Can. Anaesth. Soc. J.* 1966, **12**, 233 (reprinted in 'Classical File', *Surv. Anesthesiol.* 1977, **21**, 210).
43 Julien R. M. and Kavan E. M. *J. Pharmacol. Exp. Ther.* 1972, **123**, 393; Grant I. S. *Anaesthesia* 1986, **41**, 1024; Nicoll J. M. V. *Anaesthesia* 1986, **41**, 927.
44 Reisner L. S. and Lippmann M. *Anesth. Analg.* 1975, **64**, 468; Johnston R. R. et al. *Anesth. Analg.* 1976, **55**, 709.
45 Virtue R. W. and Payne K. W. *Anesthesiology* 1958, **19**, 562.
46 Lecky J. N. and Cohen P. S. *Anesthesiology* 1970, **33**, 371.
47 Stock J. C. L. and Strunin L. *Anesthesiology* 1985, **63**, 424.
48 Gilbert A. and Lereboullet P. *Semaine Médicale, Paris* 1901, **71**, 241; Quinn N. W. and Gollan J. L. *Br. J. Oral Surg.* 1975, **12**, 285.
49 Boomsma F. et al. *Anaesthesia* 1990, **45**, 273–278.
50 Nunn J. F. *Br. J. Anaesth.* 1990, **65**, 155.

Intravenous anaesthesia

The ideal intravenous agent reliably and pleasantly induces full anaesthesia within one arm–brain circulation time, is free from side-effects and wears off in a few minutes. It must be capable of infusion to maintain anaesthesia without problems.[1]

Intravenous anaesthetic agents may be used for:

1 the induction of anaesthesia;
2 as the sole agent for operations (TIVA);
3 to supplement volatile anaesthesia or regional analgesia;
4 for sedation.

The injection of a potent drug into the bloodstream cannot be readily withdrawn, whereas inhalation agents can be more easily eliminated.

Technique of intravenous cannulation

1 Sedation helps in the anxious patient and makes it easier to find suitable veins.
2 Amethocaine gel or EMLA are useful, especially in children.
3 The veins are made as prominent as possible by the use of a venous tourniquet. Applied near the site of injection, the tourniquet steadies the vein proximally, while the anaesthetist's finger, by stretching the skin, steadies it distally. This is very important in thin, elderly people whose veins, although prominent, very readily slip about beneath the skin and may 'run away' from the point of the needle. Nitroglycerin ointment may aid venepuncture by increasing skin vasodilatation. The arterial supply must not be occluded; pulsation is the guide to the position (and avoidance) of an artery. Moreover, the veins will not distend unless blood is flowing into the limb. In hypotension, a blood-pressure cuff may be needed for accurate squeezing of a limb. Some NIBP units have a venous stasis mode.
4 When the skin has been well cleaned with an antiseptic, the cannula is inserted so that it comes to lie between the skin and the vein wall. The point is now advanced and the vein wall is pierced at a different level from the skin puncture. This tends to prevent transfixion of the vein and lessens haematoma formation when the cannula is withdrawn. With the

needle point within the lumen of the vein the cannula is advanced over it. A few drops of local analgesic can be injected into the dermis with an intra-dermal needle before larger cannulae are inserted. Otherwise the tip of the needle is pressed on to the skin to blanch it, for 10 s, before the needle is advanced though the skin, or the needle is inserted immediately after a sharp localized slap or a cough.

Course of anaesthesia

Before any anaesthetic, the stomach and bladder should be empty. When an intravenous anaesthetic is given the following should be at hand in case of need:

1 a laryngoscope;
2 tracheal tubes and laryngeal mask airway;
3 oxygen;
4 a mask and reservoir bag;
5 a tilting table;
6 suction apparatus;
7 suitable syringes and cannulae;
8 Association of Anaesthetists' 'minimal monitoring';
9 resuscitation kit.

Control of the airway is of primary importance in intravenous anaesthesia. Occasionally a pharyngeal airway or a nasopharyngeal tube is necessary, but these should only be used if the airway becomes obstructed without them, as they may stimulate pharyngeal reflexes which upset the smooth course of the anaesthesia. They may also cause laryngospasm. *See* Table 2.4.1.

2,6 DI-ISOPROPYLPHENOL: PROPOFOL (DISOPROFOL; DIPRIVAN)

First reported use in 1977.[2] Propofol is normally a 1% formulation in an oil and water emulsion containing 10% soya bean oil, 1.2% egg phosphatide and 2.25% glycerol. A newer solvent is medium and long-chain triglyceride emulsion.[3]

The induction dose is 1–2.5 mg/kg. The effective blood concentration for anaesthesia (EC_{90}) is 3.4 μg/ml with 67% N_2O.[4] For sedation, a bolus dose of 0.2 mg/kg i.v., or infusion at 1 mg/kg/h, with target blood level of 1–1.5 μg/ml.[5]

Resistance to the anaesthetic effects of propofol is occasionally encoun-tered. Such patients may require co-induction with either short-acting opioids, or modest increase of propofol dosage, both for induction and infusion, requiring intervention in target controlled infusion (TCI) by the anaesthetist.

Quality of anaesthesia is good but myoclonic movements have been observed,[6] (as with many intravenous agents other than thiopentone.) Emergence is more rapid than with thiopentone, without hangover (assessed by the Steward Score), although a central anticholinergic type of response has been reported.[6]

Pharmacokinetics

Rapid distribution ($T\frac{1}{2}\alpha$ 2–8 min), and elimination ($T\frac{1}{2}\beta$ 56–109 min) as glucuronide, with renal excretion. Highly lipophilic. ED95 is 3–4 μg/ml. Post-anaesthesia performance of mental, manual and mechanical tasks is back to normal within 1–2 h. Cumulation in a 'third compartment' is extremely slight, and takes many hours or days to develop. Clearance is dependent on hepatic blood flow, but clinical equilibration with the recommended infusion dose is slower in fat patients than in the lean. Faster distribution in pregnancy.[7]

Pharmacodynamics

Dose-related surgical anaesthesia. Respiratory depression, dose-related, at blood concentrations above 10 μg/ml.

Cardiovascular effects

1 Arterial hypotension, usually preventable by vascular volume loading or by mild head-down tilt. This hypotension is greatest in untreated hypertension. Systolic pressure reductions of 50% have been seen with 2 mg/kg boluses of propofol. It must be used with caution in the hypovolaemic patient and in those anaesthetized in postures other than the supine horizontal.
2 Myocardial depression. The left ventricular dP/dt falls at propofol concentrations above 10 μg/ml (overdose range). At anaesthetic concentrations, cardiac output rises slightly, with a reduction of cardiac work and MVO_2.[8] There is no evidence of myocardial regional oxygenation imbalance. Many workers have found no evidence of myocardial depression in humans or animals.
3 Bradycardia (about 10 bpm on average) is probably due to central vagal activity. Asystole has been claimed to occur rarely. The atrial–His interval lengthens about 10% from 80 ms. The sinus node recovery time (SNRT) lengthens about 20% from 1000 ms. Very rarely, atrioventricular (AV) block develops, so premedication with an anticholinergic drug may be desirable, especially in beta-blocked and Ca^{2+}-channel blocked patients. Glycopyrronium or atropine are very suitable.
4 Reduction of systemic vascular resistance (SVR) of up to 30% in humans on bolus doses of 2 mg/kg.
5 Variable reductions in blood catecholamines.

6 In the sick sinus syndrome, propofol may be associated with brief periods of atrial flutter.

7 In hypertrophic obstructive cardiomyopathy (HOCM), propofol 1 mg/kg given slowly over 4 min with an opioid, has given good cardiovascular stability and increased cardiac output.

Respiration

Respiratory depression, dose-related. Less risk of laryngospasm and broncho-spasm than thiopentone.[9]

Cerebral

Reduction of $CMRO_2$ without reduction of cerebral perfusion pressure (CPP), potentiated by sevo-flurane.[10]

Interaction with volatile anaesthetics

Reduction of MAC, up to 100%, when full TIVA doses are infused.

Side-effects

Nausea and vomiting 1–2% (less than with most other induction agents). Pain on injection, more so in small peripheral veins. Pain reduced by mixing with local analgesics or diluting the drug with an equal volume of saline, or cooling the drug.[11] Slow eye-opening on emergence.[12]

Cerebral

Propofol reduces the duration of the fit in electroconvulsive therapy.

Myotonic effects

These have been classified as (i) minor, i.e. twitches of hands and feet; (ii) major, resembling a convulsion, or opisthotonus. These effects have not endangered life and are short-lived except in patients with dystrophia myotonica.[13] They may occur after anaesthesia. Many anaesthetists avoid the use of propofol in epileptic patients, although others argue that there is no sound basis for this action (*see* Sneyd, J. R. *Br. J. Anaesth.*, **82,** 168–169, 1999)

Anaphylaxis is rare.

Interactions

The half-life of alfentanil is prolonged.[14] Interaction with fentanyl is more complex.[15]

Clinical use

(Note: propofol is drawn up just prior to use. Toxic shock has occurred when the drug was contaminated with Staphylococcus aureus, incubated for several hours (overnight?) in a hot environment and then administered intravenously.)

1 As an induction agent.
2 Propofol infusion for maintenance of anaesthesia (TIVA). The maintenance infusion rate (MIR) is initially 10 mg/kg/h, falling to 8 mg/kg/h after some minutes and then to 6 mg/kg/h.[16] Target-controlled infusions (TCI) are used for this, e.g. 3.5–4 μg/ml, using age and weight.[17] For management of TIVA, *see below.*
3 For control of status epilepticus.[18]
4 For sedation in critically ill patients 1–5 mg/kg/h (blood level 1–5 μg/ml) with rapid offset, and very slight accumulation, enabling earlier discharge from intensive care units.
5 To reduce pruritis due to epidural morphine (target blood level 1 μg/ml).

THIOPENTONE SODIUM BP: THIOPENTAL USP (PENTOTHAL; TRAPANAL; PENTHIOBARBITAL; INTRAVAL; NESDONAL; FARMOTAL)

This is sodium ethyl (1-methyl butyl) thiobarbiturate. It is the sulphur analogue of pentobarbitone. Introduced commercially as pentothal sodium in 1935.

It is a yellow amorphous powder, soluble in water (and alcohol), diluted to a 2.5 % solution with pH 10.8–11. To prevent formation of free acid by CO_2 from the atmosphere, 6% anhydrous sodium carbonate is added to the powder, which is prepared in an atmosphere of nitrogen. In solution it is not very stable, but can be used for 24–48 h. The oil/water coefficient is 4.7.

Average anaesthetic dose 3–5 mg/kg i.v. giving effective blood concentration of 7 μg/ml. It is largely protein bound.

Pharmacodynamics

The central nervous system

It causes sedation, hypnosis, anaesthesia and respiratory depression, and is anticonvulsant. There is useful retrograde amnesia. The cerebral cortex and the ascending reticular-activating system are depressed before the medullary centres. Cerebral blood flow, intracranial pressure, cerebral metabolism and O_2 consumption are reduced leading to 'cerebral protection' (*see* 'Neuro-anaesthesia', Chapter 4.1).

Respiratory system

Depression, depending on the dose and rate of injection, antagonized by surgical stimuli and potentiated by opioids. The sensitivity of the respiratory centre to CO_2 is reduced. Transient apnoeas on induction are common and are treated by gentle manual intermittent positive pressure ventilation (IPPV).

Cardiovascular system

Myocardial contractility is reduced, but this is compensated by tachycardia. *Reduction of peripheral vascular resistance (PVR and SVR),* leading to pooling of blood in the periphery, causing reduction in preload and cardiac output, particularly in hypovolaemia and untreated hypertension. The drug is especially dangerous when the heart cannot compensate for changes in vascular haemodynamics, e.g. beta-blockade, constrictive pericarditis, tight valvular stenosis, complete heart block.

Hypotension, depending on rate and amount of drug injected, due to vasodilatation in skin and muscle. Blood pressure falls are likely to be greater in hypertensive or hypovolaemic patients and in those with cardiac or adrenocortical insufficiency.

Larynx

Increased sensitivity to stimuli. Laryngeal spasm may occur.

Eyes

Pupils first dilate, then contract. Reaction is lost with surgical anaesthesia. It reduces intraocular tension.

Loss of eyelash reflex is an excellent sign of adequate induction of anaesthesia.

Pregnant uterus

Thiopentone has no effect on its tone. It crosses the placental barrier, achieving its maximal concentration in fetal blood a few minutes after its injection into the mother.

Kidney

A powerful stimulator of antidiuretic hormone (ADH) secretion.

Pharmacokinetics

After injection of an anaesthetic dose of thiopentone, the blood level reaches 7–10 μg/ml within a minute, then falls rapidly and the patient regains consciousness due to the rapid redistribution of the drug to viscera, lean body mass (muscles etc.). It rapidly crosses the blood–brain barrier due to its low degree of ionization and its high lipid solubility. Equilibrium between plasma and brain is established 1 min after intravenous injection.

Distribution follows a bi- or tri-exponential model, first phase 2–4 min, second phase 40–50 min. Acumulation occurs rapidly.

Elimination half-life is 9 h (hepatic extraction ratio 0.15). Renal disease is not a contraindication to its use, although uraemia potentiates and prolongs thiopentone narcosis. Eliminated more rapidly in the young than in the old so the old require smaller doses.

Miscellaneous effects

It passes into the breast milk shortly after injection. Induction of liver enzymes which metabolize warfarin and related anticoagulants. Rarely, localized muscular spasm with pronation of the forearm receiving the injection which can be lessened by narcotic analgesics.

Causes muscular necrosis if injected into muscular tissue.

Males need more than females; the fat need more than the thin; the young need more than the old.

Complications

Local complications

PERIVENOUS INJECTION

This may cause pain, redness and swelling; haematoma formation; bruising; rarely ulceration (due to alkalinity of the solution). It may lead to median nerve injury if injection is made into the medial side of the antecubital fossa. Should solution be deposited outside the vein, 10 ml of normal saline can be injected into the area. This dilutes the thiopentone solution and aids absorption. Heparinoid cream is gently rubbed into the area hourly for several hours to prevent thrombonecrosis.

INTRA-ARTERIAL INJECTION

Symptoms
When it occurs the patient usually, but not always, feels severe burning pain down the limb. It can be avoided by injecting 2 ml of solution, and inquiring as to any pain experienced by the patient. Only if this is absent should the main injection proceed. Accidental injection into arterial cannulae and arteries around the ankle and back of hand may occur.

Late signs
May include: (i) ulcers or blisters; (ii) oedema of forearm and hand. Oedematous areas may recover, the cause of such cases being spasm rather than thrombosis. Gangrene following the intra-arterial injection of 2.5% solution is extremely rare.

Immediate symptoms and signs of intra-arterial thiopentone.

These may include:

1 Pain during injection.

2 A white hand with cyanosed fingers due to arterial spasm, which may be accompanied or followed by arterial thrombosis.

3 Patches of skin discoloration in the limb.

4 Onset of unconsciousness may be delayed beyond the usual.

Thiopentone may be accidentally injected into abnormal arteries on the back of the hand, or into arterial cannulae.

Pathology

1 The changes in pH of thiopentone which occur when it is mixed with blood in an artery result in precipitation of solid crystals of thiopentone which are swept along and eventually block small vascular channels at arteriolar and capillary levels. The crystals remain in the small vessels and their irritant properties cause a local release of noradrenaline with subsequent vascular spasm. Thus, the more of the drug injected, the greater the effect.

2 The essential lesion is arterial thrombosis, and it may not become complete for 5 days. Some of the morbidity of the intra-arterial injection of thiopentone is due to the thrombosis of the small arteries supplying nerves, and so interfering with their conduction of motor impulses.

3 Endothelial damage may be a factor.

Treatment

1 Heparin, 1000 units, is given via the cannula into the artery.

2 Though cannula in the artery inject:
   (a) papaverine 40–80 mg in 10–20 ml of saline;
   (b) prostacyclin infusion 1 μg/min;
   (c) dexamethasone injection 8 mg to reduce oedema of the arterial wall;
   (d) tolazoline (Priscol) 5 ml of 1% solution, or as a continuous drip (if available); this is a noradrenaline antagonist;
   (e) phenoxybenzamine (if available), either (0.5 mg i.a. which does not appreciably affect the general circulation or as a drip diluted with saline 50–200 μg/min;
   (f) urokinase has been suggested.[19]

3 Cancel the operation (unless it is life-saving).

4 Possibly continue volatile anaesthesia as an effective method of securing vasodilatation if the above methods are not available.

5 Perform a brachial plexus or stellate ganglion block to remove all vasoconstrictor impulses.

Key points of treatment for intra-arterial thiopentone

1 Leave cannula in the artery.
2 Dilution of injected thiopentone with heparin and saline.
3 Relief of arterial spasm and the pain it causes.
4 Prevention of thrombosis.
5 Later treatment of such symptoms as may arise (including surgical referral).

---

6 Elevate limb, wrap in sterile towels, keep it warm and monitor radial pulse, condition of fingers.
7 The oral, longer-acting anticoagulants may be necessary for the 2 weeks following.
8 Consider fasciotomy (vascular surgery referral) and hyperbaric oxygen.
9 Information – patient and staff, documentation, plastic surgery referral.

THROMBOPHLEBITIS

This is due to chemical irritation of the vein wall. It may follow the injection or be postponed for 7–10 days. It should be treated by heat, elevation, anticoagulation and rest.

INJURY TO NERVES

Injury to a nerve produces an immediate intense shooting pain in the distribution of the nerve. The area should be generously infiltrated with a local analgesic or saline solution and a neurological opinion sought.

AUTOERYTHROCYTE SENSITIZATION SYNDROME

The painful bruising syndrome.[20]

General complications

1 *Respiratory depression*, and airway obstruction. Laryngeal spasm is more common than with propofol. Oxygen is administered by gentle manual IPPV via a mask. In partial spasm this may be sufficient. If the spasm does not resolve within 30 s, suxamethonium 20–30 mg i.v. may be required to relax the spasm, with or without intubation.
2 *Circulatory collapse*. This is usually due to a relative overdose causing vasodilatation and myocardial depression. It may also be due to anaphylaxis. Treatment: raise the legs; give oxygen by IPPV; infuse fluids fast intravenously, administer inotropes. ALS may be needed.

3 *Coughing:* a sign of regurgitation, salivation or over-light anaesthesia. Hiccup occasionally seen.
4 *True cutaneous allergy* can occur either in the form of a scarlatiniform rash or as true angioneurotic oedema. Photosensitivity to thiopentone in patients recently exposed to sunlight has been reported.
5 *Severe anaphylactic reactions (allergy). See below.* These reactions, although very rare, are dangerous. They may take the form of cutaneous manifestations (rashes, weals, flushes, oedema), cardiovascular collapse (hypotension, tachycardia), bronchospasm, laryngospasm and muscle rigidity or abdominal pain.

Conditions requiring special precautions

1 Acute intermittent porphyria. Barbiturates may precipitate lower motor neuron paralysis and perhaps death, and are absolutely contraindicated. If suspected, the urine should be tested for porphyrins. It has been suggested that not all patients with porphyria are sensitive to barbiturates. *See also* Chapter 3.2.
2 A history of thiopentone anaphylaxis, which has a high mortality.
3 Shock, hypotension, hypovolaemia, dehydration, severe anaemia and uraemia. Very small doses (0.5–1 mg/kg) are required. The drug causes vasodilatation and reduces cardiac output. Preoxygenation is important. (This also denitrogenates the lungs and allows N_2O to exert its analgesic effects more quickly, so reducing the need for thiopentone.)
4 Poor cardiac reserve. The biggest risk is when this is asymptomatic. A high index of suspicion should be maintained for this condition. Thiopentone should be used with extreme caution – if at all – in cases of constrictive pericarditis, tight valvular (e.g. aortic) stenosis and complete heart block. There is sudden perfusion of the drug into coronary vessels in right-to-left shunt.
5 Patients with respiratory disease.
6 Patients with respiratory obstruction or status asthmaticus.
7 Patients with acute inflammation about the mouth, jaw and neck, trismus, Ludwigs angina. Loss of the airway may prove lethal.
8 Cases of dystrophia myotonica – it causes severe respiratory depression and prolonged apnoea may follow even small doses.
9 Alcoholics taking disulfiram (Antabuse) and patients suffering from poisoning with dinitro-orthocresol (DNC), a weed killer (barbiturates and DNC have a synergistic depressant effect on cellular respiration).
10 Hyperkalaemic familial periodic paralysis.
11 Huntington's chorea. *See* Chapter 3.2.

Methohexitone 1–2 mg/kg, is similar to thiopentone.

ETOMIDATE (HYPNOMIDATE)

The commercial preparation is presented in 10-ml ampoules containing 2 mg/ml of the drug dissolved in water with 35% propylene glycol. The pH is 8.1.

Pharmacokinetics

Dose: 0.2 mg/kg. Etomidate distributes equally between red blood cells and plasma and the protein binding is 76.5%. Only 2.5% of the injected dose remains in the circulation 2 min after administration, at which time peak concentrations are found in the brain and major organs.

Metabolism: by plasma and liver esterases. In the rat model, it is potentially porphyrogenic.[21]

Histamine release has not been reported.

Pharmacodynamics

Surgical anaesthesia in one arm–brain circulation, duration 3–5 min. Repeated doses are not cumulative.

Central nervous system

Cerebral blood flow, intracranial and intraocular pressure are reduced.

Cardiovascular system

Myocardial contractility is stimulated, with mild peripheral and coronary vasodilatation, making it most suitable for patients with poor cardiac function or hypotension.

In the young it causes some hypertension on induction (less so in the elderly).

Respiratory system

Respiratory rate slows and tidal volume rises for a brief period following induction. Respiration may then be shallow, but apnoea is likely to be brief and is less common than after thiopentone. Coughing and hiccup are uncommon.

Alimentary system

Postoperative nausea and vomiting occur.

Table 2.4.1

Drug	Propofol	Thiopentone	Methohexitone	Etomidate
Induction dose (mg/kg)	1–3	3–5	1.5	0.2
Repeat dose (mg/kg)	0.5	2	0.5	0.1
Duration	2 min	5 min	3 min	2 min
Clearance	1.8 l/min			

Side-effects

Etomidate may, very rarely cause an anaphylactoid reaction.[22]

Pain at the site of injection, occurring in a quarter to a half of patients, is reduced by the addition of 0.1% lignocaine.

Muscle movements, not associated with epileptiform discharges. The origin of these movements therefore probably lies in deep cerebral structures or the brain stem; decreased by opioids and increased by even mild reflex stimulation. It potentiates both types of muscle relaxants.[23]

Etomidate infusion suppresses the secretion of cortisol and aldosterone for up to 22 h following its termination and is not now recommended.[24]

THE BENZODIAZEPINES

These are used for premedication, co-induction, sedation (e.g. in endoscopy) and to prevent unpleasant dreams with ketamine. Sedation with these drugs needs care![25]

Continuous infusion may be used in the intensive care unit, usually with opioids.

Pharmacodynamics

The onset of these drugs is in minutes if given intravenously.

Central nervous system

Inhibition at γ-aminobutyric acid (GABA) receptors. Relieves tension and anxiety. Causes drowsiness and controls convulsions. Not analgesic. Their effects summate with those of other sedatives including alcohol. Can be safely given to patients receiving monoamine oxidase inhibitors. Thought to depress the limbic system and the amygdala where fear, anxiety and aggression are generated. Causes anterograde amnesia (for about 10 min after

---

Co-induction of anaesthesia

A combination of two or more synergistic or additive induction agents to produce anaesthesia using smaller doses of each drug.

Drugs used: midazolam, propofol, alfentanil, fentanyl, thiopentone, etc.

Advantages
If drugs act on same receptor, group, there is potentiation of anaesthetic effect with reduced side-effects. Potentially cheaper!

Disadvantages
1 Interactions: interference with binding, distribution, action, metabolism or excretion of each other, e.g. fentanyl and propofol; opioid and benzodiazepine.
2 Differing onset times and durations of different drugs.

---

intravenous injection, sometimes much longer after oral doses). Used to control drug-induced dyskinesias. Do not cause nausea or vomiting. Do not increase cerebral blood flow and can be used in patients with head injury.

Respiratory system

Cause a slight depression of breathing, usually not serious, except in the elderly and when combined with opioids or barbiturates.

Cardiovascular system

Myocardial depression and hypotension not common but can cause collapse in patients with critical cardiac function.

Muscular system

Potentiate non-depolarizing relaxants and reduces the amount of relaxation due to suxamethonium. Relieve muscle spasm and spasticity.

Pharmacokinetics

They bind to plasma proteins with distribution to muscle and fat, in hours (much longer in preterm neonates). Benzodiazepines are potentiated and prolonged by inhibition of their metabolism by cimetidine.

Excretion of metabolites is mostly in the gut and urine.

Clinical uses

Have been given orally, intramuscularly, intravenously, epidurally or rectally. There is great variation of response to these drugs.

Assessment of adequacy of sedation is by Verrill's sign[26] when the upper eyelid droops to halfway across the pupil.

Rapid injection can cause apnoea.

Midazolam (Hypnovel)

This is a water-soluble benzodiazepine which can be used for premedication, induction of anaesthesia, and sedation.

Pharmacokinetics: 95% bound to plasma albumin. Distributed as two-compartment model. $T\frac{1}{2}\beta$ 1.45 h. Metabolized by hepatic P450 to 1- and 4-hydroxymethyl midazolam. Severe accumulation occurs in hepatic failure.

Pharmacodynamics: onset of action in 1–2 min, duration 1–2 h. Sedation dose 0.01–0.1 mg/kg, anaesthetic induction dose 0.15–0.3 mg/kg. Infusion rate for sedation 2–5 μg/kg/min.

Transient apnoea has been observed with a dosage of 0.15 mg/kg which is not sufficient to induce anaesthesia reliably in unpremedicated subjects. Anterograde amnesia and drowsiness are common. It can be used with fentanyl as a cardiovascular-stable anaesthetic, reversible by flumazenil.[27]

Cardiovascular stability is reasonable, with 10% falls of arterial pressure in 10% of subjects, and some tachycardias.

Temazepam

Mainly used in premedication of patients of all ages, oral dose 0.5 mg/kg; onset 10–20 min, duration 0.5–4 h.

Diazepam

Used as intravenous sedative and amnesic for endoscopy, as anticonvulsant, and orally as anxiolytic. Dose: 0.05–0.2 mg/kg i.v., 0.1–0.2 mg/kg orally. May also be given rectally and intramuscularly. Duration 1–2 h.

Lorazepam (Ativan)

May be given orally or by injection. Duration 12 h (occasionally several days). Oral dose 1–5 mg or may be given intramuscularly, dose 2–4 mg.

Antagonists

Flumazenil is the specific antagonist at GABA-controlled chloride channels. Adult dose: 0.1–0.5 mg, given slowly intravenously or intramuscularly. Onset 1–5 min; duration 1–3 h. Side-effects: these mainly arise from reversal of benzodiazepine effects, e.g. appearance or reappearance of convulsions, return of anxiety and respiratory responsiveness. Successfully reverses benzodiazepine–fentanyl anaesthesia.[27]

SHORT-ACTING NARCOTIC ANALGESICS (OPIOIDS)

See Table 2.4.2.
Note: for other opioids, *see* Chapter 1.6.

Alfentanil (Rapifen)

First used in 1981. Adult dose for supplementary analgesia without apnoea: 5–10 μg/kg; dose for suppressing the 'stress response': 50–100 μg/kg. Infusion dose: 0.5–1 μg/kg/min (30–60 μg/kg/h) if no other opioids have been given. Onset: 30–60 s. Duration: 5–10 min, doubled by propofol.

Pharmacokinetics:[28] 90% bound to plasma proteins, only moderately lipid soluble, biexponential decay, $T_{\frac{1}{2}}\alpha$ 5 min, $T_{\frac{1}{2}}\beta$ 95 min (63 min in children), hepatic extraction ratio 0.4–0.7, elimination half-life 130 min.

Side-effects: bradycardia, nausea and vomiting (short-lived).

Particularly suitable as a supplement to anaesthesia in short procedures and in day-case surgery. May also be used in repeated dosage or continuous infusion in major surgery. Large dose alfentanil (70 μg/kg) is effective as a pre-emptive analgesic, reducing morphine requirements for up to 48 h after surgery.[29]

Remifentanil

Formulation in glycine and water, this formulation is not used in central neural blockade.

Adult infusion dose for co-induction of anaesthesia: 0.5–1 μg/kg/min (maintained for 5 min). Maintenance infusion rate (spontaneous respiration) 25–100 ng/kg/min. Dose for suppressing the 'stress response': 5–10 μg/kg in ventilated patients. Onset: 30–60 s after bolus (blood–brain equilibration half-time 1.3 min), but an infusion over 6 min is regarded as a more reliable way to achieve a plateau concentration. Elimination half-life 6–11 min (degraded by non-specific plasma and tissue esterases). Offset: 3–5 min after cessation of infusion.

Pharmacokinetics: not subject to changing context-sensitive half-time and has a reliable offset, no matter how long it has been infused. Clearance 40–70 ml/kg/min, $T\frac{1}{2}\alpha$ 3–5 min, it is hydrolysed by plasma and tissue esterases.

Effective blood levels 1 ng/ml for analgesia, 30 ng/ml for stress-response suppression.

Particularly useful as a supplement to anaesthesia in short procedures and in day-case surgery. May also be used in continuous infusion in major surgery, neurosurgery (where rapid wake-up is important) and for sedation. To prevent metabolic and endocrine responses to surgery, higher doses are necessary, starting before the operation, without fear of prolonged postoperative sedation. Rapid cessation of analgesia has to be catered for.

Fentanyl citrate (Phentanyl; Sublimaze)

Effects: intense analgesia, respiratory depression which precedes the analgesia, miosis, nausea and vomiting, which outlast the analgesia, bradycardia, various effects on smooth muscle, depending on the dose used, and addiction.

Adult dose: 0.025–0.1 mg. Respiratory depression is managed by IPPV, or antagonized by naloxone. Infusion dose of fentanyl to prevent postoperative stress response: 4–10 μg/kg/h. Onset: respiratory depression in 30–60 s, analgesia in 5–10 min (dose related). Duration 30–60 min. Terminal half-life 3–6 h (1–7 h in neonates). Fentanyl undergoes enterohepatic recirculation with rebound effects at 3–5 h after injection. (These effects do not exceed the initial ones, but delayed respiratory depression following apparent recovery of respiratory activity after fentanyl has been reported). Fentanyl is mostly destroyed in the liver and about 10% excreted in the urine.

Interactions: with diazepam it causes serious hypotension. With midazolam it causes serious respiratory depression and hypoxia.[30] It attenuates the hypertension resulting from ketamine. It potentiates anaesthetics (including midazolam) reducing dosage and minimum alveolar concentration (MAC). Intravenous boluses of fentanyl can cause a cough.[31]

Large doses of fentanyl may result in muscular rigidity, making IPPV difficult, but a relaxant will overcome this effect.

Fentanyl is highly lipophilic and is absorbed from the epidural and other fatty spaces very fast giving blood levels similar to the intravenous route.[32]

Context-sensitive half-time

The duration of fentanyl (and thiopentone, and to a lesser extent, midazolam, sufentanil and alfentanil) is extended by giving larger doses or for a longer time, as infusion, possibly because redistribution occurs slower than clearance once the volume of distribution is fully occupied.[33] This limits the usefulness of these drugs where very rapid emergence is required, e.g. in neurosurgery and the intensive therapy unit (ITU). This effect is not seen with remifentanil.

Table 2.4.2

Drug	Alfentanil	Fentanyl	Sufentanil
Bolus dose (analgesia)	5–10 μg/kg	1 μg/kg	1 μg/kg
Bolus dose (stress suppression)	50–100 μg/kg	10 μg/kg	5 μg/kg
Onset	0.5 min	1–4 min	1–4 min
Duration	5–10 min	30 min	30 min
$T_{\frac{1}{2}}\beta$	95 min	2–4 h	2–3 h

Sufentanil

Dose for supplementary analgesia: 1 μg/kg; dose for suppressing stress response: 5–20 μg/kg; infusion dose: 0.01 μg/kg/min. Onset: 1–4 min.[34] Duration: 30–60 min.

Pharmacokinetics: highly lipophilic, 90% bound to plama glycoprotein and albumin; biexponential decay, $T_{\frac{1}{2}}\beta$ 164 min (53–55 min in children[35]). Metabolized by O-demethylation and N-dealkylation.

Pharmacodynamics: intense analgesia with good cardiovascular stability even at 'stress-response inhibiting doses'.

A powerful respiratory depressant.[36] (For effects on cerebral circulation and metabolism, *see* Milde L. M., Milde J. H. and Gallagher W. J. *Anesth. Analg.* 1990, **70**, 138.)

The side effects of opioids are troublesome. An acetylcholine receptor blocker, ABT 594, as powerful an analgesic as morphine but acting on other receptors is being investigated.[37]

BUTYROPHENONES

Droperidol (Dehydrobenzperidol; Droleptan; Inapsine)

Pharmacodynamics: the butyrophenones cause mental detachment, absence of voluntary movements (catatonia), a dopaminergic inhibitory effect on the chemoreceptor trigger zone controlling nausea and vomiting and weak α-adrenergic receptor blocking action (sometimes causing hypotension). The butyrophenones compete with GABA at postsynaptic receptor sites.

Pharmacokinetics: dose: 0.1 mg/kg. Onset of effect 3–20 min after intravenous injection. Duration of effect up to 12 h. Large doses may cause extrapyramidal dyskinesia which can be overcome by antiparkinson agents (other than levodopa); diazepam or promethazine.

THE PHENOTHIAZINE DERIVATIVES

This group of drugs includes, among hundreds of others, the following:

Promethazine hydrochloride BP (Phenergan, Atosil)

Pharmacodynamics:

1 it is a powerful hypnotic in its own right (especially in children) and potentiates barbiturates and narcotic analgesics, possibly by an influence on liver
cells.
2 Powerful antagonism to histamine by its effect on H1 receptors.
3 It is a potent depressant of upper respiratory tract reflexes and is a bronchodilator.
4 It has slight atropine-like activity.
5 It is said to increase sensitivity to pain.
6 It antagonises 5-hydroxytryptamine.

It is particularly useful as a premedication, especially in asthmatics.
It is supplied as 2.5% solution and as tablets, 25 mg, and elixir, 1 mg/ml.
Dose for premedication: 0.2–1 mg/kg.

Trimeprazine tartrate BPC (Vallergan)

Also used as premedication in children, but occasionally causes restlessness.
Dose for premedication: 2 mg/kg but more has been used.

Promazine hydrochloride BP USP (Sparine)

A useful antiemetic and sedative in ITU and neuroanaesthesia.
Average adult dose: 25–50 mg i.m. 8-hourly.

Prochlorperazine maleate BP USP (Stemetil, Compazine)

Excellent antiemetic. Dose: 12.5–25 mg i.m. or p.o.
Has been used to control vertigo after inner and middle-ear operations.

DISSOCIATIVE ANAESTHESIA

Ketamine (Ketalar; Ketaject)

Ketamine is 2-*o*-chlorophenyl-2-methylaminocyclohexanone hydrochloride.
It is a white crystalline substance with a characteristic smell. Readily soluble
in water, pH 3.5–4.1 in 10% solution. Supplied in 1, 5 and 10% solutions.

Pharmacodynamics

Ketamine is rapidly absorbed after oral, intramuscular or intravenous administration. The injection of a therapeutic dose of ketamine produces a state of dissociative anaesthesia. The sleep produced is somewhat different from that of conventional anaesthesia. It occurs within minutes of intramuscular or intravenous injection due to NMDA receptor blockade and lasts for up to 15 min. Other NMDA blockers include memantine and dextromethorphan. Analgesia is a marked feature and extends into the postoperative period.[38]

CARDIOVASCULAR SYSTEM

Systolic and diastolic blood pressures are raised (attenuated by fentanyl) and pulse rate increases by myocardial stimulation and systemic and pulmonary vasconstriction. The chronotropic effect is not blocked by verapamil or beta-blockade. There is a rise in plasma noradrenaline which can be reduced by prior administration of droperidol. It has an antidysrhythmia effect.

RESPIRATORY SYSTEM

Respiration is not depressed, except by large doses, and is usually mildly stimulated. The airway is not obstructed except under deep ketamine anaesthesia. The prevention of aspiration under ketamine, while good, cannot be guaranteed.

ALIMENTARY SYSTEM

Nausea and vomiting occur and require prophylaxis. Salivation may be troublesome unless prevented by atropine or glycopyrronium.

OCULAR

Some rise of intraocular pressure may occur, but this is transient and ketamine has been recommended for tonometry in children. Eye movements and nystagmus may occur.

SKIN

Transient erythema has been reported in 15% of patients and is of little consequence.

CEREBRAL

Increases cerebral blood flow and intracranial pressure with marked regional variations.[39] Dreaming, hallucinations and delirium occur.

Phonation may take place in light ketamine anaesthesia.

LIMBS

Non-purposeful movements are seen in light ketamine anaesthesia.

Pharmacokinetics

It is converted to water-soluble norketamine by N-demethylation and hydroxylation of the cyclohexanone ring. These are excreted in the urine. $T_{\frac{1}{2}}\beta$ 153 min., Vd 2.3 l/kg.

Clinical uses

Dose: 1–2 mg/kg, i.v. and supplementary doses of 0.5 mg/kg, or 10 mg/kg i.m. Intravenous infusion rate: 40 μg/kg/min. There is a small amount of cumulation. Onset: 1 min (i.v.) and 10 min (i.m.) (shorter in children).

Ketamine is a rapidly acting parenteral anaesthetic causing sedation, profound analgesia, catalepsy, some increase in striated muscle tone, mild cardiovascular stimulation, but only slight diminution of pharyngolaryngeal reflexes. Less efficient as a visceral analgesic. It increases salivation so that atropine should always be used. Intravenous injection should take 60–120 s. Has been employed:

1 as the sole agent for minor operations;
2 as an induction agent before general anaesthesia;
3 when airway control is difficult;
4 for certain neurological radiodiagnostic and therapeutic procedures in children to abolish movement;
5 when maintenance of blood pressure is important, e.g. in states of shock and in some poor-risk patients and in the elderly;
6 for dressing of burns, skin debridement, skin grafts, etc.;
7 for dealing with mass casualties;
8 when intramuscular injection is more convenient than intravenous.
9 to produce analgesia at subanaesthetic doses;
10 for induction of anaesthesia in small children.

A 0.1% solution in 5% dextrose has been given as a slow intravenous drip for postoperative pain relief and for analgesia in patients in the intensive care unit.[41]

Interactions: it potentiates propofol and the speed of onset of rocuronium (compared to thiopentone).

Duration: 3–10 min (i.v.) and 10–30 min (i.m.), longer in the elderly.

Used in Bier's technique for intravenous regional analgesia, it produces analgesia in the arm, unfortunately followed by unconsciousness a few minutes after release of the tourniquet[41] and extradurally, 4 mg in 10 ml of 5% dextrose in water when it is reported to give good pain relief after operation without side-effects.[42]

Ketamine has been used safely in porphyria.[43]

Ketamine produces only transient hormonal changes which are minor in comparison with those superimposed by surgery. Ketamine analgesia is partially reversed by naloxone.

Ketamine has been used for intradural analgesia in war surgery.[44]

Adverse reactions

Hypertension, tachycardia, rashes.

Dreams: vivid unpleasant dreams occur, and occasionally true hallucinations. The incidence of these emergence phenomena increases with age, being about 5% under 5yrs of age, and 50% in adulthood. They can be reduced by:

1 leaving the patient without stimulation in the recovery period;
2 use of opiate and hyoscine premedication;
3 injection of droperidol (2.5–7.5 mg i.m. or i.v.) towards the end of surgery;
4 small amounts of midazolam, lorazepam or thiopentone.

These dreams occur during surgery as well as after it. 4-aminopyridine, 0.3 mg/kg, aids recovery from ketamine.

TOTAL INTRAVENOUS ANAESTHESIA (TIVA OR INFUSION ANAESTHESIA)

This technique became practicable in the early 1970s with the advent of non-barbiturate induction agents[45] and became widespread with the discovery of propofol.

It may be used for general anaesthesia or sedation during regional blockade. It may be used alone or in combination with gaseous anaesthetics.

The following agents have been used: propofol, propanidid, ketamine, S-ketamine and short-acting opioids. A good combination (allowing rapid recovery) is propofol (10–4 mg/kg/h) and remifentanil (0.1 μg/kg/min) infusion. With practice, satisfactory spontaneous respiration is easily achievable.

Table 2.4.3 Compares inhalational anaesthesia and TIVA.

Precautions needed with total intravenous anaesthesia[46]

1 Machine check before use.
2 Battery backup is important, for failure of mains supply.
3 Empty syringe warning is important.
4 Blocked (e.g. by a tap) delivery pipe warning is important.
5 Full resuscitation equipment required.
6 The delivery pipe/dedicated intravenous cannula – union may be 'pull-detachable' to prevent the cannula from being pulled out of the vein.
7 The intravenous cannula should be kept in sight to monitor this.

Table 2.4.3 Comparison of TIVA with inhalation anaesthesia.

Potency values	Inhalation MAC 50 & MAC 95	TIVA MIR 50 & MIR 95
Types of patient:		
Alcoholics	Resistant	Resistant
Elderly patients	Sensitive	Sensitive
Respiratory failure	Difficult	Easier
Difficult airway	Difficult	Difficult
Complications:		
Airway obstruction	A risk	A risk
Apnoea	A risk	A risk
Cross-infection	A risk	A risk
Awareness	Risk in alcoholics etc.	Risk in alcoholics etc.
Caused by	Empty vaporizer	Empty syringe
	Disconnections	Disconnections
	Machine failures	Machine failures

8 Caution about using mixtures of intravenous agents – they may interact or have different lengths of action.
9 A proper syringe refill system for use during the anaesthetic must be organized before starting.
10 *Respiratory monitoring is essential;* e.g. with mask and bag system using air or O_2/N_2O as the fresh gas. Note: pulse oximetry alone is not a monitor of respiration.
11 Normal minimal monitoring.

Awareness may be a problem when relaxants are used, as with a 'volatile' technique. Depth of anaesthesia monitoring with bispectral index is simple and practical.

Monitoring depth with infusion anaesthesia

1 The pattern of movement of the bag on the breathing system.
2 Bispectral index.
3 Spectral edge frequency.
4 The isolated arm technique: a response to asking for a squeeze of the anaesthetist's hand implies wakefulness.
5 Lower oesophageal contractions.
6 Frontalis electromyogram (EMG).
7 The elecetroencephalogram (EEG) (*see* 'Awareness', Chapter 2.8). The changes are somewhat specific to each individual agent, but has been used to automatically control propofol infusion.
8 Sensory evoked potentials (SEP).

Factors contributing to unplanned awareness

POOR EQUIPMENT:
  Wrong drug in vaporizer
  Leak at vaporizer
  Leaks in machine/system
  Leak in O_2-powered ventilator
  Lack of agent monitor
  Failure of agent monitor
  Use of circle system
  Lack of awareness monitor

POOR TECHNIQUES:
  Vaporizer run out
  Forget to turn vaporizer on
  Forget O_2 flush on
  Lack of analgesia
  Lack of premedication
  Reliance on opioids
  Reliance on N_2O
  Reliance on relaxants
  Total intravenous anaesthesia
  Miscalculation of dose of anaesthetic
  Delay due to difficult intubation etc

DIFFICULT PATIENTS:
  Natural variation in resistance to anaesthetic
  Past history of awareness
  Addicts
  Alcoholics
  Young patients
  Very sick and emergency cases

SOME OPERATIONS:
  Caesarean section
  Bronchoscopy
  Cardiopulmonary bypass.

SEDATION TECHNIQUES – 'SEDOANALGESIA'

This is a combination of regional analgesia and light sedation, perhaps aided by some forms of sensory deprivation, e.g. ear muffs, eye shades, etc. Propofol infusion is popular, with target blood level of 1–1.5 μg/ml.[47] Most of the agents in this chapter have been mentioned as having sedative actions. Because of the side-effects of all these drugs, and the need to monitor and control the patient's physiology during surgery, these techniques need as much care from the anaesthetist as a full general anaesthetic.[48]

SOME TYPES OF ADVERSE DRUG REACTION

1 Immediate: Type II and III: direct activation, not requiring antibody generation (dextran, althesin, haemaccel and other plasma expanders).
2 Complement activation (prior exposure necessary).
3 Histamine release, e.g. thiopentone, morphine, suxamethonium, atracurium, mivacurium.

Antibodies: innate; acquired – IgG is the most abundant immunoglobulin in body fluids, complement binding, active against microorganisms and toxins, producing type II reaction; IgE non-complement binding produces type I reaction with anaphylaxis, especially in atopic patients. activated by thiopentone.[49]

If in doubt about a history of allergy to anaesthetic drugs, the anaesthetist can conduct preanaesthetic intradermal skin testing using dilutions of 1/1000; except for morphine and induction agents (1/100).

A flare greater than 5 mm indicates significant allergy.

Adverse drug reactions during anaesthesia

Due to:

1 overdose;

2 intolerance;

3 side-effects;

4 hypersensitivity;

5 allergy and anaphylaxis.

These may also be due to 'non-anaesthetic' drugs (Parker S. D., Curry C. S. and Hirshman C. A. *Anesth. Analg.* 1990, **70**, 220). Perianaesthetic rashes are not uncommon (Desmueles H. *Anesth. Analg.* 1990, **70**, 216).

Treatment: adrenaline is far better than ephedrine and antagonizes all the mediators of hypersensitivity and anaphylaxis: histamine, SRS-A, prostaglandins, serotonin, bradykinin. Proprietary intramuscular adrenaline self-injectors are available.

REFERENCES

1 Sasada M. and Smith S. *Drugs in Anaesthesia and Intensive Care.* Oxford University Press, Oxford, 1997.
2 Kay B. and Rolly G. *Acta Anaesthiol. Belg.* 1977, **28,** 303.
3 Doenicke A., Roizen M. F. et al., *Anesth Analg.* 1997, **85,** 1399–1403.
4 Spelina K. R., Coates D. P., Monk C. R., Prys-Roberts C., Norley I. and Turtle M. J. *Br. J.Anaesth.* 1986, **58,** 1050
5 Irwin M. G., Thompson M. and Kenny G. N. C. *Anaesthesia* 1997, **52,** 525–530.
6 Saunders P. R. I. and Harris M. N. E. *Anaesthesia* 1990, **45,** 552–7, Mather S. J., Edwards N. D. and Biswas A. *ibid,* 1096.
7 Gin T. and Gregory M. A. *Br. J. Anaesth.* 1990, **64,** 148.
8 Vermeyen K. M., Erpels F. A., Janssen L. A., Beeckman C. P. and Hanegreefs G. H. *Br. J. Anaesth.* 1987, **59,** 1115.
9 Pizov M. R., Ron R. H. and Weiss Y. S. *Anesthesiology,* 1997, **82,** 111–116.
10 Heath K., Gupta S. and Matta B. F. *Anesth. Analg.* 1997, **85,** 1284–1287.
11 McCirrick A. and Hunter S. *Anaesthesia* 1990, **45,** 443–444.
12 Marsch S. C. U. and Schlaefer H. G. *Anesth. Analg.* 1990, **70,** 127.
13 Speedy H. *Br. J. Anaesth.* 1990, **64,** 110.
14 Gepts E. et al. *Anaesthesia* 1988, **43** (suppl.), 8–13.
15 Dixon J. and Roberts F. L. et al. *Br. J. Anaesth.* 1990, **64,** 142.
16 Roberts F. L., Dixon J., Lewis G. T. R., Tackley R. M. and Prys-Roberts C. *Anaesthesia* 1988, **43** (suppl), 14.
17 Gepts E. *Anaesthesia* 1998, **53** (suppl 1), 4–12.
18 Mackenzie S. J. et al. *Anaesthesia* 1991, **45,** 1043–1045.
19 Corser G. et al. *Anaesthesia* 1985, **40,** 51.
20 Hales P. *Anaesth. Intensive Care* 1981, **9,** 390.
21 Harrison G. G., Moore M. R. and Meissner P. N. *Br. J. Anaesth.* 1985, **57,** 420–423.
22 Sold M. J. *Anaesthesia* 1985, **40,** 1014.
23 Fragen R. J. et al. *Br. J. Anaesth.* 1983, **55,** 433.
24 Ledingham I. McA. and Watt I. *Lancet* 1983, **1,** 1270 & Moore R. A. and Allen M. C. *Anaesthesia* 1985, **40,** 124.
25 ASA Task force. *Anesthesiology* 1996, **83,** 459–461.
26 Verrill P. *Br. Dent. J.* 1969, **127,** 85.
27 Kaukinen S., Kataja J. and Kaukinen L. *Can. J. Anaesth.* 1990, **37,** 40.
28 Robbins G. R et al. *Can. J. Anaesth* 1990, **37,** 52.
29 Griffin M. J. et al. *Anesth. Analg.* 1997, **85,** 1317–1321.
30 Bailey P. et al. *Anesthesiology* 1990, **73,** 826–830.

31 Boher H., Fleischer F. and Werning P. *Anaesthesia* 1990, **45**, 18.
32 Loper K. A. et al. *Anesth. Analg.* 1990, **70**, 72.
33 Hughes A., Glass P. and Jacobs J. *Anesthesiology* 1992, **76**, 334–341.
34 Hickey P. R. and Hansen D. D. *Anesth. Analg.* 1984, **63**, 117–124.
35 Davis P. J. et al. *Anesth. Analg.* 1987, **66**, 203–208.
36 Bailey P. L. et al. *Anesth. Analg.* 1990, **70**, 8.
37 *Science* 1998, **279**, 32–33.
38 Ngan Kee W. D. and Shaw K. S. *Anesth. Analg.*1997, **85**, 1294–1298.
39 Hougaard K. et al. *Anesthesiology* 1974, **41**, 562.
40 Idvall J. et al. *Br. J. Anaesth.* 1979, **51**, 1167.
41 Amiot J. F. et al. *Anaesthesia* 1985, **40**, 899.
42 Islas J. A. et al. *Anesth. Analg. (Cleve.)* 1985, **64**, 1161.
43 Capouet V., Dernovoi B. and Azagra J. S. *Can. J. Anaesth.* 1987, **34**, 388–390.
44 Bion J. F. *Anaesthesia* 1984, **39**, 1023.
45 Boulton T. B. and Rushman G. B. *The Intermittent Administration of Propanidid for Dental Outpatients. Anaesthesiologie und Wiederbelebung.* Springer-Verlag, Heidelberg, 1973.
46 Donenfeld R. F. *Anesth. Analg.* 1990, **70**, 116.
47 Irwin M. G., Thompson M. and Kenny G. N. C. *Anaesthesia* 1997,**52**, 525–530.
48 Malviya S., Voepel-Lewis T. and Tait A. R. *Anesth. Analg.* 1997, **85**, 1207–1213, ASA Task force. *Anesthesiology* 1996, **83**, 459–461.
49 Ewan P. W. Treatment of anaphylactic reactions: *Prescribers' J.* 1997, **37**, 125–132.

Muscle relaxants

There has been a strong move in the world of anaesthesia towards production of 'clean' drugs, i.e. a simple action, without side-effects. In this respect, the ideal world and the real world are still well apart and side-effects of drugs are a daily concern for the practising anaesthetist. However, much progress has been made with 'cleaner' muscle relaxants.

Muscle relaxants used in anaesthesia can be classified as: (i) non-depolarizing agents (tachycurares), and (ii) depolarizing agents (leptocurares). Under certain circumstances depolarizing agents can exert a non-depolarizing effect, the so-called dual or biphasic block.

Muscular relaxation can also be produced centrally by deep general anaesthesia or peripherally by local nerve block. Most relaxants in clinical use are highly ionized and therefore are confined to the extracellular fluid.

PHYSIOLOGY OF THE NEUROMUSCULAR TRANSMISSION

Acetylcholine synthesis, storage and release

Acetylcholine (ACh) crosses the junctional cleft and becomes fixed at lipoprotein receptors on the junctional folds of the end-plate membrane and permits entry of sodium, which causes a sudden depolarization with exit of potassium from the muscle fibre. The depolarization passes along the membrane of the muscle fibre and is the final stimulus for causing the contraction of the contractile part of the muscle fibre. Meanwhile the released ACh is hydrolysed by acetylcholinesterase in the region of the motor end-plate. Thus, when the excited muscle fibre has come out of its refractory state it will not become excited again by a depolarized end-plate unless a new nerve impulse has arrived and released a new supply of ACh.

Depolarization causes Ca^{2+} to enter the nerve terminal. Increased permeability of the special sodium (Na^+) channels in the neuromuscular junction to Na^+ is the trigger, which leads to the propagating action potential. Na^+ enters the fibre, then K^+ leaves, as the action potential proceeds. A change of resting potential of 20 mV is adequate to initiate this process. Fresh ACh is synthesized in the axoplasm of the nerve terminal from choline obtained from the extracellular fluid (ECF) and is transferred to vesicles ready for use. This process may be defective in the shocked, acidotic or toxaemic patient, making reversal of relaxants impossible. Acetylcholine exists in the nerve terminals in two forms: storage and releasable. Acetylcholine release is a self-potentiating process, leading to greater release and giving access to the storage granules for further and subsequent release. Relaxant drugs act on the postjunctional receptors of the neuromuscular junction, and also the prejunctional receptors on the last part of the nerve fibre, where they prevent this self-potentiating release of ACh, causing the characteristic 'fade' seen on neuromuscular monitoring during partial relaxation.

Acetylcholine release and receptor stimulation in response to a nerve action potential is far greater than that required to elicit a single muscle fibre contraction. This large 'safety factor' means that up to 70–80% of the receptors can be occupied before surgical relaxation develops, and, conversely, reversal can be clinically adequate, even though many receptors are still blocked. Postoperative introduction of drugs which interact with relaxants may cause paralysis to redevelop.[1]

There are (at least) three receptors at the neuromuscular junction (two in the muscle and one in the nerve ending), which respond to ACh, by opening an ion channel: prejunctional, postjunctional and extrajunctional.

Prejunctional and preterminal receptors

Prejunctional nicotinic receptors control an ion channel that is specific for Na^+, which is essential for synthesis and mobilization of transmitter. These receptors contain protein subunits and are blocked by curare, resulting in 'fade' and exhaustion. They are also blocked by aminoglycoside and polymyxin antibiotics. The action of polymyxin which is due to competition with Ca^{2+}, does not produce 'fade', can be reversed by Ca^{2+} administration and is made worse by neostigmine. Corticosteroids, barbiturates, anticonvulsants, antidysrhythmics, beta-blockers and lithium may also cause this effect, thus potentiating muscle relaxants. Prejunctional block due to relaxants is quite different from that due to Mg^{2+} or aminoglycoside and polymyxin antibiotics.

In addition, there is evidence for a second population of preterminal nicotinic receptors situated more centrally than the prejunctional receptors.

Postjunctional receptors

These receptors are 8–9 nm in diameter with a central pit. The mouth of these special sodium channels is surrounded by five protein moieties, two of which (α) are cholinoceptors which respond to ACh or depolarizing relaxants, causing the other three subunits to rotate to a new conformation with opening of the channel. Na^+ and Ca^{2+} move into the muscle and K^+ moves out.[2] Nondepolarizing blockers bind to α subunits, preventing access of ACh, blocking the channel closed. (Depolarizing relaxants block the channel open, with initial stimulation, e.g. muscle fasciculations.) There are several hundred thousand receptors in each neuromuscular junction. Other drugs blocking these receptors are: local analgesics, aminoglycoside and polymyxin antibiotics, barbiturates, procainamide, quinidine, disopyramide.

Other reactions in postjunctional receptor channels include desensitization, physical channel blockade and blockade of intracellular mechanisms.

RECEPTOR DESENSITIZATION

The response to prolonged application of ACh to the motor end-plate is a decline in response to a new steady state. This waning in response is termed receptor desensitization or receptor downregulation. May represent a safety mechanism that prevents overexcitation. Occurs within the receptor molecule, agonist binding fails to cause an opening reaction. The rate of receptor desensitization is hastened by agonists (carbachol, suxamethonium, decamethonium), barbiturates, ACh esterase inhibitors (neostigmine, edrophonium, pyridostigmine), Ca^{2+} channel blockers (verapamil), local analgesics (procaine), phenothiazines (chlorpromazine), phencyclidine, volatile anaesthetics, aminoglycoside antibiotics, substance P, alcohol and caffeine.

PHYSICAL CHANNEL BLOCKADE

A large number of different drugs, as well as muscle relaxants, are capable of blocking ion channels at the neuromuscular junction. This prevents normal flow of ions and thus depolarization. May be caused by local analgesics (on the Na^+ channel of nerve), and Ca^{2+} antagonists (on the Ca^{2+} channels of heart and blood vessels). This blockade can occur in two modes, blocked when open and blocked when closed. Physical block by a molecule of an open channel (by cationic drugs only) relies on the channel being open in the first place, and the development of this is proportional to the frequency of channel opening. Provided its molecular size is small enough and its concentration is high enough, any drug may enter and occlude open ion channels. This mechanism may explain the synergy that occurs with certain drugs such as local anaesthetics and antibiotics and muscle relaxants. In addition the difficulty in antagonizing profound neuromuscular blockade may be due to open channel block by the muscle relaxant.

Hexamethonium, tricyclic drugs, and naloxone may cause physical blockade of a closed channel. Muscle relaxants, e.g. decamethonium and suxamethonium, have been known to cause physical channel blockade.

BLOCKADE OF THE INTRACELLULAR MECHANISM

For example by entry of decamethonium or dantrolene.

Phase II block involves the above mechanisms at different subphases (*see below*).

Extrajunctional receptors

These appear all over the surface of the muscle fibre, when the muscle is denervated or deprived of nerve stimulation, by injury, stroke, disuse, and 3 weeks to 3 months after major burns.[3] They are similar to, but more responsive than, junctional receptors to depolarizing agents, and less responsive to non-depolarizing agents.[4] When these receptors are present in large numbers, suxamethonium causes substantial flow of ions across the membrane producing hyperkalaemia, which is difficult to suppress by prior non-depolarizing drugs (tubocurarine can act as an agonist on these receptors). They are present before birth and in infancy, without causing problems for the anaesthetist.

Alpha-adrenergic receptors have also been found on the nerve terminals. They may be involved in the improved muscle performance seen when adrenaline levels are high.

Characteristics of muscle

A skeletal muscle fibre is a very long cell, and may run the whole length of the muscle. There are many myofibrils in each cell, with neuromuscular junctions extending throughout the length of the muscle. The external ocular muscles are different, having multineuronal innervation of fibres and a tonic response to suxamethonium.

For clinical relaxation, the human diaphragm requires 90% receptor occupancy, while the tibialis anterior needs only 20%. An average value is around 70%. Adductor pollicis may thus still be completely paralysed, even after the patient has resumed normal respiration. This is significant, since adductor pollicis is often used for monitoring. (*See also* Bowman W. C. In Adams A. P. and Cashman J. N. (eds) *Recent Advances in Anaesthesia and Analgesia – 20*. Churchill Livingstone, Edinburgh, 1998; Bowman W. C. *Pharmacology of Neuromuscular Function*. Wright, London, 1990.)

CHARACTERISTICS OF MUSCLE RELAXANTS

Molecular properties necessary for neuromuscular blocking activity

The characteristics of a drug which determine its performance as a muscle relaxant include the following:

1 Its electrostatic characteristics (particularly the position and number of its quaternary nitrogen groups). An interonium distance of 1.1 nm (as in pancuronium) was thought to be an effective spatial arrangement, allowing the second nitrogen to repel incoming ACh electrostatically. That a bond is formed between a non-depolarizing relaxant and a neuromuscular post-junctional cholinoceptor is shown by the fact that the effect of tubocurarine is not proportional to its plasma concentration, but continues after decline of this level. (However, depolarizing relaxants do show the 'washout phenomenon'.) The high level of ionization of relaxants means that they

are confined to the extracellular space, and undergo no renal tubular reabsorption.

2 Its steric nature, i.e. the way it fits the neuromuscular receptors. Receptor occupancy varies between one relaxant and another, and the steeper the occupancy/concentration profile, the more rapid is a drug's onset and wear-off characteristic. Atracurium is faster than tubocurarine.

3 The balance between its hydrophilic and hydrophobic characteristics.

4 Its optical isomerism (e.g. l-tubocurarine is ineffective).

Features of non-depolarizing neuromuscular blocking drugs

1 Do not cause muscular fasciculation.

2 Mostly mono- or bis-quaternary salts with interonium distances of 0.7–1.4 nm, and high electrostatic characteristics, i.e. very hydrophilic.

3 Relatively slow onset (1–5 min).

4 Reversed by neostigmine and other anticholinesterases.

5 Effects reduced by adrenaline and acetylcholine. Also by suxamethonium (but not in myasthenics).

6 The relaxed muscle is still responsive to other (mechanical and electrical) stimuli.

7 In partial paralysis, neuromuscular monitoring shows: 'fade'; post-tetanic facilitation followed by exhaustion; and depression of muscle twitch.

8 Potentiated by volatile agents, Mg^{2+} and hypokalaemia.

9 Slow dissociation constant at receptors.

10 Mild cooling antagonizes their effects.

11 Greater cooling (below about 33°C) potentiates them.

12 Repeated tetanic bursts cause their effect to wear off.

13 Acidosis increases duration and degree of non-depolarizing block.

Features of depolarizing (Phase I) neuromuscular blocking drugs

1 Cause muscular fasciculation (but not in myasthenic humans and in some other species). Extraocular muscles exhibit a tonic response.

2 The depolarized muscle fibres are unresponsive to other stimuli. The Na^+ channels are blocked open.

3 Repolarization is interfered with. The resting membrane potential is held up until phase II block develops, when it returns to −70 mV.

4 Not reversed by neostigmine and other anticholinesterases.

5 In partial paralysis, the neuromuscular monitoring shows: depression of muscle twitch; no 'fade' but a well-sustained response; and no post-tetanic facilitation (*see below*).

6 Potentiated by isoflurane, enflurane, ACh, respiratory alkalosis, hypothermia and Mg^{2+}.

7 Antagonized by ether, halothane, acidosis and non-depolarizing relaxants.

8 Fast dissociation constant at receptors. There is little or no bond between drug and receptor.
9 Repeated or continuous use leads to 'phase II block' (*see below*).

MONITORING NEUROMUSCULAR FUNCTION[5]

General principles

The electric stimulus is a rectangular pulse of 0.2 ms of supramaximal intensity (100–200 mV, transcutaneous). Any superficially located peripheral motor nerve may be used, but it must be remembered that different muscle groups have different sensitivities to neuromuscular blocking drugs. The ulnar nerve is the most popular for stimulation, the elbow or the wrist being convenient sites, while avoiding the twin dangers of: (i) having the stimulating electrodes too close to the recording electrodes, and (ii) directly stimulating the long flexors of the forearm.

If an electromyogram (EMG) is not available, a useful measure can be made by watching or feeling the fingers and thumb or by using an electrocardiogram (ECG), with electrodes on the thenar and hypothenar eminences and the back of the hand. For a tetanic burst, 50 Hz is adequate. A negative response to stimulation may mean that: the neuromuscular junction is blocked; the stimulator is not working; or the ulnar nerve is not in its usual position.

The neuromuscular transmission monitor compares well with the old force transducers. Paraesthesia after neuromuscular twitch monitoring has been described postoperatively.[6] (*See also* Jones R. M. et al. *Issues in Clinical Anaesthesia: Residual Neuromuscular Block*. Gardiner-Caldwell Communications, Macclesfield, 1995.)

Patterns of electrical stimulation

Five patterns of electrical nerve stimulation are used in clinical anaesthesia; single twitch, tetanic, train-of-four, post-tetanic count and double burst stimulation.

Single twitch and tetanic stimulation

In the absence of complete paralysis due to *non-depolarizing* block the single twitch and tetanic stimulation lead to a successive fade in the response. Following a tetanic stimulus (50–100 Hz), a single-twitch stimulus causes an increased response, i.e. post-tetanic facilitation (thought to be due to release of increased quanta of ACh for a few seconds). Post-tetanic facilitation is followed by a period of post-tetanic exhaustion due to depletion of readily available ACh (Figs 2.5.1 and 2.5.2).

In contrast, with *depolarizing agents* there is a well-sustained response to successive stimuli following both a single-twitch stimulus and fast tetanic stimuli. There is no post-tetanic facilitation.

Train-of-four stimulation[7]

Four stimuli are given in succession, the resulting contractions give as much information as a tetanic burst, and may be repeated more frequently. It is less painful than tetanic stimulation. The ratio of the amplitude of the fourth evoked response to that of the first is used as a measure of neuromuscular transmission and compares well with clinical tests of recovery.[8] The fourth is eliminated at about 75% depression of the control, the third at 80% and the second at 90%. Absence of all four indicates complete block (Figs 2.5.2 and 2.5.3).

A T_4/T_1 ratio $> 60\%$ is equivalent to being able to raise the head from the bed and having normal respiratory function tests.[9] A T_4/T_1 ratio $> 75\%$ is equal to being able to cough properly, open the eyes and protrude the tongue on command.

Post-tetanic count

The post-tetanic count (PTC) is a method of evaluating an intense non-depolarizing neuromuscular block. The number of single-twitch responses

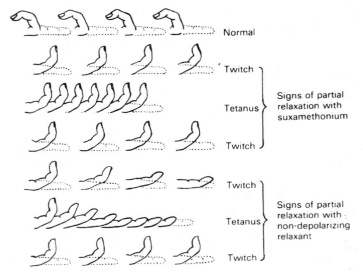

Figure 2.5.1 Finger twitch response to ulnar nerve stimulation

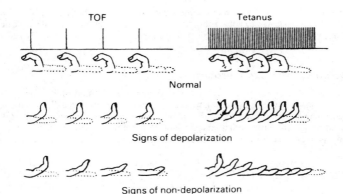

Figure 2.5.2 Finger twitch response to 'train-of-four' and tetanic stimulation of ulnar nerve

to nerve stimuli at 1 Hz following a 5-s tetanus at 50 Hz is an indication of recovery from a relaxant, when the 'train-of-four' (TOF) stimulation shows nothing.[10]

Commonly, one to five twitch responses occur.

Double burst stimulation[11]

Double burst stimulation (DBS) is more sensitive than TOF for manual detection of small degrees of non-depolarizing block. Two short 50-Hz bursts,

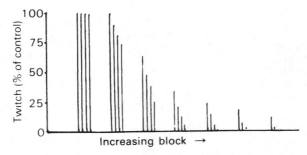

Figure 2.5.3 Measured responses to 'train-of-four' stimuli during progressive non-deplorazing relaxation. At 80% block (reasonable abdominal relaxation), T4 disappears. At 90% block (excellent abdominal relaxation) T2 has disappeared

separated by 750 ms, each burst containing three stimuli. At T_4/T_1 of 0.5, the second burst shows a 50% reduction in force (estimated manually). (For monitoring in tetraparesis, *see* Fiacchine F. et al. *Anaesthesia* 1990, **45,** 128.)

Evaluation of evoked response

The evoked response of the ulnar nerve to electrical stimulation can be evaluated visually, by touch (tactile), mechanomyographically (force displacement transducer), electromyographically or by accelerography. (Accelerography is based on the principle that at fixed mass the force developed in the adductor pollicis muscle is directly proportional to the acceleration of the finger.[12])

NON-DEPOLARIZING RELAXANTS[13]

Note that from a clinical point of view, it is the responsibility of patients to tell the anaesthetist about muscle weakness or wasting. Such conditions have a large impact on the effect of non-depolarizing relaxants.

Pharmacokinetics

Poorly bound to plasma proteins, and excepting atracurium, eliminated unchanged by the kidneys, and to a smaller extent in the bile (except gallamine). Biliary excretion increases in renal failure. The drugs are concentrated in the kidneys, liver and cartilage. Early hepatic uptake lowers the plasma

Table 2.5.1 Pharmacokinetic data.

	Distribution Volume (l/kg)	Plasma Clearance (ml/kg/min)	Excretion Urinary (%)	Biliary (%)
Alcuronium	0.32	1.3	80–85	15–20
Atracurium	0.09	6.6	10	–
Cis-Atracurium	0.15	4.5–5.7	15	–
Doxacurium	0.22	2.7	25–30	–
Gallamine	0.2	1.3	95	< 1
Metocurine	0.47	1.2	43	2
Mivacurium	0.2–0.27	55	< 10	–
Pancuronium	0.24	1.8	40	10
Pipecuronium	0.35	3.0	38	2
Rocuronium	0.21	2.9	9	54
Tubocurarine	0.30	2.3	45	–
Vecuronium	0.20	5.3	15	40

concentration of these drugs (except gallamine and atracurium). These pharmacokinetics are altered in liver disease, increasing the terminal elimination half-life ($T\frac{1}{2}\beta$) by about 50%.[14]

Absorption and excretion

Absorbed when administered intravenously, intramuscularly, subcutaneously, intraperitoneally, sublingually and per rectum. In practice, nearly always given intravenously, occasionally intramuscularly. Most of them are metabolized in the liver, and excreted by the kidneys. Plasma proteins, especially gamma-globulins, have the power of binding competitive relaxants and this influences their fate in the body, and there seems to be a positive correlation between the relaxant requirements and the serum level of gamma-globulin, e.g. in cirrhosis of the liver and other hepatic disorders. Atracurium undergoes Hofmann elimination and hydrolysis in the plasma and elsewhere in the body. It has been recommended as the non-depolarizing agent of choice in patients with renal impairment.[15]

Pharmacodynamics

The drugs have neither anaesthetic nor analgesic properties when given in clinical doses.

Effect on motor end-plate

Act by preventing the adsorption of ACh to the cholinergic receptors and so prevent the changes in the end-plate which cause muscular tone and contraction. Therapeutic doses produce the following effects in sequence: ptosis, imbalance of extraocular muscles with diplopia (which rarely may last several days), relaxation of muscles of the face, jaw, neck and limbs, and, finally, abdominal wall and diaphragm.

Effects on respiration

Paralysis of the muscles of respiration causing apnoea; the diaphragm, being less sensitive than other muscles, is usually the last one to be paralysed.

Effects on circulation

There may be hypotension with tubocurarine, hypertension with pancuronium, tachycardia with gallamine and skin flushing with atracurium.

Synergy of relaxants

This is potentiation of one by another, when used together.[16,17] For example, one-fifth of the usual dose of tubocurarine or pancuronium will double the effect of atracurium.

Histamine release[17]

Any of these drugs may release histamine at the first injection. Tubocurarine is the most likely to do so, and vecuronium probably the least likely. A second injection on the same day will not do so (owing to the great rapidity with which the histamine release develops tachyphylaxis). Development of true allergy with antibody formation, may of course occur in days or weeks following exposure to any drug.

Gastrointestinal system

The cardiac sphincter is probably not relaxed completely and still has an opening pressure of 25 cmH$_2$O.

Clinical use

Following induction of anaesthesia the relaxant is injected intravenously. The patient's lungs are gently inflated with N$_2$O, O$_2$ and volatile agent. Care must be taken not in inflate the stomach. After 1–3 min, when the effect of the muscle-relaxant drug is maximal, intubation of the trachea is carried out. Artificial ventilation is maintained, and additional doses of muscle relaxant are given as required.

During thiopentone-N$_2$O-O$_2$- relaxant anaesthesia the following clinical signs often indicate the need for more relaxant:

1 hiccup, due to contraction of the periphery of the diaphragm (may be seen on a capnograph);
2 rigidity of the abdominal wall;
3 increased resistance to inflation of the lung (in the absence of respiratory obstruction), i.e. decreased compliance;
4 bucking or coughing on the tracheal tube;
5 as indicated by neuromuscular monitoring.

Conversely analgesic supplements may be required if:

1 the patient moves his skeletal muscles in response to the surgical stimulus, e.g. face, limb or neck muscles, especially swallowing or frowning;
2 rise of blood pressure and pulse;
3 sweating, unexplained by other causes, occurs;
4 there is reflex response to surgical stimuli, e.g. hiccups.

Many anaesthetists routinely administer an intravenous or inhalation supplement to prevent possible awareness.

Whenever muscle relaxants are used, it is of paramount importance to see that the patient is breathing reasonably deeply before leaving the operating table. A relatively large number of patients may have a defect in neuromuscular transmission on their arrival in the postoperative room. Respiratory depression at the end of the operation should be treated either by artificial ventilation until the tidal volume becomes normal or, more usually, by the injection of neostigmine with atropine. The use of a nerve stimulator to monitor the proper recovery of the neuromuscular junction can be employed. (*See also* Hunter J. M. *N. Engl. J. Med.* 1995, **332,**1691.)

Clinical signs of incomplete reversal

1 Shallow respiration.
2 Jerky respiration.
3 'Tracheal tug' and 'see-saw' respiration where, as the abdomen moves out, the chest moves in.
4 Cyanosis.
5 A restless, frightened, struggling patient, who says that he or she cannot breathe.
6 Diplopia.
7 Inability to raise head or extrude tongue.

Management of incomplete reversal

Artificial ventilation is given with a mask and oxygen, while the degree of incomplete reversal is assessed.

If mild (T_4/T_1 ratio $> 50\%$ and respiration is almost adequate) more neostigmine or other anticholinesterase is given.

If severe (T_4/T_1 ratio $< 50\%$ and/or respiration is obviously inadequate) the patient is sedated, intubated and artificial ventilation continued with a ventilator for at least an hour; acid–base status is determined, and corrected. The serum electrolytes are estimated and normalized. Reassessment is performed using a nerve stimulator.

Alternative diagnoses are considered: overdose of inhalation agents, opioids, antibiotics, barbiturates, renal failure, botulism, myasthenia gravis, myasthenic syndrome, adrenal failure, hypothermia, renal failure, overdose of relaxant.

Infants and children tolerate muscle relaxants well if the dosage is suitably adjusted to their general condition and body weight (*see* Chapter 4.2).

CHOICE OF NON-DEPOLARIZING RELAXANT

Anaesthetists use the relaxants with which they are familiar. However, the following suggestion for preferred relaxants may help the tyro.

1 In renal failure: vecuronium or atracurium.
2 In hepatic failure: atracurium.
3 In myasthenia gravis (if relaxants are essential): one-tenth of the normal dose of atracurium.
4 In short cases: atracurium, rapacurium or mivacurium.
5 In obstetrics: any relaxant except gallamine.

6 In arterial surgery (to maintain arterial pressure): pancuronium.
7 To deliberately reduce blood pressure: tubocurarine.
8 For 'rapid sequence induction' (without using suxamethonium): rocuronium or rapacurium.

Occasionally some residual paresis of the muscles of accommodation persists for 24 h after operation, making reading difficult.

The drugs must be used with special care if given to the same patient on two occasions within 24 h, as a cumulative effect may occur

Benzylisoquiniliniums

Atracurium besylate[17]

Atracurium is a bis-benzylisoquinolinium compound with a mol. wt 1243. pH of solution 3.5, stored at 4°C in refrigerator.

PHARMACOKINETICS

Absorption: from intramuscular and intravenous routes.
   Distribution: throughout ECF. No effective crossing of the placenta.[18]
   Metabolism: Hofmann degradation and alkaline ester hydrolysis in the plasma and elsewhere in the body (producing a monoquarternary alcohol at first). Elimination half-life for atracurium is 20 min. The resulting tertiary amine, laudanosine, has slow renal elimination and crosses the blood–brain barrier.[19] This increases the minimum alveolar concentration (MAC) of halothane by 30% in high concentrations (unlikely to be found in clinical situations). Mean half-life for the monoquarternary alcohol is 39 min, that for laudanosine is 234 min.

PHARMACODYNAMICS

Dose: 0.5 mg/kg i.v. as initial bolus; top ups 0.3 mg/kg i.v.; average infusion 0.5 mg/kg/h. Potentiated by enflurane and isoflurane, less so by halothane.
   Infants are slightly more resistant than adults. Dose for premature neonates is 0.3 mg/kg.
   Speed of onset: 1–2 min. This can be halved by the 'priming technique', where 0.1 mg/kg is injected 3–5 min before the main dose (unpleasant for patient and not recommended).
   Duration: 20–40 min, even in anephric patients;[20] the elderly and severely ill.[21] Duration doubled at 25°C.[22]
   Quality of reversal: extremely good with neostigmine or edrophonium.
   Side-effects: no vagolytic effects on the heart, may allow bradycardia to occur.[23] Angioneurotic oedema has occurred. Histamine release does not occur when the drug is injected slowly over 75 s, or when less than 0.6 mg/kg is injected.
   The clinical signs sometimes following atracurium (e.g. flushing of the skin, maculopapular, pruritic rash, suggestive of mediator release from mast cells in

the presence of IgE) do not correlate with plasma histamine levels, nor with complement C_3 conversion. These effects are, however, abolished by pre-treatment with cimetidine 4 mg/kg i.v. and chlorpheniramine 0.1 mg/kg or phenylhydramine 0.3 mg/kg.[24] Intraocular pressure shows no change or a fall, intracranial pressure is unaltered.

Atracurium is suitable in anephric patients (the relaxant of choice). It is suitable for patients with atypical cholinesterase; organophosphorus poisoning;[25] and in myasthenia gravis.[26] It is suitable for Caesarean section; in intermediate duration cases and in long cases with intermittent injection or continuous infusion.[27,28] The recommended infusion rate is 0.5 mg/kg/h with cessation at 15 min before the estimated end of the operation. Simple neuromuscular monitoring is desirable but not essential. It is suitable when tourniquets are to be used.

Cis-*atracurium besylate*[29,30]

Cis-atracurium (the 1R-*cis*, 1'R'*cis* isomer) is the purified form of one of the 10 stereoisomers of atracurium. Presented as 5 mg/ml *cis*-atracurium in 32% benzenesulphonic acid solution w/v. Stored in non-freezing refrigerator.

Cis-atracurium is approximately three times more potent than atracurium on a molecular weight basis.

PHARMACOKINETICS

Absorption: i.v. route.

Distribution: the volume of distribution is similar to the racemate.

Metabolism: undergoes Hoffman elimination to form laudanasine and monoquaternary acrylate. Does not undergo hydrolysis by plasma esterases. The laudanasine levels are much lower than after atracurium. Mean clearance 4.5–5.7 ml/min/kg. EC_{50} 1.4 mg/l and elimination half-life 25–29 min. Recovery index (T_1 25–75%) is 13 min in adults and 10 min in children.

Since *cis*-atracurium's elimination is an organ-independent process there are only minor differences in pharmacokinetics between healthy patients and patients with liver and renal disease. Duration: 30 min.

PHARMACODYNAMICS

Dose: 0.15 mg/kg i.v.; average infusion rate 0.18 mg/kg/h reducing to 0.06–0.12 mg/kg/h (lower doses for children).

Speed of onset: the onset of an equipotent dose is slightly slower than atracurium, consistent with the inverse relationship between potency and speed of onset.

Duration: the clinically effective duration of action and recovery times are similar to those with an equipotent dose of atracurium.

Side-effects: shows little if any cardiovascular or histamine-like effects. No evidence of accumulation with repeat dosing. Elderly patients respond to *cis*-atracurium much the same as younger patients.

Mivacurium chloride[29,31]

The structure of mivacurium resembles that of atracurium and doxacurium, but in common with doxacurium the ether oxygen moiety and the carboxyl group do not have the relationship that permits Hoffman elimination. Exhibits stereoisomerism, hence presented as a racemic mixture. A short acting muscle relaxant, metabolized by plasma cholinesterase.

PHARMACOKINETICS AND PHARMACODYNAMICS

Metabolized by plasma cholinesterase at 75% of the rate of suxamethonium. Metabolism by plasma cholinesterase implies that residual neuromuscular blockade seldom requires antagonism. The products of hydrolysis are eliminated in the bile and urine. Anephric patients may be more sensitive.

Ideal for use by continuous intravenous infusion. Bolus dose 0.1–0.2 mg/kg; average infusion rate for maintenance of block 0.24–0.48 μg/kg/h.

Onset time is reported as 3.5 min with a duration of 10–20 min. The duration of action is approximately twice that of suxamethonium and half to one-third that of comparable doses of atracurium or vecuronium.

Recovery is rapid, but duration is dose dependent. The duration of action may be prolonged when plasma cholinesterase is low, in hypermagnaesaemia, hypokalaemia, when a second dose is given, and when mivacurium is given following another non-depolarizing relaxant.

Major cardiovascular side-effects have not been reported, although there may be some histamine release, some fall of arterial pressure and some fall in heart rate. Transient decreases in arterial pressure following mivacurium in doses greater than 0.15–0.2 mg/kg. Hypotension is due to histamine release.

Doxacurium

The most potent neuromuscular blocking drug currently available. Hence, it has a slow onset and very long duration of action with potential for cumulation.

PHARMACOKINETICS AND PHARMACODYNAMICS

Exhibits significant (30%) renal elimination, hence prolonged effects in patients with renal disease.[32] Cumulative potential difficult to ascertain because repeat dosing is rarely needed.[32] Antagonism by anticholinesterase is satisfactory provided considerable spontaneous recovery has taken place.

Dose: 0.03 mg/kg, peak onset 4–6 min,[33] duration 1 h.

Vascular side-effects are minor.[34] No significant cardiovascular effects. No histamine release.

Tubocurarine chloride

Was once the main non-depolarising relaxant. It had pre- and postjunctional components, was enhanced by inhalation agents, and by previous injection of suxamethonium. It lasted about 40 min, and showed cumulation. It caused histamine release and blockade of sympathetic ganglia.

Gallamine triethiodide

PHARMACODYNAMICS AND PHARMACOKINETICS

Blocks cardiac muscarinic (M2) receptors without affecting muscarinic receptors in the gut or peripheral tissues (M3). Causes prolonged tachycardia. Allergic reactions have been reported following its use.[35] It passes the placental barrier. About 80% is excreted by the kidneys, and so it should not be used in patients with renal disease.

Dose: 1–2 mg/kg.

Aminosteroids

Vecuronium bromide

The molecule has two rings, A and D. The D ring is similar to pancuronium. The A ring is modified by a tertiary nitrogen at 2B, giving less stability in solution, a shorter time course and lack of cumulation *in vivo*.[36] The solution (pH 4) is stable for 24 h at 25°C. Mol. wt 638.

PHARMACOKINETICS

Absorption: from intramuscular or intravenous route.

Distribution: throughout the ECF. The lipophilic effect of the single quarternary nitrogen enhances rapid uptake into hepatocytes. No effective crossing of the placenta.

Metabolism: theoretically in the liver with excretion in the urine.

PHARMACODYNAMICS

Dose: 0.1 mg/kg as initial intravenous bolus (adults, infants and elderly); average infusion 0.2 mg/kg/h. Potentiated (but not much extended) most by enflurane, > isoflurane > halothane. Potentiated and prolonged by previous suxamethonium.

Speed of onset: 1–2 min (can be shortened by preloading with a small dose, 6 min before the main dose).

Duration: 10–20 min (much longer with higher doses), not influenced by renal failure. Side-effects: no effect on vascular system in clinical doses.

Rocuronium[29]

A rapid-onset, de-acetoxy analogue of vecuronium. Possession of a tertiary nitrogen at the ring end of the molecule minimizes the cardiovascular effects.

PHARMACOKINETICS

The volume of distribution is 0.21 l/kg. The elimination half-life is 1.4 h. Mean clearance 2.9 ml/min/kg. Exhibits predominantly biliary excretion, 10% of a dose is excreted in urine but clearance is decreased in renal failure. Volume of distribution and elimination half-life significantly increased in patients with hepatic disease. Does not undergo hydrolysis by plasma esterases. Main metabolite is 17-desacetylrocuronium which has weak neuro-muscular blocking action.

PHARMACODYNAMICS

Dose: 600 μg/kg i.v. bolus: average infusion rate 300–600 μg/kg/h.

Twenty per cent more potent than vecuronium on a molecular weight basis. The onset of an equipotent dose is twice as rapid but the duration is similar. Whilst the time to 80% block (for intubation) is more rapid than with any other nondepolarizing relaxant the overall time to 100% block is similar to vecuronium.

Exhibits no significant cardiovascular effects even in large doses. No significant histamine release with doses up to four times the ED95.

Pipecuronium[29]

A long-acting steroid analogue of pancuronium with quaternary nitrogen at the 2 and 16 positions hence greater interonium distance. Twenty to twenty-five per cent more potent than pancuronium. Presented as 4 mg powder/ampoule, solution stable 24 h at 4°C.

PHARMACOKINETICS

Two-compartment model. Concentrated in kidney, liver and spleen; 85% is excreted by the kidneys.[37] Hence, very prolonged effect in renal failure in which case volume of distribution is increased and clearance is reduced. Metabolized by deacetylation.

Does not cross the placenta. Cumulation occurs. Potentiated by enflurane. Similar to pancuronium.[38]

PHARMACODYNAMICS

Dose: 0.05 mg/kg i.v. bolus. Slow onset (~3 min) and long duration 1–2 h. Duration and speed of recovery are comparable with pancuronium. As with doxacurium significant spontaneous recovery should have taken place before attempting antagonism with anticholinesterase. Reversibly inhibits serum cholinesterase.

Has no significant effect on circulation, and does not release histamine.

Pancuronium bromide

A long-acting bis-quaternary amino-steroid, devoid of hormonal activity.

PHARMACODYNAMICS AND PHARMACOKINETICS

Can cause stimulation of the myocardium[39] with rise in pulse rate and blood pressure. In addition to neuromuscular blockade also blocks cardiac muscarinic (M2) receptors and neuronal noradrenaline reuptake (reuptake I). It causes noradrenaline release. It can release histamine from the tissues.

It becomes strongly bound to gamma-globulin and moderately bound to serum albumin, so less than 13% of the dose is unbound and active. Thirty per cent is excreted by the kidney, 25% excreted in bile (one-third of this as hydroxylated drug). Not cumulative. It should be avoided in renal failure and total biliary obstruction.

Does not cross the blood–brain barrier. An insignificant proportion of it crosses the placental barrier. Safe in patients susceptible to malignant hyperpyrexia.

Dose: 0.05–0.1 mg/kg i.v. bolus. Duration: 20–30 min.

Rapacurium

1.5–2.5 mg/kg, has a similar time course to suxamethonium, if it is reversed by neostigmine.

Antagonists to non-depolarizing relaxants (anticholinesterase drugs)

Neostigmine

Prevents the normal hydrolysis of ACh thus allowing it to accumulate and compete with the neuromuscular blocking drug at the receptor site.

PHARMACOKINETICS AND PHARMACODYNAMICS

Partly broken down by serum cholinesterase and partly excreted unchanged by the kidneys. Renal failure reduces the clearance of this drug by up to four times.[40] Binds to the esteratic subsite of cholinesterase with its carbonate group.

Neostigmine is also a depolarizer and can cause on its own a depolarizing type of block due to build-up of ACh. Phase II block can eventually result. The amount needed to cause paralysis by persistent depolarization is much greater, normally, than that required to antagonize a clinical dose of non-depolarizing relaxant. It does not always reverse block due to aminoglycoside antibiotics; or Phase II block following suxamethonium.

When injected into a conscious patient it may cause muscular fasciculations and severe colic. In addition, it is a direct stimulant of cholinergic effector cells. It has nicotinic effects and has a direct stimulant action on muscle. In small doses it stimulates and in larger doses it depresses autonomic ganglia.

It also has muscarinic properties (from Amantia muscaria) which are blocked by atropine, e.g. bradycardia, intestinal peristalsis and spasm, bronchial and salivary secretion and bronchospasm, stimulation of the sweat glands, contraction of the pupil and contraction of the bladder. Renal excretion accounts for 50% of its clearance.[41]

Adult dose is 2.5–5 mg, with atropine 1.5 mg or glycopyrronium 0.5 mg. Duration: 2 h.

Edrophonium

It has, like neostigmine, anticholinesterase, depolarizing and direct stimulating actions on the motor end-plate. It may cause fasciculation. Much quicker in onset than neostigmine. Small doses (0.15 mg/kg) are not as long lasting as neostigmine, consequently recurarization may follow; although this is not seen with larger doses (1.0 mg/kg) or following repeated injection of 20 mg at 3-min intervals. It is rapidly metabolized, in small doses but not in large doses when its pharmacokinetics are similar to pyridostigmine and neostigmine.[42] Its pattern of reversal suggests that it acts at prejunctional receptors.

Dose: 0.5–1.0 mg/kg i.v. bolus with atropine 0.6 mg or glycopyrronium 0.2 mg.

Pyridostigmine

Used in treatment of myasthenia gravis. Its duration of action (6 h) makes it especially suitable for reversal of relaxants in cases of renal failure where the excretion of the relaxant may be delayed.

Dose: 10 mg. It is capable of penetrating the blood–brain barrier.

Physostigmine salicylate

An alkaloid obtained from the West African calabar bean. An anticholinesterase with a tertiary amine structure which can cross the blood–brain barrier. Used to treat the anticholinergic syndrome produced by atropine, hyoscine and other related alkaloids. It does not adequately antagonize neuromuscular block in doses up to 4 mg.

Clinical uses of anticholinesterase drugs

Successful antagonism of neuromuscular blockade

In the average case, towards the end of the operation, $PaCO_2$ should be normalized. Atropine and neostigmine are given. Clinical signs of adequate relaxant reversal by neostigmine:

1 return of normal tidal exchange measured either by an anemometer or by the flowmeters of the anaesthetic machine using a Ruben or other non-rebreathing valve;
2 ability to cough;
3 ability to open eyes and keep them open;

4 presence of tone in the masseters;
5 ability to raise the head from the pillow or to lift arm;
6 return of full muscular activity shown after electrical nerve stimulation.

Unsuccessful antagonism of neuromuscular blockade

If neostigmine does not reverse the block, as assessed by nerve stimulator, the following factors should be considered.

1 Has enough time been allowed since the last dose of relaxant? Twitch height using a nerve stimulator may take up to 15 min to recover, or up to 30 min when height is initially less than 20% of control;
2 Has too much relaxant been given, e.g. in renal failure and elderly patients?
3 What is the acid–base and electrolyte status?
4 What is the temperature?
5 Is the patient receiving other drugs which might make antagonism difficult, e.g. aminoglycosides?
6 Has excretion of the relaxant been impeded?

Failure to breathe after full reversal may be due to low CO_2 levels, opioid depression, breath-holding, other causes of respiratory depression (e.g. cerebral).

Breathing can be stimulated by moving the tube within the trachea and by application of a suction catheter to the carina. Artificial ventilation must be carried out until the patient can ventilate him- or herself adequately. Low blood pressure and poor tissue perfusion may retard reversal.

It is of fundamental importance that the anaesthetist should not leave patients until they are able to ventilate themselves adequately and their muscular power has returned. If this is not so, artificial ventilation should be continued.

For paediatric dosage *see* Chapter 4.2.

DEPOLARIZING RELAXANTS

Suxamethonium chloride, succinylcholine

The dicholine ester of succinic acid. The active part of the molecule is the cation, formed by the succinic radical with a quaternary ammonium group at each end of the molecular chain. If these end-groups contain three methyl groups (CH_3), the substance is a suxamethonium compound; if two methyl and one ethyl (C_2H_5), then it is an ethonium compound, hence suxamethonium and suxethonium. Solutions deteriorate in hot environments. Hydrolysis occurs at room temperature. The drug should be stored at 4°C.

Pharmacokinetics

Absorption: intravenous, intramuscular or subcutaneous.
  Distribution: throughout the ECF, and slightly across the placenta.

Metabolism: first-order pharmacokinetic elimination by hydrolysis to succinyl monocholine, then to choline and succinic acid by plasma cholinesterase. Dibucaine number (DN) 75–85. This is the percentage inhibition of cholinesterase by 10^{-5} molar solution of dibucaine (cinchocaine). The 'fluoride number' (FN) is the percentage inhibition of cholinesterase by 5×10^{-5} molar sodium fluoride. Urea inhibition has also been used. Plasma cholinesterase is found in plasma but not in red cells; also in the liver, brain, kidneys and pancreas. It also hydrolyses ester-linked local analgesics and other drugs. Plasma cholinesterase is a lipoprotein synthesized in the liver. Failure of its action due to abnormality or deficiency prolongs the action of suxamethonium. Of the population 94% are normal E^u/E^u genotypes with normal enzyme activity and a DN of 75–85. Three abnormal genes exist: E^a (atypical) homozygotes comprise 0.03% of the population; E^f (fluoride-resistant) homozygotes comprise 0.0003% of the population; E^s (silent) homozygotes comprise 0.001% of the population. Normal serum cholinesterase level about 80 units/ml.

ABNORMALITIES OF SUXAMETHONIUM METABOLISM

1 *Abnormal plasma cholinesterase (inherited).*[43]
  (a) Atypical cholinesterase: Mendelian recessive E^a/E^a homozygotes (1 per 3000 of population) have 1–2-h apnoea, during which Phase II block develops (DN 16–25). Heterozygotes (1 per 25 of population) have little or no disturbance (DN 50–65), with apnoeas up to 10 min.
  (b) Fluoride-resistant cholinesterase: homozygotes have 1-h apnoea, with Phase II block (DN 16–25). Heterozygotes have 10-min apnoea (DN 50–65).
  (c) Silent gene: all the possible combinations of heterozygotes exist (1 in 25 of the population, with apnoeas around 10 min).
2 *Plasma cholinesterase deficiency.*
  (a) Acquired: after X-ray therapy, after organophosphorus poisoning, in hyperpyrexia, in cardiac failure, in hepatic failure, uraemia, hypoproteinaemia due to malnutrition or plasmapheresis, e.g. in lupus erythematosus, myasthenia gravis, Goodpasture's syndrome, and Rh incompatibility, in trophoblastic disease, pregnancy, puerperium, the newborn (50% of adult levels), myxoedema, asthma, obesity and following treatment with: cyclophosphamide, ecothiopate, procainamide, quinidine, phenothiazines, ketamine, trimetaphan, pancuronium, monoamine oxidase inhibitors, oral contraceptives (20–30% reduction) and metrifonate (antibilharzial drug).
  (b) Congenital: presents unexpected danger to the patient. Hydrolysis proceeds only at the rate of 5% per hour. Inherited absence due to the silent gene E^s. Homozygotes have 1–2-h apnoea, and Phase II block develops in the course of this. Heterozygotes have normal DN and FN but only half the normal plasma cholinesterase activity.
3 *Plasma cholinesterase antagonism:* by anticholinesterases (e.g. neostigmine), and tacrine.

4 *Plasma cholinesterase excess:* the result is shortening of the duration of activity of the drug.
   (a) Acquired: in obesity, toxic goitre, nephrosis, depression, psoriasis, and alcoholism.
   (b) Congenital: the C_5 variant.

Pharmacodynamics

DOSE, ONSET, DURATION

Dose: 1 mg/kg (2–3 mg/kg neonates less than 10 weeks of age). Onset in 10–30 s. Duration of bolus 1–5 min. Average dose for intubation 25–100 mg. By infusion 4–10 mg/min as 0.1% solution.

MUSCULAR SYSTEM

Phase I block preceded by muscle fasciculation (*see above*), potentiated by isoflurane, anticholinesterases, magnesium and lithium.

Phase II block accompanies the prolonged action of suxamethonium, whether due to infusion or to abnormal cholinesterase activity. This development is slightly potentiated by enflurane and rather less so by halothane. The development has four stages:[44]

Stage A: depolarizing block which may last 30–50 min.

Stage B: non-depolarizing block develops quite quickly.

Stage C: a plateau 30-min period of no change.

Stage D: a 'wearing-off phase' up to 2 h long.

In infants, Phase II block may not be associated with prolonged paralysis.

Reversal Phase II block has been reversed by neostigmine and other anticholinesterases, but the results are not consistent, and therefore this approach is not in routine use. A test dose of edrophonium can be used as a pointer to the likely response.

Side-effects

PROLONGED APNOEA

After a single dose of suxamethonium the commonest causes are as follows.

1 Atypical serum cholinesterase. Homozygotes for the atypical gene show this. A heparinized sample of blood and a full clinical history will be required. Over 25% of patients with suxamethonium apnoea have normal enzymes.[45]
2 Dehydration and electrolyte imbalance leading to the development of dual block at a very early stage.
3 An overdose of the relaxant drug, i.e. total of more than 1 g in an infusion.
4 A low serum cholinesterase level in the blood. This seldom causes prolonged apnoea if 50 mg is not exceeded, a dose adequate for most patients requiring a single injection, e.g. for intubation or electroconvulsive therapy (ECT). It is unlikely to be the cause of apnoea prolonged beyond 20–30 min, if the serum cholinesterase level is more than 25 units. Apnoea

due to a low cholinesterase value may be reversed by a blood transfusion as even stored blood contains 30 units/ml cholinesterase and retains 80% of its cholinesterase activity after storage for 25 days at 6°C. Half a litre of fresh blood restores the serum cholinesterase level by 10 units/ml; half a litre of stored blood restores it by 5 units/ml. Reconstituted plasma is also useful as it contains 36–40 units/ml. Cholinesterase activity can be measured in patients who have undergone plasmapheresis and in whom the use of suxamethonium is contemplated.

5 An excessive formation of succinyl monocholine. Hydrolysis of succinylcholine takes place in two stages, succinyl monocholine being the intermediate product.[46] This has between 5% and 20% the relaxing effect of the parent compound, but as it is hydrolysed rather slowly by both acetyl and serum cholinesterase, it may accumulate in the bloodstream, but only if relatively large amounts of suxamethonium (more than 0.5 g) have been used, e.g. as intravenous infusion.

6 Phase II block (dual block).[47]

Other causes of prolonged apnoea:

1 Central depression of the respiratory centre by a narcotic analgesic, thiopentone, or volatile anaesthetics.

2 Hypocapnia: in this case respiration will recommence if the CO_2 level is allowed to rise above 6 kPa (45 mmHg).

3 Hypercapnia: very high CO_2 levels (> 13 kPa) can paralyse the respiratory centre and cause apnoea.

4 Depression of the lung stretch receptor mechanism during controlled respiration. This will usually yield to raising the end-tidal CO_2 for short periods.

5 Reflex laryngeal apnoea. Due to the presence of a tracheal tube. Removal of the tube or deflation of the cuff leads to restoration of spontaneous respiration.

6 Head injury and acute rise of intracranial pressure.

7 There are some gravely ill patients who breathe again only with difficulty once they become apnoeic. In such patients it may be wise not to abolish voluntary respiration at all.

8 Metabolic acidosis can cause a clinical picture similar to that of myoneural block. The cause of prolonged apnoea is not always fully understood.

DIFFERENTIAL DIAGNOSIS BETWEEN HYPOPNOEA DUE TO CENTRAL DEPRESSION AND THAT DUE TO PERIPHERAL PARALYSIS WHEN NERVE STIMULATOR IS NOT AVAILABLE

1 Central depression. Breathing slow, reasonably deep. No tracheal tug; no pause at end of inspiration.

2 Peripheral paralysis (myoneural block). Breathing jerky, shallow and of normal rate. Pause after inspiration and again after expiration (Morton's rectangular breathing).[48] Tracheal tug.

MANAGEMENT OF UNEXPECTEDLY PROLONGED APNOEA AFTER SUXAMETHONIUM

1 Artificial ventilation and sedation are maintained until monitoring shows the block to have worn off.
2 A blood sample is taken for cholinesterase analysis.
3 Fresh frozen plasma or cholase may be administered to correct the deficiency.
4 Near relatives are screened and if positive, issued with warning cards or bangles.

MANAGEMENT OF KNOWN OR SUSPECTED SUXAMETHONIUM SENSITIVE PATIENTS

1 Suxamethonium is avoided if possible.
2 If suxamethonium is indicated for the anaesthetic sequence, (e.g. for ECT) it may be given to documented heterozygotes only, in very small test doses, e.g. 0.05–0.1 mg/kg, when it produces a normal response. A normal dose of 1 mg/kg, when given to a heterozygote, produces apnoea for 10 min, and very rarely up to an hour.
3 In homozygotes, a rapid-onset, short-acting, non-depolarizing drug may be used (e.g. mivacurium).

Hyperkalaemia

Potassium is released from muscles following suxamethonium injection, causing a rise of serum potassium of 0.2–0.4 mmol/l. Much greater hyperkalaemia occurs after burns (3 weeks to 3 months), tetanus and spinal cord injuries. Also in patients with upper and lower motor neurone lesions, congenital cerebral palsy, Duchenne's muscular dystrophy, wasting secondary to chronic arterial insufficiency, and severe intra-abdominal infection. This great release is the result of extrajunctional receptor stimulation (*see above*).

Raised intraocular pressure

(This may be important in the presence of a perforating eye injury.) Suxamethonium, 1 mg/kg, raises the pressure an average of 7 mmHg, partly as a result of tonic contraction of the extraocular muscles, with return to normal pressure in 10 min, caused by absorption of aqueous humour (the extraocular muscles may remain contracted for 30 min, upsetting the calculations used in squint correction). The lens is left nearer the corneal endothelium, with greater risk of damage during lens extraction and implants. Some workers view its use in severe glaucoma with reserve.

Muscle pain

The pain is influenced by age, sex and physical fitness. It is suggested that uncoordinated muscle contractions that precede paralysis are the cause of the pain but this is probably not so.[49] Pains are more frequent in women and middle-aged patients than in those at the extremes of age and in men. The incidence is reduced during pregnancy. The longer the interval between the injection of an intravenous barbiturate and suxamethonium, the more intense the postoperative discomfort. Pains may be delayed until the third or fourth postoperative day. Post-suxamethonium sore throat may be a muscle-produced pain and not due to trauma.

Pain is less frequent in patients who are muscularly 'fit' than in the 'unfit' and when the injection is given slowly.

Prevention of muscle pains:

1 Pre-curarization, the intravenous injection of a small dose of a non-depolarizing relaxant 3 min before the suxamethonium. Muscle fasciculations may also be reduced by intravenous injection of suxamethonium, 10 mg, and injection of the rest of the dose after a 1-min interval, or when it is given in a drip at a rate of less than 2 mg/s.

2 Intravenous injection of lignocaine 2–6 mg/kg following thiopentone and 3 min before the relaxant. This also prolongs apnoea. Intravenous lignocaine may cause significant sinus bradycardia or even asystole. It restricts increase in serum potassium and decrease in serum calcium.[50]

It is suggested that the muscle-spindle injury as shown by the creatinine phosphokinase level is produced by suxamethonium given intermittently, especially if the patient is receiving halothane. This may result in myoglobinuria which may, among other things, give a positive Haemostix reaction in urine. Visible fasciculations are not constantly related to the severity of any subsequent symptoms.[51]

These muscle pains may not be prevented by atracurium.[52]

EFFECT IN MALIGNANT HYPERPYREXIA

Suxamethonium is one of the drugs most commonly implicated in this condition. Incidence 1 in 100 000 adult anaesthetics. It then causes muscle rigidity, not relaxation. *See* Chapter 2.8. Suxamethonium is best avoided in children with Duchenne muscular dystrophy because of the risk of malignant hyperpyrexia.[53]

DYSTROPHIA MYOTONICA

Suxamethonium exacerbates this with body rigidity preventing respiration and intubation.

CARDIOVASCULAR SYSTEM

Bradycardia and cardiac arrest may occur on the second, or even the first injection. Prevented by prior atropine or gallamine. Cardiac arrest due to hyperkalaemia may occur when suxamethonium is given to patients with existing hyperkalaemia, 3-week-old burns, crush injuries, widespread denervation, or tetanus. The treatment is standard CPR with lignocaine to prevent dysrhythmias, and measures to reduce serum potassium.

Suxamethonium may cause a rise in blood pressure, perhaps due to ganglion stimulation, a nicotinic response.

CENTRAL NERVOUS SYSTEM

Muscarinic effects may occur.

ALIMENTARY SYSTEM

Muscarinic effects, salivation and gastric secretion. Increase in intragastric pressure to more than 20 mmHg, due to severe muscle fasciculation. The cricopharyngeal sphincter loses its tone.

PLACENTAL BARRIER

Small amounts of this highly polarized drug do in fact reach the fetus, but are without effect on the baby. Excellent for operative obstetrics and Caesarean section.

ANAPHYLAXIS

True anaphylaxis without previous exposure, has been reported, with bronchospasm, hypotension, acute circulatory collapse,[54] pharyngeal and facial oedema, and a positive transfer (Prausnitz–Kustner) reaction.
   Incidence 1:5000 and rising.

Prevention of some side-effects

(Except perhaps rise of intraocular pressure.)

1 'Self-taming' by 10 mg suxamethonium injected a minute before induction of anaesthesia (unpleasant for the patient).
2 Pre-curarization 3 min before induction of anaesthesia; vecuronium 0.5 mg, or other non-depolarizing drug.

See also under 'muscle pains'.

Use of different relaxants in the same patient

The effects of different non-depolarizing relaxants are additive (faster onset, more intense block, and longer duration). In general, depolarizers should not be used after non-depolarizers. Only if the effects of the first drug have worn off should one of the other group be used.

Some factors influencing neuromuscular block

In disease

1 *Myasthenia gravis and myasthenic syndrome* (*see* Chapter 3.1) and any type of generalized muscle weakness.
2 *Liver and kidney disease.*
3 *Electrolyte imbalance.* Particularly changes in potassium.
4 *Connective tissue diseases* may show increased sensitivity to non-depolarizing relaxants.
5 *Dystrophia myotonica. See above.*

6 *Hypothermia* potentiates the effects of depolarizing and tends to diminish the activity of non-depolarizing relaxants. The action of atracurium may be prolonged, perhaps as a result of slowing of the Hofmann elimination process.

7 *Repeated plasmapheresis* may lead to progressive depletion of serum cholinesterase.

Effects of drugs

1 *Aminoglycoside antibiotics*. Neomycin, streptomycin, kanamycin, gentamicin, tobramycin, bacitracin, colimycin, polymixin, clindamycin and colistimethate, if given parenterally or intraperitoneally, may cause a non-depolarizing block which will be potentiated by non-depolarizing relaxants. It is not always reversed by neostigmine. Tetracycline and penicillin show no neuromuscular blocking activity.

2 *Ecothiopate eye drops* are an anticholinesterase used in the treatment of glaucoma. Apnoea from an intubating dose of suxamethonium may be prolonged. The effects of ecothiopate drops may last for 3 weeks.

3 *Aprotinin (Trasylol)*. Slightly reduces the serum cholinesterase activity of the blood, but unless its level is already very low from other causes, prolonged apnoea is very unlikely.

4 *Metriphonate*, used in the treatment of urinary schistosomiasis, reduces serum cholinesterase.

5 *Lithium salts*. A raised blood lithium level potentiates the effects of anaesthesia and relaxants; at least two doses should be omitted before anaesthesia. Delayed onset and prolongation of suxamethonium block may result. Potent diuretics may increase this toxicity of lithium. Similarly, significant preoperative dehydration is to be avoided as this may cause lithium toxicity.

FURTHER READING

Bowman W. C. *Pharmacology of Neuromuscular Function*. Wright, London, 1990.
Bowman W. C. In Adams A. P. and Cashman J. N. (eds) *Recent Advances in Anaesthesia and Analgesia – 20*. Churchill Livingstone, Edinburgh, 1998.

REFERENCES

1 Standaert F. G. *Clin. Anesthesiol.* 1985, **3,** 243.
2 Guy H.R. *Biophysical J.* 1984, **35,** 249.
3 Stya M. and Axelrod D. J. *J. Neurosci.* 1984, **4,** 70.
4 Azar I. *Anesthesiology* 1984, **61,** 173.

5 Jones R. M. *Anaesthesia* 1985, **40,** 964; Pearce A. C. Neuromuscular blockade monitoring. In Atkinson R. S. and Adams A. P. (eds) *Recent Advances in Anaesthesia and Analgesia – 16.* Churchill Livingstone, Edinburgh, 1989.
6 Sia R. L. and Straatman N. J. A. *Anaesthesia* 1985, **40,** 167.
7 Roberts D. V. and Wilson A. *Br. J. Pharmacol.* 1968, **34,** 229; Ali H. H. et al. *Br. J. Anaesth.* 1970, **42,** 967; Lee C. M. *Anesth. Analg. Curr. Res.* 1975, **54,** 649; Zeh D. W. and Katz R. L. *Anesth. Analg. Curr. Res.* 1978, **57,** 13; Ali H. H. and Savarese J. J. *Anesthesiology* 1976, **45,** 216.
8 Miller R. D. *Anesthesiology* 1976, **44,** 318.
9 Ali H.H. et al. *Br. J. Anaesth.* 1971, **43,** 473; Ali H.H. et al. *Br. J. Anaesth.* 1975, **47,** 570.
10 Viby-Mogensen J. et al. *Anesthesiology* 1981, **55,** 458.
11 Engbaek J. et al. *Br. J. Anaesth.* 1989, **62,** 274.
12 Jensen E. et al. *Acta Anaesth. Scand.* 1988, **32,** 49.
13 Norman J. *Clin. Anesthesiol.* 1985, **3,** 273.
14 Duvaldestin P. et al. *Clin. Anesthesiol.* 1985, **3,** 293.
15 Miller R. D. *Can. Anaesth. Soc. J.* 1979, **26,** 83.
16 Wong K. C. *Fed. Proc.* 1969, **28,** 420
17 Jones R. M. *Anaesthesia* 1985, **40,** 964.
18 Skarpa P. et al. *Br. J. Anaesth.* 1983, **55,** 275; Flynn P. J. et al. *Br. J. Anaesth.* 1984, **56,** 599.
19 Chapple D. J. and Miller A. A. *Br. J. Anaesth.* 1987, **59,** 218.
20 Hunter J. M. et al. *Br. J. Anaesth.* 1982, **54,** 1251.
21 Rowlands D. E. *Br. J. Anaesth.* 1983, **55,** 123 and 125.
22 Flynn P. J. et al. *Br. J. Anaesth.* 1984, **56,** 967.
23 Bellis D. J et al. *Anaesthesia* 1990, **45,** 118.
24 Aldrete J. A. *Br. J. Anaesth.* 1985, **57,** 929
25 Baraka A. et al. *Br. J. Anaesth.* 1984, **56,** 673.
26 MacDonald A. M. et al. *Br. J Anaesth.* 1984, **56,** 651; Bell C. F. et al. *Anaesthesia* 1984, **39,** 961.
27 Pearce A. C. et al. *Br. J. Anaesth.* 1984, **56,** 973.
28 Eager B. M. et al. *Br. J. Anaesth.* 1984, **56,** 447.
29 Mirakhur R.K. *Drugs* 1992, **44,** 182.
30 Jones R. M. Savareses J. J. and Van Aken H. (eds) *Curr. Opin. Anesthesiology* 1995, **9,** Suppl. 1.
31 Savarese J. J. et al. *Anesthesiology* 1988, **68,** 723–732; Stoops C. M. et al. *Anesth. Analg.* 1989, **68,** 333.
32 Cashman J. N. et al. *Br. J. Anaesth.* 1990, **64,** 186.
33 Basta S. J. et al. *Anesthesiology* 1988, **69,** 478.
34 Murray D. J. et al. *Anesthesiology* 1988, **69,** 472; Bracey B. J. et al. *Can. Anaesth. Soc. J.* 1989, **36,** S117.
35 Walmsley D. A. *Lancet* 1959, **2,** 237; Evans P. J. D. and McKinnon I. *Anaesth. Intensive Care* 1977, **5,** 239; Fisher M. McD. *Anaesth. Intensive Care* 1978, **6,** 62.
36 Buzello W. and Noldge G. *Br. J. Anaesth.* 1982, **54,** 1151.
37 Caldwell J. E. et al, *Anesthesiology,* 1988, **70,** 784.
38 Caldwell J. E. et al, *Br. J. Anaesth.* 1988, **61,** 693.

39 Pratila M. G. and Pratilas V. *Anesthesiology* 1978, **49,** 338; Smith G. et al. *Br. J. Anaesth.* 1970, **42,** 923.

40 Cronnelly R. *Clin. Anesthesiol.* 1985, **3,** 315.

41 Cronnelly R. et al. *Anesthesiology* 1979, **51,** 222.

42 Cronelly R. et al. *Clin. Pharmacol. Ther.* 1980, **28,** 78.

43 Viby-Mogensen J. *Cholinesterase and Succinylcholine.* Laegeforenningens Forlag, Kobenhavn, 1982.

44 Viby-Mogensen J. *Anesthesiology* 1981, **55,** 429.

45 Viby-Mogensen J. and Hanel H. K. *Acta Anaesthiol. Scand.* 1978, **22,** 371.

46 Whittaker J. P. and Wijesundera S. *Biochem. J.* 1952, **52,** 475.

47 Zaimis E. *J. Physiol.* 1953, **122,** 238.

48 Morton H. J. V. *Proc. R. Soc. Med.* 1945, **38,** 441.

49 Verma R. S. *Anaesthesia* 1982, **37,** 688.

50 Chatterji S. et al. *Anaesthesia* 1983, **38,** 867.

51 Collier C. B. *Anaesth. Intensive Care* 1980, **8,** 26.

52 Budd A. *Anaesthesia* 1985, **40,** 642.

53 Rosemberg H. and Heiman-Patterson T. *Anesthesiology*, 1983, **59,** 362.

54 Youngman P. R. and Wilson J. D. *Lancet* 1983, **2,** 597.

Chapter 2.6

Intubation and ventilation

Indications for intubation

1 *To maintain airway* if otherwise difficult because of anatomy, position of patient, operation site (e.g. head neck or chest), or liability to laryngeal spasm (e.g. haemorrhoidectomy etc.).

2 *To allow intermittent positive-pressure ventilation (IPPV):*

    (a) if relaxation is needed, e.g. many abdominal operations;

    (b) in thoracic operations where suctioning can also be easily carried out;

    (c) to minimize the dose of volatile agent and/or allow large doses of narcotics;

    (d) in infant anaesthesia where respiration is easily depressed and intubation halves the anatomic dead space;

    (e) in respiratory failure.

3 *To prevent aspiration* of stomach contents or blood and debris from operations on the head and upper airways.

Tracheal insufflation in animals was described by Andreas Vesalius (1514–1564) of Padua in 1555.

The larynx is the organ of voice, the sphincter between the pharynx and trachea. It extends from the root of the tongue to the trachea (Fig. 2.6.1) and lies opposite C.3-6 vertebrae; higher in children and in females. It is covered by the depressor muscles of the hyoid bone, by the thyroid gland and by the cricothyroid muscles. Composed of the following cartilages, joined together by ligaments; thyroid, cricoid, two arytenoid, two corniculate (Santorini), two cuneiform (Wrisberg) and the epiglottis.

The cavity of the larynx extends from the super laryngeal aperture to the lower border of the cricoid cartilage. The piriform fossa is a recess, on each side, bounded by the aryepiglottic fold medially and the thyroid cartilage and thyrohyoid membrane laterally. Beneath its mucosa lie twigs of the internal laryngeal nerve, which may be blocked by topical local analgesics. The depression between the dorsum of the tongue and the epiglottis is divided

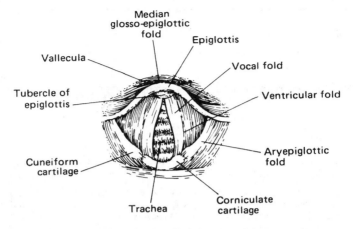

Figure 2.6.1 A laryngoscopic view of the interior of the larynx. (From *Gray's Anatomy*, by kind permission of Professor T.B. Johnston.)

into two valleculae by the glosso-epiglottic fold. The epiglottis is not essential for swallowing, breathing, or phonation.

The superior laryngeal aperture is wider in front than behind, and slopes downwards and backwards. Bounded anteriorly by the epiglottis; laterally by the aryepiglottic folds containing the two small nodules on each side, cuneiform anteriorly and the corniculate posteriorly; posteriorly by the arytenoids. This view is seen at laryngoscopy. The vestibule of the larynx is the superior part of the cavity of the larynx and extends from the aryepiglottic folds to the vestibular (ventricular) folds. Each of the latter is a ridge formed by the vestibular ligament and extends from the angle of the thyroid cartilage anteriorly, backwards along the side cavity of the larynx to the cuneiform cartilage. The vesticular folds are the false cords, the space between them is the rima vestibuli, while a depression on the side-wall of the larynx between the vestibular fold and the vocal fold (false and true cords) is the saccule of the larynx.

The vocal cords (folds) stretch from the thyroid cartilage anteriorly, to the arytenoid cartilage of the corresponding side posteriorly. The space between the cords is the glottis. It is bounded in front by the intermembranous part of the cords (the vocal folds); behind, by the intercartilaginous part. The glottis is the narrowest part of the larynx in adults and measures about 2.3 cm from front to back in males, 1.7 cm in females. In children, the narrowest part is found just below the cords at the cricoid ring. The shape and width of the glottis vary with phonation and respiration and the tone of the muscles controlling it. When these are in spasm, the glottis is obliterated.

The mucosa of the upper part of the larynx is lined by squamous cells like the oropharynx; the cords are covered by a thin layer of mucosa, closely adherent to them, white in colour. The lower larynx is lined by ciliated epithelium with mucous glands and goblet cells.

The extrinsic muscles are the thyrohyoid and the sternothyroid and the inferior constrictor of the pharynx. The first elevates, the second depresses the larynx while the third constricts the pharynx.

The intrinsic muscles

Those which open and close the glottis

1 The posterior (open) and lateral crico-arytenoids (close).
2 The interarytenoid. During inspiration, cords abduct. On expiration they return nearly to the midline. On phonation they actually touch.

Those controlling the tension of the cords

1 The cricothyroids are tensors of the cords.
2 The posterior crico-arytenoids.
3 The thyroarytenoids are relaxers of the cords.
4 The vocales.

Those controlling the inlet of the larynx

1 The aryepiglottics.
2 The thyroepiglottics. In laryngeal spasm both the true and the false cords are adducted.

Nerve supply (from the vagus)

All sensory nerve impulses from the larynx reach the nucleus solitarius in the medulla.

The superior laryngeal branch of the vagus arises near the base of the skull and divides into the internal laryngeal nerve, the sensory supply to both surfaces of the epiglottis and to the larynx down to the vocal cords and the motor external laryngeal nerve which supplies the cricothyroid muscle and the inferior constrictor of the pharynx, the division taking place slightly below and anterior to the greater cornu of the hyoid bone. The external laryngeal nerve may be injured during ligation of the superior thyroid vessels at thyroidectomy, causing temporary huskiness of voice. The recurrent laryngeal branch supplies the remaining intrinsic muscles and is sensory to the mucosa below the cords.

The recurrent laryngeal nerve carries abductor and adductor fibres, but if it is injured abductor paralysis is greater than adductor paralysis. With bilateral injury there is respiratory difficulty as the cords lie together and speech is difficult with a valve-like obstruction and inspiratory stridor. Complete paralysis of both recurrent nerves inactivates both abductor and adductor muscles. The tensing action of the cricothyroid muscles still maintains cords in adduction.

Paralysis of one cord may be symptomless but paralysis of both is serious and may require surgery.

Paralysis of both recurrent and superior laryngeal nerves together produces the cadaveric position. In this, also seen when relaxants have had a full effect, the cords lie midway between abduction and adduction; they are not under tension due to cricothyroid paralysis.

Topical analgesia of the larynx may, by paralysing twigs from the external laryngeal nerves going to the cricothyroids, cause both a temporary alteration in the appearance of the cords and in the voice.

Arterial supply: Laryngeal branches of the superior and inferior thyroid arteries which accompany the nerves.

ANAESTHETIC AGENTS IN RELATION TO TRACHEAL INTUBATION

Induction agents alone

Intubation is possible under propofol 1–2 μg/kg, with alfentanil 10–20 μg/kg. or remifentanil 1–2 μg/kg.

Intravenous induction followed by progression to deep inhalation anaesthesia with spontaneous respiration can also be used (although respiratory and cardiovascular depression may occur).

Sevoflurane is popular in children, and useful in the difficult intubation case where awake intubation is not possible.[1] Laryngoscopy and intubation are well facilitated by this agent alone.

Induction agents and suxamethonium 0.5–1.5 mg/kg i.v.

Onset in seconds and profound relaxation makes intubation quick and atraumatic. Offset after a few minutes is an additional safety factor in failed intubation. Suxamethonium can be given 3 mg/kg i.m. or by sublingual injection in an emergency.

Non-depolarizing relaxants

Vecuronium, mivacurium, cis-atracurium or atracurium take up to 90 s to produce relaxation adequate for intubation, during which time gentle face-mask ventilation is applied. Rocuronium is significantly faster, but has a longer duration (a problem in failed intubation, but early reversal is usually easy!) Rapacurium has a time-course similar to suxamethonium.

Relaxants should never be given unless the anaesthetist is confident of his or her ability to ventilate the lungs using a face mask.

RAPID-SEQUENCE INDUCTION OF ANAESTHESIA

Preoxygenation, induction agent and suxamethonium are the norm, with cricoid pressure. A trained assistant (ODA), running suction, tilting table, selection of tested cuffed endotracheal tubes, laryngoscopes and gum-elastic bougies are at hand. Cricoid pressure is only released when the endotracheal cuff is safely inflated.

Rocuronium 1 mg/kg with thiopentone has been used successfully in rapid-sequence induction. Good intubating conditions are obtained faster if ketamine is the induction agent.[2]

CONTENTS OF THE INTUBATION TROLLEY

Apparatus

Endotracheal tubes

The tube number is the internal diameter in millimetres. Most tubes are made of semi-rigid polyvinyl chloride (PVC), e.g. Portex. The toxicity of the PVC is tested by implantation in rabbit muscle (IT = 'implantation tested') or by cell culture. Z79 is the committee in the US that approves anaesthetic equipment. Red rubber, silicone and PVC are all flammable in concentrations of O_2 and N_2O that are used clinically.

There are many types of tubes for special purposes. A *microlaryngeal tube* is a 5-mm tube with an adult-sized cuff for microlaryngeal surgery. *Wire-reinforced* silicone rubber tubes resist kinking and are available down to 2.5 mm. *RAE preformed nasal* and oral tubes (Ring, Adair, Elwyn),[3] up-facing and down-facing, are widely used in upper extremity surgery.

Inflatable cuffs[4]

Nearly all endotracheal tubes have cuffs to prevent leakage between the endotracheal tube and the trachea – leakage of gas out during inspiratory phase of IPPV, and of gastric contents, blood and mucus into the lungs. Available on tubes down to about 5 mm. The integrity of the cuff should be tested before use. The tube to the pilot balloon enters the shaft of a nasal tube much nearer its proximal end than for an orotracheal tube.

Cuffs are of low-volume, high-pressure, or high-volume, low-pressure type. Pressure on the tracheal wall is likely to be less than cuff pressure, but may be nearly equal if the cuff is floppy.

Cuff pressure may be monitored and should not exceed 30 cmH_2O or 22 mmHg. to prevent ischaemic damage to the tracheal mucosa. It is important that cuffs should not be inflated more than the minimum needed to prevent audible leakage of gas when the reservoir bag is compressed. Over-inflation causes, at least, a sore throat; at worst, necrosis of the tracheal mucosa. This is an area for constant vigilance. Leakage past low-pressure cuffs has been reported.[5]

The rise in pressure that occurs as N_2O diffuses into the cuff may be minimized by inflation with normal saline, filling the cuff with anaesthetic gas mixtures, or the use of a pressure limiting device or a foam-filled cuff.

Laryngoscopes

The Macintosh laryngoscope blade is short, curved and Z-shaped on cross-section. Its tip enters the vallecula, lifts the base of the tongue and the epiglottis, so that the cords can be visualized. Both aspects of the epiglottis are supplied by the internal branch of the superior laryngeal nerve. A version made of acetyl co-polymer can be boiled but not autoclaved. The Magill blade is straight and the tip designed to elevate the epiglottis from behind.

While the blade of each instrument is designed to be inserted into the right side of the patient's mouth (moving the tongue over to the left) there is a blade available for the left side.[6]

Full-size blades can be used for quite small children, but neonates and babies may require special straight blades, e.g. the Oxford infant blade.

A paraglossal straight-blade intubation has been recommended.[7]

The Polio laryngoscope can be used on patients in iron-lung respirators, its Macintosh-type blade makes an angle of approximately 135 degrees with the handle. Other blades may help with a difficult intubation.[8]

The McCoy blade has a hinged tip, actuated by a lever which is positioned alongside the length of the handle, on the opposite side to the blade. After insertion (with the hand further clockwise round the handle than usual), pressing the lever elevates the hinged tip, after it is in the vallecula, especially useful in grade 3 intubations, and in combination with cricoid pressure (Fig. 2.6.2).[9]

The Bullard intubating laryngoscope is useful when the neck is immobile and mouth opening restricted. It has fibreoptics, suction and intubation channels, and is made in adult and paediatric versions.[10]

Intubating forceps

Magill's forceps, made in two sizes, are commonly used. A modification with an antero-posterior grip has been described.[11]

First used to introduce gum-elastic catheters for insufflation anaesthesia.

Lubricants

A water-soluble lubricant applied to the tube, with or without local analgesic (e.g. 2–4% lignocaine), may reduce trauma but not necessarily the incidence of sore throat (about 50%).

Topical analgesia

Analgesic solution may be sprayed onto the superior laryngeal aperture, the cords and the mucosa of the larynx and trachea using metered-dose aerosols. They can become a source of infection. Lignocaine 3 mg/kg should not be exceeded.

OROTRACHEAL INTUBATION UNDER DIRECT VISION

Assessment of difficulty of intubation: predictive factors

1 History of rheumatoid arthritis (also carries risk of damage to the spinal cord by odontoid peg during extension of the head); arthritis of the temporomandibular joints.

2 Known history of difficult intubation: high Cormack & Lehane scores from previous laryngoscopies.

3 Poor mouth opening (< 3 fb) or a long, high arched palate and narrow mouth, as in Marfan's syndrome.

4 High Mallampati score.[12]

5 Thyromental distance < 6 cm.[13]

6 Small mandible size, inability to protrude jaw, overhanging upper front teeth.

7 Neck stiffness or injury (cervical X-rays are important here), burns, contractures at the front of the neck, bony spicules on the spinous processes of the cervical vertebrae, use of hard collars in neck injuries; reduced atlanto-occipital distance, atlanto-odontoid distance (> 3 mm).[14] Also a short muscular neck with a full set of teeth.

8 Dental caps and crowns, awkward or loose front teeth.

9 Very large breasts or gross obesity.

10 Hypertrophy of the posterior one-third of the tongue.

11 Subglottic stenosis, following previous prolonged intubation or tracheostomy.

12 Trismus.

13 Known or suspected laryngeal obstruction.
Soft tissue X-ray of neck is needed here. Tumours of the mouth or larynx, laryngocele (pathological enlargement of the saccule of the larynx),[15] epiglottic cyst.[16]

14 Congenital abnormalities
Abnormalities of the face or neck (*see* Chapter 3.2), e.g. Achondroplasia, where there may be a kyphosis between C2 and C3,[17] Pierre–Robin and Treacher–Collins syndromes, acromegaly (*see* Chapter 3.2), Klippel–Fiel syndrome.

15 Previous suxamethonium masseter spasm (if rapid sequence induction is needed).

Mallampati scores

1 Soft palate, uvula and pillars visible

2 Pillars obscured but posterior pharyngeal wall visible below soft palate

3 Soft palate only visible

4 Soft palate not visible

Various radiological predictors of difficulty have also been suggested.

1 Increased distance between the mental symphysis and the lower alveolar margin which requires wide depression of the lower jaw during intubation.
2 A ratio of effective mandibular length to its posterior depth that is less than 3.6.
3 Reduction in the radiological distance between the occiput and the posterior tubercle of C1 or the C1/C2 intergap.[18] Attempts to extend the head on the neck will then result in anterior bowing of the cervical spine and anterior displacement of the larynx.
4 C1/C2 interspinous gap.

Sagittal magnetic resonance images of the upper airways may be valuable in specialized cases.

Technique (*see* Fig. 2.6.1)

A small pillow should usually be placed under the occiput to flex the neck and extend the atlanto-occipital joint. This straightens the path from the upper incisors to the larynx. Loose, filled or capped teeth, especially upper incisors, may be protected from the laryngoscope blade by a guard. General anaesthesia is induced by an intravenous or inhalational agent. No hypoxia will occur for up to 4 min of apnoea provided pure oxygen has been breathed for the previous 3 min. A little more intravenous agent or the introduction of a volatile agent may be needed while waiting for a non-depolarizing relaxant to take effect. Relaxation must be good, and can be monitored by stimulator on the facial nerve. Alternatively deep inhalational anaesthesia may be established (in the stage 3 plane 2 or below, with complete suppression of reflexes). Less harm is done by getting the patient a little too deep than by using force in a patient with active reflexes and rigid neck muscles. Absence of reflexes and adequate muscular relaxation are necessary for laryngoscopy in all but expert hands.

The suppression of laryngeal reflexes by propofol has encouraged some to use this (2.5 mg/kg), with alfentanil 30 μg/kg[19] or lignocaine 1.5 mg/kg,[20] to allow intubation with no muscle relaxant. This is not recommended for the inexperienced.

The curved blade may be the easier to use if the patient has a full set of teeth, and may cause less stretching of the faucial pillars and less bruising than a straight blade. It is inserted from the right side of the patient's mouth to prevent the tongue blocking the view of the larynx, while watching the blade tip as it is advanced alongside the tongue towards the midline. When the epiglottis is seen, the tip is inserted firmly but not forcibly into the vallecula and is used to lift the base of the epiglottis forwards to reveal the cords. Backward pressure on the thyroid cartilage by an assistant may help bring the cords into view. A curved tube is easier to insert than a straight one. A gum-elastic bougie[21] may be very helpful for intubations with Cormack & Lehane scores of 2–4, with its tip curved anteriorly, passed into the trachea and used

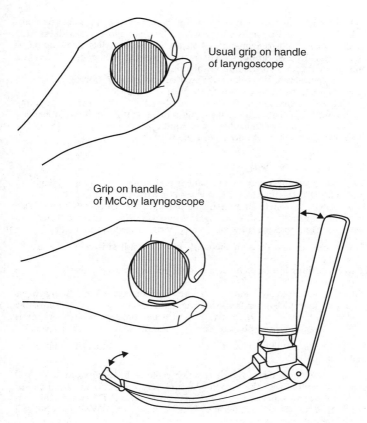

Usual grip on handle
of laryngoscope

Grip on handle
of McCoy laryngoscope

Figure 2.6.2 A McCoy laryngoscope.

as an introducer. Passage of the tube over the bougie may be helped by keeping the laryngoscope in the mouth, and by rotating the tube 90 degrees anticlockwise as the bevel reaches the larynx.[22] An angioscope may be inserted down a bougie for visual insertion.[23]

Grading of difficulty has been proposed according to the amount of the larynx exposed at laryngoscopy.[24]

The incidence of difficulty: 1 in 300 adult non-obstetric surgical patients.[25]

It may be unwise to abolish spontaneous respiration in these patients before checking that manual ventilation is possible using a face mask. Leaks around a face mask may prevent manual ventilation in patients with facial deformities.

Even a beard may cause a major leak. Intubation equipment should be available wherever anaesthesia is given: two working laryngoscopes with assorted blades, Magill forceps, gum-elastic bougies, malleable stylets, oro- and naso-pharyngeal airways, various sizes of tracheal tubes, suction apparatus, and an emergency kit for transtracheal ventilation.

More specialized, less frequently used equipment (e.g. fibreoptic laryngo-scopes) should be kept centrally in the theatre complex.

Many of the anatomic difficulties listed above will still be present after any operation, and will also add to the dangers of extubation until the patient can maintain the airway. Difficulties (and solutions) should be recorded in the notes for the benefit of future anaesthetists.

Is the tube correctly placed in the trachea?

This is vital to the safety of the patient and requires life-long vigilance to guarantee that the tube is in the trachea every time.

It is easy to wrongly intubate the oesophagus, no matter how experienced the anaesthetist. It must be recognized immediately. The anaesthetist can only be certain that the tube has been correctly placed in the trachea if:

1 it is seen to pass through the cords and it is still visible in front of the arytenoids;
2 tracheal rings can be seen when a fibreoptic bronchoscope is passed down the tube;
3 CO_2 is present and continues to be present in the expired gas. Stomach gas may contain CO_2 after face-mask ventilation, although ventilation of the stomach reduces the level of CO_2 after a few breaths. If capnography is not available, a disposable colorimetric CO_2 detector has been described.[26]

Other tests of tube placement which require some familiarity include the following:

1 The oesophageal detector device; which exploits the rigidity of the tracheal wall compared with the oesophagus, and does not allow the distal end of the tube to be blocked when suction is applied – SCOTI (sonomatic confirmation of tracheal intubation) is less efficient than Wee's oesophageal intubation detector device.[27]

   The self-inflating bulb oesophageal intubation detector device is effective in normal individuals but may give false negatives in the morbidly obese and late pregnancy.[28]
2 Auscultation for air entry over the trachea and the absence of a gurgle over the epigastrium when the reservoir bag is squeezed.
3 Palpating the tube in the larynx through the mouth or at the front of the neck.
4 The use of a lighted stylet down the tube whose light shines through the front of the neck.

The feel and movements of the reservoir bag, auscultation of the chest and observation of its movements, though useful, may all be unreliable. Bag movement can seem just like respiratory movement even when the tube is in the

---

Immediate complications of intubation

1 Hypertension and tachycardia. Nicardipine 10–30 μg/kg has been used (Song D. et al. *Anesth. Analg.* 1997, **85,** 1247–1251.)

2 Kinking tube or biting.

3 Disconnection of anaesthetic circuit from the tube.

4 Blockage of tube by blood, mucus, etc.

5 Accidental extubation.

6 Obstruction by the inflated cuff, especially if a weak portion herniates over the tip of the tube.

7 Obstruction by apposition of the bevel of the tube against the tracheal wall.

8 Intubation of the right bronchus if tube is too long. Diagnosed by low O_2 saturations, absence of air entry into left lung, and jerky breathing or bucking. Average distance between central incisors and carina is 27 cm in an adult male and 23 cm in a female. The tip of the tube moves about 4 cm caudad as the neck moves from full extension to full flexion.

In the newborn, 5 cm separates the gums from the cords, and a similar distance separates the cords from the carina.

---

oesophagus. Oximetry is not a particularly useful early warning sign of oesophageal intubation, especially if preoxygenation has taken place. The results of unrecognized oesophageal intubation can be brain damage or death.[29]

If the clinical state of the patient should deteriorate after intubation or if there is any doubt whatsoever about tube placement, the tube should be removed and the patient ventilated by face mask. A face mask may even be used with the open tube in place if the anaesthetist is unwilling to remove it. '*When in doubt, take it out.*'

Key points in rapid sequence induction

1 Preoxygenate

2 Check suction/scopes/tubes

3 Induction agent and then relaxant

4 Cricoid pressure; 0.5–1 kg. wt.

5 Intubate and inflate cuff

6 Check seal and remove cricoid pressure

7 Continue anaesthesia

The anaesthetist must also be convinced that all parts of each lung are being ventilated, by auscultation over the trachea, each upper zone and each axilla. Causes of diminished air entry into one lung are endobronchial placement of tube, pneumothorax, bronchial obstruction by gastric contents, blood, secretions, tumour, etc.

Technique of blind orotracheal intubation

This is very occasionally necessary when abnormal anatomy precludes the use of a laryngoscope when the nasal route is undesirable, or in animals and birds. There are five methods. The patient should be deeply anaesthetized.

1 An assistant draws the tongue forwards while the anaesthetist stands facing the patient and on his or her left, passes two fingers of the left hand over the dorsum of the tongue and hooks the epiglottis forwards. The tube, which must be fully curved, is guided by these two fingers into the glottis. Curved introducers may help.
2 The anaesthetist stands in the usual place at the head of the table and inserts the left thumb into the patient's mouth with the fingers on the patient's chin. The tip of the thumb makes contact with the back of the tongue. This gives good control of the forward and backward movement of the lower jaw. The tube is guided into the glottis with the right hand.
3 The tube, which must not be too fully curved, can be passed 'blind' through a prop held in the mouth, with the head in full extension.
4 Via an ordinary laryngeal mask; either a small (6 mm) tracheal tube is inserted straight through the laryngeal mask into the trachea, or a bougie is inserted, the laryngeal mask removed and the tracheal tube railroaded over the bougie into the trachea.[30] A special intubating laryngeal mask (ILMA) with tubes is available and normally very efficient.[31] A threaded 15-mm tube connector has been developed for this.[32]
5 Light-guided intubation via laryngeal mask.[33]

NASAL INTUBATION

Indications

1 When an oral tube is in the surgeon's way, e.g. in dental extraction and operations on the tongue.
2 In the presence of crowns or other dental work vulnerable to damage by a laryngoscope.
3 In the patient in whom direct laryngoscopy is likely to be difficult, or has failed. The anaesthetist will not succeed with blind intubation in these cases unless he is practised in the technique.

Technique for blind nasal intubation

The distance between nares and carina averages 32 cm in males and 27 cm in females, i.e. 4–5 cm further than from incisors to carina. Extreme gentleness should prevail. It is a knack, only acquired by practice. The experienced worker employs tubes of the size, shape and consistency to suit the individual technique.

1 The nares should be examined for patency by listening to the patient's breathing with each naris occluded. Nasal polypi should be excluded. The nasal mucosa may be constricted by 4% cocaine spray, 1% ephedrine, or 3% lignocaine and 0.25% phenylephrine.
2 Select the largest size of tube which should pass atraumatically through the larger naris: for a big man up to 8 mm, for a small woman between 5 and 7 mm. The position of the patient's head depends on the curve of the tube: the greater the curve, the more flexed should be the head. Magill advised the position adopted 'when sniffing the morning air', the head on a single pillow, with slight extension of the atlanto-occipital joint.
3 The anaesthetist may attempt nasal intubation with the patient apnoeic after muscle relaxation, or under deep inhalational anaesthesia. Some find blind intubation easier in the paralysed patient since reflex laryngospasm does not occur.
4 The well-lubricated tube, with its concavity directed to the patient's feet, is inserted into the naris initially upwards for 2–3 cm, to clear the inferior turbinate, then directly backwards. Movement of the bevel by rotation of the tube may assist easier passage, at this stage and when the tube enters the nasopharynx.
5 If the patient is breathing spontaneously, the opposite nostril may be occluded so that all breathing is taking place through the tube. The jaw should be slightly elevated to lift the epiglottis from the posterior pharyngeal wall. If the right naris is used the head should be inclined slightly to the right, and vice versa. The anaesthetist should listen carefully to the respiration. The breath sounds conducted through the tube become maximal when its tip is immediately above the glottis. If the tube does not enter the larynx, its direction may be adjusted by rotation of the tube, rotation of the neck or digital movement of the larynx to meet the advancing tube. Should the tube enter the oesophagus it can be partially withdrawn and its tip directed anteriorly by increased extension of the neck or by using a tube with a larger curvature. Occasionally the tip of the tube impinges on the anterior commissure of the larynx, when it will often enter the larynx if the neck is flexed or a tube of lesser curvature is used. As the tube passes the cords there may be some coughing or breath-holding in the lightly anaesthetized patient, even when muscle relaxants have been employed. In the patient who is not paralysed the tube may enter the trachea during the explosive cough which may follow spasm of the cords. In the case of failure to intubate through one naris, success may be achieved through the other, or with a tube of different curvature.

6 Normal free breath sounds at the proximal end of a tube of reasonable length show that it is in the trachea. If the tube can be inserted fully and no breath sounds heard, it is probably in the oesophagus. Normal breathing through the tube, while the lower jaw is pushed backwards, suggests successful intubation. Capnography confirms this.

Difficulties

If unsuccessful, blind intubation should not be persisted in or trauma may result. Tubes, which must be supple and rather soft, should always be handled gently and not forcibly rammed down the patient's throat. Difficulty may be encountered if the tube is not sufficiently curved. A radius of curvature of 10 cm is suitable. The tube tip may catch in the vallecula, between the base of the tongue and the epiglottis, when rotation of the tube should allow it to slip down the lateral wall of the pharynx. It may also catch in a pyriform fossa, lateral to its correct position. This is likely where the nose is asymmetric, and is overcome by rotating the tube, by moving the larynx laterally to meet the tube or by rotating the patient's head.

If blind intubation fails, a laryngoscope may be inserted and the tube guided into the trachea by the Magill intubating forceps, or a wire hook in the oropharynx to guide the tube backwards or forwards.

A prominent arch of the atlas vertebra may cause obstruction and perhaps its overlying mucosa to be torn. To overcome this a small suction catheter may be threaded through the endotracheal tube and tension kept on it as it is delivered through the mouth, thus displacing the tip of the tube.

Epistaxis, though messy, seldom interferes with the anaesthesia or causes postoperative discomfort. Partial obstruction of a nasotracheal tube by an avulsed piece of turbinate may occur.[34]

The tube may be compressed by nasal spurs and a deviated septum. Nasal intubation has been followed by bacteraemia in 12% of children[35] and in 17–21% of adults.[36]

Requirements for fibreoptic intubation

1 Good O_2 supply; good fibrescope with suction channel and tracheal tube ready mounted. Good light source.

2 Good patient position.

3 Vasoconstricted and analgesic nasal passages.

4 Empty pharynx (starved patient or previous removal of blood or debris in trauma cases).

5 Reduction of laryngeal reflexes (e.g. by local analgesia).

> **Reasons for failed fibreoptic intubation**
> 1 Poor local analgesia.
> 2 Excessive blood or secretions.
> 3 Epiglottis touching posterior pharyngeal wall.
> 4 Abnormal airway anatomy.
> 5 Inability to advance endotracheal tube.
> 6 Fibrescope stuck in endotracheal tube.

FIBREOPTIC LARYNGOSCOPY AND INTUBATION

This is the method of choice for the intubation of an awake patient under topical analgesia, perhaps supplemented with sedation,[37] but can also be used in anaesthetized patients either breathing spontaneously, with controlled ventilation, or with percutaneous transtracheal jet ventilation.[38]

Many find the technique more difficult in the anaesthetized patient, and oral intubation more difficult than nasal, although split chimney oral airways make it easier while breathing anaesthetic gases, or under light propofol infusion (e.g. 1.5 μg/ml). The patient's head and cervical spine are extended, to lift the epiglottis. Full monitoring is begun. The patients must be able to oxygenate themselves or to be oxygenated during this procedure.

The instrument is used as an introducer for the tracheal tube for babies, a 3-mm tube may be passed over the smallest laryngoscope, or a guide wire passed through the suction channel into the trachea as an introducer.

The use of an armoured tube will ensure that it does not compress the fibrescope after insertion (making its withdrawal from the tube impossible).

Possible indications for awake intubation:

1 difficulty in intubation by other methods, e.g. congenital abnormalities of head and neck, rheumatoid arthritis, ankylosing spondylitis;
2 upper airway obstruction with difficult access to larynx, although not where the airway is contaminated with blood etc.;
3 bronchopleural fistula.

The following methods of local analgesia may be used after the airway is dried by glycopyrronium or atropine:

1 sucking an amethocaine 60-mg lozenge;
2 cocaine applied to the nasal mucosa (maximum dose 3 mg/kg);
3 spraying lignocaine into the mouth, pharynx, cords and trachea through the laryngoscope;
4 bilateral superior laryngeal nerve block, either percutaneously,[39] or via the pyriform fossae with Krause's forceps;
5 transtracheal injection of 2–4% lignocaine 2 ml;
6 inhalation of lignocaine via a nebulizer.

Sedation for fibreoptic intubation

The patient should be able to breathe and protrude the tongue on command.

Intravenous agents with very short half-lives are ideal (but these may also cause airway obstruction[40]), e.g. low-dose propofol infusion (which also reduces laryngeal reflexes), in a bolus dose of 0.2 mg/kg. i.v., or infusion at 1 mg/kg/h, with target blood level of 1.5 μg/ml. Midazolam 2.5 mg with remifentanil, or alfentanil 50–250 μg i.v., fentanyl 25–50 μg i.v. and droperidol are used. If recall of the intubation is felt to be undesirable, midazolam is preferred.

See also Ovassapian A. *Fiberoptic Airway Endoscopy in Anesthesia and Critical Care.* Raven Press, New York, 1990; Pierce A. In Adams A. P. and Cashman J. (eds) *Recent Advances in Anaesthesia – 19.* Churchill-Livingstone, Edinburgh, 1997.

FAILED INTUBATION DRILL

Incidence 1 in 2300 non-obstetric surgical cases. Persistent attempts at intubation of a difficult case is often unproductive and can even be disastrous. It may be better to admit defeat at a relatively early stage. A plan of management must be adopted that ensures *oxygenation of the patient without aspiration of gastric contents.* This 'failed intubation drill' is most commonly needed in obstetric anaesthesia. Difficulty with tracheal intubation is one of the most important factors leading to deaths attributed to anaesthesia.

Tunstall's drill for the patient at high risk of aspiration[41] is as follows.

1 Call for senior help.
2 Maintain oxygenation by face mask.
3 Minimize aspiration by:
   (a) keeping cricoid pressure applied;
   (b) possibly tilting the patient head down in the left lateral position;
   (c) aspirating pharynx if needed.
4 Possibly pass a gastric tube to empty stomach (but this may encourage regurgitation) and instill 20 ml 0.3 mol/l sodium citrate; remove gastric tube.
5 (a) Then either wake the patient up and consider alternative methods of intubation, or regional analgesia[42] used, or
   (b) establish spontaneously breathing inhalational anaesthesia if the operation is urgent (cricoid pressure can be used with a laryngeal mask in place).

The *intubating laryngeal mask* (ILMA) may be used at this point.[43] Not all workers agree with turning of the patient into the lateral position which may be impractical and make ventilation difficult, or with the passage of a gastric tube which may itself provoke vomiting. Total intravenous anaesthesia (TIVA) may be useful, also ketamine (with atropine and benzodiazepine).

6 Local infiltration of incision if relaxation is needed.

Other techniques to aid difficult intubation

1 Difficulties due to gross obesity or late pregnancy may be overcome with a polio laryngoscope.
2 An epidural catheter or a guide wire may be passed retrogradely through the cricothyroid membrane up to the pharynx and out through the mouth or nose, and used as an introducer for a tracheal tube.[44]

If all efforts at intubation fail, and the airway is obstructed, transtracheal ventilation may be life-saving. A 14-G intravenous cannula or needle is thrust into the trachea through the cricothyroid membrane. It takes only seconds to do this. The luer connection is connected to the barrel of a syringe into which is thrust a cuffed tracheal tube. This is connected to the anaesthesia system and manual ventilation given.

A modified bronchoscope injector has been used but could cause surgical emphysema.

A standard resuscitation bag may provide adequate ventilation through a 12-G cannula. Following this, insertion of a 4-mm mini-tracheostomy tube or other commercial cricothyrotomy kits should allow relatively easy ventilation. In the situations where this is needed, the neck itself is often highly abnormal, e.g. with haematoma, making insertion more difficult.

With all these methods there must be a clear expiratory pathway to prevent dangerously high airway pressures, if necessary through a second needle or cannula in the cricothyroid membrane.[45]

EXTUBATION

Selective extubation may be performed in theatre or with the patient awake (e.g. in the recovery ward) as appropriate to the emergency risks, the age, respiratory and cardiac diseases.

Extubation coughing, hypertension and tachycardia (which can pose as much risk as intubation) may be lessened by lignocaine, 60 mg instilled down the tube or 1 mg/kg i.v. or by substituting a laryngeal mask for the tracheal tube while still anaesthetized.[46]

Pharyngeal secretions are removed by suction and the patient allowed to breathe 100% O_2 before extubation. The airway must then be watched carefully. It may be more safely managed in the lateral head-down position.

Post-extubation laryngeal spasm has been managed by:

1 giving O_2 by manual ventilation via a face mask;
2 doxapram 1.5 mg/kg;[47]
3 topical analgesia;
4 lignocaine injected intravenously;[48]
5 injection of a small dose of suxamethonium and ventilation with O_2; reintubation may be required.

A sample protocol for extubation in recovery, high-dependency or intensive therapy units

1 Adequate respiration in rate (>6 bpm) and depth.

2 Clear airway above the larynx – it should have been suctioned.

3 Pure O_2 given for 2 min before extubation.

4 Other parameters must be satisfactory, e.g. SpO_2, arterial pressure.

5 The tape securing the tube is removed, the cuff is deflated, and with full expansion of the lungs, the tube is removed.

6 Continued monitoring of SpO_2, BP, respiratory rate and depth, $ETCO_2$, etc.

Laryngeal spasm may result in acute pulmonary oedema, as may other causes of upper airway obstruction,[49] possibly due to low alveolar pressures encouraging fluid transudation.

Difficulty in extubation is unusual, but may be caused by the cuff failing to deflate or becoming distorted, or the tube accidentally becoming sutured in place. Airway obstruction after extubation may be due to a haematoma in the neck, tracheomalacia, throat packs, other foreign bodies and tumours.

REFLEX RESPONSES TO LARYNGOSCOPY, INTUBATION AND EXTUBATION[50]

During light general anaesthesia, direct laryngoscopy and intubation cause an increase in heart rate and arterial pressure, and dysrhythmia in up to 90% of patients because of afferent stimulation of the vagus and a sympatho-adrenal response.

Hypertensive subjects show an exaggerated response. Endorphin release also occurs on intubation.[51]

These reflexes are of significance in patients with coronary artery disease, raised intracranial pressure, intracranial aneurysm or open eye surgery.

There is no influence of the type of laryngoscope blade used.[52]

The responses are less under deep general anaesthesia, adequate topical analgesia, and with smooth blind nasal and fibreoptic intubation.[53]

These responses may be minimized by:

1 fentanyl at conventional doses of 2–6 μg/kg,[54] or high doses of up to 50 μg/kg;

2 alfentanil 10–40 μg/kg;[55]

3 lignocaine 1–1.5 mg/kg i.v. or by inhalation – this is not always effective, and is best given 4 min before laryngoscopy;[56]

4 vasodilators such as sodium nitroprusside 1–2 μg/kg, isosorbide dinitrate 80 μg/kg[57] or alpha-blockers;
5 premedication with clonidine 5 μg/kg,[58] or mivazerol;[59]
6 esmolol 50–100 μg/kg;[60]
7 induction with propofol;[61]
8 verapamil 0.1 mg/kg i.v.,[62] nifedipine 10 mg sublingually a few minutes before induction[63] or diltiazem 0.2–0.3 mg/kg 1 min before laryngoscopy;[64]
9 enalapril 5 mg orally 4 h preoperatively, or captopril 12.5–25 mg sublingually 25 min preoperatively.[65]

Intraocular and intracranial pressures may double at tracheal intubation especially if suxamethonium is employed.

Suction

Hypoxia and atelectasis may occur during bronchial suction.

Catheter sizes are expressed in FG (French gauge). Division by 3 gives the approximate external diameter in millimetres. Lengths vary between 38 and 61 cm. If its external diameter is less than half the internal diameter of the tracheal tube, a significant negative pressure will not develop in the lungs during suction.

ENDOTRACHEAL ABSORPTION OF DRUGS[66]

The following drugs are well absorbed, especially if diluted in 10 ml normal saline: adrenaline, isoprenaline, lignocaine, atropine, diazepam and naloxone.

COMPLICATIONS AFTER INTUBATION

Direct trauma

To the lips, teeth, gums, eyes, nose, uvula, throat and larynx, resulting in hoarseness, dysphagia, sore throat, etc. Sore throat may also result purely from suxamethonium muscle pain.

Teeth are occasionally damaged, and a guard may be helpful.

If a tooth is knocked out it must be found to prevent it from falling into the trachea. If a radiograph shows it to be in a bronchus, it should be removed bronchoscopically. It should be handled only by the crown and placed in saline as reimplantation may be possible.

Nasal intubation may dislodge nasal polyps, cause epistaxis, damage turbinates, or cause ulceration of turbinates if intubation is prolonged.

Tears in the mucosa of the pharynx, oesophagus, larynx or trachea may result in extensive surgical and mediastinal emphysema. Retropharyngeal abscess has been reported.

A haematoma may form in the cords, especially the left, or in the supra-glottic region, which may result in dysphonia and dysphagia but usually clears up in a few days. It bears no constant relationship to the difficulty of intubation. The arytenoids may be dislocated,[67] or more serious damage done to the laryngeal muscles and ligaments.

Permanent alteration of the voice has been reported in 3% of patients after intubation.[68]

Subtle voice changes can be quantified by laryngeal acoustics.[69]

Nerve injuries

Recurrent laryngeal nerve palsy has been reported following intubation and results in a paralysed cord. Most commonly due to the surgery, but other possible causes include stretching of nerve if the neck is extended during intubation or extubation, and inflation of the cuff within the larynx.[70]

Idiopathic palsy of the recurrent nerve, a transient cranial mono-neuropathy, can occur with a reasonable chance of good recovery.[71]

The law of F. Semon (1849–1921) states that in a disorder of the laryngeal motor nerves, the abductors of the cords are the first and occasionally the only muscles affected.[72]

Bilateral cord paralysis, perhaps due to pressure of the inflated cuff on the laminae of the thyroid cartilage and the recurrent nerves,[73] may occur.

Increasing airway obstruction results, which requires face-mask continuous positive airway pressure (CPAP) or reintubation.

Lingual nerve palsy due to acute compression or stretching in its course from the medial surface of the mandible to the underside of the tongue has occurred, especially on the right. The prognosis is good.[74]

Fracture-subluxation of the cervical spine

A risk from extension of the atlanto-axial joint in fractures, malformations or abnormal fragility of the cervical spine (as in rheumatoid arthritis and Down's syndrome), where muscle tone has been abolished by relaxants. Cervical collar with in-line fixation may be needed.

Infections

Sinusitis and otitis media may result from nasotracheal intubation. The bronchial tree may also become contaminated.

Tracheal rupture during anaesthesia

This has occurred in both adults and neonates, and not necessarily associated with trauma.[75]

Ignition of the tube during laser surgery

See otorhinolarygology Chapter 4.1.

Acute glottic oedema

This rarely follows long- or short-term intubation, especially in a patient with acute laryngitis. More serious in children because of the small larynx and loose submucosal tissue in the subglottic region.

Presents up to several hours after extubation with hoarseness, cough, choking, restlessness, stridor, ashy grey pallor, and the signs of upper airway obstruction, i.e. inspiratory indrawing at the suprasternal notch, epigastrium, intercostal spaces or around the clavicles.

Sedation is contraindicated. Humidification and nebulized racemic adrenaline may be useful. Reintubation with a smaller tube may be needed, or even tracheostomy.

Ulceration and granuloma formation in the larynx[76]

Rarely, a contact ulcer may form in the mucosa over the prominent tip of the vocal process of one or both arytenoids in the posterior third of the rima glottidis, or in the subglottis of children after prolonged intubation.

In the trachea, tracheomalacia, fibrosis and stenosis may result.

If hoarseness persists for more than a week after intubation, laryngoscopy should be performed. A contact ulcer will heal if the voice is completely rested. A granuloma may need ENT referral for excision.

Ventilator-associated pneumonia

This is a multifactorial situation, often difficult to diagnose in the presence of adult respiratory distress syndrome (ARDS). The clinical pulmonary infection score (CPIS) (temperature, white blood-cell count (WBC), volume and nature of tracheal aspirate) and radiological variables and blind bronchial bacteriological sampling are helpful.[77]

THE LARYNGEAL MASK AIRWAY (LMA)

See Brain A. I. J. *Br. J. Anaesth.* 1983, **55,** 801; Brain A. I. J. et al. *Anaesthesia* 1985, **40,** 356; Brain A. I. J. *The Intavent Laryngeal Mask Instruction Manual.* Henley-on-Thames: Intavent International, 1990; Brimacombe J. and Brain A. J. *The Laryngeal Mask Airway – A Practical Guide.* Media Publishing, London, 1997.

This airway is a cuffed mask designed to fit closely over the laryngeal aperture. It is made in several sizes: size 1 for babies up to 6.5 kg, size 2 or 2.5 for children over 6.5 kg, sizes 3 for small and 4 or 5 for large adults.[78] Before use, the cuff should be deflated and lubricant applied. After induction of anaesthesia with propofol (which depresses laryngeal reflexes), or the establishment of sufficiently deep inhalational anaesthesia, it is introduced blindly into the hypopharynx. If passage is blocked by the epiglottis, insertion may be easier with the aperture facing backwards, and the mask then rotated when in the pharynx. It is best not inserted immediately after thiopentone only, as laryngeal reflexes are very active. The cuff is inflated with about 2–4 ml (size 1), 10 ml (size 2), 20 ml (size 3) and 30 ml (size 4–5) of air. It forms a seal around the larynx, and allows spontaneous ventilation or gentle IPPV without intubation of the trachea or oesophagus. If the epiglottis is folded downwards by the tip of the mask on insertion, the airway may be obstructed. *The seal does not always prevent aspiration of stomach contents,*[79] indeed, the opening of the oesophagus may be included within the cuff. Gastric distension may occur if used for IPPV with airway pressures over about 2 kPa. A bite-block is useful protection against occlusion during emergence. It is best removed when protective reflexes have fully returned, and the patient has started to swallow. Suction is usually not needed. Reinforced tubes are available.

It provides a relatively secure, hands-free airway in place of a face mask or tracheal intubation for routine anaesthesia in both adults and children,[80] although a careful watch for obstruction must still be kept. It is valuable in many operations, where the airway may give difficulties, e.g. radiotherapy[81] and dental extractions[82] in children. It causes only a small rise in heart rate, blood pressure, and intraocular pressure comparable with those seen after insertion of an oropharyngeal airway. Cricoid pressure is effective with an LMA.[83]

It may be easy to insert in those patients in whom laryngoscopy and tracheal intubation is difficult, and has even been used for emergency Caesarean section when intubation proved impossible.[84] In the latter case a cuffed tube in the oesophagus may help prevent regurgitation and aspiration. Both adult sizes will allow a 6-mm cuffed endotracheal tube to be passed through it blindly into the trachea,[85] and an intubating model is available with special endotracheal tubes.

The laryngeal mask airway has a role in airway management by paramedics.[86]

It is autoclaved between uses.

See also Brodrick P. M. et al. *Anaesthesia* 1989, **44,** 238; Maltby J. R. et al. *Can. J. Anaesth.* 1990, **37,** 509.

VENTILATION OF THE LUNGS

It is possible to institute IPPV if a sufficient depth of anaesthesia is reached with a volatile agent. This was introduced by Arthur E. Guedel (1883–1956) and David Treweek of Los Angeles in 1934,[87] using ether ('ether apnoea'). Waters in 1936 was the first to use the term 'controlled respiration'. This is easier if the PCO_2 is lowered. IPPV is now usually performed with the help of muscle relaxants. Many tragic accidents have occurred when ventilator tubing has become disconnected, or ventilators have failed, and a ventilator disconnection alarm, usually operating by sensing the intermittent rise in airway pressure, should be used.

Effects of intermittent positive-pressure ventilation

Dead space

There is little change in anatomic dead space. Although the functional residual capacity falls on induction of anaesthesia, which should reduce anatomic dead space, there is also a mild bronchodilator effect of volatile agents. By contrast, alveolar dead space increases considerably, from zero to about 70 ml in an adult. More of the lungs are under zone 1 conditions, where the capillaries are squashed by the higher intra-alveolar pressures. The ratio of physiological dead space to tidal volume (Vd/Vt) increases from a normal value of 0.3 to about 0.4–0.7 in ventilated anaesthetized subjects. This ratio increases if there is lung pathology.

Compliance

Anaesthesia, with or without IPPV, produces about a 50% reduction in lung compliance.

Shunt

This is reduced by IPPV, which tends to hold alveoli open. There is also a fall in mixed venous oxygen saturation, due to a fall in cardiac output (see below), and this results in little improvement in arterial oxygenation in patients with normal lungs. Patients with abnormal lungs often show less reduction in cardiac output, as the airway pressure is less easily transmitted to the pleural cavity, and satisfactory oxygenation may be achieved using a lower inspired O_2 concentration.

Hyperventilation

This results in a respiratory alkalosis. This shifts the haemoglobin dissociation curve to the left, increasing its affinity for O_2, causes cerebral vasoconstriction and decreases cardiac output. Increases in postoperative reaction times have been seen. Intracranial and intraocular pressure is reduced. There may also be a reduced blood flow to the placenta.

Cardiovascular changes

Right atrial pressure is raised, and so venous return and cardiac output are decreased. This has been appreciated since Cournand's classic paper.[88]

There is venoconstriction in an attempt to compensate. An increased secretion of aldosterone and antidiuretic hormone (ADH) may result in sodium and water retention. The increase in mean alveolar pressure acts to lessen any tendency for transudation of fluid into the alveoli, and may reduce pulmonary oedema.

Oxygen consumption

This is reduced because of abolition of respiratory work.

These changes with IPPV tend to be greater if positive end-expiratory pressure (PEEP) is applied. There will also be a rise in cerebral venous and intracranial pressures in parallel with increase in mean intrathoracic pressure.

Pulmonary barotrauma may result from excessive airway pressures if they are transmitted to the alveoli. Positive end-expiratory pressure of $20\,cmH_2O$ or more is associated with a high incidence of barotrauma. The alveolar–capillary membrane is disrupted, and air enters the interstitial

---

Complications of IPPV in operating theatres

Failure to produce respiration
Leaks in breathing system.
Disconnections.
Unexpected failure of ventilator.
Too great a dead space.

Pulmonary barotrauma
Too large tidal volume.
Too high inflation pressure

Dilution of anaesthetic gases, with awareness
Leakage of driving gas into anaesthesia system.
Entrainment of room air by ventilator.
Failure of delivery of anaesthesia gases into patient system.

Hyperventilation
Hypocapnia.
Hypotension.

Hypoventilation
Hypoxia.
Hypercarbia.

Cross-infection

space. Subcutaneous emphysema, pneumothorax (which is likely to be a tension pneumothorax), pneumomediastinum or gross hyperinflation of the lungs may result. Seldom should an airway pressure of 40 cmH$_2$O be exceeded, although during a severe bout of coughing an intrabronchial pressure of 100 cmH$_2$O has been recorded. The danger of pneumothorax is increased if there are fractured ribs, and IPPV is safer with a chest drain in place.

High-frequency positive pressure ventilation

High-frequency positive pressure ventilation (HFPPV) can range from the use of low tidal volumes at a frequency of 1–2 Hz, to jet ventilation (up to about 5 Hz), up to the use of tidal volumes well below the dead space but at frequencies up to 40 Hz, which is then called high-frequency oscillatory ventilation (HFOV).[89] Conventional ventilators may be used up to a frequency of about 2 Hz. Above this, Venturi or high-frequency solenoid valves must be used.

The technique can be applied using a narrow-bore insufflation tube, either by itself or passed down the centre of a tracheal tube, or through a specially designed tracheal tube. It may have a place in the management of anaesthesia for bronchoscopy, resection of tracheal stenosis, or in a patient with a large air leak due to bronchopleural fistula. It is also used in intensive therapy.

TRACHEAL INTUBATION IN INFANTS AND CHILDREN[90]

Induction with a volatile agent (e.g. sevoflurane or halothane[91]), or an intravenous agent is used. Suxamethonium 1–2 mg/kg i.v. may be used. In *neonates*, awake intubation may raise anterior fontanelle pressure threefold and this may put a preterm baby at risk of intraventricular haemorrhage.[92]

The *child's* larynx differs from the adult, as follows.

1 It is more anterior and higher: the rima glottidis is opposite the C3/C4 interspace in the infant, in adults one space lower.
2 The epiglottis is relatively longer and V-shaped, instead of flat as in the adult. It makes an angle of 45 degrees with the anterior pharyngeal wall while in adults it lies closer to the base of the tongue.
3 The narrowest part of the larynx is at the level of the cricoid cartilage, which is not distensible (the cords form the narrowest part in adults), i.e. the paediatric larynx is funnel-shaped. A tracheal tube may be passed through the glottis, but be held up at the cricoid ring, causing trauma and oedema. If this occurs, a smaller tube should be substituted.
4 A child's laryngeal reflexes are very active.
5 The morbidity from long-term intubation, even up to 6 weeks or more, is small.[93]

Less flexion of the cervical spine for laryngoscopy is needed than in adults,[94] and in infants it is unhelpful to have the head on a pillow because of the relatively large head. Uncuffed tubes are normally used below the age of about 10 years.

The tip of a straight laryngoscope blade is inserted from the right side of the mouth, pushes the tongue to the left, and is placed deep (posterior) to the epiglottis to lift it forwards. At birth, the trachea averages 4 cm long and 6 mm wide.

The length of the trachea (cm) is roughly age in years divided by 4 plus 4. In children under 3 years, the main bronchi come off the trachea at an equal angle.

Size of tubes

Length

In the neonate an orotracheal tube should be 10–11 cm long. It is a common error to insert them too far. Length (cm) of orotracheal tube in older children is age divided by 2 plus 12. Nasotracheal tubes are 3 cm longer, or may be calculated (in cm) from three times the internal diameter (mm) plus 2.[95]

Internal diameter

For neonates internal diameter of tube is 2.5–3.0 mm; 3.0–3.5 mm for 1–3 months; 3.5–4.0 mm up to 1 year; 4.0–4.5 mm up to 2 years; 4.5–5.0 mm up to 4 years; 5.5 up to 6 years; 6.0 up to 8 years; 6.5 up to 10 years; 7.0 up to 12 years. A rough guide is to use a tube that is the size of the distal phalanx of the patient's little finger. Formulae for internal diameter: up to 6 years, age divided by 3 plus 3.5; over 6 years, age divided by 4 plus 4.5. Smaller sizes should be readily available in case of the occasional subglottic stenosis (more common in the presence of imperforate anus). In small children and infants it is important to confirm by auscultation that the tracheal tube is not too long (and has reached either main bronchus). SpO_2 persistently around 85% is highly indicative of this.

REFERENCES

1 Mostafa S. M. and Atherton A. M. J. *Br. J. Anaesth.* 1997, **79,** 292–293.
2 Baraka A. S, Sayyid S. S. and Assaf B. A. *Anesth. Analg.* 1997, **84,** 1104–1107.
3 Ring W. H. et al. *Anesth. Analg.* 1975, **54,** 273.
4 Latto I. P. In Latto I. P. and Rosen M. (eds) *Difficulties in Tracheal Intubation.* Baillière Tindall, Eastbourne, 1985, p.48.
5 Oikonnen M. and Aromaa U. *Anaesthesia* 1997, **52,** 567–569.
6 Pope E. S. *Anaesthesia* 1960, **15,** 326.
7 Henderson J. J. *Anaesthesia* 1997, **52,** 552–560.

8 McIntyre J. W. R. *Can. J. Anaesth.* 1989, **36,** 94.
9 Randell T., Maattanen M. and Kytta J. *Anaesthesia* 1998, **53,** 536–539.
10 Borland L. M. and Casselbrant M. *Anesth. Analg.* 1990, **70,** 105.
11 Magill I. W. *Br. Med. J.* 1920, **2,** 670; Libermann H. *Anaesth. Intensive Care* 1978, **6,** 162.
12 Mallampati S. R. et al. *Can. Anaesth. Soc. J.* 1985, **32,** 429; Samsoon G. L. T. and Young J. R. B. *Anaesthesia* 1987, **42,** 487.
13 McIntyre J. W. R. *Can. J. Anaesth.* 1987, **34,** 204.
14 White A. and Kander P. L. *Br. J. Anaesth.* 1975, **47,** 468.
15 Divekar V. M. et al. *Can. Anaesth. Soc. J.* 1979, **26,** 141.
16 Kloss J. and Petty C. *Anesthesiology* 1975, **43,** 380.
17 Berkowitz I. D. et al. *Anesthesiology* 1990, **73,** 739.
18 Nichol H. C. and Zuck D. *Br. J. Anaesth.* 1983, **55,** 141.
19 Saarnivaara L. and Klemola U.-M. *Acta Anaesthesiol. Scand.* 1991, **35,** 19.
20 Mulholland D. and Carlisle R. J. T. *Anaesthesia* 1991, 46, 312.
21 Macintosh R. R. *Br. Med. J.* 1949, **1,** 28.
22 Dogra S. et al. *Anaesthesia* 1990, **45,** 774.
23 Stanley G. D. and Appadurai I. R. *Anaesthesia* 1998, **53,** 609–610.
24 Cormack R. S. and Lehane J. *Anaesthesia* 1984, **39,** 1105.
25 Williams K. N. et al. *Br. J. Anaesth.* 1991, **66,** 38.
26 O'Flaherty D. and Adams A. P. *Anaesthesia* 1990, **45,** 653.
27 Lockey D. J. *Anaesthesia* 1997, **52,** 242–243; Wee D. M. *Anaesthesia* 1988, **43,** 27.
28 Lang D. J., Wafai Y. and Salem M. R. *Anesthesiology* 1996, **85,** 246–253.
29 Green R. A. In *Anaesthesia Review 4.* Churchill Livingstone, London, 1987, 147; Utting J. E. *Br. J. Anaesth.* 1987, **59,** 877.
30 Heath M. L. and Allagain J. *Anaesthesia* 1991, **46,** 545; Kapila A., Addy E. V., Verghese C. and Brain A. I. J. *Br. J. Anaesth.* 1995, **75,** 228–229.
31 Brain A. I. J. et al. *Br. J. Anaesth.* 1997, **79,** 704–709.
32 Liban J. B. *Anaesthesia* 1998, **53,** 606.
33 Hung O. R. *Anesth. Analg.* 1997, **85,** 1415.
34 Boysen K. *Anaesthesia* 1985, **40,** 1024.
35 Berry F. A. et al. *Pediatrics* 1973, **51,** 476.
36 McShane A. J. and Hone R. *Br. Med. J.* 1986, **292,** 26 and 410.
37 Pierce A. In Adams A. P. and Cashman J. (eds) *Recent Advances in Anaesthesia – 19.* Churchill Livingstone, Edinburgh, 1997.
38 McLellan I. et al. *Can. J. Anaesth.* 1988, **35,** 404.
39 Gotta A. W. and Sullivan C. A. *Br. J. Anaesth.* 1981, **53,** 1055.
40 Shaw I. C., Welchow E. A., Harrison B. J. and Michal S. *Anaesthesia* 1997, **52,** 582–585.
41 Tunstall M. E. *Anaesthesia* 1976, **31,** 850; Tunstall M. E. and Sheikh A. *Clin. Anaesthesiol.* 1986, **4,** 171.
42 Lyons G. *Anaesthesia* 1985, **40,** 759.
43 Chadwick I. S. and Vohra A. *Anaesthesia* 1989, **44,** 261; Reynolds F. *Anaesthesia* 1989, **44,** 870; McClune S. et al. *Anaesthesia* 1990, **45,** 227; Brain A. I. J. et al. *Br. J. Anaesth.* 1997, **79,** 704–709.
44 Harmer M. and Vaughan R. S. *Anaesthesia* 1980, **35,** 921
45 Craft T. M. et al. *Br. J. Anaesth.* 1990, **64,** 524.

46 Koga K., Asai T., Vaughan R. and Latto I. P. *Anaesthesia* 1998, **53,** 540–544.
47 Owen H. *Anaesthesia* 1982, **37,** 1112.
48 Gefke K. et al. *Acta Anaesthesiol. Scand.* 1983, **27,** 111.
49 Lang S. A. et al. *Can. J. Anaesth.* 1990, **37,** 210.
50 Thomson I. R. *Can. J. Anaesth.* 1989, **39,** 367.
51 Lehtinen A.-M. *Br. J. Anaesth.* 1984, **56,** 247.
52 Cozanitis D. A. et al. *Can. Anaesth. Soc. J.* 1984, **31,** 155.
53 Pierce A. In Adams A. P. and Cashman J. (eds) *Recent Advances in Anaesthesia* – 19. Churchill Livingstone, Edinburgh, 1997.
54 Van Aken H. et al. *Anesthesiology* 1988, **68,** 157.
55 Crawford D. C. et al. *Br. J. Anaesth.* 1987, **39,** 707.
56 Laurito C. E. et al. *Anesth. Analg.* 1988, **67,** 389; Wilson I. G. et al. *Anaesthesia* 1991, **46,** 177.
57 Hatano Y. et al. *Acta Anesthesiol. Scand.* 1989, **33,** 214.
58 Ghignone M. et al. *Anesthesiology* 1986, **64,** 36.
59 McSPI Europe Research Group. *Anesthesiology* 1997, **86,** 346 and 363.
60 Helfman S. M. et al. *Anesth. Analg.* 1991, **72,** 482.
61 Harris C. E. et al. *Anaesthesia* 1988, **43** (suppl.), 32.
62 Nishikawa T. and Namiki A. *Acta Anesthesiol. Scand.* 1989, **33,** 232.
63 Indu B. et al. *Can. J. Anaesth.* 1989, **36,** 269.
64 Mikawa K. et al. *Anaesthesia* 1990, **45,** 289.
65 McCarthy G. J. et al. *Anaesthesia* 1990, **45,** 243.
66 Greenbaum R. *Anaesthesia* 1987, **42,** 927; Editorial. *Lancet* 1988, **1,** 743.
67 Frink E. J. and Pattison B. D. *Anesthesiology* 1989, **70,** 358.
68 Kark A. E. et al. *Br. Med. J.* 1984, **289,** 1412.
69 Priebe H.-J. et al. *Anesth. Analg.* 1988, **67,** 219.
70 Hahn F. W. et al. *Arch. Otolaryngol.* 1970, **92,** 226; Ellis P. D. M. *Anesthesiology* 1977, **46,** 374.
71 Blau J. N. and Kepadia R. *Br. Med. J.* 1972, **4,** 259.
72 Semon F. *Arch. Laryngol.* 1881, **2,** 197.
73 Gibbin K. P. and Eggiston M. J. *Br. J. Anaesth.* 1981, **53,** 1091.
74 Loughman E. *Anaesth. Intensive Care* 1983, **11,** 171.
75 Smith B. A. C. and Hopkinson R. B. *Anaesthesia* 1984, **39,** 894; Correspondence, *Anaesthesia* 1985, **40,** 211 and 212; Gaukroger P. B. and Anderson G. *Anaesth. Intensive Care* 1986, **14,** 199.
76 Keane W. M. et al. *Ann. Otol. Rhinol. Laryngol.* 1982, **91,** 584; Balestrieri F. *Otolarnygol. Clin. North Am.* 1982, **15,** 567.
77 Kirtland S. H. et al. *Chest* 1997, **112,** 445–457.
78 Berry A. M., Brimacombe J. R., McManus K. F. and Goldblatt M. *Anaesthesia* 1998, **53,** 565–570.
79 Griffin R. M. and Hatcher I. S. *Anaesthesia* 1990, **45,** 1039.
80 Mason D. G. and Bingham R. M. *Anaesthesia* 1990, **45,** 760.
81 Grebenik C. R. et al. *Anesthesiology* 1990, **72,** 474.
82 Bailie R. et al. *Anaesthesia* 1991, **46,** 358.
83 Braude N. et al. *Anaesthesia* 1989, **44,** 551; Hickey S. et al. *Anaesthesia* 1990, **45,** 629.

84 Chadwick I. S. and Vohra A. *Anaesthesia* 1989, **44,** 261; Reynolds F. *Anaesthesia* 1989, **44,** 870; McClune S. et al. *Anaesthesia* 1990, **45,** 227.
85 Heath M. L. and Allagain J. *Anaesthesia* 1991, **46,** 545.
86 Davies P. R. F. et al. *Lancet* 1990, **336,** 977.
87 Guedel A. F. and Treweek D. M. *Curr. Res. Anesth. Analg.* 1934, **13,** 263. Reprinted in 'Classical File', *Surv. Anesthesiol.* 1970, **14,** 405.
88 Coumand A. et al. *Am. J. Physiol.* 1948, **152,** 162; Morgan B. C. et al. *Anesthesiology* 196, **27,** 584.
89 McEvoy R. D. *Anaesth. Intensive Care* 1985, **13,** 178.
90 Mather S. J. and Hughes D. G. *A Handbook of Paediatric Anaesthesia.* Oxford University Press, Oxford, 1996.
91 Bacher A. and Burton A. W. *Anesth. Analg.* 1997, **85,** 1203–1206.
92 Friesen R. H. et al. *Anesth. Analg.* 1987, **66,** 874.
93 Black A. E. et al. *Br. J. Anaesth.* 1990, **65,** 461.
94 Westhorpe R. N. *Anaesth. Intensive Care* 1987, **15,** 384.
95 Yates A. P. et al. *Br. J. Anaesth.* 1987, **59,** 524.

Production of ischaemia during operations and control of arterial pressure

Bleeding is due to cutting blood vessels!

Some patients bleed very little with a normal blood pressure and the relationship between arterial pressure and bleeding is not as clear as was once thought.

INCREASED BLEEDING DURING SURGERY

Surgical and traumatic bleeding may be exacerbated by the following.

1 Respiratory obstruction.
2 Hypercapnia.
3 Venous congestion.
4 Unnecessary production of tachycardia by atropine and other vagolytic drugs.
5 Conditions causing a rise in the basal metabolic rate, e.g. thyrotoxicosis.
6 Haemostasis disorders, e.g. idiopathic thrombocytopenic purpura (and platelet inactivation due to aspirin), anticoagulants, haemophilia (*see also* Chapter 3.1), coagulopathy due to:
   (a) massive blood transfusion;
   (b) citrate intoxication;
   (c) incompatible blood transfusion: (*see also* Chapter 1.2);
   (d) hypothermia.
7 The capillary hyperaemia of acute and chronic inflammation.
8 Trauma to the blood in extracorporeal circuits.

Causes of venous congestion

1 Coughing.

2 Posture.

3 Heart disease.

4 Lung disease.

5 Overtransfusion and overinfusion.

6 Raised expiratory resistance in the anaesthetic system.

ISCHAEMIA DURING OPERATIONS

In addition to the total ischaemia produced in the limbs by tourniquets (*see below*), relative ischaemia may be produced by:

1 reduction of *venous* bleeding by elevating the part to be operated on, e.g. head-up in mastoid or facial surgery, Trendelenberg position in varicose vein surgery;

2 reduction of *capillary* bleeding by local injection of vasoconstrictors, e.g. adrenaline, vasopressin, etc.;

3 reduction of *arterial* bleeding by reducing pulse rate, arterial pressure and $PaCO_2$, (by intermittent positive-pressure ventilation (IPPV));

4 drugs to reduce transfusions: aprotinin, tranexamic acid (but not desmopressin).[1]

A comprehensive ischaemic technique may use all of these approaches. The production of adequate ischaemia does not usually demand hypotension.

REDUCTION OF A RAISED ARTERIAL PRESSURE

Produced by the following.

1 Reduction of peripheral vascular resistance by drugs:
   (a)   volatile agents, especially isoflurane;
   (b)   nitroprusside and nitrites (*see below*).

2 Reduction of peripheral vascular resistance by spinal blockade (*see* Chapter 5.3).

The 'normal' systolic pressure during sleep is often little above 80 mmHg.
   Blood pressure should be monitored continuously or frequently by the most accurate method available. A systolic pressure of 60–80 mmHg (MAP 50 mmHg) is the average limit for tissue autoregulation. Below this limit, flow falls linearly with pressure. Hypertensive patients have the auto-regulation curve shifted to the right.

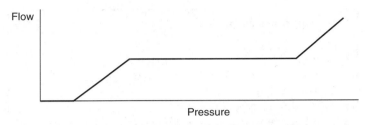

Figure 2.7.1 Autoregulation of organ blood flow

Renal blood flow

Glomerular filtration decreases with the fall in blood pressure and ceases at MAP 50 mmHg. Renal perfusion sufficient to meet the metabolic needs of the kidney does not suffer until the pressure is much lower, and as the pressure rises, function returns. Acute tubular necrosis is a risk at MAP 20 mmHg for more than a few minutes.

Cerebral blood flow

Normal autoregulation (Fig. 2.7.1) maintains this down to MAP 40 mmHg. From 40 to 20 mmHg., the flow falls linearly. Below 20 mmHg., cerebral blood flow is completely inadequate.

Coronary blood flow

This is autoregulated down to diastolic 40 mmHg in the normal heart. Low arterial pressure reduces cardiac work and the demand of the myocardium for oxygen so that myocardial perfusion remains adequate. Below diastolic 40 mmHg the heart is unlikely to be able to raise arterial pressure and vaso-pressors, intravenous infusion or the cautious use of ephedrine would be needed. Myocardial ischaemia is likely at diastolic pressure of 20 mmHg. In coronary atheroma, the autoregulation band is moved to the right.

VASODILATORS

Sodium nitroprusside

Physical and chemical properties

A commercial preparation (Nipride) is freeze-dried and presented as 50 mg dry powder in a sealed ampoule. Dissolved in 500 ml 5% dextrose for clinical use (100 or 200 μg/ml). Such solutions are unstable and must be protected from light (10% decrease in potency in 3 h, 50% in 48 h in bright light).

Appearance of blue colour suggests undue breakdown and such solutions should be discarded.

The solution should be prepared immediately before use.

Pharmacodynamics

Direct fourth-order small-arteriolar vasodilatation.

Cardiac output is usually maintained, and here there is a major difference from the effect of other drugs. Tissue perfusion is unlikely to be compromised. Moderate tachycardia is frequent, probably due to stimulation of baroreceptor reflexes. Renal blood flow is increased. It is a cerebral vasodilator which tends to maintain cerebral blood flow and oxygenation as the blood pressure drops.

(Sodium nitroprusside is safe in a dose up to 10 μg/kg/min. High dosage can cause fatal cyanide intoxication.)

Pharmacokinetics

Sodium nitroprusside is rapidly broken down in the blood stream, probably both in the plasma and in the red cells, with the production of the active agent, NO, and hydrocyanic acid which is then conjugated with thiosulphate to form thiocyanate. Overdosage leads to accumulation of free cyanide ions, so that dosage must be strictly controlled. Thiocyanate levels can be measured as a monitor of toxicity during prolonged administration of nitroprusside, though it rises too slowly to be a useful index of overdose during short-term infusions. Thiocyanate is excreted in the urine. A small amount of cyanide is excreted after combination with vitamin B_{12} to form cyanocobalamin, but this is not clinically important.

Toxic reactions: there have been some case reports of cardiovascular collapse and severe metabolic acidosis after administration of large doses of sodium nitroprusside in resistant patients, hypothermia, or those with hepatic or renal failure. It is likely that such patients have suffered acute cyanide poisoning, the metabolic acidosis being a result of histotoxic hypoxia.[2]

It has been suggested that the minimal lethal dose of nitroprusside for short-term infusions is about 200–300 mg, whereas a dose of more than 20 mg/day is rarely necessary.[3]

Nitroprusside should be avoided when normal cyanide metabolism is inhibited as in liver or renal failure, Leber's optic atrophy[4] and tobacco amblyopia.

Treatment of overdose

1 Stop the infusion.
2 Monitor temperature, blood gases, renal output, electrocardiogram (ECG), arterial pressure.

Indications for nitroprusside

1 Neurosurgery – rarely for cerebral aneurysms and arteriovenous malformations.

2 Phaeochromocytoma.

3 Scoliosis surgery.

4 Aortic surgery.

5 Cardiopulmonary bypass, to decrease afterload in the immediate postoperative period.

6 To control hypertension in intensive care.

7 Acute hypertensive crises to reduce cardiac workload.

8 Management of ergot overdose.

---

3 Fluid replacement should be adequate. If severe metabolic acidosis is confirmed, 25 ml 50% sodium thiosulphate should be given intravenously over 3–5 min. If there is no improvement 20 ml (300 mg) of cobalt edetate is recommended at 1 ml/s.[5]

Clinical use

A separate intravenous infusion should be set up containing 100 μg/ml in 5% dextrose. The maximum safe dose should be calculated as 1.5 mg/kg and never exceeded. An electronic drip controller or 'Dial a Flow' should be used and T-piece or two-way tap systems avoided.

An initial infusion rate of 0.5 μg/kg/min is recommended in the healthy adult. Response is usually seen within 30 s and thereafter arterial pressure changes determine the infusion rate; 10 μg/kg/min should not be exceeded. Arterial pressure begins to rise within 1 min of the cessation of the infusion and is normally complete within 5–10 min. Direct arterial pressure is monitored.

The return of normal blood pressure should take place within a few minutes of turning off the infusion. Colloid infusion or a pressor agent may be required.

During long-term use, plasma thiocyanate levels may be monitored to avoid overdose. Levels should not exceed 1.7 mmol/l (10 mg%).

Nitroglycerin: glyceryl trinitrate (Nitrostat)

First used for the treatment of angina by William Murrell (1853–1912) of London, in 1879.[6]

The raw material of dynamite. This has been infused intravenously at a rate of about 20 μg/min. Its action is similar to that of nitroprusside, but it is claimed that the course of hypotension is smoother with fewer peaks and troughs of arterial pressure.

Pharmacodynamics

A direct venodilator, cerebral and coronary vasodilator. Intracranial pressure rises.

Its solutions are absorbed by polyvinyl chloride containers and tubing so that polythene or glass must be used.

Clinical use

Many workers employ a 0.1-mg/ml solution with an initial pumped rate of 10 μg/min. Hypotensive effects come on more slowly and last much longer than when sodium nitroprusside is infused. A power-driven syringe pump may be used.

OTHER HYPOTENSIVE AGENTS

1 The volatile agents, e.g. isoflurane, are predominantly vasodilator. Isoflurane preserves cerebral and coronary perfusion, even in severe hypotension.
2 Beta-blockers: act by producing bradycardia.
   (a) Propranolol: a β_1 and β_2 blocker; dose 0.035 mg/kg i.v., repeated until the pulse rate is at the required rate; onset in one circulation time, duration about 45 min. Dangerous bronchospasm may occur in the asthmatic patient.
   (b) Metoprolol: a cardioselective beta-blocker (may be safer in asthma), dose 0.1 mg/kg, onset in one circulation time, duration 1–1.5 h. It is also satisfactory when used with halothane.
   (c) Labetalol: this reduces arterial pressure by reducing cardiac output and heart rate and decreasing peripheral resistance. Alpha and beta receptors are blocked so that hypotension is produced without tachycardia. Dose: 5–25 mg i.v. Should marked bradycardia occur, atropine may be given, and this may result in a rise of arterial pressure. If this fails, a catecholamine (ephedrine or adrenaline) bolus injection or infusion will reverse the competitive block. Duration: 1–2 h.
3 Nifedipine 10 mg and congeners. They act rapidly, especially when given sublingually but are less predictable than labetalol.
4 Fenoldepam: an arteriodilator which stimulates DA1 and DA2 receptors, has been used in acute and chronic heart failure and for control of hypertension after coronary artery bypass graft (CABG).

There may be overswing from use of any antihypertensive technique and the arterial pressure becomes unstable, with risk of severe hypotension.

A '**hypotension drill**' must be worked out to cope with unexpected severe falls of systolic pressure (e.g. <60 mmHg)

1 Run the intravenous drip at full speed. Volume-loading the circulation with 1–2 litres of colloid restores stability.

2 Reduce any volatile agent, stop any vasodilator infusion.

3 Inject atropine if bradycardia has become severe (<50 bpm).

4 Inject ephedrine, 10 mg i.v., or adrenaline 1 μg/kg repeated as necessary.

5 Level the patient, if head-up, and raise legs.

6 Increase FiO_2 to 100% and maintain faultless normoventilation.

7 Continuously monitor arterial pressure and function of organs.

The anaesthetist is warned against production of hypotension at the request of a surgeon where this may *affect the safety of the patient*.

TOURNIQUETS

Tourniquets during operations on limbs are the responsibility of the operating surgeon. Care must be taken that they are properly padded. Pneumatic tourniquets using a Bourdon-type pressure gauge are not always well maintained with the risk of unduly high pressures causing nerve damage. The surgeon is informed after each hour of tourniquet time has passed. Three hours is the absolute maximum. Application of tourniquets to the lower limbs raises the central venous pressure. Tourniquets may cause sickling in patients with sickle-cell trait and disease. Pressures: 1.5× systolic in arm, 2× systolic in leg.

REFERENCES

1 Lanpacis A. and Fergusson D. *Anesth. Analg.* 1997, **85,** 1258–1267.

2 Cole P. V. *Anaesthesia* 1978, **33,** 473.

3 *See also* Vesey C. J. et al. *Br. J. Anaesth.* 1976, **48,** 651; Cole P. V. In Hewer C. L. and Atkinson R. S. (ed.) *Recent Advances in Anaesthesia and Analgesia – 13.* Churchill Livingstone, Edinburgh, 1979.

4 Leber T. *Arch. Ophthalmol.* 1871, **17,** 249.

5 Bryson D. D. *Lancet* 1978, **1,** 92.

6 Murrell W. *Lancet* 1879, **2,** 80.

Complications of anaesthesia[1]

All techniques of anaesthesia rarely result in complications, morbidity and even mortality. This need not signify negligence or blame. Most often they are due to the condition of the patient. The inevitable rare possibility of such sequelae should play a major part in the decision-making about anaesthetic technique for an individual patient.

RESPIRATORY COMPLICATIONS

Upper airway obstruction

Diagnosed by the presence of an inadequate tidal volume, with:

1 excessive abdominal movement, together with retraction of the chest wall and the supraclavicular, infraclavicular and suprasternal spaces;
2 use of accessory muscles of respiration;
3 noisy breathing, i.e. stridor (unless obstruction is complete);
4 high airway pressure during intermittent positive-pressure ventilation (IPPV);
5 ultimately cyanosis, although this is a late sign if a high inspired O_2 concentration is used.

The extreme negative intrathoracic pressures generated by upper airway obstruction may result in acute pulmonary oedema. This is sometimes mistaken by anaesthetists for aspiration.[2]

Upper airway obstruction may be due to one of the following.

1 *Obstruction at the lips.* Especially in edentulous patients, and corrected by the use of an oro- or nasopharyngeal airway.
2 *Obstruction by the tongue or soft palate.*[3] The tone in the genioglossus muscles helps hold the tongue away from the posterior pharyngeal wall. The activity of these muscles (which is maximal during inspiration) is abolished by anaesthesia, and the tongue approximates against the posterior pharyngeal wall ('swallowing the tongue'). The soft palate can do the same. Once this has happened, the suction created by inspiration

makes the obstruction worse. It may be especially dangerous in the recovery phase. Much less likely to occur if the patient is nursed in the lateral position. Remedied by lifting the jaw up and forwards, a manoeuvre first described in 1874.[4] At the same time the head is extended on the spine at the atlanto-occipital joint. Alternatively, an oropharyngeal airway (size 3 for men, size 2 for women) is inserted and usually restores the airway.[5] A laryngeal mask airway may also be used. It may be necessary to resort to tracheal intubation.

3 *Obstruction above the glottis.* Due to a swab, tooth, foreign body, saliva, vomitus, blood or oedema. The obstructing material must be removed by the fingers, gravity, swabbing or suction. Very rarely, dislocation of the epiglottis or cysts or tumours of the epiglottis are encountered.

4 *Obstruction at the glottis.* This is due to:
   (a) laryngeal spasm, a sphincter-like closure of the aryepiglottic folds;
   (b) impaction of the epiglottis into the larynx (which may be corrected under direct vision with a laryngoscope);
   (c) incomplete reversal of muscle relaxants, which prevent cord abduction;
   (d) foreign bodies, e.g. teeth, vomitus (when laryngoscopy is needed).

Laryngeal spasm commonly results from intense surgical stimulation under anaesthesia that is too light, e.g. dilatation of the cervix or the anus. This can lead to dangerous hypoxia. Temporary cessation of surgical stimuli may be necessary, or the administration of a small dose of suxamethonium (or a non-depolarizing relaxant) to permit artificial ventilation of the lungs. The passage of a tracheal tube ensures that the condition will not recur. This is a powerful reason to always have suxamethonium drawn up before induction of any anaesthetic.

If a patient with upper airway obstruction is *in extremis*, a very large intravenous cannula (12 G or 14 G) can be inserted through the cricothyroid membrane, or a mini-tracheostomy performed to allow ventilation with oxygen. More desperate devices have been used, such as the spike of a 'giving-set' which enters a fluid container, or even the shell of a ball-point pen.

5 *Faults of apparatus:*
   (a) misplacement, kinking or other obstruction of a tracheal tube and connectors;
   (b) absence of gas flow to patient due to empty cylinders or disconnection.

Capnography is valuable to confirm that the tracheal tube is correctly placed in the trachea. It may be necessary to remove all the anaesthetic apparatus, including the tracheal tube, and ventilate the lungs with O_2 by a face mask. If the oxygen has failed, then the lungs may be ventilated with air, using a self-inflating bag, or even with the anaesthetist's expired air.

Bronchospasm

The patient's lower airways are excessively responsive due to the following:

1 Asthma.
2 Surgical stimulation, or airway stimulation, e.g. intubation, under light anaesthesia. Carinal stimulation by a tube that is too long is particularly effective at producing bronchospasm.
3 Drug reaction (*see below*).
4 Respiratory infection.
5 Pulmonary oedema.
6 Severe reduction in lung volume as in a tension pneumothorax.

Management

Diagnosis of cause. Prevention by:

1 smooth induction and maintaining anaesthesia at suitable depth;
2 spraying larynx and trachea with lignocaine when airway instrumentation is anticipated;
3 administration of bronchodilator drugs with premedication. Broncho-dilators: salbutamol 4 μg/kg over 1 min i.v., ephedrine 10–30 mg i.v., or aminophylline 250 mg i.v. slowly.

An adrenaline infusion 1–10 μg/min may be considered. Corticosteroids, e.g. hydrocortisone, 100 mg i.v. may be given but will not have an immediate action.

Coughing

Usually due to inadequate depth of anaesthesia when volatile agents are used and when patient has chemical (e.g. heavy smoking) or infective inflammation of the upper airways, but may also be due to irritation of the larynx from regurgitated gastric material, saliva or the use of artificial airways. Less common with propofol than with thiopentone. Best controlled by deepening anaesthesia or use of a muscle relaxant. All airway complications are more common in smokers, and have even been shown to be more common in children who are passive smokers at home.[6]

Hiccup

Intermittent spasm of the diaphragm, accompanied by sudden closure of the glottis.

Causes

Stimulation of sensory phrenic nerve endings, which are connected with the coeliac and other intra-abdominal autonomic plexuses. The vagus may also act as part of the afferent arc of the reflex. Thus, through these pathways, hiccup may arise from impulses in any abdominal or thoracic viscus. May also be via central stimulation of the medulla, as in alcoholic intoxication, uraemia, encephalitis.

Treatment

1 Deepening of anaesthesia.
2 Giving a muscle relaxant in relatively large doses.
3 Nasopharyngeal stimulation by use of suction catheter or ice-cold saline.

Sputum retention and atelectasis

Caused by inadequate coughing due to pain, residual neuromuscular block, or sedatives. The impairment of mucociliary transport in the lungs after inhalation of cold, dry gas mixtures may play a part. Most common after upper abdominal operations, especially if oblique or transverse incisions are not used. Commoner in the obese, smokers, and those with pre-existing lung disease.

Diagnosis

1 Rapid breathing, 30–60 per min.
2 Tachycardia.
3 Dilatation of alae nasi.
4 Slight cyanosis if breathing air.
5 Restricted movements, quiet breath sounds, decreased resonance over affected area of the lungs which is often the dependent part.
6 Radiographic shadows like those in bronchopneumonia.

Elevation of a hemi-diaphragm is very common after upper abdominal operations, in absence of clinical atelectasis. *Massive collapse* causes pain in the chest of sudden onset, dyspnoea, cyanosis, fever, tachycardia and mediastinal shift. Untreated atelectasis will lead to hypoxaemia and infection.

Treatment

Physiotherapy and encouragement of coughing, with appropriate use of analgesics (e.g. narcotics, Entonox). When problems are anticipated, continuous extradural block or other regional technique is helpful. If sputum cannot be coughed out, other measures must be considered such as aspiration of a sputum plug via a tracheal tube or bronchoscope, or mini-tracheostomy. Postoperative doxapram is used by some workers.

Ventilation/perfusion mismatching causes the O_2 saturation to fall after general anaesthesia, even when respiratory function is normal. It is influenced by the site of operation, smoking, age, the presence of cardiorespiratory disease and obesity. This is readily treated by O_2 administration, which may have to be continued for some days.

Aspiration pneumonitis

See below, 'Vomiting and regurgitation'.

Sleep apnoea

Due either to airway obstruction, or to central respiratory depression.[7] The latter is also called Ondine's curse (named from the water sprite in German mythology who killed her victims by stopping respiration), a term first used in connection with anaesthesia by Severinghaus,[8] and has followed surgery to the cervical cord.[9] Obstructive sleep apnoea is also a problem in children with large adenoids and tonsils. These patients may present for surgery unrelated to their ENT problems, and they need special consideration in the postoperative period.[10]

Rapid eye movement (REM) sleep does not occur during or immediately after general anaesthesia. During the following 2 or 3 days there is an increased amount of REM sleep to compensate. Even during normal REM sleep there can be periods of obstructive or central apnoea, lasting for up to 10 s. Postoperatively, on the second and third nights, these periods of apnoea are increased in length and more frequent, more so if opiates are given. They are associated with hypertension, tachycardia, hypoxaemia and hypercarbia. Myocardial ischaemia may occur.

Management of sleep apnoea patients

Preoperatively

Assess SpO_2 at night and correct with continuous positive airway pressure (nCPAP).

Assess airway/intubation difficulty.

Has the patient had failed treatment for sleep apnoea?

During anaesthesia

Regional techniques if at all possible.

Prepare for fibreoptic intubation.

No long-acting relaxants or opioids.

Postoperatively

Regional techniques for analgesia.

Extubate wide awake/sitting up.

O_2/nCPAP for 5 nights in HDU with full monitoring.

Those who are susceptible include those with preoperative history of sleep apnoea (often with daytime sleepiness), and the obese snoring patient. The airway should be carefully assessed, as very difficult intubation is common. *Regional techniques are used if at all possible*, and opiates and long-acting relaxants avoided. Extubate the trachea with the patient wide awake, and sitting up. Postoperatively, there is a strong case for monitoring the oxygen saturation or blood gases in a high-dependency unit for several days, giving oxygen continuously,[11] and considering the use of continuous positive airway pressure (CPAP).

Pulmonary barotrauma

Occurs if excessive airway pressures are transmitted to the alveoli, or if the lungs are at risk because of disease (especially emphysema) or fractured ribs. The alveolar–capillary membrane is disrupted, and air enters the interstitial space. Subcutaneous surgical emphysema in the neck, pneumothorax (which is likely to be a tension pneumothorax), pneumomediastinum or gross hyperinflation of the lungs may result. Mediastinal emphysema often causes a crushing sound when the stethoscope is applied to the left border of the heart, Hamman's sign.[12] Radiologically there may be a small air space running parallel to the left or right border of the heart.

Pneumothorax commonly occurs when the pleura is accidentally opened during operations such as cervical sympathectomy, rib resection and nephrectomy. The lungs should be inflated to expel air as the hole is closed. Pneumothorax also occurs as a complication of anaesthetic techniques such as intercostal and brachial plexus blocks, or central lines.

Deep venous thrombosis and pulmonary embolism

Risk factors

Deep venous thrombosis (DVT) in the legs and pelvis is more common in those over 40 years old, with a previous history of DVT, the immobilized, patients on oestrogen-containing oral contraceptives, those with carcinoma, and patients after certain operations, e.g. pelvic surgery, hip surgery and varicose veins. Those with Leiden factor V mutation and similar conditions present a high and recurrent risk.

Symptoms of pulmonary embolism

Very varied, and include unexplained fever, faintness, dyspnoea, substernal discomfort, pleural pain and haemoptysis. Onset may coincide with getting up or straining at stool. Typically, the sudden onset of pain in chest during the second postoperative week. This may be small and ephemeral or large and fatal.

Signs of pulmonary embolism

Tachycardia, rise in central venous pressure (CVP), hypotension, cyanosis, gallop rhythm, pleural rub, signs of consolidation. *Radiographs of chest* may show linear shadows, effusion. There is pulmonary oligaemia if the embolus is large. Electrocardiogram (ECG) may show an S wave in limb Lead I, a Q wave in Lead III and T-wave inversion in Lead III; representing right heart strain. A *ventilation/perfusion scan* is sometimes undertaken to confirm the diagnosis.

If it occurs during an operation, there is increasing desaturation and hypotension. This classically occurs with:

1 the detachment of a venous clot in the leg following the application of an Esmarch bandage;
2 change in the patient's position;
3 hypernephroma;
4 amniotic fluid in obstetric patients.

Treatment

A small embolus is not treated as such, but anticoagulants prevent the deep venous thrombosis extending and resulting in further emboli. Venography and ligation of veins may be appropriate. Fibrinolytic therapy is used for the larger embolus, or even immediate pulmonary embolectomy on cardiopulmonary bypass.

Prevention[13]

Thrombi in the veins of the calf are common, but are only likely to cause pulmonary embolism when they extend into the iliofemoral veins or if they originate in pelvic veins. Deep venous thrombosis usually starts before, during or very soon after operation.

There is reduced fibrinolytic activity and increased platelet adhesiveness after operation (except prostatectomy). Regional techniques such as extradural or intradural anaesthesia reduce the incidence of DVT, although it is not certain whether this results in a reduction in mortality due to pulmonary embolism.

Preventative measures include:

1 early ambulation;
2 elevation of the legs during operation;
3 intermittent pneumatic compression of the calf, replacing the normal muscle pump effect;
4 elastic support stockings;
5 a heel cushion on the operating table, preventing pressure on calf veins;
6 low-dose subcutaneous heparin (*see below*);
7 the use of colloid rather than crystalloid, especially dextran 70;
8 stopping oral contraceptives containing oestrogen for 4 weeks before major surgery.

9 Warfarin 2–5 mg daily.
10 Desirudin 15 mg twice daily.
11 Aspirin 75 mg daily.

Low-dose heparin or elastic support stockings are commonly used. Although low-dose heparin does not usually increase intraoperative bleeding much, the use of regional blocks should only be undertaken where there is a clear advantage and activated partial thromboplastin time (APTT) ratio is < 1.5. This applies particularly to the use of extra- and intradural blocks where a haematoma can cause a disastrous paraplegia. *See* Chapter 5.3.

Heparin

First discovered in 1916 by a medical student in Baltimore.[14] It potentiates the action of antithrombin III, and so inhibits activated factors IX, X, XI, XII and thrombin.

For DVT prophylaxis, sodium or calcium heparin 5000 units can be given subcutaneously 2 h before operation and 8- or 12-hourly afterwards for 7 days. Thrombocytopenia may result from an immune-mediated reaction in a patient who has been on heparin for more than 5 days, and so the platelet count should be monitored in such a patient, and the heparin stopped if it is lowered.

Low-molecular-weight heparins have the advantage of a once-daily dose regimen, and may be more effective in certain types of surgery, e.g. hip replacement. Examples are dalteparin and enoxaparin. They act more specifically on factor Xa, and so are claimed to cause less bleeding tendency than unfractionated heparin. Dalteparin is given as 2500 units 1–2 h before surgery, and continued daily. These doses can be doubled if the risk of DVT is high.

CARDIOVASCULAR COMPLICATIONS

Cardiac dysrhythmias

May be associated with:

1 cardiac pathology;
2 hypercapnia or hypoxia;
3 toxins, malignant hyperpyrexia, drugs (e.g. adrenaline), anaphylaxis etc.;
4 electrolyte imbalance.

The following are examples.

Sinus tachycardia: the underlying cause (pain, hypovalaemia etc) should be treated.
Sinus or nodal bradycardia: usually responds to small dose of atropine (0.1-mg increments).

Atrial ectopics, occasional ventricular ectopics are usually benign and require no specific treatment other than correction of hypercapnia if present and reduction in concentration of inhalation agent.

Supraventricular tachycardia is usually serious. Paroxysmal tachycardia may be terminated by use of vagotonic manoeuvres, such as carotid sinus massage, eyeball pressure. Then use drugs such as: verapamil 5–10 mg or adenosine 3 mg (and then 6 or12 mg if needed). Adenosine is less of a myocardial depressant.[15] Alternative drugs are esmolol 40 mg over 1 min, or amiodarone 300 mg over 15 min. If these fail then synchronized defibrillation should be used starting with 100 J.

Ventricular tachycardia is serious. this can not only impair cardiac output, but may proceed to ventricular fibrillation. Treatment is with synchronized defibrillation (100–200 J), lignocaine 50–200 mg, correction of the potassium and magnesium concentrations, and perhaps amiodarone.[16]

Atrial fibrillation: digoxin 0.5 mg i.v. is the drug of choice for controlling the ventricular rate. Esmolol 40 mg is an alternative.

Myocardial ischaemia and infarction

See Chapter 3.1 for the factors that predispose to cardiac risk during and after surgery.

Stroke

This has an incidence of approximately 0.2% after general surgery in patients without known cerebrovascular disease. It occurs typically from 2 to 10 days postoperatively. The causes are uncertain, but include emboli when in atrial fibrillation, thrombosis due to hypotension and the hypercoagulable state that occurs after surgery, and obstruction to a vertebral artery when the neck is rotated. The choice of anaesthetic agent is probably of little importance.[17] *See* Chapter 4.1 'Anaesthesia for vascular surgery'.

Hypertension in the immediate postoperative period

Possible causes are:

1 pain or full bladder;
2 hypercapnia;
3 confusion after anaesthesia;
4 unsuspected phaeochromocytoma (extremely rare);
5 vasoconstriction after cardiopulmonary bypass and other vascular surgery;
6 thyroid crisis.

The risks are mainly of extra myocardial O_2 demand. There is often an associated tachycardia, which will also impair coronary filling. These two factors may lead to myocardial infarction. A history of hypertension should be taken into consideration when assessing postoperative blood pressure. If an obvious cause cannot be treated, it may be useful to administer a vasodilator drug such as hydralazine 10 mg i.v. or nifedipine 10 mg sublingually with full monitoring and facilities to correct hypotension.

Air or gas embolism

Causes

Surgical: operations involving injury to veins in the neck, thorax, breast and pelvis; operations on the brain and cord in the sitting position; operations on the heart; laparoscopy. Gas embolism may complicate irrigation of semi-closed cavities with hydrogen peroxide (e.g. the mastoid).

Diagnostic and therapeutic injection of air into peritoneal cavity, pleural cavity, large joints, urinary bladder, tissue spaces, e.g. the perinephric area and nasal antra, uterus and tubes.

Accidental entrance of air during intravenous techniques.

Results

These depend on how much gas enters the circulation, and how fast it enters. If air enters the veins in any quantity it will cause a hissing sound in the wound and it will go to the right heart and lung, causing an air-lock obstruction in the pulmonary artery. This may result in a loud continuous precordial murmur, the so-called 'mill-wheel murmur'. There may be sudden cyanosis, hypotension, engorged neck veins, tachycardia, irregular gasping respiration, and cardiac arrest. Early diagnosis is aided by an oesophageal or precordial stethoscope, a Doppler probe on the precordium; and monitoring of end tidal CO_2, which falls abruptly.

Treatment

1 Prevent further entrance of air into the circulation, by compressing veins to raise venous pressure; tilting the patient so that the entry site is below the heart; flooding the wound with saline.
2 Place the patient on his or her left side so that bubbles are kept away from the mouth of the pulmonary artery.
3 Give 100% O_2 and stop administration of N_2O which is more soluble in blood than nitrogen and so will increase the size of the emboli.
4 Insert a CVP catheter to aspirate directly from the right heart.
5 Compression in a hyperbaric chamber is valuable in air embolism in divers.

COMPLICATIONS RESULTING FROM POSTURE

Trendelenburg position

Friedrich Trendelenburg (1844–1924) first used his tilt in 1880 when Professor of Surgery at Rostock to facilitate urological operations.

This head-down position is generally well-tolerated in anaesthetized patients breathing spontaneously. However, in short, stout patients, especially if there is an abdominal mass, pressure on the diaphragm may reduce lung volumes considerably, and IPPV is preferred except in very brief operations. Cyanosis occurs in the face and neck of plethoric patients in this position due to venous stasis, even with adequate ventilation.

If the arm has to be abducted, this should not be at greater than a right angle, with the elbow slightly flexed and pronated, to prevent pull on the brachial plexus, and the head turned to the side of the arm. The arm should not drop down below the plane of the body (*see below*).

The increase in cerebral venous pressure will cause a fall in cerebral perfusion, particularly if the patient is hypotensive. Prolonged head-down tilt can cause cerebral oedema and retinal detachment. Raising the legs, while keeping the body horizontal, is a better way of improving venous return.

Prone position

The functional residual capacity is greater than in the supine position. A pillow should be placed under each shoulder and another under the pelvis, so that breathing is not unduly interfered with and so that all pressure is completely removed from the abdomen and the IVC. This prevents the extradural veins becoming unduly distended. A cuffed tracheal tube may be wise in case regurgitation of stomach contents should occur, although some experienced anaesthetists use a laryngeal mask airway (or even a face mask) with success. Skeletal injury readily occurs when turning the unconscious patient. Particular care should be taken when moving the arms that a shoulder is not dislocated. Corneal abrasions are common (*see below*). Retinal arterial occlusion and blindness from pressure on the eye have been reported.[18]

Lithotomy position

When the lithotomy position is required, both legs should be moved together to avoid strain on the pelvic ligaments. If the patient is arranged so that the anterior superior iliac spines are on a level with the break in the table, he or she will be in a good lithotomy position when the legs are supported on the stirrups. The knee should be outside any metal supports, to avoid pressure on the lateral popliteal nerves. If the hips are very flexed, sciatic nerve stretch may occur. Bilateral compartment syndrome has occurred after $7\frac{1}{2}$ hours of surgery in the lithotomy position.[19] *See also* Chapter 4.3 'Gynaecology'.

Lateral position

This impairs spontaneous respiration, especially if a bridge is also used. In the lateral position with an anaesthetized patient breathing spontaneously, more ventilation goes to the upper lung while more blood flow goes to the lower lung, thus causing mismatch and impaired gas exchange. This is made worse by IPPV. (*See* Chapter 4.1 'Thoracic surgery'). Care should be taken with the position of the arms to try and prevent nerve compression (*see below*).

Supine position

Pressure on and stretching of nerves of the arm, particularly the ulnar nerve at the elbow, must be avoided. The elbow should be padded, and the forearm supinated which provides more protection for the ulnar nerve. Legs should be flat on the table, and not crossed. The tendo Achillis must not rest on the unpadded edge of the table. A soft pad, raising heels from the table, avoids pressure on the calf veins, and so may lessen the incidence of venous thrombosis.

Backache is not infrequent after operations performed in the supine position in patients with lumbar lordosis. It can often be prevented by the use of an inflatable wedge, as a lumbar support.

Changes of position of the head and neck

A patient with a decreased cardiac output or carotid artery disease is at risk of reduced cerebral blood flow, if changes in position alter the relationships of the vertebral arteries to surrounding bony structures. This is likely on rotation of the head, or hyperextension of the neck at the atlanto-occipital joint. This can be tested for at the preoperative examination. Full extension may result in a faint. Patients with cervical pathology may have nerve symptoms following immobilization from any cause, including surgery.

Moving the patient

The reflexes that maintain blood pressure are greatly reduced in an anaesthetized patient, who therefore reacts adversely to minor changes in body posture. This is particularly true if also hypovolaemic, or under spinal anaesthesia. All movements should be smooth and gentle, not jerky and rough.

Position in bed

The patient should lie in the semi-prone position until his or her reflexes return. This is maintained by a pillow between the bed and the chest; the upper knee is flexed. This helps to maintain a free airway by causing the tongue to fall away from the posterior pharyngeal wall; it also helps to prevent aspiration of vomitus into the air passages. The patient should not be placed in a head-up position until it is quite certain that the cardiovascular system is able to maintain an adequate circulation through the brain. Otherwise syncopal reactions and even death may occur.

See also Martin J. T. and Warner M. A. *Positioning in Anesthesia and Surgery*, 3rd edn. Philadelphia, W.B. Saunders, 1997.

VOMITING AND REGURGITATION

The anaesthetist constantly faces the problem of the aspiration of material from the alimentary canal into the lungs during induction, maintenance and recovery from anaesthesia.

Vomiting

Some patients are very prone to vomiting and should inform the anaesthetist of this risk beforehand.

The act of vomiting is preceded by salivation, rapid breathing, pallor, sweating, tachycardia and severe discomfort.

The vomiting centre is closely related to the respiratory and vasomotor centres and the salivary and vestibular nuclei, in the dorsolateral border of lateral reticular formation. The chemoreceptor trigger zone lies superficial to the true vomiting centre in the area postrema of the fourth ventricle. It has many dopamine receptors.

A pressure of 40 cmH$_2$O is needed to lift the contents of the stomach into the mouth in the upright position. While the glottis goes into spasm during the expulsive phase, it soon relaxes, so that aspiration of stomach contents into the bronchial tree is almost bound to happen in the unconscious supine patient. Vomiting is more likely in very light anaesthesia, especially if the base of the tongue or pharynx is stimulated by airways etc. Vomiting also may harm skin flaps, the abdominal wall or other areas recently operated on, as well as raising the intraocular or intracranial pressure. *See below* for the prevention of nausea and vomiting.

Regurgitation

Being a passive act, regurgitation may be silent and unheralded, and so more dangerous than vomiting. The major mechanism preventing regurgitation is the barrier pressure, i.e. the difference between intragastric pressure and the pressure exerted by the lower oesophageal sphincter. It is more likely if the stomach is full, if the patient is head-down, or if there is an indwelling gastric tube.

The mechanics of regurgitation

The cardiac sphincter is both a sphincter and a valve. It remains closed because of:

1 a muscular sphincter;
2 folds of thickened mucosa in the oesophagus;
3 the angle at which the oesophagus joins the fundus of the stomach;
4 the pinch-cock action of the crus of the diaphragm (in two-thirds of patients the right crus only).

Its activity is controlled by the vagus and sympathetic nerves. It is made incompetent by:

1 anatomical abnormality, e.g. hiatus hernia;
2 a gastric tube;
3 passage of anaesthetic gas from above during attempts at IPPV;
4 attempts at active respiration in the presence of upper airway obstruction;
5 atropine or hyoscine – this effect may be antagonized by metoclopramide or domperidone 10 mg which themselves increase the tone.

The cricopharyngeal sphincter is at the upper end of the oesophagus at the level of C6 and is composed of striated muscle (the rest of the oesophagus has smooth muscle). Its action is both voluntary and reflex. Its integrity is affected by both anaesthetics and relaxants. It normally acts as a sphincter, but as a valve when paralysed, when it tends to obstruct the passage of fluids from the pharynx to the oesophagus, but not in the reverse direction.

The normal intragastric pressure is 5–7 cmH$_2$O and double this in late pregnancy. This is well below the pressure required for reflux through the cardia. Even when the stomach is distended the pressure is unlikely to be greater than 18 cmH$_2$O unless there is contraction of the abdominal muscles. Measurements of intragastric pressure during the fasciculation following suxamethonium are usually not greatly increased, but in about 12% of patients a rise greater than 19 cmH$_2$O occurs.

Dangers of aspiration of stomach contents

1 Laryngeal spasm, reflex vagal bradycardia, atelectasis, bronchopneumonia and lung abscess. Foreign material gravitates into the dependent apex of the lower lobe with the patient lying supine, and into the dependent upper lobe with the patient on his side: these are the commonest sites of abscess formation. Clinical onset may be mild, after a latent period of 2–10 days, simulating early bronchopneumonia. The earliest X-ray sign is a patch of consolidation; later a fluid level may be seen. An abscess is treated by postural drainage and antibiotics.
2 Aspiration of acid gastric contents causes a chemical trauma to bronchial and alveolar epithelia – acute exudative pneumonitis or *Mendelson's syndrome*.[20] He described this in obstetric patients, but it is not confined to them. Greatest risk is said to be when a volume of more than 25 ml with a pH of less than 2.5 is aspirated. This is based on primate data, and has not been confirmed in humans. Following immediately, or after an interval of a few hours, the patient shows cyanosis, dyspnoea, bronchospasm, hypotension and tachycardia. There are crackles and wheezes in the

lungs, with a characteristic radiographic appearance of irregular mottled densities. In severe cases acute pulmonary oedema causes a rapid death.

Prevention of acid aspiration syndrome

There is no foolproof method, but the following are well-established.

1 Avoid heavy preoperative sedation, which may result in aspiration of stomach contents in the ward before or after operation.
2 Ensure an empty stomach by:
   (a) adequate preoperative starvation;
   (b) emptying it via a gastric tube, but this is not always reliable;
   (c) metoclopramide 10 mg to hasten gastric emptying;
   (d) induction of vomiting by apomorphine, 0.5 mg increments until vomiting occurs. This is unpleasant!
3 Inhibition of secretion of acid gastric juice by H_2 antagonists, e.g. ranitidine 150 mg orally the night before and on the morning of operation, or 50 mg i.v. Nizatidine is an alternative. Famotidine is available orally, but not in an intravenous preparation.
4 Neutralization of gastric contents by antacids, e.g. sodium citrate (15–30 ml of 0.33 mol/l solution). Its efficacy may be improved by turning the patient to promote mixing.
5 Rapid-sequence induction of anaesthesia: adequate preoxygenation (100% for at least 3 min), intravenous induction agent in a predetermined dose, suxamethonium 1.0–1.5 mg/kg (avoiding pretreatment with a non-depolarizing relaxant). When suxamethonium is contraindicated rocuronium has been advocated as an alternative. When intravenous induction is contraindicated, inhalational induction may be substituted.

   Cricoid pressure is used to prevent regurgitation by occluding the oesophagus between the cricoid cartilage and the vertebrae, as recommended by Sellick.[21] It should be applied as the patient loses consciousness, using the tips of the first two fingers and thumb of an assistant to apply pressure on the cricoid cartilage. The pressure required is said to be 40 newtons, but this is probably too great. The neck is extended and the other hand placed behind the neck to steady it. This method must not be used during active vomiting as it may lead to oesophageal rupture. It also distorts the appearance of the glottis. Cricoid pressure, to be safe, must ensure that the onset of unconsciousness, the achievement of full muscular relaxation and the application of firm cricoid pressure are timed to occur simultaneously. It should not be released until the cuff of the tracheal tube is inflated.
6 Use a regional block technique, and allow the patient to remain awake and with full protective reflexes.
7 Awake intubation of the trachea. Topical analgesia of the upper airways and fibreoptic endoscopy will enable a tube to be inserted into the trachea in the conscious patient.
8 After operation, lay the patient on his or her side and extubate in that position.

Treatment of acid aspiration

Prevent further aspiration by tilting the head downwards or turning the patient on one side. Use suction and give O_2. Tracheal suction may be sufficient in mild cases, whereas in others suction through a bronchoscope will be required. Further treatment is supportive: bronchodilators, antibiotics and physiotherapy. Steroids are no longer recommended by most anaesthetists.

Postoperative nausea and vomiting[22]

Postoperative nausea and vomiting (PONV) may be central from causes acting on the brain stem and higher centres; peripheral, from causes acting on the gut; and vestibular. It can be influenced by the following:[23]

1 *Type of patient*. Some patients are prone to PONV, e.g. those who suffer from travel sickness. Suggestion, and the example of surrounding patients, are important factors. Suitable preoperative reassurance is important. Postoperative nausea and vomiting is more frequent in women than in men, and in the young (especially children) than in the old.
2 *Anaesthetic agent and technique*. Narcotic analgesics cause PONV in some patients. This is still true when patient-controlled analgesia is used, even if an antiemetic is included in the mixture.[24] More common with inhalational techniques, especially for prolonged operations and when N_2O[25] is used. All regional blocks usually cause less PONV. Hypoxia is a potent cause of PONV. Less common with propofol than with barbiturates.
3 *Condition of stomach*. Vomiting is likely unless the stomach is empty, e.g. in those patients who have not complied with fasting instructions.
4 *Type of operation*. Vomiting is frequent after gynaecological, abdominal, eye, ear, throat and brain surgery.

Treatment and prevention

Prevent the factors above, when possible, and consider giving an antiemetic, such as the following.

1 *Phenothiazines*. Act as dopamine antagonists on the chemoreceptor trigger zone, e.g. prochlorperazine 12.5 mg i.m.; promethazine 25 mg. The latter has antianalgesic effects.
2 *Antihistamines*. Cyclizine 50 mg i.m. Can be given slowly intravenously, but causes a tachycardia. It has been added to morphine in an effort to prevent nausea and vomiting – 50 mg to morphine 10 mg (Cyclimorph).
3 *Dopamine antagonists*. Metoclopramide 10 mg acts both centrally and peripherally. It speeds gastric emptying time and increases the tone of the lower oesophageal sphincter. Will not relieve sea-sickness. Domperidone 10 mg crosses the blood–brain barrier very slowly and so does not usually cause neurological or psychological side-effects.

4 *Butyrophenone derivatives*, e.g. droperidol 1–5 mg, but is also effective for PONV in much smaller doses, e.g. 0.25–1 mg. Has a specific effect on the chemoreceptor trigger zone. May cause severe dysphoria.
5 *Anticholinergic drugs.* Hyoscine 0.4 mg. Inhibits the muscarinic activity of acetylcholine on the gut and may also have a central action.
6 *5-HT₃ antagonists.* Ondansetron 4–8 mg i.m. or i.v. is useful for high-risk patients. It is effective and potentiates other antiemetics. Expense is the only real disadvantage, as it is relatively free of side-effects. May be used in children above 2 years old (dose 0.1 mg/kg). It may also be given orally in adults in a dose of up to 16 mg. It is widely used in chemotherapy and radiotherapy. Granisetron is an alternative.
7 *Clonidine* reduces the amount of opiate required, and so lessens PONV.
8 *Acupuncture.* The P6 acupuncture point is 5 cm proximal to the wrist crease, between the tendons of the palmaris longus and the flexor carpi radialis of the right forearm, 1 cm below the skin, i.e. on 'the pericardial meridian'.[26]

NEUROLOGICAL COMPLICATIONS

Abnormal muscle movements and convulsions

Several types of abnormal muscular action may occur during anaesthesia.

1 Clonus: usually occurring in light anaesthesia and disappearing when anaesthesia is deepened. Commonly seen in the legs and may be stopped by raising thighs, leaving legs unsupported or by a small dose of muscle relaxant.
2 Epilepsy.
3 Convulsions due to hypoxia.
4 Convulsions due to local analgesic drugs, e.g. lignocaine, bupivacaine. Treat with intravenous thiopentone, midazolam or diazepam.
5 Involuntary muscle movements with some induction agents, e.g. etomidate.
6 Enflurane, and methohexitone cause increased activity on electroencephalogram (EEG) and epileptiform seizures have been reported.
7 Propofol has been associated with convulsions, which can be delayed for hours or even days after anaesthesia.
8 Severe myoclonus (wrongly called shivering) after halothane or other volatile agents may be mistaken for a convulsion.
9 Eclampsia.

Delayed recovery from anaesthesia

This may be due to the following.

1 *Drugs used during operation* in relative overdosage, e.g. phenothiazine derivatives, narcotic analgesics, thiopentone, volatile agents.

2 *Disturbances of physiology resulting from anaesthesia*, e.g. hypercapnia, a hypoxic episode during anaesthesia, electrolyte and acid–base disturbances, fainting (especially in the dental chair), induced hypotension, hypothermia.
3 *Disturbances resulting from surgery*, e.g. haemorrhage, fat embolism, air embolism, operative trauma in brain surgery.
4 *Patient's disease*, e.g. cerebrovascular accident, myocardial infarction, myxoedema, hypopituitarism, hypoglycaemia, hyperglycaemic coma, adrenal deficiency, uraemia, liver failure, an occult and undiagnosed brain tumour.
5 *Drugs taken before operation*, e.g. monoamine oxidase inhibitors (with pethidine during operation), sedatives.
6 T*he central anticholinergic syndrome* – may be treated with physostigmine 1–2 mg (*see* Chapter 1.1).
7 *Septicaemia* presenting in the early postoperative period.

Peripheral neuropathy

First recognized in 1894 by Budinger[27] as being due to malposition of the patient with consequent stretching and compression of nerves.

Aetiology

These are more common in patients with existing risk factors for neuropathy (e.g. diabetes, multiple sclerosis), and in operations lasting more than 30 min.

1 Stretching and compression of nerves, as a result of unphysiological positions. This is combined with abolition of pain and discomfort which would otherwise act as a warning.
2 Injection of substances into or around nerves. Irritation may be chemical, a result of direct needle or surgical trauma, or due to bacterial contamination or haematoma.
3 Use of tourniquets; if excessive pressure is allowed over a nerve trunk.

Pressure for upper-limb ischaemia need only exceed arterial blood pressure by 50–75 mmHg.

Specific neuropathies

BRACHIAL PLEXUS[28]

Stretching can occur as a result of:

1 extension and lateral flexion of head to opposite side;
2 abduction, external rotation and extension of the arm;
3 suspension of the arm from a bar when the patient is in lateral position;
4 extreme abduction of the arms above the head with the patient supine;
5 suspension by wrists to prevent slipping of patient in Trendelenburg position.

Compression can occur:

1 when shoulder braces are used with Trendelenburg position – if placed too medially the clavicle may be depressed so that the plexus has to traverse a longer and more devious course;

2 with the arm abducted in the Trendelenburg position the plexus may be depressed and stretched over the head of the humerus – shoulder braces, placed too laterally, may further depress the head of the humerus and with it the plexus;

3 the patient's abnormal anatomy – the plexus may be deviated posteriorly by the tendon of pectoralis minor or by the tip of the coracoid process in the obese patient undergoing cholecystectomy with gallbladder bridge inserted. *Various congenital anomalies* may render plexus more vulnerable, e.g. hypertrophy of scalenus anterior or scalenus media, cervical rib, anomalous derivation of the plexus and abnormal slope of the shoulder.

The entire plexus may be injured or the upper roots only. It is less common for the lower roots to be affected alone. Involvement may be restricted to one cord.

To avoid stretching the plexus, the following measures should be taken.

1 Shoulder braces are best avoided, with the patient supported on a non-slip mattress.

2 Arm-board must prevent backward displacement of arm.

3 Hyperextension and external rotation of elbow must be avoided.

Prognosis is good, but recovery may take months. The deltoid, biceps and brachialis are the muscles usually affected.

RADIAL NERVE

Can be injured due to stretching if the arm is allowed to sag over the side of the table. Can be compressed by use of a vertical screen support. Causes wrist-drop.

ULNAR NERVE

Can be damaged if the elbow is allowed to fall over the sharp edge of the table so that the nerve is compressed against the medial epicondyle of the humerus. Injury has also been reported as a result of full flexion of the elbow when the arm is placed in front of the chest. The nerve is stretched around the medial epicondyle of the humerus. If the elbow is extended, it is best to supinate the forearm to provide more protection to the nerve. Injury causes hypothenar weakness, and later 'claw hand'. Relatively minor trauma to the ulnar nerve may cause severe disability.[29]

MEDIAN NERVE

May be damaged as a result of technically perfect intravenous injections in the cubital fossa, as a result of direct needle trauma or extravasation of drugs. Results in inability to oppose thumb and little finger.

LATERAL POPLITEAL NERVE

Compression between the head of the fibula and a badly placed lithotomy pole damages the nerve and may result in foot-drop. This is the most frequently damaged nerve in the lower limb.

SAPHENOUS NERVE

Compression can occur between lithotomy pole and medial tibial condyle, when the leg is suspended lateral to the pole. Sensory loss results along the medial side of the calf.

SCIATIC NERVE

Can be traumatized by intramuscular injections in the buttock. It may be damaged in emaciated patients, lying on a hard table with opposite buttock elevated, as for hip-pinning. Paralysis of all muscles below knee, and perhaps of hamstrings results, with sensory loss. Has also been affected in a high lithotomy position, with the thighs excessively flexed.[30]

PUDENDAL NERVE

Can be compressed against a poorly padded perineal post during hip-pinning with traction to legs. The nerve is pressed against the ischial tuberosity. Causes loss of perineal sensation and faecal incontinence.

FEMORAL NERVE

Can be damaged by use of a self-retaining retractor during lower laparotomy. Causes loss of flexion of hip and loss of extension of knee. Sensation is lost over the anterior thigh and anteromedial aspect of the calf.

SUPRAORBITAL NERVE

Can be compressed by a metal endotracheal connector or tight head harness. Causes photophobia, forehead numbness and pain in the eye.

FACIAL NERVE

Can be compressed between fingers and ascending ramus of mandible. Causes facial paralysis. Buccal branch has been injured by tight harness, and paralyses orbicularis oris.

ABDUCENS NERVE WITH OTHER CRANIAL NERVES

Has followed spinal analgesia. See Chapter 5.3.

MANAGEMENT

Refer to neurologist for conduction studies for degree and place of block. Treat contributing factors, e.g. diabetes.

Postanaesthetic excitement

Most common in children; after operations for cataract and in the strong and fit. Made worse by premedication with sedative but non-analgesic drugs, and operations causing great pain or a full bladder. Psychiatric abnormalities may be the cause. Analgesics should be given in adequate dosage for pain. Small doses of intravenous benzodiazepines may be required. Large doses will cause apnoea.

Paralysis following intra- or extradural analgesia

See Chapter 5.3.

Extrapyramidal side-effects

Caused by phenothiazines, butyrophenone derivatives, metoclopramide, large doses of methyldopa and rauwolfia alkaloids, levodopa. There may be acute dystonia, painless spasmodic contractions; akathesia, uncontrolled restlessness, pseudoparkinsonism, persistent tardive dyskinesia, grimacing, pulling faces, etc.

Treatment

Withdraw the drug. For acute dystonic states, promethazine 25 mg i.v., procyclidine 10 mg i.v. or benztropine 2 mg i.v. (may cause the anticholinergic side-effects of dry mouth, blurred vision and constipation) or diazepam 10 mg i.v.

Awareness of surgery during general anaesthesia

Awareness during anaesthesia is not all-or-nothing, but a spectrum which ranges from full consciousness of the surroundings, through awareness of pain, auditory awareness, to unconsciousness with some movement to strong stimuli.[31]

CONSCIOUS AWARENESS WITHOUT AMNESIA

Pain felt and conversations overheard and remembered. Meaningful sounds (whose input is directed to the dominant cerebral hemisphere) are more easily remembered afterwards. Incidence of awareness with pain is about 1 in 10 000 elective general anaesthetics,[32] but it is more common to have awareness without memory of pain.

CONSCIOUS AWARENESS WITH AMNESIA

Obedience to spoken command during surgery which is not remembered. Detectable by the isolated arm technique. Amnesia appears to develop very early as anaesthesia deepens.[33]

SUBCONSCIOUS AWARENESS

Purposeful limb movements but no response to spoken command. More often caused by sensory input from the non-dominant side of the body. Subconscious awareness is not usually remembered afterwards, but may be exposed later by hypnosis (implicit memory). The extent to which subconscious awareness matters is not known.[34]

PSEUDO-AWARENESS

A patient becomes conscious of sounds and other sensations in the postoperative room, and wrongly assumes they are occurring during surgery.

Causes of awareness[35]

1 Patients who have an inborn or acquired resistance to anaesthesia.
2 Faulty technique (including a technique relying on O_2, N_2O and opiates only).
3 Faulty equipment (empty vaporizer, O_2 flush left on, failure of N_2O supply, etc).
4 Incautious derogatory comments by surgeons and others are more likely to be registered and remembered.
5 Justified administration of very light anaesthesia in a very sick patient.

Auditory awareness is the most common clinically, closely followed by awareness of intubation (when the induction agent is wearing off, yet before an adequate amount of inhalational agent has been taken up). It may be reasonable to warn patients of possible auditory awareness if they are at particular risk, yet be reassured that there will be no pain.

Detection of awareness during anaesthesia

CLINICAL DETECTION

Movement and phonation in the unparalysed patient; in the paralysed patient look for sweating, reactive pupils, hypertension, tachycardia and lacrimation. These show a fairly poor correlation with purposeful responses to surgery, and the connection between cortical and autonomic function in a conscious patient is not well maintained during adequate anaesthesia. The 'isolated arm technique'[36] enables an otherwise paralysed patient to respond by squeezing the anaesthetist's hand if awareness develops. This may be useful for research, but not for routine clinical practice.

Factors contributing to awareness during anaesthesia

Equipment:

Gas supply:
  Failure of N_2O.
  Gas leaks.
  Failure to flush a circle system.
  Oxygen flush left open.

Vaporizer:
  Empty.
  Not turned on.
  Wrong agent in it.
  Leak of gas at O-ring seal.

Ventilator:
  Mixing of driving gas with respired gases.

Monitors:
  No agent monitor.
  No N_2O monitor.
  No adequate monitor of awareness.

Technique:
  Insufficient sedation, premedication.
  Total intravenous anaesthesia.
  Miscalculation of doses of intravenous drugs.
  Difficult intubation.

Patients:
  Resistance to anaesthesia.
  Alcoholism.
  Very sick cases.
  Emergencies.

Surgery:
  Obstetrics.
  Cardiopulmonary bypass.
  Bronchoscopy.

ELECTROENCEPHALOGRAM

The raw EEG is transformed into a spectrum of power as a function of frequency. The median frequency is reduced to 5 Hz by anaesthesia. Spectral edge frequency also shows reductions, but cannot accurately predict depth of anaesthesia.[37] The bispectral index is probably the most promising index derived from the EEG.[38] It has been used with some success during inhalational[39] and intravenous propofol anaesthesia.[40]

RESPIRATORY SINUS ARRHYTHMIA

Diminishes with increasing depth of intravenous or inhalational anaesthesia, but the variability of response is great.[41]

EVOKED POTENTIALS

Auditory, visual or somatosensory. These show changes related to depth of anaesthesia, but are difficult to interpret reliably.[42] They are affected differently by different anaesthetics. Volatile agents affect the latencies of the responses, but the intravenous agents and opiates do so much less.

FRONTALIS ELECTROMYOGRAM

Reduction of tonic frontalis EMG activity with deepening anaesthesia, and an increase with strong stimuli, e.g. skin incision and intubation. Too unreliable for routine use.[43]

LOWER OESOPHAGEAL CONTRACTIONS

Decrease in rate and pressure from several times a minute during consciousness to zero at about 2 MAC, but are an unreliable sign of awareness.[44]

Prevention of awareness

It is most important to check all aspects of the anaesthetic machine thoroughly and to understand the various causes of awareness. It would seem unwise to rely solely on N_2O and opiates to provide protection against awareness. Even benzodiazepines may not be entirely satisfactory in this regard,[45] but are convenient as premedicants. It is best to rely upon adequate amounts of either propofol, thiopentone or a volatile agent.

Ear plugs (for the patient!) and headphones playing soothing music have a useful place here. The use of volatile agent monitors with alarms is likely to help prevent some cases of awareness. If anaesthesia must be discontinued to save the patient's life during surgery, it is worth considering giving diazepam or midazolam to impair hearing and memory formation. If it is thought likely that awareness has occurred inadvertently, regain anaesthesia immediately with a full dose of propofol or thiopentone, reassure the patient verbally, and talk to the patient after surgery. Counselling may be needed.

If a patient complains of operative awareness some time later, listen, establish the facts, do not disbelieve what the patient says, and arrange suitable psychological counselling. It may be helpful to have a witness to your conversation. Make full notes.

MALIGNANT HYPERPYREXIA OR HYPERTHERMIA

Described as a familial disease in an Australian family by Denborough et al. in 1960.[46]

Malignant hyperpyrexia (MH) is associated with arthrogryposis multiplex congenita, osteogenesis imperfecta, congenital ptosis and strabismus, hernias, kyphoscoliosis, cleft palate, and Duchenne muscular dystrophy. (Suxamethonium is avoided because of cardiac effects and risk of malignant hyperpyrexia.)[47]

In MH, heat production exceeds heat loss in the body to cause a rise of temperature of at least $2°C/h$. It is inherited as an autosomal dominant with incomplete penetrance and generation skipping, possibly due to a defect in the gene responsible for calcium channels on chromosome 19. It is characterized by cyanosis, mottled rash, muscle rigidity or masseter spasm (after suxamethonium, although this is not always associated with MH), hypercapnia (an early sign), hyperventilation, hyperkalaemia, metabolic acidosis, dysrhythmias, diffuse intravascular coagulation, and pyrexia (a relatively late sign). There is haemolysis, and a raised creatine phosphokinase (e.g. 80 000 U) and transaminases. Heat production is up to 2000 kJ/h. Exhaustion and cardiac failure cause death in 70% if untreated.

Pathophysiology

The primary lesion is in the sarcoplasmic reticulum of the skeletal musculature, where an enzyme system controls the movement of calcium ions.[48] A sudden rise in intracellular calcium leads to the hypermetabolic state.

It is precipitated by drug administration, particularly anaesthetics, but also monoamine oxidase inhibitors, phenothiazines, amide local analgesics (lignocaine) and tricyclic antidepressants. The most commonly implicated anaesthetics are suxamethonium and halothane. Most others (except perhaps N_2O) have caused it on rare occasions.[49] This includes sevoflurane and desflurane.[50]

Incidence

About 1 in 8000 in the UK. Age distribution: 19 months to 70 years. It becomes more severe after puberty. The affected patient is commonly a young athletic male. In Denmark there was one case of fulminant hyperpyrexia in 250 000 anaesthetics but there was suspicion of it in 1 in 16 000 patients who received all types of anaesthetics and in 1 in 4200 when both suxamethonium and a volatile agent were employed. Of those who received suxamethonium, 1 : 12 000 developed spasm of the masseters.[51]

Management

This is a medical emergency, and action must be taken immediately.

1 Withdraw volatile anaesthetic agents and hyperventilate with O_2. The severity of the condition is dose related, so early cessation of the anaesthetic is of the utmost importance.
2 Cool the patient with ice, wet sheets, fan, cold water gastric and peritoneal lavage.
3 Get help.
4 Measure the temperature, blood gases, and electrolytes. Insert an arterial line. Acidosis is corrected with bicarbonate.
5 Give dantrolene 1–2 mg/kg, and repeat up to 10 mg/kg. This takes time (and several pairs of hands) to reconstitute, and the resultant solution contains mannitol.
6 Hyperkalaemia can be corrected with glucose 50% (1 litre) and insulin 100 units.
7 Promote a diuresis.
8 Give dexamethasone 20 mg, methylprednisolone 10 mg/kg or other steroid.
9 Abandon the operation if possible.

An emergency pack for this condition should be kept in the theatre refrigerator, containing methylprednisolone, 8.4% sodium bicarbonate, 50% glucose, dantrolene and insulin.

The prognosis is worse with late identification, or if further suxamethonium or volatile agent has been given in a misguided attempt to abolish rigidity. Successful treatment brings about reversal of effects in 30–60 min. Continuing close monitoring is needed in case symptoms reappear some hours after successful treatment. Further dantrolene may be needed. The creatine phosphokinase (CPK) should be measured, and analgesia will be needed for muscle pains.

Dantrolene is a muscle relaxant acting by reducing calcium release from the sarcoplasmic reticulum, and uncoupling the excitation–contraction sequence. Weakness may be caused by doses over 4 mg/kg. Supplied in an ampoule containing dantrolene 20 mg, mannitol, 13 g, buffered to a pH of 9.5 with sodium bicarbonate. Reversal, if necessary, by germine monoacetate 0.5 mg/kg and transiently by neostigmine 0.04 mg/kg. 4-amino-pyridine may produce a slow, incomplete reversal.[52]

Management of anaesthesia in a patient susceptible to malignant hyperpyrexia

In patients known to have MH, a technique using intravenous induction, N_2O, O_2, opioid, and non-depolarizing relaxant is safe, as is regional blockade with bupivacaine. A vapour-free anaesthetic machine with new hoses is best. If a special machine is not kept, it is sufficient to run O_2 through for 2 h or so, remove all vaporizers and fit a new breathing circuit. Full monitoring, cooling and treatment facilities should be available.

If trigger agents are avoided, preoperative oral dantrolene (1 mg/kg 6 or 8-hourly for 24 h) should not be needed. It can cause nausea, vomiting, weakness and confusion.

Investigation of patient and relatives

Postoperative counselling is mandatory. Muscle biopsy, with exposure in vitro, should be performed by a recognized MH unit (University of Leeds Department of Anaesthesia). Affected persons should wear a bracelet stamped with the name of the disease and known triggers.

ACCIDENTAL HYPOTHERMIA

This may occur during long operations, e.g. vascular surgery with massive blood transfusion, and can be minimized by operating in a warm theatre, warming intravenous fluids and the use of a high-efficiency warming blanket. The critical theatre temperature is about 21°C.

Accidental hypothermia can also occur in the newborn and in the aged, and secondary to such conditions as myxoedema, hypopituitarism, adrenal failure, drug overdose, apparent drowning and as a result of coma, immobility or exposure.

Physiological effects

Cardiovascular system

Dysrhythmias occur at temperatures below 30°C; spontaneous ventricular fibrillation may be seen, but is not likely above 28°C. More likely with hypokalaemia or sudden changes in pH and PCO_2. There is a progressive bradycardia and fall in cardiac output and blood pressure. Stroke volume is little affected and coronary blood flow is well maintained. Electrocardiogram changes include lengthening of the QRS complex, prolongation of the PR interval, elevation of the ST segment, T-wave depression and the appearance of a J wave (small positive wave on the downstroke of the R which may appear at about 30°C). Vasoconstriction of skin vessels occurs. Blood viscosity is increased. Blood clotting is impaired, and the platelet count drops rapidly.[53]

Respiratory system

The O_2 dissociation curve is shifted to the left so that liberation of O_2 to the tissues is hindered. More dissolved O_2 is carried in the plasma. Breathing is depressed.

Acid–base balance

Acidosis tends to occur. This is partly respiratory due to hypoventilation, and partly metabolic due to increased formation of lactic acid with the inadequate circulation, and its decreased breakdown due to impaired liver function. Abnormal renal function prevents correction of acidosis.

Measurement of pH presents some difficulties. Laboratory estimations are carried out at 37°C, so a correction factor must be added of 0.0147 pH unit per °C fall in temperature.[54] Direct PCO_2 measurement presents similar problems, but blood gas machines allow for temperature corrections. Base excess measurements require no temperature correction.

Central nervous system

Cerebral O_2 consumption is 39% of normal at 30°C, and 35% at 28°C.[55] The cerebral cortex can tolerate the acute hypoxia due to complete circulatory arrest for 5–10 min at 28°C, 20 min at 20°C, and 50 min at 15°C.[56] There is a reduction in cerebral blood flow, brain volume and intracranial pressure. Consciousness is usually lost between 28°C and 30°C.

Metabolism

With each fall of 1°C, metabolism is reduced by 6–7%. The functions of the liver and kidneys are depressed during hypothermia so that drugs must be given in small amounts. Utilization of glucose is depressed, and continued intravenous infusion of glucose solution may result in a high blood-glucose level, not affected by insulin. Metabolism of substances like heparin, lactic acid and citrate is inhibited. The ECG change of QT prolongation is an indication for the administration of calcium gluconate or chloride. Renal blood flow, glomerular filtration and selective reabsorption are diminished. Below 30°C there is a secretion of dilute urine.

Electrolytes

There may be a rise in serum potassium. The cold heart is more sensitive to potassium, so small changes are of significance.

The neuromuscular junction

Duration and magnitude of block by depolarizing drugs are increased, the effect of non-depolarizing drugs is reduced.

Rewarming

Must be undertaken with care as there is a danger of burning the patient if rewarming is overzealous. Rewarming can be expedited by use of a mattress with circulating fluid, by the use of warm blankets, metal foil reflective blankets, warm water or warm air. A temperature higher than 40°C should not be used. Support of the cardiac output may be needed.

Dexamethasone 8 mg i.m. is used.

ANAPHYLACTIC REACTIONS IN ANAESTHESIA

Adverse reactions to anaesthetics contribute increasingly to anaesthetic morbidity and to a smaller degree to anaesthetic mortality. The precise incidence of anaphylaxis during anaesthesia is uncertain, but has been estimated to be 1 in 6000 anaesthetics in France,[57] and between 1 in 10 000 and 1 in 20 000 in Australia.[58] These figures suggest about 175 to 1000 such reactions per year in the UK.

Anaphylaxis is a result of drug-specific IgE attaching to receptors on the surface of basophils and mast cells, and then, on further exposure to the drug, cross-linking of this IgE activates the cells and powerful mediators are released. These cause the clinical signs. The mediators include histamine, prostaglandins, leukotrienes and platelet-activating factor. An *anaphylactoid reaction* is when the drug precipitates the release of these mediators directly, without IgE being involved, and is clinically indistinguishable from anaphylaxis.

Adverse drug reactions during anaesthesia

Due to:

1 overdose;

2 intolerance;

3 recognized side-effects;

4 wrong drug or diluent;

5 anaphylactoid (the drug directly causes mediator release);

6 allergy and anaphylaxis (the drug causes mediator release via IgE antibody).

5 and 6 are clinically indistinguishable.

Not always due to anaesthetic drugs.[59]

Minor rashes during anaesthesia are common.[60]

There is no reliable screening test for allergy to particular drugs, and therefore no method of predicting anaphylaxis in any particular patient. Some have used the RAST (radioallergosorbent test), which measures drug-specific IgE antibodies in the blood. It is not considered a very sensitive test, and suxamethonium is the only anaesthetic drug for which the test is currently available.

Clinical manifestations of anaphylaxis

About three times more common in women than in men. It is no more common in atopic individuals (those with eczema, allergic asthma or hay fever). There is often no record of any previous exposure to the drug. Reactions normally occur within minutes of exposure to the drug, and the dose given may be very small. This suggests that the common practice of giving a small 'test dose' before the main dose of a drug such as penicillin has no validity. Anaphylaxis does not occur in response to inhalational agents.

The signs may be delayed by 30–60 min, and this is particularly likely with an allergy to latex. In practice most cases are manifest soon after induction, whereas latex allergy presents well into the period of surgery. Latex allergy is associated with allergies to certain foods, such as banana, avocado, kiwi fruit and chestnut.[61] In a patient known to be sensitive to latex, all equipment in contact with the patient must be chosen to be latex-free. This will include gloves, airways, tubes, breathing circuits, monitoring apparatus, intravenous equipment, etc.[62]

There may be:

1 cardiovascular collapse (severe hypotension, absent pulses, hypoxia, tachycardia, dysrhythmias);
2 bronchospasm, laryngospasm, chest tightness, coughing, abdominal pain;
3 laryngeal oedema;
4 cutaneous manifestations, including facial oedema, flushing, erythema, urticaria, weals and generalized oedema;
5 nausea, abdominal pain and diarrhoea.

Hypotension which is resistant to treatment should arouse the suspicion of anaphylaxis.

Clinical management

1 Withdraw all likely responsible drugs, stop anaesthesia if possible.
2 Administer O_2, ensure airway.
3 Elevate legs if possible.
4 Give intravenous adrenaline in a bolus dose of 50–100 μg (1 μg/kg) which can be repeated as needed up to 1 mg.
5 Rapid intravenous infusion of crystalloid or colloid, at least 2 litres, is likely to be required (up to 25% of plasma volume may have been lost).

6 Consider need for intermittent positive-pressure ventilation (IPPV), further drug therapy: bronchodilators (aminophylline 250 mg slowly or salbutamol 250–500 μg), antihistamines (chlorpheniramine 10–20 mg i.v.), steroids (hydrocortisone 100–300 mg) and bicarbonate if there is an acidosis.
7 Consider need for further infusion of adrenaline 4–8 μg/min, or further vasoconstrictors, e.g. methoxamine.
8 Beware of extubation if laryngeal oedema is present.

Adrenaline is the mainstay of treatment. If intravenous access is not available, it may also be given intramuscularly (0.5–1.0 mg, or 0.5–1.0 ml of 1 : 1000), or intratracheally (10 ml of 1 : 10 000). The dose should be titrated against the response. Note that it may need to be continued by intravenous infusion after the immediate crisis.[63]

Further management

1 Take 10-ml blood samples in plain glass tubes 60 min after the reaction for estimation of tryptase released by mast cells.
2 Take a urine sample for measurement of methylhistamine (a metabolite of histamine);
3 Contact the referral immunology laboratory for advice, to help confirm the diagnosis and further management.
4 Write full clinical notes, and send a 'yellow card' adverse drug reaction notification to the Committee on Safety of Medicines.
5 Arrange for skin tests to be performed at a suitable later date.
6 Communicate the plan and any conclusions to the patient's general practitioner, and suggest safe drug combinations for future anaesthesia.
7 Explain the situation to the patient, and arrange for a warning card and bracelet.

The normal plasma level of tryptase is under 1.0 ng/ml. The level may be raised as much as 14 h after an anaphylactic reaction, and blood samples can yield reliable results even if taken post-mortem. The serum may be separated and stored safely at $-20°C$ for later analysis if necessary.

Skin-prick testing is probably the most reliable test of sensitivity to drugs, but must be done by someone experienced in its interpretation. Neat and 1 : 10 dilutions are used, together with positive (histamine) and negative (phenol saline) controls. A positive result is a weal to the 1 : 10 dilution which is more than 2 mm larger than the negative control.

ELECTRICAL HAZARDS

Surgical diathermy

Diathermy is a radio-frequency (about 3 MHz) power oscillation (used continuously for cutting, and in 20-msec bursts at a lower frequency for coagulation) with the patient forming part of the circuit, producing intense heat (over 1000°C) at the small electrode which the surgeon uses in the wound, and only slight warmth in the area of the large earth-plate. The power used is 50–400 W and the current through the patient about 200–400 mA, but may be 2 A during urological resection. Fortunately radio-frequency AC is very poor at causing ventricular fibrillation.

The apparatus may cause explosions, or interfere with monitors and cardiac pacemakers. Poor contact of the earth-plate with skin may cause burns. A broken earth-plate lead may cause the patient to earth him- or herself to part of the operating table and thus acquire a burn. A sparking earth-plate lead may ignite a spirit-based skin preparation. Unintended use when the active electrode is touching the wrong part of the patient, or a surgeon or assistant may also cause a burn. Bipolar diathermy, where the current just passes from one blade of a forceps to the other, uses less power and interferes least with monitors and pacemakers.

Electrocution

Mains frequency (50 Hz in the UK, 60Hz in the US) is particularly effective in producing ventricular fibrillation. Dry skin resistance may be $1 \text{ M}\Omega/\text{cm}^2$, which can be reduced to 500Ω by electrode jelly. One milliamp AC or 5 mA DC gives a tingling feeling in the skin; 15 mA AC or 75 mA DC causes muscle contraction; over 70 mA AC or 300 mA DC may cause ventricular fibrillation (this current need only flow for less than 20 ms). As little as 44 μA may cause ventricular fibrillation if applied direct to the heart.[64] Direct current flowing through skin can destroy tissue giving a punched-out open sore. Execution by the electric chair uses a current of 5–10 A.[65]

Safety precautions

The patient should be isolated from earth if possible, perhaps incorporating a transformer in the power supply. He or she should be protected from the metal of the table which is capacitively coupled to earth at diathermy frequencies. The current between any electrode and earth should not be more than 10 μA (for ECG, etc.). Diathermy should make an audible noise when activated, and the electrode sheathed when not in use. Earth-free solid-state or battery-powered diathermy sets are preferred. With any monitoring or diathermy equipment, leakage current between mains supply and patient circuit must not exceed 0.1 mA; if it does, the mains should be automatically isolated with an alarm. Household earth leakage circuit breakers are not suitable for use with anaesthetic equipment.

Fires and explosions

For the interesting history of these accidents, *see* Macdonald A. G. *Br. J. Anaesth.* 1994, **72**, 710.

Flammable anaesthetic agents (such as diethyl and divinyl ether, ethyl chloride and cyclopropane) are not used in many countries, and so the elaborate precautions needed to minimize the possibility of sparks in operating theatres are often unnecessary. Halothane, enflurane and isoflurane are non-flammable and non-explosive at room temperature in either air or O_2 at normal concentrations. In a 30%/70% O_2/N_2O mixture these volatile agents can only be ignited at concentrations above 4.75%, 5.75% and 7.0% respectively, and so can be regarded as nearly non-flammable under clinical conditions.

Electrical medical equipment used between 5 and 25 cm of any potential leak of flammable anaesthetic agents must be 'anaesthetic-proof' (AP), designated by a symbol of a green dot or band bearing the letters AP inside an inverted triangle. Equipment used within 5 cm of a potential leak, or used within the gas circuit, must be anaesthetic-proof category G equipment (APG).

Nitrous oxide, as well as air and O_2, supports combustion strongly. Mixtures corresponding exactly with the chemical equation, so that combustion is complete (*stoichiometric*) are most easily ignited and generate the most powerful deflagrations. There are limits of flammability, when the mixture becomes too weak, or the O_2 content too low. A source of heat sufficient to raise a vapour to its ignition temperature is required to generate an explosion.

Flammable substances include:

1 alcohol-based skin preparation solutions, which can pool in skin creases;
2 intestinal gases such as hydrogen and methane, which have been ignited by diathermy;
3 hydrogen produced by diathermy applied to the bladder;
4 tracheal tubes, ignited by diathermy in the mouth.

Sources of ignition:

1 *Heat:* from hot surfaces, wires, thermocautery.
2 *Electric current:* either in normal use, e.g. diathermy, monitors, sparks from electric motors, switches, etc; or as a result of faulty short-circuits.
3 *Static electricity:* produced by non-conductive materials such as artificial fibres, especially in a dry atmosphere.
4 *Lasers:* in or near the airway may ignite vapours or plastic equipment.
5 *Spontaneous*, e.g. when a rapid pressure rise heats up a gas. Any oil or grease in contact with N_2O or O_2 may ignite when a cylinder is opened. Lubricants must not be used, and cylinder valves opened slowly.

MISCELLANEOUS COMPLICATIONS

Ophthalmological complications

1 *Corneal abrasions:*[66] a common injury, especially in the prone position, and can lead to permament damage.[67] Prevented by adhesive tape sealing

the lids, soft contact lenses, or instilling aqueous gel or paraffin-based ointments into the conjunctival sac before anaesthesia. The latter are not recommended because of a significant morbidity (pain and inflammation). Abrasions can be diagnosed if a drop of 0.5% amethocaine is put into the eye, followed by fluorescein, when the abraded cornea will take up the stain. Treatment consists of a firm pad and bandage.

2 *Acute glaucoma* (closed angle): in susceptible patients who will complain of pain in and around the eye of a different nature to that due to foreign bodies or abrasions. The eye is red, the cornea cloudy and the pupil dilated on the affected side. There may be nausea and vomiting. Treatment in emergency: acetazolamide 500 mg or 10% mannitol i.v.; pilocarpine drops 0.5% into the conjunctival sac. Skilled ophthalmic help needed urgently.

3 *Vitreous haemorrhage:* has followed hypotensive techniques.

4 *Retinal infarction and blindness:* from pressure of an anaesthetic mask on the eyeball, or from a misplaced head support in the prone position. The blindness may be transient, but can be permament. May also result from spasm of basilar arteries.[68] Transient blindness can follow glycine absorption after transurethral surgery.

5 *Retinal emboli.*

6 *Ocular displacement:* this has occurred during IPPV in the head-down position, due to increased venous pressure.

Spontaneous rupture of tympanic membrane

This has been reported in a previously fit patient receiving N_2O and O_2.[69]

Minor sequelae

These are often the cause of considerable discomfort to the patient. They include trauma to lips, gums and teeth, sore throat, pharyngeal or laryngeal abrasions, superficial thrombophlebitis or just simple ecchymosis following intravenous injections, backache following lithotomy position, nausea and vomiting and an occipital bald spot following pressure during prolonged surgery and for which a special pillow may be preventive. They are disappointingly common, yet may often be avoided by greater care in the handling of the unconscious. These sequelae following minor surgery can cause considerable distress.

HAZARDS TO MEDICAL AND NURSING STAFF

Previous concerns about increased incidence of malignancy in theatre staff are now considered unfounded. Anaesthesia is a stressful occupation, particularly when a patient suffers a major and unexpected complication during surgery. Anaesthetists are more prone to suicide than many of their fellow doctors.

Other hazards include exposure to radiation, and injuries incurred as a result of lifting patients.

Reproduction

Some studies have shown that staff exposed to trace concentrations of waste anaesthetic gases suffer from increased rates of spontaneous abortion, and fetal abnormalities. This has even been shown in partners of male staff. All these findings have been contradicted in other surveys, have not established a causal link, and the consensus view is there is no significant risk.[70] Reduced fertility has also been reported in dental assistants exposed to N_2O.[71] Nitrous oxide is the only anaesthetic agent that has been shown to be teratogenic in experimental animals, and is known to affect DNA synthesis through inhibition of methionine synthetase.

Regulations exist in many countries to limit waste anaesthetic agents in the atmosphere of operating rooms, in the UK through COSHH (Control of Substances Hazardous to Health). Maximal suggested levels in different countries range from 2 to 50 ppm for the volatile agents (for isoflurane it is highest in the UK), and from 25 to 100 ppm for N_2O, although these values may be difficult to achieve in areas such as recovery, or if there are substantial leaks in breathing circuits.[72]

Measures to reduce pollution

1 Adequate ventilation of operating theatres.
2 Disposal of waste gases to outside air. For active scavenging an appropriate device is essential to prevent negative pressure being transmitted to the patient circuit.
3 The use of low-flow (e.g. 1 l/min) or completely closed breathing circuits.
4 Total intravenous anaesthesia.
5 The use of regional analgesia, combined with intravenous sedation if needed.
6 Careful filling of vaporizers with antispill devices at a time when few staff are present in the room.

Even trace concentrations well above those that are now regarded as acceptable in the operating theatre have no measurable effect on the performance on anaesthetists.[73] It is common sense, however, to keep the concentration as low as possible.

Blood-borne viruses[74]

These include hepatitis B, C and D and the human immunodeficiency virus (HIV) which causes acquired immune deficiency syndrome (AIDS). The hepatitis B virus (HBV) and HIV are the ones of major concern to anaesthetists, but all these diseases are transmitted by contact with infected blood and many other body fluids, and entry into the anaesthetist's body through a cut, skin abrasion or needlestick injury. The carrier state in a patient is obviously an indication for very careful safeguards, and should not affect surgical or obstetric care.

Hepatitis B: the incidence of the carrier state of hepatitis B is about 0.2% in UK, 5% in the Eastern Mediterranean and 10% in those of SE Asia. The presence of the surface (Australia) antigen and the Be antigen are associated with the infectious virus. Patients under high suspicion of being infectious include those who:

1 have liver disease, acute or chronic;
2 have undergone haemodialysis;
3 are immunosuppressed;
4 are immigrants or visitors from countries where carriers are common, especially if they have received blood transfusions there;
5 have received blood from paid donors;
6 are inmates of prisons or other institutions;
7 are drug addicts, prostitutes or homosexuals;
8 have tattoos.

There is a high risk of transmission of HBV through a needlestick injury, up to 30%.

Human immunodeficiency virus: the incidence in the UK is uncertain, and varies greatly in different areas of the country. It is around 0.1% overall, but considerably higher in London and some other cities. The above list of patients at higher risk for hepatitis B also applies to HIV. It is particularly common in homosexuals and intravenous drug addicts. The risk of transmission through needlestick injury is considerably lower than for HBV, and is probably very much less than 1%.

A few patients will be known to be virus carriers, but most carriers will not be known to the hospital. Routine screening for HBV is not practical. Testing for HIV cannot be done without full consent of the patient because of the life-style implications of a positive test, and in any case cannot exclude a patient who is in the 3-month window between infection and seroconversion. It is therefore wise to regard all patients as potentially infectious and take 'universal precautions'. These include the following:

1 Wearing gloves during venipuncture, putting up drips, inserting airways and tracheal intubation and extubation. The reasons why anaesthetists do not always wear gloves are largely invalid.[75]
2 Not resheathing needles, but disposing of them in a proper 'sharps' box.
3 Proper sterilization of reusable equipment, and the proper disposal of single-use equipment by incineration. Hepatitis B virus and HIV are killed by autoclaving, ionizing radiation and immersion in hypochlorite, formaldehyde or glutaraldehyde.
4 Biopsy specimens and blood, etc. must be sent to the laboratory in sealed containers.

5 Breathing circuits should present no risk, as the viruses are not transmitted by air-borne spread, but it is common practice to use a bacterial and viral filter placed between the circuit and the patient to prevent contamination with secretions.

6 Washing the floor and all contaminated surfaces with hypochlorite solution.

Anaesthetists should be protected by immunization against hepatitis B, which is safe and effective, followed by measurement of the antibody response. Boosters may be needed at 5-year intervals. Short-term protection against HBV (in case of a needlestick injury) can be provided for someone who has not been immunized by giving HBV immunoglobulin. There is no vaccine against HIV yet, and accidental exposure to this virus needs expert advice from an occupational health physician.[76] Antiviral drugs such as zidovudine are usually given.

If an anaesthetist is a carrier of one of these viruses he or she must seek medical advice. There are many examples of transmission of HBV from doctor to patient, but very few for HIV. These have all occurred during invasive surgical procedures, which are not normally performed by anaesthetists. The infected anaesthetist is very likely to be able to carry on his or her practice, provided that appropriate medical advice has been sought and followed.

Addiction and the anaesthetist

Anaesthetists are an at-risk group because of the relatively easy access they have to addictive drugs. Anaesthetists who have been addicted to opioid drugs should be carefully counselled and may even be advised to change to another specialty.

REFERENCES

1 Chopra V. et al. *Anaesthesia* 1990, **45,** 3; Gravenstein P. *Manual of Complications during Anesthesia.* Lippincott, Philadelphia, 1991.
2 Sulek C. A. *Curr. Rev. Clin. Anesth.* 1992, **13,** 9; Lang S. A. *Canad. J. Anaesth.* 1990, **37,** 210.
3 Drummond G. B. *Br. J. Anaesth.* 1991, **66,** 153.
4 Heiberg J. *Med. Times Gaz.* 1874, Jan. 10th.
5 Guedel A. E. J. *Am. Med. Assoc.* 1933, **100,** 1862.
6 Skolnick E. T. et al. *Anesthesiology* 1998, **88,** 1144.
7 Boushra N. N. *Can. J. Anaesth.* 1996, **43,** 599; Rosenberg-Ademsen S. et al. *Br. J. Anaesth.* 1996, **76,** 552.
8 Severinghaus J. W. and Mitchell R. A. *Clin. Res.* 1962, **10,** 122.
9 Vella L. M. et al. *Anaesthesia* 1984, **39,** 108.
10 Warwick J. P. and Mason D. G. *Anaesthesia* 1998, **53,** 571.
11 Powell J. F. et al. *Anaesthesia* 1996, **51,** 769.

12 Hamman L. *Trans. Assoc. Am. Physicians.* 1937, **52,** 311.
13 Bullingham A. and Strunin L. *Br. J. Anaesth.* 1995, **75,** 622; Wheatley T. and Veitch P. S. *Br. J. Anaesth.* 1997, **78,** 118; Best A. J. et al. *Ann. Royl. Coll. Surg. Eng.* 1998, **80,** 350.
14 McLean J. *Am J Physiol.* 1916, **41,** 250.
15 *Drug Therap. Bull.* 1993, **31,** 49.
16 Chamberlain D. *Br. J. Anaesth.* 1997, **79,** 198.
17 Kam P. C. A. and Calcroft R. M. *Anaesthesia* 1997, **52,** 879.
18 Lincoln J. P. and Sawyer N. P. *Anesthesiology* 1966, **22,** 800.
19 Tuckey J. *Br. J. Anaesth.* 1996, **77,** 546.
20 Mendelson C. L. *Am. J. Obstet. Gynec.* 1946, **52,** 191.
21 Sellick B. A. *Lancet* 1961, **2,** 404; *Anaesthesia* 1982, **37,** 213.
22 See also supplement *Br. J. Anaesth.* 1992, **69,** IS, 685.
23 Kortilla K. *Acta Anaesthesiol. Scand.* 1998, **42,** 493.
24 Woodhouse A. and Mather L. E. *Anaesthesia* 1997, **52,** 770.
25 Hartnung J. *Anesth. Analg.* 1996, **83,** 114.
26 Dundee J.W. et al. *Lancet* 1990, **i,** 541.
27 Budinger K. *Arch. Klin. Chir.* 1894, **47,** 121.
28 Cooper D. E. et al. *Clin. Orthop. Rel. Res.* 1988, **228,** 33.
29 Stoelting R. K. *Anesth. Analg.* 1993, **76,** 7.
30 Warner M. A. et al. *Anesthesiology* 1994, **81,** 6.
31 Bailey L. R. and Jones J. G. *Anaesthesia* 1997, **52,** 460.
32 Jones J. G. *Br. J. Anaesth.* 1994, **73,** 31.
33 Andrade J. et al. *Consciousness and Cognition* 1994, **3,** 148.
34 Bonke B. et al. *Br. J. Anaesth.* 1986, **58,** 957.
35 Ranta S. O-V. et al. *Anesth. Analg.* 1998, **86,** 1084.
36 Tunstall M. E. *Br. Med. J.* 1977, **1b,** 1321.
37 Dwyer R. C. et al. *Anesthesiology* 1994, **81,** 403.
38 Leslie K. et al. *Anesth. Analg.* 1995, **81,** 1263.
39 Sebel P. S. et al. *Anesth. Analg.* 1997, **84,** 891.
40 Struys M. et al. *Anaesthesia* 1998, **53,** 4; Schraag S et al. *Anaesthesia* 1998, **53,** 320.
41 Pomfrett C. J. et al. *Br. J. Anaesth.* 1994, **72,** 397.
42 Schwender D. et al. *Acta Anaesthesiol. Scand.* 1996, **40,** 171.
43 Chang T. et al. *Anesth. Analg.* 1988, **67,** 521.
44 Raftery S. et al. *Br. J. Anaesth.* 1991, **66,** 566.
45 Schwender D. et al. *Canad. J. Anaesth.* 1993, **40,** 1148.
46 Denborough M. A. et al. *Lancet* 1960, **2,** 15; *Br. J. Anaesth.* 1962, **34,** 395.
47 Rosenberg H. and Heiman-Patterson T. *Anesthesiology* 1983, **59,** 362.
48 Cheah K. S. et al. *Acta Anaesthesiol. Scand.* 1990, **34,** 114.
49 McGuire N. and Easy W. R. *Anaesthesia* 1990, **45,** 124.
50 Allen G. C. and Brubaker C. L. *Anesth. Analg.* 1998, **86,** 1328.
51 Ording H. *Anesth. Analg. (Cleve.)* 1985, **64,** 700.
52 Lee C. et al. *Anesthesiology* 1981, **54,** 61.
53 Easterbrook P. J. and Davis H. F. *Br. Med. J.* 1985, **291,** 23.
54 Rosenthal T. B. *J. Biol. Chem.* 1948, **173,** 25.
55 Stone H. H. et al. *Surg. Gynecol. Obstet.* 1956, **103,** 313.
56 Treasure T. *Ann. R. Coll. Surg.* 1984, **66,** 235.

57 Laxenaire M-C. et al. *Ann. Fr. Anesth. Reanim.* 1993, **12,** 91.
58 Fisher M. McD. and Baldo B. A. *Europ. J. Anaesthesiol.* 1994, **11,** 263.
59 Parker S. D. et al. *Anesth. Analg.* 1990, **70,** 220.
60 Desmueles H. *Anesth. Analg.* 1990, **70,** 216.
61 Kam P. C. A. et al. *Anaesthesia* 1997, **52,** 570.
62 Dakin M. J. and Yentis S. M. *Anaesthesia* 1998, **53,** 774.
63 Association of Anaesthetists. *Anaphylactic Reactions associated with Anaesthesia – 2.* Association of Anaesthetists, London, 1995.
64 Hull C. J. *Br. J. Anaesth.* 1978, **50,** 647.
65 Jones G. R. N. *Lancet* 1990, **335,** 713.
66 White E. and Crosse M. M. *Anaesthesia* 1998, **53,** 157.
67 Gild W. M. et al. *Anesthesiology* 1992, **72,** 204.
68 Johnson R. C. and Moss P. J. *Anaesthesia* 1981, **36,** 954.
69 White P. F. *Anesthesiology* 1983, **59,** 369.
70 Buring J. E. et al. *Anesthesiology* 1985, **62,** 325; Halsey M. J. *Anaesthesia* 1991, **45,** 486.
71 Rowland A. S. et al. *N. Engl. J. Med.* 1992, **327,** 993.
72 Barker J. P. and Abdelatti M. O. *Anaesthesia* 1997, **52,** 1077.
73 Rice S. A. *Clin. Anaesthesiol.* 1983, **1,** 507.
74 Layon A. J. et al. *Can. J. Anaesth.* 1997, **44,** 689.
75 Harrison C. A., Rogers D. W. and Rosen M. *Anaesthesia* 1990, **45,** 831.
76 Greene E. S. et al. *Anesth. Analg.* 1996, **83,** 273.

Section 3
THE PATIENT

Medical diseases influencing anaesthesia

Anaesthesia is a very safe procedure in the fit, healthy patient, although risk is increased when systemic disease is present. The 1987 confidential enquiry into perioperative deaths (CEPOD)[1] concluded that only 3 deaths resulting from some half a million operations (1 in 185 000) were solely due to anaesthesia. Anaesthesia can never be entirely safe, if only because patients may have significant disease without any symptoms. Some problems will also be encountered due to what amounts to a patient's self-abuse (e.g. smoking, obesity).

The anaesthetist's responsibility is to recognize risk factors and to advise surgeons and patients that they should be corrected before elective surgery. The anaesthetist may be asked to help in this process if the time and facilities are available. This is more important in the case of emergency surgery where time is short and speedy correction is necessary. The anaesthetist must give an accurate and honest risk assessment to the patient, and therefore needs current morbidity and mortality figures. Common sense is an invaluable tool in these situations. Any such assessment of risk may call for invasive preoperative monitoring to measure extent of dysfunction, especially in the elderly.

THE ELDERLY PATIENT

Assessment of risk in the elderly

There may be a difference between chronological and biological ages, e.g. a 90-year-old may be as healthy and resilient as many 70-year-olds. The surgical team need to assess the operative risk and decide whether the operation should be postponed for medical treatment to improve the patient. Although surgical mortality and morbidity rise with age, this is because concurrent disease is more common in the elderly, and not because of age itself.[2] Even the over 90s may present a relatively small risk.

The elderly patient presents two sets of problems:

An increased incidence of concurrent diseases

These may be multiple, for which the patient may be taking many drugs. The pathology may be 'hidden', e.g. painless peritonitis, apyrexial septicaemia, silent myocardial infarction, hence the need for minimum routine tests of full blood count, urinalysis, urea and electrolytes, and electrocardiogram (ECG).

Altered pathophysiology

GENERAL

Slower mental and physical recovery from trauma or surgery. Slower wound healing, weaker tissues, tendency to bed sores. Fragile skin and veins. Many physiological capacities reduce by 1% per year over the age of 40. Muscle weakness is common with the need for lower doses of relaxants.

Poor adaptation to hospital diet. Malnutrition, e.g. relative starvation, obesity, anaemia, vitamin deficiency, hypoproteinaemia. Osteoporosis, loss of teeth and jaw substance. Osteoarthritis and Paget's disease are common.

Slower metabolic rate, making it easier to hyperventilate. Cerebral vessels still react to a lowered PCO_2 and severely decrease brain perfusion.

NERVOUS SYSTEM

Preoperative cognitive deficit, making history-taking difficult. (Memory assessment by the Camden Scale: What is your name? When were you born? Where do you live now? Who is the reigning monarch? Who is the prime minister? What is the date/day of the week today?) Less ability to 'process' data. Confusion resulting from the upheaval of hospital admission. Deafness, especially high tones, with resulting difficulty in communication, and less compliance with instructions. Less elasticity of lens of eye.

Neurones are lost at up to 50 000 per day, especially in some areas, e.g. neocortex, spinal motor neurones. Nerve conduction is slowed. Pain threshold is increased. Autonomic function impaired: postural hypotension, less homeostasis in temperature control, tendency to urinary retention and constipation (exacerbated by anticholinergics and opioids).

CARDIOVASCULAR

Less elastic arteries with a rise in arterial pressure, especially systolic. Less homeostasis of vascular pressures, and intolerance to hypotension. Lowered blood volume, stroke volume and cardiac index (by 1% per year over 40). Longer circulation time. Haemoglobin slightly lower. Conduction blocks and arrhythmias more common. Deep venous thrombosis (DVT) more common. Reduced vascular stability is a particular problem during spinal or epidural analgesia. The small changes in venous return resulting from intermittent positive-pressure ventilation (IPPV), vasodilator drugs, haemorrhage, etc have a major effect in the elderly, and must be carefully managed by the anaesthetist.

RESPIRATORY

Vital capacity drops, residual volume rises with age. Closing volume rises and may exceed functional residual capacity. Less elastic recoil of lungs. Ventilation/perfusion mismatch results in a lowered PaO_2. Increase in physiological dead space. Laryngeal sensitivity is reduced and silent aspiration of gastric contents can occur. Chest-wall rigidity due to opiates is more common. It is less easy to detect lung pathology in the elderly by clinical examination.

BODY FLUIDS

Glomerular filtration rate declines 1% per year after 40 years. Slight rises in urea (up to 10 mmol/l) and creatinine (up to 160 μmol/l). Reduced body water. Water excretion and conservation less efficient. Patients with fractured neck of femur are often dehydrated.

Pre- and postoperative sedation

Elderly people may be confused, especially postoperatively.[3] Common causes are cerebral hypoxia due to cardiorespiratory disease, and deafness. Sedatives will make this worse. To produce sleep, alcohol is useful for those accustomed to it, or benzodiazepines. Hyoscine is best avoided. Postoperative cognitive deficit is as common as preoperative cognitive deficit (POCD).

Anaesthesia[4]

There is a steady reduction with age in the requirements for inhalational and intravenous anaesthetic requirements.[5] Minimum alveolar concentration (MAC) reduces by about 6% per decade throughout adult life,[6] and is lessened by about 20% at 70 years, and 30% at 90 years. Renal and hepatic excretion of drugs is slower. Protein binding and volumes of distribution are often altered. Intravenous agents are well tolerated, if dosage is kept low and they are given slowly. Etomidate is useful as it tends to maintain arterial pressure. Non-depolarizing relaxants are not as well reversed in the elderly (especially if hypothermic).

Early postoperative ambulation is usually desirable to prevent venous thrombosis, while rapid recovery of the cough reflex helps prevent postoperative atelectasis. A common cause of death is pulmonary embolism.

In elderly people with emphysema, general anaesthesia, maintaining spontaneous respiration, has given good results. Good speedy operating is useful at all times, but is especially valuable in the elderly. Postoperative hypoxaemia increases with age. Oxygen therapy usually corrects this, and is given routinely until the patient has a good saturation on room air (hours or days if needed).

Extra- and intradural analgesia is often suitable for operations below the umbilicus, but close attention must be paid to prevention of hypotension and hypothermia. Ephedrine is sometimes less effective in the elderly, and phenylephrine or metaraminol are useful alternative vasoconstrictors.[7] As with the younger patient, it is difficult to find evidence that any particular anaesthetic technique provides better morbidity and mortality. The skill of the anaesthetist is foremost.

PREGNANCY

Spontaneous abortion or premature labour may result following general anaesthesia for surgical conditions unconnected with pregnancy, but these risks diminish with gestational age. The incidence of fetal abnormalities is not increased.[8] Ideally, surgery should be postponed until 6 weeks post-partum. If this is not possible, the second trimester is satisfactory. If anaesthesia is necessary in an emergency, it should be remembered that in the last two trimesters the $PaCO_2$ is normally 4 kPa (30 mmHg), and that both cardiac output and blood volume are increased. The fetal heart may be monitored from about 18 weeks. Active involvement of an obstetrician is important.

The lower oesophageal sphincter becomes increasingly incompetent throughout pregnancy, and does not return fully to normal until 6 weeks post-partum.[9] Even in early pregnancy opiate premedicants are best avoided, and from the second trimester onwards consideration must be given to intubation to protect against aspiration. In a pregnancy of over 16 weeks, aortocaval compression syndrome can more than halve the maternal cardiac output and cause fetal hypoxia. Whether regional block or general anaesthesia is undertaken, such patients should be anaesthetized in the lateral position or with a wedge under the right side. Prophylaxis against DVT should be given. The reduction in plasma proteins can increase the toxicity of local anaesthetics.

Anaesthetics are not teratogenic in clinical practice, even N_2O which has a known effect on nucleic acid synthesis.[10] Ranitidine is not teratogenic. Known teratogens include warfarin, anticancer agents. Some drugs can harm the fetus in a variety of other ways, e.g. steroids, antithyroid drugs, warfarin in late pregnancy, tetracycline, streptomycin, sulphonamides. Benzodiazepines are associated with an increased incidence of cleft lip/palate. Non-steroidal anti-inflammatory drugs (NSAIDs) may cause premature closure of the ductus *in utero*. Other drugs, e.g. all narcotics, sedatives and anaesthetics, cross into breast milk. The pH of milk is lower than that of plasma, and drugs that are weak bases can reach high concentrations.

For Obstetric anaesthesia, *see* Chapter 4.3 'Obstetrics'.

HIATUS HERNIA

This abnormality, often unsuspected, may result in regurgitation during induction or maintenance of anaesthesia, most commonly in middle-aged obese patients or those in late pregnancy. Such patients tend to have a reduced barrier pressure (difference in pressures between the lower oesophageal sphincter and stomach).

Hiatus hernia is suggested by retrosternal pain, burning or reflux into the pharynx induced by gravity. The anaesthetist should treat such patients as suffering from acute intestinal obstruction to reduce the likelihood of regurgitation and aspiration. Preoperative administration of an H_2 antagonist (ranitidine 150 mg orally, 50 mg i.m.) or antacid (0.3 mol/l sodium citrate, 15–30 ml) may be helpful. Metoclopramide 10 mg i.m. can be given to increase lower oesophageal sphincter tone.

CARDIOVASCULAR DISEASE

Patients with organic heart disease who compensate sufficiently to carry on their daily jobs usually tolerate anaesthesia well, provided it is carefully administered and overdosage, hypoxia, hypercapnia and hypotension avoided. Attention should be paid to the heart rate. Above about 100 bpm, the shortened diastolic interval reduces coronary perfusion time.

The following cardiovascular conditions should be carefully sought, as they are particularly hazardous under anaesthesia and can cause sudden death, especially if there is inadvertant hypoxia, hyper- or hypotension:

1 recent myocardial infarction or unstable angina;
2 aortic stenosis;
3 heart block with Stokes–Adams attacks;
4 untreated hypertension;
5 myocarditis or cardiomyopathy (*see below*), which may be silent and not evident from an ECG.

If the cardiac output is low, the circulation time is prolonged. Intravenous drugs take longer to act, and if suxamethonium is used it should be given in larger doses (e.g. 100 mg or more). In a digitalized patient arrhythmias may occur following suxamethonium.

Cardiac risk factors

Several attempts have been made to quantify the operative risk to patients with heart disease.[11] The best known is still the Goldman index,[12] in which scores were given thus: third sound or gallop rhythm (11); myocardial infarction within last 6 months (10); any arrhythmia, or at least 5 ventricular ectopic beats per minute (7); age over 70 years (5); emergency surgery (4); aortic stenosis (3); abdominal or thoracic operation (3); poor general condition (3). A total over 13 correlated with a poor prognosis (11% life-threatening complications), and above 26, perioperative mortality was over 50%. Others have found heart failure and poor ventricular function to be adverse factors.[13] Such scoring systems are of little value when considering an individual patient.[14]

Coronary artery disease

Preoperative assessment[15]

Up to 15% of these patients have no abnormalities on routine examination nor on their resting ECG. An exercise ECG (the changes in the ST segment relative to increase in heart rate) is more sensitive. Echocardiography gives useful non-invasive information on myocardial function. Nuclear imaging of the ventricles and coronary perfusion, and coronary angiography are little used before most non-cardiac surgery. Prior coronary artery bypass grafting may be considered in some patients, although the overall risk of the two operations may well be higher. Drug therapy for angina, heart failure or hypertension should not be stopped before surgery.

Management

A risk of reinfarction persists for up to a week after operation. Control of arrhythmias and cardiac failure are required in addition to good analgesia. A balance of myocardial O_2 supply and demand must be struck. Oxygen supply depends on saturation of an adequate haemoglobin concentration, sufficient diastolic blood pressure and a slow pulse rate. Demand is reduced by preventing undue increases in systolic pressure and pulse rate.

Transoesophageal 2-dimentional echocardiography is very expensive but probably the best technique for detecting abnormalities of heart-wall motion and thus intraoperative ischaemia, although there is little objective evidence that its use results in an improved outcome. It requires considerable training and experience to interpret the signals correctly.[16]

Careful haemodynamic control and prevention of intraoperative ischaemia can reduce postoperative infarction.[17] Nifedipine and nitroglycerin are useful coronary vasodilators. Nitrates, nifedipine and nitroprusside reduce afterload and control postoperative hypertension. Tachycardia and hypertension due, for example, to laryngoscopy, atropine or inadequate analgesia may decrease coronary filling by shortening diastole. The use of opiates or beta-blockade may be needed. The short action of esmolol is particularly useful. The cardiac rate/systolic pressure product is a rough index of myocardial O_2 demand (upper acceptable limit 20 000 in normal patients, 12 000 in those with coronary disease). Isoflurane is a coronary vasodilator. In about a quarter of patients[18] with coronary disease the anatomic pattern of abnormalities may allow isoflurane to 'steal' coronary blood from the diseased areas, but other evidence suggests that it can also lessen ischaemic damage in the myocardium.[19]

Haemodynamic stability and oxygenation should be ensured in the post-operative period. Obstructive sleep apnoea may cause large drops in O_2 saturation and myocardial ischaemia, particularly when opiates are given.

Myocardial infarction

First pre-mortem diagnosis by Adam Hammer (1818–1878) in 1878.[20]
Operation within 3 months of cardiac infarction carries a 25–50% risk of
reinfarction, most likely to occur on the third postoperative day. Operation
3–6 months after infarction carries a 10–25% risk of reinfarction, reducing
to about 5% for operation 6 months or more after infarction. Upper abdominal and thoracic operations carry the highest risk. The incidence is not related
to the type of general anaesthetic used. These considerable risks must be
balanced against those of not undertaking the operation proposed. The
degree of ventricular impairment may be a more important prognostic
factor than the presence of recent infarction. Occasionally a treatable cause
of myocardial infarction may be found, e.g. polycythaemia.

Hypertension

The problems for the anaesthetist relate to: larger than normal rises in blood
pressure in response to stress, sympathetic stimuli and to some drugs;
atheroma and thrombosis in the coronary and cerebral arteries; renal failure;
left ventricular hypertrophy and stiffness, needing a high filling pressure and
reasonable time for filling; sensitivity to nodal rhythm; tendency to hypotension, especially after epidural block. The blood volume is reduced in
untreated hypertensive patients.

Preoperative assessment

Treatable causes of hypertension should be sought (endocrine, renal, coarctation, etc.), as should secondary effects of hypertension on the heart
(ischaemia, hypertrophy, failure), lungs (oedema), brain (ischaemia), kidneys
(uraemia) and the eyes. Assessment will include an ECG. Medication is continued up to the time of surgery. If untreated, operation is delayed if possible
to allow adequate control of blood pressure. A high blood pressure in an
anxious patient who has just been admitted is not necessarily associated
with a risk of postoperative infarction.[21] Subsequent blood-pressure readings
should be normal in such patients. Persistent lability of blood pressure in the
anxious patient may present a similar risk to the known hypertensive.[22] Even
a single dose of a beta-blocker such as atenolol[23] or nifedipine may be helpful
in preventing postoperative myocardial ischaemia. A diastolic pressure over
110 mmHg constitutes a serious risk.

Management

Most moderately hypertensive patients present few problems provided care is
taken with the maintenance of blood pressure and flow to coronary, cerebral
and renal circulations. Normal autoregulation may be diminished. Minimal
doses of anaesthetic agents are indicated, and intravenous fluids help lessen
any fall in blood pressure after induction. Tracheal intubation may raise the

blood pressure greatly, especially the systolic value and cause myocardial ischaemia and arrhythmias. This can be reduced by prior administration of opiates or beta-blockers (e.g. atenolol 25–50 mg orally the evening before the operation, or esmolol 10–20 mg i.v. before induction). Most different anaesthetic techniques have been used successfully. Ketamine can increase cardiac work dangerously. Hypertensive patients react badly to rapid changes of posture.

Postoperatively

Severe rises of blood pressure may occur in response to pain or a full bladder. Even a small haemorrhage may cause severe hypotension.

Cardiac failure

Congestive heart failure may present with dyspnoea, orthopnoea, raised venous pressure, gallop rhythm or atrial fibrillation. These patients present serious risks. Diagnosis of the cause and vigorous preoperative treatment are required. Many anaesthetic agents make cardiac failure worse, whereas opioids, benzodiazepines and phenothiazine premedicants are well tolerated. Local analgesic techniques are sometimes preferred. Spinal anaesthesia, however, has profound effects on the cardiovascular system, and will require close monitoring and early prevention of hypotension.

If operation cannot be delayed and general anaesthesia is necessary, the following points should be borne in mind:

1 The tachycardia normally seen on induction may be absent. Transient asystole is sometimes seen after suxamethonium, less likely after prior atropine.
2 Pulmonary oedema increases respiratory work, so paralysis and IPPV may be indicated. Nitrous oxide (usually safe in this condition) may then suffice with minimal volatile agent.
3 Ketamine, while maintaining blood pressure, increases left ventricular work and myocardial O_2 demand.
4 Invasive monitoring of RA and LA pressures may be needed which should be kept as high as the preoperative values.
5 Inotropes, e.g. dobutamine 2–10 $\mu g/kg/min$, and the reduction of afterload with vasodilators may be needed to maintain cardiac output.

Heart block

A term introduced by W.H. Gaskell (1847–1914), first described in 1691 by Gerbezius. Stokes–Adams attacks described by W.M. Stokes (1804–1878) and R. Adams (1791–1875).[24]

Heart block may be congenital or due to ischaemia, valvular disease, previous cardiac surgery, or myocarditis. *Right bundle branch block* may be of little significance, whereas *left bundle branch block* usually indicates significant cardiac disease. *Bifascicular block* of the right bundle and the anterior fascicle of the left is less hazardous than once thought, unless it is symptomatic.

First-degree block is a lengthening of the PR interval to more than 0.2 s. *Second-degree block* has missed beats with a normal PR interval (Möbitz type II) or a progressively lengthening PR interval (Wenckebach). Wenckebach is more benign and usually responds to atropine or isoprenaline. A pacemaker is not usually needed unless there are Stokes–Adams attacks or cardiac failure. Möbitz type II may progress to third-degree or complete block under anaesthesia.

In *complete heart block* the idioventricular rate is about 35 bpm, and hypotension usually occurs. The cardiac output is relatively fixed. In either Möbitz type II or complete heart block, general anaesthesia is seldom indicated until a pacemaker has been inserted. It is important to maintain cardiac output and avoid excessive vasodilatation with induction agents, blood loss, sudden postural change and pacemaker damage. Safety precautions include a standby external pacemaker and readily available drugs such as ephedrine and isoprenaline. Halothane and neostigmine should be used with caution.

Sick sinus syndrome

A severe sinus bradycardia or even sinus arrest which may be associated with episodes of paroxysmal supraventricular tachycardia. It may be more serious under anaesthesia. It can be demonstrated by carotid sinus massage. Patients may need a temporary transvenous pacing wire inserted preoperatively.

Presence of an indwelling pacemaker

The type of pacemaker is described by a five-letter code:

1 chamber paced (Ventricle, Atrium or Dual);
2 chamber sensed;
3 response to a sensed wave (Triggered or Inhibited);
4 programmable functions;
5 antitachycardia functions.

The anaesthetist should discover the indications for its insertion and the date of its last check.

Diathermy can damage the pacemaker circuits, cause ventricular fibrillation by currents induced in pacing leads, inhibit the pacemaker, switch it into a fixed rate mode or reprogramme it entirely. If possible diathermy is best avoided, but an operation may be undertaken safely provided that the active diathermy electrode is kept at least 15 cm from the pacemaker and the indifferent diathermy plate placed as far away from the pacemaker as possible and in a direction which ensures that the diathermy dipole will be at right angles to that of the pacemaker system. Diathermy should be used in short bursts and with the lowest possible power. Bipolar systems are safest. AC and DC electric motors seldom cause problems. Cellular telephones may cause temporary interference. External magnets should not be used as these usually allow complex reprogramming. Magnetic resonance imaging (MRI) may cause permanent damage. Pacemakers that sense physiological variables and change their rate are common, and are best converted into fixed rate mode. Suxamethonium-induced muscle fasciculations have inhibited a demand pacemaker,[25] as has TENS and peripheral nerve stimulators. Defibrillation may increase the pacing threshold.

Automatic implantable cardioverter defibrillator

This device has been used for the treatment of recurrent ventricular arrhythmias since 1980. It should usually be deactivated before anaesthesia surgery, either by the use of an external magnet or by using its programming device. This prevents it discharging in response to an inappropriate signal such as shivering, fasciculations, diathermy, etc. The use of diathermy warrants the same precautions as with pacemakers.[26]

Supraventricular arrhythmias

In *atrial fibrillation*, the ventricular rate should be controlled preoperatively by digitalization (0.0625–0.5 mg/day). Other possible drugs include beta-blockers or amiodarone (200–400 mg/day). Cardioversion may be needed. *Paroxysmal supraventricular tachycardia* may respond to vagal manoeuvres such as a Valsalva manoeuvre, carotid sinus massage or eyeball pressure. Verapamil (40–120 mg t.d.s.), beta-blockers and adenosine (0.05–0.25 mg/kg i.v.) are useful. In *Wolff–Parkinson–White syndrome* there is an accessory bundle of Kent between the atria and ventricles which may form part of a circular conduction pattern and cause tachyarrhythmias. Disopyramide (300–800 mg/day), beta-blockers and amiodarone are all useful. Digoxin and verapamil may exacerbate it. Some patients require extensive electrophysiological study and transcatheter or surgical ablation of the abnormal bundle.[27]

Ventricular ectopic beats

Present in up to 50% of normal patients if the ECG is monitored for 24 h. Usually indicate underlying pathology if they increase in frequency on exercise. Hypokalaemia or hypoventilation should be corrected. Controlled if necessary by lignocaine, beta-blockers or withdrawing halothane. Amiodarone is used for refractory ventricular arrhythmias.[28]

Cardiomyopathy

General anaesthesia is likely to be dangerous, and the same considerations apply as for cardiac failure (*see above*). Hypertrophic obstructive cardio-myopathy is worsened by catecholamines and responds to beta-blockers. A slow infusion of propofol has also been used successfully.

Congenital and rheumatic heart disease

Patients with damaged or defective endocardium, e.g. valve disease, ventri-cular septal defect, mitral leaflet prolapse with a systolic murmur are at risk of subacute bacterial endocarditis and need antibiotic cover for certain oper-ations, especially dental extractions, obstetric and gynaecological procedures, and endoscopies of the gut, urinary or respiratory tracts. Amoxycillin 3 g orally or 1 g i.m. (plus gentamicin 120 mg i.m. for special risk patients) is recommended. Erythromycin 1.5 g orally, clindamycin 600 mg orally or vancomycin 1 g slowly i.v. may be used for those allergic to penicillin. *See* The Endocarditis Working Party of the British Society for Antimicrobial Chemotherapy *Lancet* 1990, **335,** 88.

Mitral incompetence

Mild reduction of systemic vascular resistance is helpful. Asymptomatic mitral valve prolapse is common, and if it causes a systolic murmur antibiotic cover is needed as above.[29]

Mitral stenosis

The patient may be on anticoagulants for arterial and venous thrombo-embolism, and digoxin for atrial fibrillation. The left ventricle requires a longer diastolic filling time, so tachycardia is undesirable, especially if there is atrial fibrillation. Mild vasodilatation is beneficial (with relief of pulmonary hypertension) but if excessive leads to severe hypotension due to the fixed cardiac output. Minimal doses of anaesthetic are desirable and inotropes may be needed. Danger of pulmonary oedema.

Aortic stenosis

Preservation of normal sinus rhythm and heart rate is very important.

Aortic incompetence

Improved by mild tachycardia and vasodilatation with moderate fluid loading to maintain the diastolic pressure. Spinal blockade however can result in serious hypotension, unless treated early.

Valve prostheses

The patients are often anticoagulated, especially for a mitral prothesis. Warfarin may be stopped up to 6 days preoperatively, heparin given peri-operatively and warfarin restarted 1–3 days later, all controlled by the inter-national normalized ratio (INR) and the activated partial thromboplastin time (APTT). For some patients their warfarin may be changed to aspirin and dipyramidole. Each patient must be considered individually. Antibiotic prophylaxis is needed as above for special risk patients.

Constrictive pericarditis

Intravenous induction agents, especially thiopentone, are likely to cause pro-found hypotension, as the heart is unable to increase its output to compensate for a drop in peripheral resistance.

THE HYPOVOLAEMIC PATIENT

Operation should not be undertaken, except in cases of grave emergency, until the patient is resuscitated. As hypovolaemia worsens, peripheral pulses dis-appear (at a systolic pressure of about 60 mmHg), then central pulses (as coma occurs), then pupils dilate, then the cardiac impulse and sounds fade before cardiac arrest.

Central venous and arterial pressure monitoring should be started. Raise the legs. Full fluid replacement (with blood, colloids or crystalloid as appro-priate) before use of vasodilator drugs is imperative. Once improvement has occurred, with central venous pressure (CVP) rising, and hands and feet becoming warm and pink, the operation need not be delayed. The systolic pressure should, if possible, be restored to at least 100 mmHg, when the blood volume is probably not less than 70% of normal.

Anaesthesia

No premedication is needed, but atropine may be given intravenously if thought necessary before induction. Vomiting may occur at induction as shock, fear and anxiety are important causes of delayed gastric emptying. Shocked and recently resuscitated patients require much less anaesthesia and fewer relaxants than normal. Light general anaesthesia with IPPV is the method of choice. High O_2 concentrations may be needed. The aim of the anaesthetic technique is to preserve blood flow to the brain, heart and kidneys. Volatile agents must be used carefully if hypotension is not to be potentiated. Inotropic support should be ready. Regional analgesia may be very satisfactory but only if hypotension can be avoided.

PULMONARY DISEASE

Coryza

Acute coryza, uncomplicated by fever or lower respiratory disease, is often regarded as a contraindication to even minor elective surgery in adults. Although this sounds like common sense, there is little evidence to support this view.[30] Blocked nostrils may require the early use of an oropharyngeal airway. It is certainly sensible to postpone major elective operations on the thorax or abdomen because of the risk of chest infection. In paediatric practice there is a low threshold to postpone surgery as children with upper respiratory infections have more reactive airways, and are more likely to have postoperative pulmonary complications and hypoxaemia, especially in younger children and those who have been intubated.[31]

Chronic obstructive airways (pulmonary) disease

Chronic obstructive airways (pulmonary) disease (COAD or COPD) includes all patients who have irreversible airflow limitation due to a combination of chronic bronchitis and emphysema.

1 *Chronic bronchitis* is defined clinically by a chronic or recurrent increase in the volume of mucoid bronchial secretion sufficient to cause expectoration. Chronic hypoxia leads to polycythaemia and cor pulmonale (blue bloater). Hypoventilation causes the arterial PCO_2 to rise and the respiratory centre becomes less sensitive. When a chest infection occurs the hypoventilation is worse. Sputum should be coughed up before anaesthesia, by postural drainage for 2 h, if necessary. Induction should strive to avoid stimulation of airway reflexes. Tracheal intubation under light anaesthesia may provoke coughing, straining and bronchospasm. Intubation will allow better tracheobronchial toilet. Pre- and postoperative physiotherapy is required.[32]
2 *Emphysema* is characterized pathologically by abnormally large air spaces distal to the terminal bronchiole with destruction of their walls. This causes loss of lung elastic recoil, overexpansion, early closure of airways during expiration and gas trapping. Ventilation is well maintained but hard work (pink puffer). The diaphragm is horizontal and flattened and pulls the lower ribs inwards during inspiration. The scalene and sternomastoid muscles assist inspiration.

Note the following points in all these patients.

1 Hypersensitivity of respiratory reflexes (bucking, bronchospasm, etc.) to irritant vapours, thiopentone, secretions and intubation.
2 Abnormal pattern of breathing may hamper the abdominal surgeon if respiration is spontaneous.
3 Dependence on hypoxia for respiratory drive, via the aortic and carotid bodies. This is nearly abolished by anaesthesia and if the patient breathes O_2-rich mixtures, CO_2 narcosis may go unnoticed.

4 Undue sensitivity to all respiratory depressants.
5 In chronic bronchitis IPPV may need high airway pressures with adverse effects on the circulation and possible barotrauma.
6 In emphysema the reduced elastic recoil prolongs expiration.
7 The disturbance of gas exchange that occurs on induction of anaesthesia is much more striking than in normal people.[33]

Dyspnoea at rest and hypoxaemia have been suggested as the best predictors of the need for postoperative IPPV in patients with severe COAD.[34]

Anaesthetic management

Preoperative care should include cessation of smoking, physiotherapy, treatment of bronchospasm or infection, loss of excess weight, and drainage of any pleural effusion. Lung-function tests (simple spirometry) help define the severity of airways obstruction, and the extent to which it responds to a bronchodilator.

PREMEDICATION

Antihistamines and benzodiazepines are well tolerated. Opiates, especially pethidine, can be used cautiously. Atropine sometimes makes sputum too thick for easy suction. A bronchodilator inhaler should be given if there is a reversible component to the airways obstruction.

ANAESTHESIA

Regional blocks can be very useful, although the patient may find it difficult to lie flat and avoid coughing for long periods. Good reasons can be advanced for preferring either spontaneous or controlled respiration. The former is particularly suitable for minor surgery, using a volatile agent. Paralysis, intubation and IPPV allow tracheal suction and the use of the smallest doses of depressant drugs. The use of relaxants need not be lead to difficulty in restarting respiration if reversal is adequate, even if the $PaCO_2$ is lower than the patient's normal level.

POSTOPERATIVE CARE

Humidified O_2 may be needed and physiotherapy should be given. Adequate pain relief by cautious doses of opiates or by regional blocks will help deep breathing, although evidence that the latter improve morbidity is scarce. Infusion of doxapram hydrochloride 1.5–4 mg/min may be a useful respiratory stimulant and help reduce lung complications in high-risk patients. Postoperative IPPV may be needed, especially in obese patients.

Asthma

A disease characterized by variable wheezing, dyspnoea or cough due to widespread airway narrowing, varying in severity over short periods of time, either spontaneously or as a result of treatment. Drugs which may cause bronchoconstriction in susceptible patients include muscle relaxants, thiopentone and beta-blockers. These effects may be due to IgE-mediated histamine release, or a non-allergic mechanism such as with prostaglandin $F_{2\alpha}$ (used for induced abortions) and beta-blockers. Up to 10% of adult asthmatics are sensitive to aspirin and other NSAIDs, and these should be used with great caution unless the patient is known not to be sensitive. Other triggers include cold, exercise and infection.

Anaesthetic management of patients with severe asthma

Except in emergency, patients with asthma should not be operated on until their lung condition is optimal as postoperative lung complications are more common. Use bronchodilators, physiotherapy, antibiotics if there is infection, and steroids to reduce bronchial oedema and spasm. Sedative premedication, especially antihistamines, are useful. Patients on large doses (> 1.5 mg/day of beclomethasone) of inhaled steroids can have suppressed adrenal function and need additional steroid cover. Regional techniques may be preferred if possible.

Volatile anaesthetics are bronchodilators and well tolerated. Nebulized salbutamol can be given during the operation. The following may make the asthma worse: intravenous thiopentone; clumsy inhalational induction of anaesthesia; tracheal intubation, especially if relaxation is incomplete or anaesthesia too light; stimulation of the upper respiratory tract by gastric acid, blood, mucus, etc. Acute bronchospasm following intubation may be treated with intravenous aminophylline 5 mg/kg (slowly) or a sympathomimetic such as ephedrine, salbutamol 200 μg or adrenaline. All beta-blockers are best avoided, but if one is essential a cardioselective one should be used such as metoprolol 2–10 mg. With careful management, the incidence of postoperative respiratory complications is very low.[35]

Restrictive lung disease

The lungs and/or chest wall are stiff, e.g. lung fibrosis and kyphoscoliosis. All lung volumes and the diffusing capacity are reduced, and the work of breathing is high. The bronchi, however, may be held open by fibrotic lung, giving a high forced expiratory volume in 1 s (FEV1.0)/forced vital capacity (FVC) ratio. There is often hypoxaemia. Patients with some restrictive diseases, e.g. severe scoliosis, may depend on ventilators in their everyday life.

High pressures are needed for IPPV, and a simple inhalational anaesthetic technique with minimal relaxants and narcotics is often satisfactory. Some operations (e.g. prostate, limbs) are well-managed with regional blocks, although these patients may not be comfortable lying flat and may not be able to control their coughing. It is easy to give too much sedation.

Negative pressure ventilation may be useful postoperatively, especially in the Kelleher rotating iron lung which aids physiotherapy and postural drainage. It supports ventilation in a way that avoids intubation and sedation, and allows the patient to eat and sleep.[36]

For a review of the problems of anaesthesia in patients who have received transplanted lungs, *see* Haddow G. R. *Can. J. Anaesth.* 1997, **44,** 182.

ANAEMIA

There is a reduction in arterial O_2 content but not in PaO_2. It should, when possible, be investigated and treated medically before operation as blood for transfusion is always in short supply. If the anaemia cannot be fully investigated preoperatively, it should not be forgotten afterwards. Many prefer not to perform elective surgery on patients with a haemoglobin concentration of less than 10 g/dl, although some evidence suggests that 8 g/dl may be a safe lower limit in otherwise fit patients provided the operation is not likely to result in a blood loss over 500 ml.[37]

The cardiorespiratory state must also be taken into consideration. Anaemia may exacerbate symptoms of atherosclerosis. Preoperative transfusion should normally be given 24 h before surgery, to allow time for depleted 2,3-diphosphoglycerate (2,3-DPG) in the stored red cells to be restored. Anaemia results in an increased 2,3-DPG which shifts the O_2 dissociation curve to the right. Smoking should be prohibited to reduce the carboxyhaemoglobin, which may represent 10–15% of total haemoglobin, but which cannot transport O_2. Even severe hypoxia may not be accompanied by cyanosis.

SICKLE-CELL ANAEMIA AND SICKLE-CELL TRAIT

First described by J. B. Herrick of Chicago (1861–1954)[38] (who also gave the first modern description of coronary thrombosis in 1912). A hereditary, autosomal recessive, haemolytic anaemia. The abnormal gene is carried by 60 million people world-wide, mainly in Africa. All patients of tropical African or West Indian descent must be considered at risk, especially children. May also occur in certain parts of Italy, Greece, the Middle East and eastern India. It is due to substitution of valine for glutamic acid at position 6 of the β chain of haemoglobin A, resulting in haemoglobin S.

In *sickle-cell anaemia* (homozygous, SS) 90% of the haemoglobin is S; in the *trait* (heterozygous, AS) 30–40% is S, the remainder being A. Haemoglobin S is vulnerable to reduction in PO_2. Should this be less than about 5.5 kPa the reduced haemoglobin forms long complex strands called 'tactoids' which distort red cells. Their increased fragility causes a haemolytic anaemia. They also tend to aggregate, block small vessels and cause infarction. In the trait, sickling occurs at a PO_2 of about 2.7 kPa. Increasing the PO_2 does not reverse the changes. Acute crises, haemolytic, thrombotic or aplastic, may interrupt the chronic state.

Normal adults have largely haemoglobin A ($\alpha_2\beta_2$), with 2.5% haemoglobin A2 ($\alpha_2\delta_2$). The neonate has 70% foetal haemoglobin (F, $\alpha_2\gamma_2$). A similar but milder anaemia occurs in SC disease in which half the haemoglobin is S and half C. In C lysine is substituted for glutamic acid at position 6 of the β chain. This is commonest in West Africa. This disease commonly presents with an infarctive crisis after childbirth or surgery.

Management

Patients with sickle-cell disease may present for surgery because of:

1 abdominal pain due to vascular lesions;
2 osteomyelitis;
3 priapism;
4 leg ulcers;
5 gallstones;
6 retinopathy;
7 general surgical diseases;
8 obstetrics.

All black people should be tested for anaemia and sickling before any anaesthetic, even if this means a delay. About 10% of British black people are at risk. If the haemoglobin is less than 11 g/dl and the sickling test positive, sickle-cell anaemia is probable.

The *Sickledex test* is a commercial macroscopic test for insoluble deoxygenated HbS. False positives may occur in dysproteinaemias. The test is unreliable below the age of 3 months. A positive test does not differentiate between the disease and the trait and haemoglobin electrophoresis is needed. If the haemoglobin concentration and blood film are normal it is likely that the trait is present. Note that anaemia can be masked by dehydration, and SC disease may not show a significant anaemia.

The following may precipitate sickling:

1 hypoxia;
2 hypothermia;
3 tourniquets (this may rule out intravenous regional analgesia);
4 acidosis and circulatory stasis;
5 dehydration.

Trait

Usually symptomless and presents no special anaesthetic risks except in major interventions such as thoracotomy, or during the use of tourniquets. However, preoxygenation, at least 30% O_2 during operation, postoperative O_2 therapy and good hydration are usually recommended.

Disease

These patients are at high risk. Adequate oxygenation and hydration and avoidance of cardiorespiratory depression at all times are mandatory.

A transfusion of red cells should be given if haemoglobin is less than 8 g/dl and major surgery is contemplated. The aim is to reduce the level of HbS to less than 30%. If the haemoglobin is unusually high, a partial exchange transfusion is needed. Administration of alkali is controversial. Sickling is more likely to occur in the presence of acidosis but the shift of the dissociation curve to the left with deliberate alkalinization lowers the venous and tissue PO_2.

Regional analgesia, with the exception of Bier's block, should be preferred to general anaesthesia where suitable. Sickling can occur during what seems to be a faultless operation. Anticoagulants may be required after surgery to prevent pulmonary embolism, especially if thrombosis, or pain in the bones is present.

Blood from a patient with sickle-cell trait can be safely donated for transfusion but not that from patients with other haemoglobinopathies.

Acute sickle-cell crisis

The thrombotic crisis is commonest. It is precipitated by infection, cold or dehydration, and presents with bone pain, usually in the back or limbs, and sometimes mimics a surgical acute abdomen. The acute pain team should be involved in management, and although intramuscular opiates can be used, patient-controlled analgesia (PCA) is preferable. Fentanyl is favoured by some. Non-steroidal anti-inflammatory drugs are useful adjuncts.[39]

THALASSAEMIA

First described in Detroit in 1925 by T. B. Cooley. Named after 'thalassa' = the sea (i.e. Mediterranean). Commonest single-gene disorder world-wide. There is reduced production of one or more of the globin chains, most commonly the β chain. Occurs in a band from the Mediterranean, through the Middle East and southern Asia, as far as New Guinea. Also in some West Africans. The patient with *homozygous β-thalassaemia* (Cooley's or Mediterranean anaemia, thalassaemia major) has high levels of fetal haemoglobin (30–90% of total), the rest being HbA_2. Anaemia results from both haemolysis and impaired erythropoesis. Regular blood transfusions are needed, and iron overload can lead to heart and liver damage. There is an increased risk of infection. *Heterozygous β-thalassaemia* is the symptom-free carrier state. *Beta-thalassaemia* can be combined with an abnormal haemoglobin, one gene being inherited from each parent, and has many variants. Haemoglobin C thalassaemia is relatively mild, but HbS thalassaemia is serious and can be clinically identical to sickle-cell disease. Haemoglobin E thalassaemia is common in SE Asia and associated with severe anaemia.

POLYCYTHAEMIA

Most commonly secondary to chronic hypoxia or an erythropoietin-secreting renal tumour, but may be a primary myeloproliferative disease (*polycythaemia vera*). The latter is rare in patients under 40 and is twice as common in males. It may be suspected in patients with a ruddy cyanosis and injected conjunctivae, especially if there is splenomegaly and pruritis. Haemoglobin level and packed cell volume (PCV) are increased. The patient should be treated before operation by myelosuppressive drugs or ^{32}P, and a normal blood picture should have been present for several months before the proposed surgery. Operations on patients with uncontrolled polycythaemia carry a high risk of reactionary haemorrhage, e.g. after dental extractions, due to platelet defects, as well as arterial and venous thrombosis. In emergency cases, repeated and voluminous phlebotomies may be helpful. Patients with a PCV over 50%, and certainly over 55%, are at risk of thrombosis. Below 48%, there is no greater risk than usual. Between these two lies an area of uncertainty where prophylaxis is wise.

See also Sosis M. B. *J. Clin. Anesth.* 1990, **2**, 31.

METHAEMOGLOBINAEMIA AND SULPHAEMOGLOBINAEMIA

Methaemoglobin is derived from normal haemoglobin when the iron in the haem group is oxidized from ferrous to ferric. If a patient appears cyanosed in the absence of heart or lung disease, the blood should be spectroscopically examined for such abnormal pigments. Cyanosis is detected with 1.5 g/dl of methaemoglobin (compared with 5 g/dl of deoxyhaemoglobin). The reading of a pulse oximeter tends towards 85% in the presence of large amounts of methaemoglobin. Symptoms rarely occur unless 20% methaemoglobin is present. Above this, fatigue, dyspnoea, headache, dizziness and even coma and death can occur. The condition can be genetic or secondary to exogenous agents, e.g. nitrites, sulphonamides, *prilocaine*, bizarre poisons, etc. Not only is the oxygen-carrying capacity of blood reduced but also the dissociation curve is shifted to the left. Treatment is with reducing agents, ascorbic acid (300–600 mg daily) or methylene blue (1–2 mg/kg i.v. of 1% solution over 5 min, or 60 mg orally t.d.s.) which convert methaemoglobin back to normal haemoglobin. In extreme cases exchange transfusion may be considered.

Sulphaemoglobinaemia at levels of 0.5 g/dl will produce cyanosis. It is usually caused by drugs, particularly sulphonamides.

HAEMOPHILIA

There are some 4000 haemophiliacs in the UK. It is a sex-linked recessive disorder, although about 30% of males with the disease give no history of blood abnormality in previous generations. Female carriers may have postoperative bleeding problems. Haemophiliacs should attend a Haemophilia Centre where an official Haemophilia Card is issued. There is no such thing, surgically, as a mild haemophiliac. The partial thromboplastin time is prolonged and the bleeding time normal. Necessary surgery is possible with good laboratory backup. About 85% have *haemophilia A* (factor VIII deficiency) and 15% *haemophilia B* or *Christmas disease* (factor IX deficiency). The levels may range from < 2% of normal (severe) to > 45% (clinically unaffected). Factor IX is stable in stored blood but factor VIII levels are halved after just one day of storage. Some patients have developed antibodies to factor VIII which makes them unsuitable for surgery. Female carriers can be detected in utero. Haemophiliac patients are at high risk of carrying the human immunodeficiency virus (HIV) and hepatitis viruses.

Operation regimen

Intramuscular injections are avoided if possible. Treatment requires the transfusion of materials rich in the deficient factor immediately preoperatively until a haemostatic level is reached (> 50% of normal values), and the maintenance of this level until healing is well advanced (a week or more for major surgery). Before an operation, patients should have their blood tested for factor VIII antibody. Elective surgery is only possible if its titre is low. The available materials are fresh frozen plasma, cryoprecipitate, factor VIII and factor IX concentrates. Tranexamic acid may also be useful. The biological half-lives of factor VIII and IX are 8–12 h and 18 h respectively. Factor VIII (or IX) levels should be monitored daily.

In minor surgery such as dental extraction, the synthetic vasopressin DDAVP may be used. Before extraction, 0.4 μg/kg i.v. plus tranexamic acid 10 mg/kg is given. The latter is continued orally three times a day for 5 days. Penicillin should be given to prevent infection of the sockets.

ANAESTHESIA IN PATIENTS WITH IMPAIRED RENAL FUNCTION

Most operations in well-hydrated patients cause minor changes in renal blood flow and glomerular filtration. The endocrine stress response to surgery and trauma includes the secretion of aldosterone, and especially antidiuretic hormone (ADH) which promotes oliguria and water retention. Most patients with mild kidney disease do well unless more than 50% of the nephron mass is damaged. Under anaesthesia some degree of autoregulation may be preserved

---

Anaesthetic problems of a patient with chronic renal failure

Fluid retention and oedema.

Hyperkalaemia.

Metabolic acidosis.

Anaemia.

Neuropathy (including autonomic and slow gastric emptying).

Hypertension.

Pericardial effusion.

Hypocalcaemia, hyperphosphataemia.

Medication, e.g. antihypertensive drugs.

Difficult veins and care needed of chronic vascular access site.

Abnormal pharmacokinetics.

Poor wound healing and increased chance of infection.

---

but function is impaired when mean arterial pressure drops below 60 mmHg. Total renal ischaemia of more than 30 min duration is likely to result in damage to the tubules.

The uraemic patient may complain of nausea, vomiting or diarrhoea. There may be electrolyte imbalance, raised serum potassium, metabolic acidosis, anaemia, hypertension, cardiac failure, bleeding tendency due to abnormal platelet function, halitosis from ammoniacal decomposition of the salivary urea, drowsiness, convulsions and coma. The blood urea may not rise above normal until the glomerular filtration rate has fallen to about 25% of normal. Symptoms due to uraemia are rare until the blood urea approaches 15 mmol/l. Vomiting, if severe and persistent, may result in hypokalaemia and hyponatraemia. Dialysis patients are on sodium and water restriction and should not be overloaded by the anaesthetist! Parenteral nutrition must restrict protein while providing essential amino acids. There may be osteomalacia and hypocalcaemia.

The anaemia is normochromic and normocytic, caused by a decreased production of erythropoietin. There is also a defect in the membranes of red cells which shorten their lives. The patients are well-adapted to their low haemoglobin levels with increased 2, 3-DPG, and seldom need transfusion with its associated hazards.

Risk factors for patients with pre-existing renal impairment include:

1 hypovolaemic hypotension;
2 liver failure or obstructive jaundice;
3 cardiac or major vascular surgery;
4 major trauma;

5 sepsis;
6 massive blood transfusion;
7 pregnancy-induced hypertension and amniotic fluid embolism.

In all cases, blood volume, pressure and renal blood flow must be maintained.

Regional analgesia may be especially suitable in uraemia, but coagulation defects should be excluded and blood pressure maintained. Duration of action of local anaesthetics may be reduced if the tissues are acidic. If general anaesthesia is preferred, consider antacid therapy, as an autonomic neuropathy may delay gastric emptying. Thiopentone is more potent due to changes in plasma proteins and pH. Propofol and benzodiazepines are not affected. Opiates are metabolized in the liver, but active metabolites such as morphine-6-glucuronide and norpethidine may accumulate as they are renally excreted. Other drugs excreted by the kidneys include digoxin, aminoglycosides, chlorpropamide and angiotensin-converting enzyme (ACE) inhibitors. A complete list is found in the *British National Formulary*. Mannitol,[40] frusemide and dopamine[41] may be useful to maintain renal function.

Suxamethonium may be safe unless the serum potassium is more than 5 mmol/l. Atracurium, rocuronium or vecuronium are suitable nondepolarizing relaxants. Enflurane is best avoided, as nephrotoxic levels of fluoride ions (peak greater than 50 μmol/l) have been seen after just 3.5 MAC-hours.[42] Sevoflurane, halothane, isoflurane and desflurane result in little or no increase in fluoride and are preferred. Isoflurane has only resulted in nephrotoxic fluoride levels after its use as a sedative in intensive care for up to 127 h (34 MAC-hours).[43]

For anaesthesia for renal transplantation *see* Chapter 4.1 'Urology'.

LIVER DISEASE

Blood supply

The average adult liver weighs 2.9 kg. Its total blood flow is normally 1.5 l/min, about 30% of which is provided by the hepatic artery which supplies 50% of the O_2 requirement. The rest comes from the portal vein. Oxygen consumption is about 55 ml/min. General anaesthesia and surgery causes a fall in hepatic blood flow which is greater than the fall in O_2 consumption, especially if the patient is hyperventilated, but this is probably not harmful. Epidural analgesia reduces hepatic arterial blood flow as the blood pressure drops.

Liver function

The blood tests used are imprecise indicators of liver function, but have a place in pre- and postoperative assessment. Abnormalities are frequently seen in asymptomatic patients, as are normal results in patients with known liver disease. Tests include the following:

1 *Bilirubin:* elevated as a result of hepatocellular damage, excess formation (haemolysis) or biliary obstruction. If direct (conjugated) bilirubin predominates there is likely to be obstruction.
2 *Transaminases:* may leak from liver cells into the bloodstream when damage occurs. Other tissues such as heart and skeletal muscle also contain transaminases, so high blood levels are not specific for liver pathology.
3 *Alkaline phosphatase:* present in bile duct cells. Blood levels are raised in biliary obstruction, but also in hepatocellular disease. Also found in other tissues.
4 *Serum albumin:* normal value is 3.5–5.0 g/dl. Half-life is about 3 weeks, so falls do not occur for some time following liver damage. Albumin levels less than 2.8 g/dl usually point to significant disease. The production of globulin is unaffected by liver disease.
5 *Prothrombin time (INR):* raised due to defective production of fibrinogen, prothrombin and factors V, VII, IX, X, XI and XIII. Also synthesis of prothrombin and factors VII, IX and X are dependent on vitamin K, which cannot be absorbed in the gut without bile salts.
6 *Glucose:* hypoglycaemia occurs in advanced liver disease.

Drug metabolism

The liver is the site of many metabolic processes including the synthesis, conjugation, oxidation, reduction and hydrolysis. Drug elimination may therefore be impaired in advanced liver disease. Low levels of serum albumin may lead to changes in protein binding, thus leaving greater quantities of drugs unbound to exert their pharmacological effects.

Anaesthesia in a patient with liver disease

1 *Drugs:* elimination of induction agents may be impaired, but this is only of significance with infusion techniques. There is likely to be a sensitivity to opiates. Resistance is shown to some non-depolarizing muscle relaxants, but biliary obstruction can prolong the effect of the steroidal relaxants. As renal problems often coexist, atracurium may be the relaxant of choice.
2 *Serum cholinesterase:* the level must be at least halved before any effects on suxamethonium elimination are seen. Problems are unusual in clinical practice.
3 *Abnormal clotting:*
   (a) decreased synthesis of factors (described above);
   (b) half-lives of coagulation factors may be shortened as a result of increased utilization (e.g. disseminated intravascular coagulation, loss into reticuloendothelial system, excessive bleeding);
   (c) abnormal fibrinogen can be produced (dysfibrinogenaemia);

    (d) thrombocytopenia;

    (e) impaired platelet function.

    Vitamin K, fresh frozen plasma and platelets may all be needed.

4　*Encephalopathy:* advanced liver disease leads to altered mental state, neuro-muscular signs, drowsiness, coma and death. High blood ammonia levels may be important in its genesis. There is always significant portal to systemic shunting. Precipitating factors include:

    (a) sedatives, which should be avoided whenever possible or small doses of midazolam used with great caution;

    (b) gastrointestinal haemorrhage or other protein load;

    (c) diuretics with disturbance of electrolyte balance;

    (d) infection;

    (e) progression of underlying liver disease.

5　*Kidneys:* there is a risk of precipitating renal failure in jaundiced patients, especially those with biliary obstruction. Urine production should exceed 30 ml/h, and mannitol administered if necessary.

Severe impairment of liver function and high operative risk is indicated by:

1　serum albumin level below 2.8 g/dl;

2　serum bilirubin over 40 μmol/l;

3　prothrombin time > 6 s longer than control;

4　grade 3 or 4 encephalopathy.

PORPHYRIA[44]

From the Greek *porphyros* = purple.

    Rare in England, prevalent in South Africa and Scandinavia. A family of inborn errors of haem synthesis. The rate-limiting enzyme of haem synthesis is the first one in the pathway, d-aminolaevulinic acid (ALA) synthase, normally inhibited by haem. When subsequent enzymes in the pathway are deficient this inhibition fails, and abnormal precursors (porphyrins) are formed in excess. The particular precursors and the clinical pattern that results depend on which of these subsequent enzymes are abnormal. All porphyrias have a high activity of ALA synthase.

    There are three acute hepatic porphyrias which can be precipitated by drugs that increase ALA synthase activity. They are all inherited as Mendelian dominants:

1　acute intermittent porphyria (common in Sweden, and the most common in the UK);

2　variegate porphyria (common in white South Africans);

3　hereditary coproporphyria, in which the predominant porphyrin in the urine and faeces is coproporphyrin.

Non-acute porphyrias (cutaneous hepatic porphyria and erythropoietic porphyrias) may be acquired or hereditary, are not sensitive to barbiturates.

The drugs that may precipitate acute attacks are barbiturates, sulphonamides, anticonvulsants, alcohol and oral contraceptives. There is doubt about lignocaine. Such attacks may also arise *de novo* or may be associated with infection or pregnancy.

Clinical features

1 *Gastrointestinal:* acute abdominal pain and vomiting. Surgeons are sometimes tempted to operate.
2 *Neurological:* peripheral neuropathy which can be bad enough to lead to respiratory failure and need IPPV, epilepsy, psychiatric symptoms, rarely coma.
3 *Cardiovascular:* tachycardia, raised blood pressure and even left ventricular failure during the active phase.
4 *Skin photosensitivity* (not seen in acute intermittent porphyria).
5 *Urine:* turns red or dark brown on standing.

Diagnosis is by spectroscopic measurement of porphyrins or their precursors, e.g. porphobilinogen in the urine or faeces. Bedside urine tests are available.

Barbiturates, including thiopentone, are absolutely contraindicated as they may precipitate the acute syndrome described above. If intravenous induction is planned, propofol, etomidate or ketamine have been used without incident, although animal experiments have not always confirmed their safety.[45] Benzodiazepines and muscle relaxants are safe. Aspirin, codeine, morphine, pethidine, fentanyl and buprenorphine are suitable analgesics. Pentazocine should be avoided. Atropine is preferred to hyoscine. Nitrous oxide, O_2, volatile agents, relaxants and their reversal agents present no danger. Medicolegal worries rather than scientific reasons make some workers avoid regional analgesia in these patients. Bupivacaine is safe,[46] whereas lignocaine may not be. Detailed drug advice may be obtained from the Porphyria Research Unit, Western Infirmary, Glasgow.

King George III and some of his descendants probably suffered from this condition.[47]

CHRONIC ALCOHOLISM

Early recognition with very careful preoperative assessment is required. Alcohol is eliminated by oxidation in the liver to acetaldehyde by the enzyme alcohol dehydrogenase. The rate of elimination is about 10 ml/h. Chronic alcoholism damages the liver but also induces drug-metabolizing enzymes, so the response to drugs is not always predictable. Alcoholic cirrhosis may be associated with hyperventilation and arterial O_2 desaturation, the latter due to shunting of blood from peri-oesophageal and mediastinal veins to pulmonary veins. There may be peripheral vasodilatation, cardiomyopathy, congestive failure. Alcoholism may also cause pancreatitis, regurgitation, nutritional and vitamin deficiencies, peripheral neuropathy and cerebral degeneration.

Anaesthesia

Alcohol should not be withdrawn while awaiting operation. Midazolam is useful for sedation. Regional analgesia should be considered but coagulation may be abnormal. Isoflurane or sevoflurane are suitable. In acute alcoholism, patients withstand trauma badly perhaps due to vasodilatation. Vasoconstrictors may be needed. To prevent withdrawal symptoms 8–10% alcohol in saline 500 ml i.v. over several hours may be helpful.

DRUG ADDICTION[48]

Narcotics

These patients may manufacture symptoms to earn surgery and postoperative morphine, or interfere with the wound to prolong their stay in hospital. There may be thrombophlebitis and multiple abscesses from unhygienic injections, so that only central veins remain for intravenous therapy. Sepsis, tuberculosis, endocarditis, hepatitis B and HIV are all common. Resistant to all sedatives. Hypotension is common in the operating theatre. Symptoms of withdrawal from narcotics include cramp, vomiting and diarrhoea, and can mimic intestinal obstruction.

Others

Nine-tetrahydrocannabinol, from *cannabis*, causes tachycardia and hypertension, exacerbated by atropine or adrenaline-containing local analgesics. *Cocaine* can cause myocardial ischaemia and cardiomyopathy. Amphetamine addiction may increase the required doses of anaesthetic agents.

ACQUIRED IMMUNE DEFICIENCY SYNDROME

First described in 1981 when Pneumocystis carinii pneumonia and Kaposi's sarcoma were reported in homosexuals in the US. The incidence has been rising rapidly since. Caused by a lymphocytotropic retrovirus (HIV) and transmitted in blood and semen, although the virus has also been found in saliva, urine and tears. Endemic in parts of Africa. Reduces the CD4 cells (part of the T4 helper lymphocyte population).

There may be a transient illness resembling glandular fever 1–2 weeks after infection, a variable symptom-free period of up to several years, and then AIDS-related complex (lymphadenopathy, fever, diarrhoea, weight loss, oral candidiasis) and finally overt AIDS with atypical pneumonias, other infections and Kaposi's sarcoma. This is invariably fatal. Most infected patients are asymptomatic carriers. Anonymous testing of over 115 000 pregnant women in inner London revealed an incidence as high as 0.49 in 1000.[49] Although testing for HIV antibody is diagnostic, seroconversion only occurs about 3 months after infection. Patient consent is essential before testing.

Certain groups are at high risk: homosexual and bisexual men, haemophiliacs, drug abusers and children of affected mothers. Patients with this condition present a hazard to staff, although seroconversion after needlestick injury is rare. Hepatitis B is transmitted more readily because of the higher replication rate of this virus. Used needles should be placed in special containers without recapping and specimen containers sealed carefully. Extreme caution in handling body fluids and excreta is advised. Many recommend the wearing of gloves with any patient when there is likely to be contact with blood or saliva.[50] Zidovudine prophylaxis may be indicated after injury to staff, and expert advice should be sought.

DIABETES MELLITUS

Insulin was isolated and first used to treat diabetics in 1922.[51] Insulin is the body's major anabolic hormone. In the type 1 (younger) diabetic there is a lack of insulin, associated with an injury to chromosome 6. In type 2 diabetes (the older patient) there is a resistance to the peripheral actions of insulin. Glucose, fat and protein metabolism are affected, and complications are widespread.

Problems include the following:

1 *High blood sugar:* which gives polyuria and thirst, likelihood of tissue infections and poor wound healing.
2 *Ketoacidosis:* severe metabolic acidosis, loss of extracellular sodium and water, circulatory collapse and coma.
3 *Cardiac disease:* coronary atheroma is common, and operative risk increased;
4 *Peripheral vascular disease:* in all major arteries, often needs surgery, which involves a higher risk than in the non-diabetic.
5 *Diabetic nephropathy:* may lead to nephrotic syndrome and uraemia.
6 *Peripheral neuropathy:* contributes to the formation of foot ulcers.
7 *Autonomic neuropathy:* can cause cardiorespiratory arrest, postural hypotension, gastroparesis and postoperative retention of urine. Sleep apnoea in diabetic patients with autonomic neuropathy may be a particular hazard if respiratory depressant drugs are given. Sudden death may occur.[52]
8 *Retinopathy and cataracts:* which often require surgery.

Diagnosed by a fasting blood sugar over 7.8 mmol/l, or a random sugar over 11.1 mmol/l. Surgical mortality is higher in diabetics but this may be related more to the complications of diabetes, especially vascular disease, rather than to the metabolic disturbance itself. Diabetes is often detected for the first time in a patient presenting for surgery.

Type 1 diabetics need insulin-replacement therapy. The different preparations of insulin are divided into short-acting (such as soluble insulin), and the medium- or long-acting. Mixtures of different types are often prescribed, but soluble insulin is used in the perioperative period. Type 2 diabetics are either controlled by attention to diet, or by oral hypoglycaemic agents. _Sulphonylureas_ mainly stimulate insulin production by the pancreas. Most have a duration of action not exceeding 12–16 h. Chlorpropamide, however, has a half-life of 36 h and a duration of action up to 60 h. Fasting hypoglycaemia may occur, and the drug should be stopped 1–2 days preoperatively. _Biguanides_ (e.g. metformin) decrease hepatic gluconeogenesis and increase tissue glucose use. Hypoglycaemia is not a problem.

Schemes of control over the time of surgery[53]

There is no single scheme to cover all cases. It is usually wiser to have a slightly increased blood sugar than to risk hypoglycaemia. The aim is to keep blood glucose around 8–10 mmol/l and to maintain the use of glucose by the cells. Problems arise from the following.

1 _Hypoglycaemia:_ probably the greatest danger, especially to the brain. Causes trembling, sweating, pallor, pins and needles in tongue and lips, hunger, diplopia, slurring of speech, confusion, fits and coma.
2 _The normal endocrine stress response to surgery and trauma:_ which involves the secretion of catabolic hormones such as corticosteroids and catecholamines, and which is normally antagonized by insulin.
3 _Starvation:_ inevitable, especially in abdominal surgery, but the resulting catabolic response with ketoacidosis is more severe in a diabetic. Ketoacidosis causes dehydration, hyperventilation, and a smell of acetone on the breath. Avoiding general anaesthesia solves most of the perioperative problems. However, even for local analgesia, the patient may have to be starved. In every case, the period of starvation should be minimized. The patient should be first on an operating list, and given an early light breakfast if scheduled for afternoon surgery.

Metabolism of the lactate in Hartmann's solution may contribute to hyperglycaemia in diabetics. Beta-blocking agents may cause hypoglycaemia. Glucocorticoids, thiazides and frusemide may worsen control of diabetes. Diabetic patients sometimes present simulating an acute abdomen.

Type 1 diabetes

The aim is: to prevent ketoacidosis, and to avoid hypoglycaemia. If the diabetes has been difficult to control, the patient should be stabilized on soluble insulin, twice daily, for 2–3 days before operation. Various regimens have been recommended for the operative period, but none has been shown to be superior.

1 The Alberti regimen[54] in which 10 units of insulin are added to 500 ml of 10% glucose, with 1 g of potassium chloride. This is infused intravenously at 100 ml/h. Many personalized versions of this regimen exist. The important features are that the insulin is given continuously and that it is balanced with the correct amount of glucose. Blood glucose and potassium is estimated at the start of the operation, every 2–3 h and postoperatively, and appropriate changes made. The Alberti regimen may be continued, with blood-glucose monitoring, until the patient starts to eat again.

2 The insulin is given by continuous intravenous infusion from a syringe driver (usually 50 units in 50 ml) at a rate which varies according to the blood sugar, while glucose is given separately. Many find this easier than regimen 1 as changes may be made more easily in response to changes in blood sugar.

3 Give half the normal dose of soluble insulin in the morning with 500 ml 5% glucose intravenously 6-hourly. Operation is carried out in the morning and at midday the remainder of the morning insulin dose is given unless blood glucose is less than 6 mmol/l. Bolus intravenous injections of 10 g glucose can be given if necessary. The evening dose of insulin can be given as usual unless blood glucose is below the level quoted above.

4 Brief minor surgery may be managed by giving neither insulin nor glucose immediately preoperatively, but giving half the normal daily requirement with a meal early postoperatively.

Type 2 diabetes

Type 2 diabetics need insulin only for major surgery, and if starvation is prolonged. For minor surgery, any oral hypoglycaemic agents can be withheld on the morning of surgery, and restarted with feeding.

The poorly controlled diabetic

There is ketosis, glycosuria, dehydration and potassium loss. These patients are difficult to manage and the advice of a diabetic physician will be valuable. Non-urgent surgery must be postponed, but operations such as drainage of abscesses or treatment of infected gangrene may be necessary to achieve control. After partial correction of acidosis with sodium bicarbonate (50 mmol if pH > 7.1; 100 mmol if pH < 7.0), regimens 1 or 2 above offer a scheme for rapid control of the situation. Hypokalaemia is corrected with potassium chloride 10–20 mmol/h, if the urine flow is greater than 1 ml/min. There is a real danger of vomiting during induction in the diabetic with ketosis.

Diabetic (ketoacidotic) coma

The following abnormalities require treatment:

1 lack of insulin;
2 dehydration;
3 loss of sodium and potassium;
4 metabolic acidosis;
5 precipitating diseases, especially infections, myocardial infarction.

Insulin has a short half-life (5 min) in the blood when given intravenously. and is best given by continuous infusion. Sodium bicarbonate should be administered in small quantities. Excessive amounts may cause a rapid drop in potassium, cardiac arrest, leftwards shift of the O_2 dissociation curve and an intracellular acidosis.

The following regimen is typical.

1 *Insulin:* 4–6 units/h by continuous intravenous infusion. Blood sugar is measured 1–2-hourly and should fall by 3–5 mmol/l/h. When the level falls below 11–14 mmol/l, insulin may be given according to a sliding scale.
2 *Fluid and electrolytes:* average deficit is water 6 litres, sodium 500 mmol, chloride 400 mmol, potassium 350 mmol, phosphate 1 mmol/l. Give 1 litre normal saline in first 30 min, 2–3 litres in the next 2–3 h, and then 500 ml/h until about 5 litres has been given. Change to 4% dextrose in 0.18% saline 500 ml 4-hourly when the blood sugar falls to 10–15 mmol/l. Measure electrolytes 2-hourly and change to 0.45% saline if serum sodium rises above 150 mmol/l. Add potassium 13–20 mmol in the first hour then 26 mmol hourly, depending on the rate of fall.
3 *Sodium bicarbonate:* only if acidaemia is severe. One hundred millimoles if pH is less than 7.0, 50 mmol if pH is between 7.0 and 7.1, preferably using isotonic (1.4%) solution.

Monitor blood sugar, urea, electrolytes, haemoglobin, PCV, arterial blood gases, ECG, urine composition and flow. Administer O_2 to maintain saturations. Nasogastric aspiration will be needed.

Other causes of coma in a diabetic

1 *Hyperosmolar, non-ketoacidotic coma:* in the older patient who is dehydrated with very high blood sugar but no ketonuria. Sodium bicarbonate is not needed and hypotonic fluids (0.45% saline), insulin and potassium are given.
2 *Lactic acidosis:* blood lactic acid levels should be determined, but the condition may be suspected when the anion gap (difference between sum of sodium and potassium ions and sum of chloride and bicarbonate ions) is greater than 20. Large amounts of bicarbonate may be needed.

3 *Hypoglycaemia:* rarely presents in true coma, but its onset is much quicker than ketoacidotic coma. If blood sugar is less than 2 mmol/l, give 20 ml of i.v. 50% dextrose.

4 *Those unrelated to diabetes:* e.g. stroke, head injury, drug overdose, etc.

SURGICAL TREATMENT OF HYPERINSULINISM

An insulinoma may be part of a multiple endocrine neoplasia syndrome. About 10% are malignant, and metastasize to the liver. When an insulinoma is to be removed a preoperative glucose load should be given and a 25–50% solution should be infused via a central line during the procedure according to blood sugar estimations performed every 15 min.[55] Surgical manipulation of the tumour can release large amounts of insulin. There should be a sustained rise in blood sugar after excision.

HYPERTHYROIDISM

The Greek word for shield gives the thyroid gland its name. The commonest cause of thyrotoxicosis is Graves' disease (diffuse toxic goitre), typically in women of 20–40 years, caused by IgG autoantibodies. If there is a goitre the anaesthetist should ask for the symptoms of thyrotoxicosis and look for atrial fibrillation and heart failure. Hyperthyroidism can occur without an enlarged thyroid. Cardiac involvement may be the presenting feature, especially in older patients. Proximal muscle weakness is also common. Treatment is with antithyroid drugs, radioactive iodine or surgery. The patient should be euthyroid before operation. An acute exacerbation, or thyroid crisis, is life-threatening. Iodine and beta-blockade are likely to be needed. For details *see* Chapter 4.1 'Endocrine'.

HYPOTHYROIDISM

Myxoedema is common (> 10%) and undiagnosed in older women. Metabolism of drugs, especially sedatives and narcotics, is slowed and respiratory depression easily produced. Usually due to primary failure of the thyroid gland with high thyroid-stimulating hormone (TSH) levels. If due to pituitary failure the adrenal cortex response to stress is also likely to be impaired. There may also be hypothermia, hypoglycaemia, muscular weakness, pericardial effusion and even coma. Such patients are poor anaesthetic risks and correction is necessary before any elective surgery. Oral T_4 takes 10 days to exert its effect. Oral T_3 acts quicker and can also be given intravenously (5–20 μg given slowly 4-hourly if needed, or continuously at up to 5 μg/h) with ECG monitoring looking for flattened T waves or ST depression. Use special caution in older patients and those suffering from angina. Steroids are also beneficial in myxoedema coma. For anaesthesia, an N_2O, O_2, volatile agent, relaxant sequence with IPPV is perhaps the most suitable technique. Mild, undiagnosed hypothyroidism in patients undergoing surgery may result post-operatively in myxoedema coma and respiratory obstruction.

DISEASES OF THE ADRENAL GLANDS

Primary adrenal failure (Addison's disease)

First described by Thomas Addison (1793–1860) of Guy's Hospital.[56] May be seen following bilateral adrenalectomy, or after destruction of the glands by tuberculosis, metastases, infarction, granuloma or autoimmune disease.

The diagnosis should be considered in unexplained cases of hyponatraemia. Patients with this complaint are susceptible to infection, sodium loss and narcotics. They are likely to be debilitated, pigmented, hypotensive, hyponatraemic, hypoglycaemic and perhaps tuberculous. They are bad anaesthetic risks as Addisonian crises are easily precipitated. These start with loss of sodium chloride in the urine and so of large amounts of water. This fluid loss is aggravated by diarrhoea and vomiting, and causes severe dehydration and circulatory failure. Adequate preoperative treatment greatly lessens the risk. Sodium chloride, glucose and hydrocortisone should be given to maintain blood volume. Postoperative hypotension is still likely and should be treated similarly. Normal cortisol production is 30 mg/day, equivalent to 7.5 mg of prednisone. For anaesthesia in Addisonian crisis, *see* Smith M. G. and Byrne A. J. *Anaesthesia* 1981, **36,** 681.

Waterhouse–Friderichsen syndrome[57]

Adrenal infarction which is usually fatal ('adrenal apoplexy'). Often associated with meningococcal septicaemia and first described by Voelcker (1861–1946) in 1894.[58] Hyperpyrexia and circulatory collapse are the usual modes of death. Rarely the condition comes to operation because of associated arterial embolism or peritonitis, when steroids must be given.

Secondary adrenal failure (adrenocorticotrophic hormone deficiency)

This may result from:

1 removal of the pituitary (hypophysectomy);
2 destruction of the pituitary, e.g. tumours, radiotherapy, Simmonds' disease (*see below*);
3 inhibition of the pituitary by steroid therapy.

May cause death if steroids are not given to replace those normally secreted in response to surgical stress.[59] (*See* Chapter 4.1 'Endocrine'.)

Cushing's syndrome

Described in 1932 by the neurosurgeon Harvey Cushing (1869–1939). Caused by cortisol overproduction, usually secondary to a pituitary adenoma. More rarely due to an adrenal adenoma or ectopic adrenocorticotrophic hormone (ACTH) production by a tumour. A similar clinical picture is frequent in patients on steroid medication. Most of the important features are due to tissue destruction: striae, fragile skin and capillaries, bruising, muscle weakness, osteoporosis, 'orange-on-matchsticks' appearance of the body. Hypertension, hypokalaemia and diabetes mellitus are common. Hypophysectomy is often performed.

Phaeochromocytoma

See Chapter 4.1 'Endocrine'.

DISEASES OF THE PITUITARY GLAND

Hyperpituitarism

In adults, acromegaly. In children and adolescents, gigantism.

Acromegaly

First described by Saucerotte (1741–1812)[60] in 1801 and by Pierre Marie (1853–1940) in 1886.[61] Due to an acidophilic or chromophobe cell adenoma of the pituitary forming after the epiphyses have fused. Slow onset with bony changes in the jaws, enlarged tongue, thickening of the mucosa of the pharynx, enlarged larynx with elongation, thickening and even calcification of the cords. There may be recurrent laryngeal nerve paralysis and laryngeal stenosis, and the cricoid may be narrowed, so making intubation difficult. Careful assessment is required, perhaps with a fibreoptic laryngoscope. Blind nasal intubation may be needed. The hands become 'spade-like' and there may be kyphosis, diabetes and an enlarged thyroid. May present as carpal tunnel syndrome. Increased mortality due to cardiac and cerebrovascular disease. Sleep apnoea is common and may be central, obstructive or mixed.

Treatment is usually by hypophysectomy, although yttrium-90 implants and drug therapy (bromocriptine and octreotide) are also used. Postoperatively, there may be upper airways obstruction and intubation may have to be continued. For *trans-sphenoidal hypophysectomy*, steroid cover must be commenced before the operation and continued. Thyroxine replacement will also be needed. There should be vigilance for diabetes insipidus. When the operation is performed for metastatic cancer, attention must be paid to preoperative anaemia, pleural effusions and bony secondaries making movement dangerous because of the possibility of fractures.

Hypopituitarism (Simmonds' disease)[62]

Morris Simmonds (1855–1925). Chronic hypopituitarism is most commonly due to a pituitary tumour or iatrogenic ablation. Ischaemic necrosis of the anterior lobe after haemorrhage in labour (Sheehan's syndrome)[63] is now rare. There may be diminished production of any of the anterior lobe hormones: growth hormone, ACTH, thyrotrophin, gonadotrophin and prolactin. The clinical picture depends on the pattern of such deficiencies. Substitution therapy may be required. General anaesthesia is liable to precipitate coma in these patients. Permanent deficit in posterior lobe hormones (oxytocin or vasopressin) is usually a result of hypothalamic disease.

CARCINOID TUMOURS

First described by Merling in 1838 and named by Obendorfer in 1907,[64] they are less malignant than carcinoma. They arise from argentaffin Kultschitzky cells of the crypts of Lieberkuhn of the gastrointestinal tract; can occur anywhere derived from the embryological foregut (including thyroid and bronchi) but 50–90% originate in the area of the appendix. These tumours neither metastasize nor secrete. Extra-appendicular tumours, however, are often malignant and about 25% of malignant carcinoids produce and secrete serotonin (5-hydroxytryptamine (5-HT)) and other hormones including bradykinin.

Carcinoid syndrome

There are big variations in the clinical manifestations. The syndrome does not occur unless there are liver secondaries with secretion into the hepatic veins. It is characterized by:

1 a growing intra-abdominal malignancy;
2 cutaneous flushes with tachycardia and fall in blood pressure, precipitated by food, alcohol and emotional stress;
3 profuse diarrhoea, nausea, vomiting and abdominal cramps;
4 wheezing.

Attacks may be precipitated by hypotension or by compressing the tumour, e.g. palpation, abdominal straining, or suxamethonium fasciculations.

Long-term manifestations are valvular fibrosis of the right side of the heart which may require surgery, weight loss, pellagra and facial telangiectasia. The disease progresses very slowly.

Diagnosis is confirmed by urinary excretion of 5-hydroxyindole acetic acid. Normal 2–9 mg/24 h; > 25 mg/24 h is diagnostic. Up to 1000 mg/24 h has been described.

Medical treatment includes antihistamines (both H_1 and H_2 blockers), α-adrenergic blockers, aprotonin, 5-HT_1 antagonists (cyproheptadine, methysergide) and 5-HT_2 antagonists (ketanserin). Cytotoxic agents are disappointing. Octreotide, a somatostatin analogue, lowers 5-HT secretion and is effective at controlling symptoms. Surgery may be for removal of primary or secondary tumour, or for heart valve replacement.

Anaesthesia may provoke acute flushing and severe bronchospasm. This is particularly likely if hypotension occurs and so spinal techniques are not recommended. Morphine may cause 5-HT release. Smooth induction of anaesthesia is desirable. Vecuronium has been recommended as the relaxant of choice.[65] Angiotensin (starting with 1.5 mg/kg) is useful for severe intraoperative hypotension. Octreotide has been used successfully to control the effects and release of 5-HT intraoperatively.[66] Careful monitoring should continue into the postoperative period. Awakening from anaesthesia may be delayed. The blood sugar should be monitored.

CONNECTIVE TISSUE DISORDERS

Polyarteritis nodosa may involve the kidneys, gut, skin, heart and lungs. Liver dysfunction may modify the response to muscle relaxants.

Systemic lupus erythematosus can result in the production of an antibody which is an anticoagulant *in vitro*, but causes thrombosis and abortion *in vivo*.

Rheumatoid arthritis

First described by Sir Alfred Garrod in 1859; a disease of modern times (since 18th century); affects 2% of men and 5% of women over 64. Still's disease is a juvenile form. Symmetrical, peripheral polyarthritis, associated with vasculitis in various organs, heart and lung involvement and peripheral neuropathy and Sjögren's syndrome (keratoconjunctivitis sicca).

Potential difficulties may arise from the following:

1 Immobility or subluxation in the cervical spine, especially atlanto-axial. The vertebral arteries may be compressed. The odontoid peg can move posteriorly on neck flexion and compress the cord. Protective muscle tone is lost during anaesthesia.
2 Temporomandibular joint arthritis making laryngoscopy difficult.

3 Crico-arytenoid joint arthritis and neuropathy of laryngeal muscles causing stridor. Thus, there may be *difficulty in intubation* together with the
need for great care after operation. Preoperative chest and cervical spine
(in flexion) radiography may be required.
4 Amyloidosis of kidneys.
5 Pulmonary fibrosis and obstructive airways disease can cause respiratory
depression and pneumonia after operation.
6 Steroid therapy.
7 Fragility of skin and veins.
8 Pericarditis, aortic regurgitation.
9 Anaemia.
10 Peripheral neuropathy.

Ankylosing spondylitis

First described by B. Connor in 1693. Usually affects young men. Often
familial. Starts in lumbar spine (radiological 'bamboo spine') and can
spread to the cervical spine and atlanto-occipital joint, where stiffness may
cause *difficult intubation*, and has led to spinal fractures. Temporomandibular
or crico-arytenoid joints may also be ankylosed. Blind intubation techniques,
awake intubation using a fibreoptic bronchoscope, the use of a laryngeal mask
airway or even tracheostomy may be needed.

Although costovertebral involvement and kyphosis restrict chest expansion,
the diaphragm compensates and lung function is good. Cardiothoracic and
abdominal surgery need not result in pulmonary complications. Take care
to ensure that adequate ventilation returns after operation. Extradural
block for hip surgery may be technically easier via the sacral than the
lumbar approach. There may be associated aortic regurgitation, iritis and
amyloidosis.

SCOLIOSIS

Usually idiopathic but may be due to congenital vertebral anomalies or to
neuromuscular disorders: polio, muscular dystrophy, etc. Malignant hyperpyrexia has been seen in these patients. May be associated with congenital
heart disease. For Harrington rod surgery, it may be necessary to wake the
patient to check cord integrity during the operation. Excessive hypotension
may reduce cord blood supply. A narcotic, N_2O, O_2, IPPV technique is
usually satisfactory. These patients have a reduced vital capacity, and
cannot increase their tidal volume. Airway obstruction is seldom a feature.
Fluoroscopic assessment of diaphragmatic movement will exclude paralysis.
Underventilation is a danger even before anaesthesia is induced, premedication must not depress respiration. Postoperatively, they require careful observation and administration of pain relief, and if necessary IPPV. Hypoxaemia
results from ventilation/perfusion inequality. Pulmonary hypertension, right

heart failure and respiratory failure can result. Ventilation by external negative pressure or nasal mask may be useful.[67]

ACHONDROPLASIA[68]

Described in 1791 by Sommering (1755–1830), Polish–German physician and by M.H. Romberg (1795–1873) in 1817. Difficulties include the fit of face masks, tracheal intubation due to abnormalities at the base of the skull, and restrictive chest wall disease. For Caesarean section, extradural block, although technically difficult, has been safely used.[69]

PAROXYSMAL MYOGLOBINURIA (OR RHABDOMYOLYSIS)

Acute episodes of muscle pain and weakness with myoglobinuria, sometimes following exercise. May be a deficiency of carnitine palmityl transferase. Rhabdomyolysis may follow the use of suxamethonium.

MYASTHENIA

The myasthenic state may be present as follows.

Myasthenia gravis

First described by Thomas Willis (1621–1675) in 1672 and Samuel Wilks (1824–1911) in 1877[70] and named pseudoparalytica myasthenica by Friedrich Jolly (1844–1904), the German neurologist, who also described its electro-diagnosis.[71] The first thymectomy for myasthenia gravis was performed by F. Sauerbruch (1845–1951) in 1911.[72]

It is a chronic disease which tends to relapse and remit, twice as common in women. It can develop any time between childhood and old age, but usually in early adulthood. The symptoms are worse in the few months following child-birth. Myasthenia gravis is an autoimmune disease in which there are circulating IgG antibodies, probably dependent on the thymus, to the acetylcholine receptor. Associated with thyrotoxicosis, collagen diseases and thymoma (in 10% of patients). While severe cases are easily diagnosed, mild ones can be overlooked and may cause anaesthetic difficulties. Ocular, bulbar and other head and neck muscles are commonly involved, with ptosis, dysphagia and easy fatigue of the jaw muscles. Weakness comes on after exercise and improves following rest. Tendon reflexes are brisk. Undiagnosed myasthenia is a cause of unsuspected weakness after relaxants.

There are also: a *neonatal form* in babies born of mysathenic mothers, which recovers spontaneously; rare *congenital non-immune forms* which show variable responses to anticholinesterases.

Tests

1 *Electromyography.* Reduction in response to a single twitch in rested muscles, and to repetitive stimuli at both high and low frequencies.
2 *Edrophonium* ('Tensilon' 10 mg i.v.). In myasthenics there is a full but temporary return of muscular power. In normal patients and myasthenics who are adequately treated there may be fasciculations, colic, salivation and diarrhoea, but muscular power is unaffected.
3 *Acetylcholine receptor antibody estimation.*

Treatment

Oral anticholinesterases, e.g. neostigmine and the longer-acting pyridostigmine, provide symptomatic relief. (Overdosage with anticholinesterases causes a cholinergic crisis, in which there is muscle weakness and fasciculation, lacrimation, sweating and colic.) Other treatments for myasthenia gravis are steroids and immunosuppressives such as azathioprine. Thymectomy is considered, particularly in the younger patient and if a thymoma is present. Plasmapheresis may produce dramatic improvement in an emergency and even maintain the patient in remission.

Preoperative preparation

The serum potassium should be normal as hypokalaemia aggravates myasthenia. Dose of anticholinesterase should be slightly reduced just before operation to avoid excess. A nasogastric tube may be in place for feeding. Sedative premedication should be minimal. Opiates should be avoided. Steroid cover is required for those receiving it regularly.

Anaesthetic management

The chief concern is to ensure adequate respiration both during and after the operation, bearing in mind the muscular weakness and bronchial secretion from neostigmine. Regional analgesia which does not depress respiration, e.g. intra- or extradural block to T10, may be suitable. Rapidly eliminated anaesthetic agents such as sevoflurane are drugs of choice, even though myasthenics are more sensitive to the neuromuscular effects of volatile agents. Relaxants can often be avoided and spontaneous respiration used, but small doses of short-acting relaxants with monitoring of the neuromuscular block may be used. Tracheal intubation may be advisable to ensure a perfect airway and to facilitate suction. Neostigmine should be administered with care to avoid overdosage. Intensive care facilities may be needed postoperatively. Mandatory minute volume ventilation may be beneficial in the postoperative period.

The muscles affected by myasthenia gravis are hypersensitive to non-depolarizing relaxants. Even myasthenics successfully treated with steroids and not requiring anticholinesterases may still show this hypersensitivity. By contrast, there is resistance to decamethonium and suxamethonium, but a dual (non-depolarizing) block may follow.

Management of myasthenic emergencies

Both myasthenic and cholinergic crises are medical emergencies which may cause severe respiratory failure, and can sometimes follow anaesthesia and surgery. A clear airway and adequate respiration must be established first, using IPPV if needed. It is advisable to withhold all drugs until the nature of the crisis has been diagnosed. The patient should be nursed in an intensive care unit. The reactions of the end-plates to neostigmine may be complex and require expert evaluation. Plasma electrolytes, particularly potassium, should be restored to normal values.

Myasthenic syndrome

A condition of proximal muscular weakness developing in a patient with small-cell bronchial carcinoma, usually in older males. More rarely associated with other cancers. May present with prolonged apnoea after anaesthesia. The condition was first described as a distinct entity by Eaton and Lambert in 1957 (the Eaton–Lambert syndrome).[73] Caused by IgG antibodies from the tumour directed against the calcium channels in the presynaptic membrane and less quanta of acetylcholine being released for each nerve impulse.

Differs from myasthenia gravis as follows:

1 It involves proximal limb muscles rather than bulbar and extraocular muscles.
2 The presence of aching muscular pains in the limbs.
3 Diminished tendon reflexes.
4 Poor response to neostigmine and other anticholinesterase medication.
5 Marked sensitivity to both depolarizing and non-depolarizing blockers.
6 Electromyographic characteristics:
   (a) reduced response to single or slow stimuli;
   (b) growth of potentials with tetanic stimulation.

Diaminopyridine is useful treatment, but can cause fits. Immunosuppression has also been used. Temporary improvement of the muscle weakness may follow surgical removal of the carcinoma. Symptoms of muscular weakness should be sought and liver function assessed if such patients are to receive relaxants. High extradural analgesia has been used.[74]

Caused by drugs

Aminoglycoside antibiotics (neomycin, streptomycin, gentamicin), tetracycline, quinidine, procainamide and beta-blockers can worsen any tendency to myasthenia. This can be diagnosed by edrophonium. Penicillamine has also precipitated myasthenia gravis.

Myalgia encephalitis (*see* Chapter 3.2).

DISEASES OF THE NERVOUS SYSTEM

Spinal analgesia and extradural block are considered inadvisable by some because future symptoms and signs may be blamed on these methods of analgesia. This blame is usually without foundation. A history of frequent headaches may also make spinal analgesia undesirable.

Epilepsy

Patients with epilepsy should be kept on anticonvulsants before, during and after operation. In susceptible patients, epilepsy may be triggered off by cholinergic drugs, methohexitone, monoamine oxidase inhibitors, phenothiazines, tricyclic antidepressants, enflurane, and sudden withdrawal of barbiturates, benzodiazepines and hypocapnia. It has also been reported after propofol.[75] Thiopentone is a good induction agent and isoflurane suitable for maintenance. If the patient is starved postoperatively, anticonvulsants must be given parenterally.

Status epilepticus may have to be treated with barbiturate anaesthesia if diazepam and phenytoin fails to bring control. Paradoxically, propofol infusion has also been used with success.[76]

Paraplegia

At the time of a spinal injury there is considerable sympathetic discharge, which can even cause neurogenic pulmonary oedema. After a few minutes, there is the stage of spinal shock (which can last up to several weeks) with hypotension, bradycardia, hypotonia, arreflexia. Tracheal intubation or suction at this time can result in severe bradycardia or asystole.

The final and lasting phase of the spinal injury is the reflex phase, with the return of reflexes and sympathetic tone. If the patient's lowest functional root is C5 he or she is totally dependent on others; if it is C7 he or she has enough use of the arms to be more independent. In patients with transection above about T7 *autonomic hyperreflexia* may result from painful stimuli, especially visceral: transurethral surgery, bladder distension, etc. This causes vasodilatation above the injury, and constriction below. Severe hypertension, bradycardia, arrhythmias and even myocardial ischaemia can occur. General anaesthesia can also precipitate this response, and spinal blockade may be preferable, although its height can be difficult to predict in these patients. About 40% of those undergoing surgery at a site innervated below the level of injury will require anaesthesia as it is difficult to be sure that the lesion of the cord is complete.

Suxamethonium may be dangerous in the period between about 3 days and 6 months (or perhaps longer) after onset of paraplegia. It releases more potassium than usual from muscles, and the extreme hyperkalaemia can cause arrhythmias or cardiac arrest, although deaths have not been reported, and successful resuscitation is the rule.[77]

Additional considerations are as follows:[78]

1 Poor autonomic control of the cardiovascular system, especially with changes in posture. Pressor drugs may be needed. The renin–angiotensin system is more active than normal, and ACE inhibitors may cause profound hypotension.
2 Deep venous thrombosis is very common.
3 Poor control of body temperature.
4 Impaired breathing and coughing, with intercostal and abdominal wall muscle paralysis. Vital capacity is a useful measure of respiratory reserve, and values below 1 litre indicate the likelihood of postoperative respiratory support.
5 Positioning on the operating table with muscle contractures, or spasms provoked by surgical stimuli.
6 Decubitus ulcers leading to chronic infection.
7 Normochromic normocytic anaemia is common.

Dystrophia myotonica

First described by Déléage in 1890 and again in 1909.[79] Inherited as an autosomal dominant. Presents in early adulthood with:

1 expressionless face;
2 wasting of masseters, sternomastoids and forearms;
3 limb weakness with inability to let go after a handshake or to relax previously contracted muscles;
4 percussion myotonia;
5 cataracts;
6 frontal baldness;
7 atrophy of gonads;
8 involvement of external muscles of the eye;
9 dysphagia.

It is a disorder of muscular fibre membranes with an abnormality of chloride conductance, resulting in calcium not being returned to the sarcoplasmic reticulum. The myoneural junction is normal. There may be respiratory muscle weakness, a low vital capacity and an increased $PaCO_2$. Cardiomyopathy, mitral valve prolapse and conduction defects are common. This disease should be sought in a young patient with cataracts (as should diabetes).

Anaesthetic management

Preoperatively: ECG, spirometry. Respiratory depressants should be avoided before, during and after operation. Thiopentone can cause apnoea, so if used should be given as careful 50 mg increments. Cardiovascular depression and arrhythmias may occur during anaesthesia and be worsened by volatile agents. Intubation is often possible without relaxants. IPPV may be required during operation and immediate postoperatively. Myotonia may be caused by diathermy or by TENS.

Non-depolarizing relaxants such as atracurium or vecuronium may be used cautiously but do not abolish myotonia. Infusion of propofol and atracurium may be suitable, although sensitivity to propofol has been reported.[80] Anticholinesterase drugs may increase the myotonia. Depolarizing relaxants are hazardous. They can cause increased muscle tone and prevent intubation. It gives place to ordinary depolarizing relaxation with injection of additional doses. Spinal analgesia does not relax myotonia but injection of local analgesic into the muscle, or parenteral dantrolene, may do so. Extradural block may be satisfactory, but shivering may induce myotonia and uterine atony in the obstetric patient can result in haemorrhage. Pharyngeal muscle dysfunction may lead to aspiration.

In obstetrics, *see also* Blumgart C. H. et al. *Anaesthesia* 1990, **45,** 26; In children, Anderson B. J. and Brown T. C. K. *Anaesth. Intensive Care* 1989, **17,** 320.

Huntington's chorea[81]

Inhalation agents are probably the most suitable. Thiopentone may cause prolonged apnoea and should be used with great care. Midazolam or propofol (+ atracurium) have been used successfully.[82] Abnormal serum cholinesterase may prolong the action of suxamethonium, although some patients respond normally.[83]

Hypokalaemic periodic paralysis

Dominant inheritance, in which attacks of generalized weakness lasting several hours may be precipitated by exercise, heavy meals or the stress of surgery. Potassium moves into the muscle cells. Thiopentone may cause temporary peripheral paralysis. Muscle relaxants may cause residual muscle weakness, but atracurium has been used without problem.

Multiple sclerosis

Disseminated sclerosis, a term used by German pathologists in 1882, was changed to multiple sclerosis in 1946. Description systematized by J. M. Charcot (1825–1893) in 1868.[84] It has been suggested that general anaesthesia may cause a relapse, but this is probably not true.[85] Nitrous oxide interferes with vitamin B_{12} metabolism, and some have suggested a link between B_{12} and multiple sclerosis. It may be wise to avoid N_2O, except in brief operations.[86] Central neural blockade is sometimes avoided on medico-legal grounds, although the justification for this is most doubtful. The relapse rate is probably no greater following intradural block than after general anaesthesia.[87] Special anaesthetic care is not usually necessary. Relapses are more common in the 3 months post-partum.

In obstetrics *see* Bader A. M. et al. *J. Clin. Anesth.* 1988, **1**, 21.

Motor neurone disease (amyotrophic lateral sclerosis)

First described by Erb (1840–1921) in 1884 and by Gowers (1845–1915) in 1902.[88] A progressive disease of the over-50s which causes degeneration of the anterior horn cells in the spinal cord and bulbar palsy.

These patients may be emotionally labile. Excitement and tachycardia should be avoided. They are sensitive to barbiturates and non-depolarizing relaxants. Both should be given cautiously and their effects carefully moni-tored. Suxamethonium is best avoided as both hyperkalaemia and contracture may occur.[89] Inhalation agents may be suitable but their concentration should be increased with care. Respiratory depressant drugs must be used sparingly. Postoperative dysphagia may lead to aspiration. Epidural analgesia has been used safely.

Duchenne muscular dystrophy

Sex-linked recessive. It is the commonest muscular dystrophy and presents in early boyhood. Heart muscle is always involved and sudden cardiac arrest may occur during anaesthesia. The patients often present for orthopaedic procedures. Suxamethonium and halothane should be avoided as some patients develop malignant hyperpyrexia.[90] Temperature and ECG should be monitored throughout.

For complications *see* Larsen U. T. et al. *Can. J. Anaesth.* 1989, **36**, 418.

REFERENCES

1 Buck N. et al. *The Report Of A Confidential Enquiry Into Perioperative Deaths.* London, The Nuffield Provincial Hospital Trust and the King's Fund, 1987.
2 Forrest J. B. et al. *Anesthesiology* 1992, **76**, 3; Edwards A. E. *Anaesthesia* 1996, **51**, 3.
3 Parikh S. S. and Chung F. *Anesth. Analg.* 1995, **80**, 1223.

4 Ward R. M. and Hutton P. *Br. Med. Bull.* 1990, **46**, 156.

5 Rampil I. J. et al. *Anesthesiology* 1991, **74**, 429.

6 Mapleson W. W. *Br. J. Anaesth.* 1996, **76**, 179.

7 Critchley L. A. H. *Anaesthesia* 1996, **51**, 1139.

8 Duncan P.J. et al. *Anesthesiology* 1986, **64**, 790.

9 Cotton B.R. and Smith G. *Br. J. Anaesth.* 1984, **56**, 37.

10 Konieczko K. M. et al. *Br. J. Anaesth.* 1987, **59**, 449.

11 Goldman L. *Anesth. Analg.* 1995, **80**, 810; Howell S. J. et al. *Br. J. Anaesth.* 1998, **80**, 14.

12 Goldman L. et al. *N. Engl. J. Med.* 1977, **297**, 845; Goldman L. *J. Cardiothorac. Anesth.* 1987, **1**, 237.

13 Pedersen T. et al. *Acta Anaesthesiol. Scand.* 1990, **34**, 144.

14 Mangano D. T. *Anesthesiology* 1995, **83**, 897; Juste R. N. *Anaesthesia* 1996, **51**, 255.

15 ACC/AHA Task Force Report. *Guidelines for Perioperative Cardiovascular Evaluation for Non-Cardiac Surgery. Anesth. Analg.* 1996, **82**, 854.

16 Townend J. N. and Hutton P. *Br. J. Anaesth.* 1996, **77**, 137; Béique F. et al. *Can. J. Anaesth.* 1996, **43**, 252; Oxorn D. et al. *Can. J. Anaesth.* 1996, **43**, 278; Kolev N. et al. (European Multicentre Study) *Anaesthesia* 1998, **53**, 767.

17 Slogoff S. and Keats A. S. *Anesthesiology* 1985, **62**, 107.

18 Buffington C. W. et al. *Anesthesiology* 1988, **69**, 721.

19 Tarnow J. et al. *Anesthesiology* 1986, **64**, 147.

20 Hammer A. *Wien. Med. Wochenschr.* 1878, **28**, 97.

21 Howell S. J. at el. *Anaesthesia* 1996, **51**, 1000.

22 Stone J. G. *Anesthesiology* 1988, **68**, 495.

23 Wallace A. et al. *Anesthesiology* 1998, **88**, 7.

24 Stokes W. M. *Dubl. Q. J. Med. Sci.* 1846, **2**, 73; Adams R. *Dubl. Hosp. Rep.* 1827, **4**, 353.

25 Finfer S. R. *Br. J. Anaesth.* 1991, **66**, 509.

26 Kam P. C. A. *Br. J. Anaesth.* 1997, **78**, 102.

27 Renwick J. et al. *Can. J. Anaesth.* 1993, **40**, 1053.

28 Baiser J. R. *Anesthesiology* 1997, **86**, 974.

29 Hanson E. W. *Anesthesiology* 1996, **85**, 178.

30 Fennelly M. E. and Hall G. M. *Br. J. Anaesth.* 1990, **64**, 535.

31 Cohen M. M. and Cameron C. B. *Anesth. Analg.* 1991, **72**, 282.

32 Selsby D. and Jones J. G. *Br. J. Anaesth.* 1990, **64**, 621.

33 Hedenstierna G. *Br. J. Anaesth.* 1990, **64**, 507.

34 Nunn J. F. et al. *Anaesthesia* 1988, **43**, 543.

35 Warner D. O. et al. *Anesthesiology* 1996, **85**, 460.

36 Patrick J. A. et al. *Anaesthesia* 1990, **45**, 390.

37 Carson J. L. et al. *Lancet* 1988, **1**, 727.

38 Herrick J. B. *Arch. Intern. Med.* 1910, **6**, 517.

39 Vijay V. et al. *Br. J. Anaesth.* 1998, **80**, 820.

40 Gelman S. *Anesth. Analg.* 1996, **82**, 899.

41 Gelman S. *Anesth. Analg.* 1998, **86**, 1.

42 Loehning R. W. and Mazze R. I. *Anesthesiology* 1974, **40**, 203.

43 Spencer E. M. et al. *Br. J. Anaesth.* 1990, **65,** 574P.
44 Jensen N. F. et al. *Anesth. Analg.* 1995, **80,** 591.
45 Harrison G. G., Meissner P. N. and Hift R. J. *Anaesthesia* 1993, **48,** 417.
46 McNeill M. J. and Bennet A. *Br. J. Anaesth.* 1990, **64,** 371.
47 Macalpine I. and Hunter R. *Br. Med. J.* 1966, **1,** 65.
48 *See also* Wood P. R. and Soni N. *Anaesthesia* 1989, **44,** 672.
49 Peckham C. S. et al. *Lancet* 1990, **335,** 516.
50 Association of Anaesthetists. *Recommendations of the Expert Advisory Group on Aids.* London: HMSO, 1990.
51 Banting F. G. and Best C. H. *J. Lab. Clin. Med.* 1922, **7,** 25.
52 Watkins P. J. *J. R. Coll. Physicians* 1998, **32,** 360.
53 Eldridge A. J. and Sear J. W. *Anaesthesia* 1996, **51,** 45.
54 Alberti K. G. M. M. and Thomas D. J. B. *Br. J. Anaesth.* 1979, **51,** 693; Thomas D. J. B. et al. *Anaesthesia* 1984, **39,** 629.
55 Muir J. J. et al. *Anesthesiology* 1983, **59,** 371.
56 Addison T. *Lond. Med. Gaz.* 1849, **48,** 517.
57 Waterhouse R. *Lancet* 1911, **1,** 577; Friderichsen C. *Jb. Kinderheilk.* 1918, **87,** 109.
58 Voelker A. R. *Middx Hosp. Rep. Med. Surg. Path. Regist.* 1894, 278.
59 Fraser C. G. et al. *J. Am. Med. Assoc.* 1952, **149,** 1542.
60 Saucerotte N. *Mélang. de Chirurg. (Paris)* 1801, **1,** 407.
61 Marie P. *Med. Rev. Paris* 1886, **6,** 297.
62 Simmonds M. *Dtsch. Med. Wochenschr.* 1914, **40,** 322.
63 Sheehan H. L. *Am. J. Obstet. Gynecol.* 1954, **68,** 202.
64 Obendorfer S. S. *Frankf. Z. Path.* 1907, **1,** 426.
65 Simpson K. H. *Br. J. Anaesth.* 1985, **57,** 934.
66 Hughes E. W. and Hodkinson B. P. *Anaesth. Intensive Care* 1989, **17,** 367.
67 Elliott M. W. et al. *Br. Med. J.* 1990, **300,** 358.
68 Berkowitz I. D. et al. *Anesthesiology* 1990, **73,**739.
69 Wardall G. J. and Frame W. T. *Br. J. Anaesth.* 1990, **64,** 367.
70 Willis T. *The London Practice of Physick.* T. Cassell, London, 1685; Wilks S. *Guy's Hosp. Rep.* 1877, **3 (Series 27),** 7.
71 Jolly F. *Neurol. Zbl.* 1895, **14,** 34.
72 Sauerbruch E. F. *Mitt. Grenzgeb. Med. Chir.* 1912–13, **25,** 746.
73 Eaton M. L. and Lambert E. H. *J. Am. Med. Assoc.* 1957, **163,** 1117.
74 Sakura S. et al. *Anaesthesia* 1991, **46,** 560.
75 Shearer E. S. *Anaesthesia* 1990, **45,** 255.
76 Mackenzie S. J. et al. *Anaesthesia* 1990, **45,** 1043.
77 Goy J. *Spinal Injuries.* In Loach A. (ed.) *Orthopaedic Anaesthesia.* Edward Arnold, London, 1994, p. 145.
78 Hambly P. R. and Martin B. *Anaesthesia* 1998, **53,** 273.
79 Steinert H. *Dtsch. Z. Nerven Heilk.* 1909, **37,** 58; Batten F. E. and Gibbs H. P. *Brain* 1909, **32,** 187.
80 Speedy H. *Br. J. Anaesth.* 1990, **64,** 110.
81 Huntington G. (1850–1916) *Med. Surg. Reporter (Philadelphia)* 1872, **26,** 317.
82 Kaufman M. A. and Erb T. *Anaesthesia* 1990, **45,** 889.

83 Costarino A. and Gross J. R. *Anesthesiology* 1985, **63,** 570.

84 Charcot J. M. *Gaz. Hôp. Civ. Milit. Paris* 1868, **41,** 554; *C. R. Soc. Biol. (Paris)* 1868, **20,** 16.

85 Bamford C. et al. *J. Can. Sci. Neurol.* 1987, **5,** 41.

86 Watt J. W. H. *Anaesthesia* 1998, **53,** 825.

87 Bouchard P. et al. *Ann. Fr. Anaesth. Reanim.* 1984, **3,** 195.

88 Erb W. H. *Dtsch. Arch. Klin. Med.* 1884, **34,** 467; Gowers W. R. *Br. Med. J.* 1902, **2,** 89.

89 Azar I. *Anesthesiology* 1984, **61,** 173.

90 Wang J. M. and Stanley T. H. *Can. Anaesth. Soc. J.* 1986, **33,** 492.

Chapter 3.2

Dictionary of key points about rare diseases

An anaesthetist faced by problems which may arise in his or her patient due to an unusual disease may find the following list useful in the choice of anaesthetic.

Aaskog–Scott syndrome Difficult intubation due to cervical spine stiffness.

Achalasia of the cardia Increased regurgitation risk.

Achondroplasia Intubation difficult, due to short cervical spine (Brimacombe J. R. and Caunt J. A. *Anaesthesia* 1990, **45,** 132). Extradural anaesthesia is possible (Wardall G. J. and Frame W. T. *Br. J. Anaesth.* 1990, **64,** 367).

Acromegaly Airway sometimes very difficult, partly due to large tongue; intubation difficult, partly due to narrow cricoid ring. Diabetes, hypertension occur. A pituitary tumour may exert local pressure effects. Posthypophysectomy, steroids required.

Addison's disease Hypovolaemia, hypotension, hyponatraemia, hypoglycaemia. Steroids are urgently required. The undiagnosed case is a trap for the anaesthetist and intensivist! T. A. Addison (1793–1860), London physician.

Adrenogenital syndrome May be mistaken for pyloric stenosis! Fludrocortisone steriod cover may be required for salt loss. Preoperative electrolyte check required. (Bongiovanni A. M. and Root A. W. *N. Engl. J. Med.* 1963, **268,** 1283, 1342, 1391.)

Aglossia–adactilia syndrome Difficult intubation due to micrognathia.

Agranulocytosis Susceptibility to infections. Haematology referral is advised.

AIDS (acquired immune deficiency syndrome) Cross-infection is guarded against. The practical problems are caused by its complications, e.g. Pneumocystis pneumonia, malnutrition. (*See also* Chapter 3.1.)

Albers–Schonberg disease Brittle bones, risk of fractures while moving or positioning patient. Anaemia, splenomegaly, hypercalcaemia. Heinrich Ernst Albers Schonberg (1865–1921), Hamburg physician.

Albright–Butler syndrome Renal calculi with renal failure, acidosis, hypokalaemia, hypercalcaemia. Cardiac arrythmias occur. (Morris R. C. *N. Engl. J. Med.* 1969, **281**, 1405.)

Albright's osteodystrophy (pseudohypoparathyroidism) Ectopic calcification, hypocalcaemia, neuromuscular excitability, convulsions. F. Albright (1900–1969), Boston physician.

Alcoholism Resistance to anaesthetics, cirrhosis, cardiomyopathy, perioperative withdrawal crisis (delirium tremens).

Alport syndrome Conduction deafness and renal failure in adult life.

Alstrom syndrome Obese, deaf and blind by 7 years of age. Diabetes and renal failure in adult life. C. H. A. Alstrom (1903), Stockholm geneticist.

Alveolar hypoventilation (Ondine's curse) Great danger of postoperative respiratory failure. Re-establishing spontaneous ventilation may be difficult. (Wiesel S. and Fox G. S. *Can. J. Anaesth.* 1990, **37**, 122.)

Amoebiasis Anaemia, dehydration, liver abscess with pulmonary complications. Toxaemia and septicaemia may be severe.

Amyloidosis Macroglossia is a feature. Unexpected cardiac or renal failure may occur. Associated with multiple myeloma, rheumatoid arthritis and chronic infections. (Welch D. B. *Anaesthesia* 1982, **37**, 63.)

Amyotonia congenita (Kugelberg–Welander disease, Werdnig–Hoffmann disease) Spinal muscular atrophy types I and II with anterior horn cell degeneration. Ventilation problems due to muscle weakness. Very sensitive to thiopentone, respiratory depressants and muscle relaxants. (Ellis F. R. *Br. J. Anaesth.* 1974, **46**, 605.)

Amyotrophic lateral sclerosis (motor neurone disease) Very sensitive to thiopentone, curare and respiratory depressants. Suxamethonium causes dangerous hyperkalaemia. (Rosenbaum K. J. et al. *Anesthesiology* 1971, **35**, 638.) Postoperative weakness may be severe. The disease is progressive.

Analbuminaemia Sensitivity to protein-bound drugs, e.g. thiopentone, curare, bupivacaine.

Andersen's disease (glycogen storage disease IV) Hypoglycaemia under anaesthesia. Dorothy H. A. Andersen (1901–1963), New York pathologist.

Andersen's syndrome Cystic fibrosis.

Anhidrotic ectodermal dysplasia (Christ–Siemens–Touraine syndrome) Difficult intubation, heat intolerance, recurrent chest infections. (Beahrs J. O. et al. *Ann. Intern. Med.* 1971, **74**, 92.)

Ankylosing spondylitis Difficult intubation sometimes. *See* Chapter 2.6.

Anorexia nervosa There is malnutrition with risk of hypothermia, hypotension, hypokalaemia, anaemia. Myocardial weakness in addition to muscle weakness.

Apert's syndrome (craniosynostosis) Difficult intubation, due to micrognathia; raised intracranial pressure, other congenital defects, e.g. VSD. (Andersson H. and Gomes S. P. *Acta Paediatr. Scand.* 1968, **57**, 47; Sumner E. and Hatch D. J. (eds) *Textbook of Paediatric Anaesthetic Practice.* Baillière Tindall, London, 1989.) Eugene Apert (1868–1940), Paris paediatrician.

Apical hypertrophic cardiomyopathy Sudden severe cardiac failure or dysrhythmia, runs in families but may be asmptomatic and unheralded. A diagnosis to be considered when there is unexpected cardiac arrest in a young patient.

Arnold–Chiari malformation Herniation of cerebellum and medulla through foramen magnum with headache, hydrocephalus, cranial nerve entrapment, torsion of brainstem, raised intracranial pressure, and signs of syringomyelia in about 50%. (Banerji N. K. and Millar J. H. D. *Brain* 1974, **97**, 157–168.) In obstetrics, a careful neuroanaesthetic may be the option open to least criticism.

Arthrogryposis (congenital contractures) Difficult veins, difficult airway, due to micrognathia and cervical spine/jaw stiffness. Scoliosis, myopathic muscles. Sensitive to thiopentone, associated congenital heart disease of 10% of patients. Possibility of malignant hyperpyrexia. (Baines D. B. et al. *Anaesth. Intensive Care* 1986, **14**, 370; Oberdi G. S. et al. *Can. J. Anaesth.* 1988, **35**, 288–290 & 612–614.)

Armadillo disease Spontaneous myokymia of arms and legs, with absent tendon reflexes, but increased tone, abolished by relaxants and phenytoin, but not by regional blockade or sleep. (Wilton A. and Graham J. G. *Hospital Update* 1990, **16**, 698–700.)

Asbestosis Pulmonary fibrosis with respiratory failure. May be on steroids, may have tuberculosis.

Asplenia syndrome Associated congenital heart disease with cardiac failure.

Ataxia–telangiectasia Immunoincompetence (IgA and IgE). Recurrent infections.

Atrial fibrillation (acute) The root cause should be elicited. Addition of a beta-blocker, verapamil or amiodarone to digoxin has been recommended if ventricular function is adequate. Cardioversion may be indicated. May be precipitated by hypokalaemia and hypotension. (Fulham M. J. and Cookson W. O. C. *Anaesth. Intensive Care* 1984, **12**, 121.)

Atrial septal defect (ASD) The shunt is usually left to right. Mitral regurgitation is common in the primum defect. The secundum defect leads to pulmonary hypertension and right ventricular hypertrophy with worsening prognosis. Antibiotic cover is usual. Decreasing systemic vascular resistance decreases the shunt, as does intermittent positive-pressure ventilation (IPPV). Right to left shunt (e.g. in hypoxia and severe systemic hypotension) causes arterial desaturation, delivery of high concentrations of intravenous agents to the coronary arteries, and transfer of emboli to the arterial side. The entrance of air into the venous circulation is meticulously avoided.

Atrioventricular block (first degree) There may be severe bradycardia requiring atropine or pacing. (Hayward R. et al. *Anaesthesia* 1982, **37,** 1190.)

Autoimmune anaemias May be on steroids. Respiration may be difficult to restart after IPPV.

Autonomic hyperreflexia *See* Hutchinson R. C. *Anaesthesia* 1986, **41,** 663.

Barlow's syndrome (click-murmur mitral valve prolapse) Bradycardia resistant to atropine, dysrhythmias responding to beta-blockade, and thromboembolism occur. Excessive tachycardia and anxiety should be avoided. Antibiotic cover is usual.

Bartter syndrome Electrolyte abnormalities occur and require correction.

Behçet syndrome Steroid cover often required. Mouth ulcers can be a problem.

Becker Syndrome *See* Duchenne muscular dystrophy.

Beckwith (Wiedemann) syndrome (infantile gigantism) Macroglossia with airway problems, severe hypoglycaemia, requiring intravenous cover during preoperative starvation. (Filippi G. and McKusick V. A. *Medicine (Baltimore)* 1970, **49,** 279.)

Beri-beri Cardiomyopathy with failure, decreased systemic vascular resistance, muscular weakness due to neuropathy. Autonomic neuropathy causes severe hypotension under anaesthesia. Memory loss and Korsakoff's psychosis are common. Careful treatment with vitamin B is highly desirable; it restores systemic vascular resistance. Digoxin is helpful in enabling the heart to cope with this.

Berylliosis Pulmonary fibrosis with respiratory failure. May be on steroids.

Blackfan–Diamond syndrome (congenital red-cell aplasia) Thrombocytopenia, anaemia, VSD. May be on steroids

Bloom's Syndrome Defect in DNA management; X-rays are more likely to damage cells, and should be restricted.

Bowen's syndrome (cerebrohepatorenal syndrome) Renal failure, hypoprothrombinaemia, sensitivity to muscle relaxants. J. T. Bowen (1857–1941) Boston dermatologist.

Bronchiolitis fibrosa obliterans Pulmonary fibrosis. May be on steroids.

Buerger's disease Bronchitis and emphysema, peripheral vascular insufficiency. Indirect arterial pressure measurements may be inaccurate (reading too high).

Bullous cystic lung disease (For suggested technique of anaesthesia *see* Normandale J. P. and Feneck R. O. *Anaesthesia* 1985, **40,** 1182.)

Burkitt's lymphoma May be difficult to intubate. Denis B. Burkitt (1911–), of Dublin, London and Uganda.

Burns Hypovolaemia, lung burns, hyperkalaemia with suxamethonium, Sepsis, severe pain, intubation problem sometimes, *see* Chapters 4.1 and 4.4.

Carcinoid syndrome Tricuspid valve malfunction, sudden bronchospasm, especially with cyclopropane and hypotension, *see* Chapter 3.1.

Cardiac tamponade Low cardiac output, high venous pressure, anaesthesia and IPPV may worsen the failure.

Cardiomyopathy May be sporadic, postviral, or run in families (Oakley C. *Br. Med. J.* 1997, **315,** 1520–1524). Often symptomless, or with dyspnoea, angina or syncope. Electrocardiography (ECG) and echocardiography are diagnostic. Patients may be on beta-blockers or DDD pacing. Transplantation may be indicated. General anaesthesia is to be avoided where possible (risk of arrhythmias and failure). This is a diagnosis to consider in unexpected failure or arrest in a younger patient.

Carpenter's syndrome (cranial synostosis with small mandible, congenital heart disease; PDA & VSD) Intubation problems. (Andersson H. and Gomes S. P. *Acta Paediatr. Scand.* 1968, **57,** 47.) George C. Carpenter (1859–1910), London paediatrician.

Central core myopathy See Congenital myopathy.

Cerebrocostomandibular syndrome Difficult intubation and respiration (cleft palate, micrognathia, microthorax, tracheal abnormalities, vertebral anomalies).

Chagas' disease (American trypanosomiasis) Hepatic failure, cardiomyopathy. (Barretto J. C. *Br. J. Anaesth.* 1979, **51,** 1189.) Carlos Chagas (1879–1934), Brazilian physician.

Charcot–Marie–Tooth disease type 1 Severe respiratory insufficiency with peripheral neuromuscular failure (Antognini J. F. *Can. J. Anaesth.* 1992, **39,** 398–400). Spinal and lower limb deformities with hyperkalaemia. Exacerbated during pregnancy (Rudnik-Schonedborn S. et al. *Neurology* 1993, **43,** 2011–2016). Suxamethonium contraindicated (Cooperman I. H. *J. Am. Med. Assoc.* 1970, **213,** 1867–1871).

CHARGE Association Difficult intubation due to micrognathia, cleft palate. Also choanal atresia, microphallus and cryptorchidism. Congenital heart disease in 70%.

Chediak–Higashi syndrome (immunodeficiency, with some albinism) Recurrent infections, thrombocytopenia, haemorrhage problems. May be on steroids. (Blume R. S. and Wolff S. M. *Medicine (Baltimore)* 1972, **51,** 247.)

Cherubism Oral airway obstruction due to macroglossia, intubation may be impossible, urgent tracheostomy may be required. Corrective surgery may be very haemorrhagic.

Choanal atresia Nasal obstruction. If bilateral, severe respiratory obstruction can be an emergency, solved by an oral airway, which is taped in place. During surgical correction, compression of the tracheal tube by Boyle–Davis gag can be a problem. The child is extubated wide awake with nasal splints in place.

Chotzen syndrome (craniosynostosis) Difficult intubation due to micrognathia; renal failure is sometimes a problem. (Andersson H. and Gomes S. P. *Acta Paediatr. Scand.* 1968, **57**, 47.) F. C. Chotzen, Breslau psychiatrist.

Christ–Siemens–Tourane syndrome (ectodermal dysplasia) Difficult intubation due to micrognathia. No hair or teeth. Defective thermoregulation due to absent sweat glands; cooling mattress should be available. Atropine etc. are avoided.

Christmas disease The problem is haemorrhage due to coagulopathy due to low factor IX, with normal factor VIII and prolonged APTT.

Chronic granuloma disease Lung problems due to granulomas.

Cleft palate Difficult intubation, respiratory obstruction may result from heavy sedative premedication, *see* Paediatric anaesthesia

Cockayne's syndrome (Cockayne E. A. *Arch. Dis. Child* 1936, **11**, 1.) An inherited autosomal recessive disorder with progressive mental and physical retardation, deafness, blindness, bony malformations, etc. Intubation may be very difficult. (Cook S. *Anaesthesia* 1982, **37**, 104.)

Congenital analgesia Sedation or general anaesthesia may still be required for surgery and abnormal responses to drugs may be present. (Layman P. R. *Anaesthesia* 1986, **41**, 395.)

Congenital myopathy (central core disease) Ventilation problem due to muscle weakness. Sensitivity to muscle relaxants. Malignant hyperpyrexia may occur. (Shuaib A. and Paasuke R. T. et al. *Medicine* 1987, **66**, 389).

Congenital trophoblastic disease Patients have a low plasma cholinesterase level and elevated chorionic gonadotrophin. (Davies J. M. et al. *Anaesthesia* 1984, **12**, 1074.)

Conn's syndrome Primary hyperaldosteronism. Hypertension, hypovolaemia (causing orthostatic hypotension), hypokalaemia (causing muscle weakness and requiring care with relaxants), metabolic alkalosis. Oedema is uncommon. J. C. Conn (1907–), Ann Arbor internist. Potassium supplements, spironolactone and antihypertensives may be needed. Enflurane is avoided if there is polyuric nephropathy.

Conjoined twins (Siamese twins) Intubation difficulties sometimes, adrenal failure, one infant may exsanguinate the other at operation, multiple anaesthetics required. Slow gas induction due to wider distribution of the agents, *see* Paediatric anaesthesia Chapter 4.2; Diaz J. H. and Furman E.B. *Anesthesiology* 1987, **67**, 965–973.

Conradi–Hunermann syndrome (chondrodystrophy and mental deficiency)
Renal and congenital heart disease are the main risk factors.

Core syndrome Muscle weakness disease with ventilation problems. *See* Congenital myopathy.

Cretinism Intubation difficulties due to macroglossia, sensitivity to anaesthetic drugs. Muscle weakness may give respiratory problems and cardiomyopathy occurs. Steroid cover may be required. Hypoglycaemia and electrolyte problems occur.

Creutzfeldt–Jacob disease Muscular incoordination and malnutrition may cause problems. For anaesthesia *see* MacMurdo S. D. et al. *Anesthesiology* 1984, **60**, 590. For diagnosis *see* Otto M. et al. *Br. Med. J.* 1998, **316**, 577–581.

Cri-du-chat disease (microcephaly, micrognathia, macroglossia) Difficult airway, difficult intubation, associated ASD & VSD (in 25%).

Crohn's disease Anaemia, toxaemia (sometimes very severe), hypoproteinaemia. May be on steroids. B. B. Crohn (1884–1983), New York physician. Attempted correction of intraoperative tachycardia may precipitate cardiac failure.

Crouzon's disease (craniosynostosis) Difficult intubation due to micrognathia, postoperative respiratory obstruction. Corrective operations very haemorrhagic. Coarctation of aorta occurs. (Andersson H. and Gomes S. P. *Acta Paediatr. Scand.* 1968, **57**, 47.)

Cushing's syndrome Diabetes, hypertension, hypokalaemia, sodium retention, obesity, thin skin. Harvey Cushing (1869–1939), Boston neurosurgeon.

Cutis laxa (elastic degeneration) Fragile skin, blood vessels, lung infections and emphysema common. Pendulous laryngeal and pharyngeal mucosa may obstruct breathing (Wooley M. W. et al. *J. Pediatr. Surg.* 1967, **2**, 325) and damage to airway mucosa with haematoma formation is a risk.

Cystic fibrosis Atropine may inspissate secretions (Lamberty J. M. and Rubin B. K. *Anaesthesia* 1985, **40**, 448). Nasal polypectomy may be required and children withstand anaesthesia well. May have chronic obstructive lung disease, airway obstruction, malnutrition and bleeding tendency and liver dysfunction. There is a risk of respiratory problems but careful humidification, bronchodilators, asepsis and antibiotics will usually avoid these. Intravenous hydration and intubation for bronchial suction are usual. Intrinsic pulmonary disease; inspissated secretions made worse by atropine etc. An important priority is prevention of accumulation of lung secretions postoperatively. Humidification and postural drainage are important. Hypoxia and hypotension are not well tolerated. Regional blockade is the anaesthesia of choice if possible. (Bose D., Yentis S. M. and Fauvel N. J. *Anaesthesia* 1997, **52**, 578–582.)

Cystic hygroma Respiratory obstruction after induction due to the soft tissue mass, often corrected by nasal airway, difficult intubation sometimes.

Dermatomyositis Mouth opening restricted, chest infections, anaemia, hypersensitivity to non-depolarizing relaxants. Steroid cover required. (Eisele J. H. In Katz E. and Kadis M. (eds) *Anesthesia for Uncommon Diseases*. Saunders, Philadephia, 1973.)

Congenital diaphragmatic hernia Usually an emergency. Discovered by failure to correct cyanosis at birth. respiratory failure due to hypoplastic lung, dyspnoea, hypoxia, acidosis, cardiac failure, pneumothorax occur. Postoperative respiratory failure usually requires intensive therapy unit (ITU) paediatrics.

Diastrophic dwarfism Difficult intubation due to micrognathia and short neck.

DiGeorge syndrome (immune deficiency, athymia) Chest infections, stridor, aortic arch anomalies with cardiac failure, hypoparathyroidism, hypocalcaemia, tetany. Fresh donor blood is irradiated to prevent graft-versus-host reaction.

Disseminated sclerosis (multiple sclerosis) Deterioration may follow pyrexia, and spinal (and other regional) analgesia although this is not proven. (Alderson J. D. *Anaesthesia* 1991, **45,** 1084–1085; Bamford C. *J. Can. Sci. Neurol.* 1987, **5,** 41–44). *See* Chapter 3.1.

Down's syndrome (mongolism, trisomy 21) Requires very large doses of sedatives and premedication. Large tongue, small mouth, neck may be stiff, with dangerous atlanto-axial dislocation. Intubation difficult and upper airway may obstruct. Risk of extubation stridor, especially after cardiac surgery. Associated congenital heart disease, esp. septal defects (in 50%). Extubation laryngeal spasm may occur. The eye is sensitive to local atropine but large doses of atropine or glycopyrronium may be required for hypersalivation. Hypoglycaemia ocurs easily. (Gallamnaugh S. C. *Br. Med. J.* 1985, **291,** 117; Powell J. F. *Anaesthesia* 1991, **45,** 1049–1051.) *See* Chapter 4.2. J. Langdon Down (1826–1896), London physician.

Drug Addiction Opioid addicts may have inaccessible veins, requiring 'gas' induction. They may arrive with considerable respiratory depression from the most recent 'fix'. Drug withdrawal (or simulated withdrawal) may occur postoperatively. They may be infected with hepatitis or AIDS. Amphetamine addicts may have adrenergic storms, while glue-sniffing causes unstable cardiovascular symptoms. Cocaine addicts may require resuscitation from overdose.

Dubowitz' syndrome Difficult intubation (microcephaly, micrognathia), also hypertelorism.

Duchenne muscular dystrophy The commonest muscular disorder in childhood. Developing muscular weakness, scoliosis, obesity and falling vital capacity lead to chronic and ultimately fatal respiratory failure. Ventilatory support after operation may be necessary (Heckmatt J. Z. *Br. Med. J.* 1987, **295**, 1014.) There is frequent cardiac involvement, with unexpected arrest (Chalkaidis G. A. and Branch K. G. *Anaesthesia* 1990, **45**, 22). Atropine, opiates and non-depolarizing relaxants may well be avoided. A simple volatile agent gives adequate relaxation. Has been associated with hyperpyrexial reactions (Ellis F. R. *Br. J. Anaesth.* 1974, **46**, 605; Lintner S. P. K. and Thomas P. R. *Br. J. Anaesth.* 1982, **54**, 1331; Rosenberg H., Heiman-Patterson T. et al. *Anesthesiology* 1983, **59**, 362). G.B.D. Duchenne (1806–1895), French neurologist. (*See* Chapter 3.1.) (Morris P. *J. Paed. Anaesth.* 1997, **7**, 1–4.)

Dygue–Melchior–Clausen's syndrome Difficult intubation due to cervical spine.

Dysautonomia (Riley–Day syndrome) *See* Familial dysautonomia.

Dystrophia myotonica Respiratory failure and infections, hypertonic muscles (unable to relax after handshake), frontal bald patch and cataracts. Cardiac involvement in a significant proportion. Prolonged muscle spasm after suxamethonium (Speedy H. *Br. J. Anaesth.* 1990, **64**, 110). Neostigmine and shivering. Hypersensitivity to respiratory depressants and non-depolarizing relaxants (which in some cases may not relax the myotonia). Associated with malignant hyperpyrexia, so halothane generally avoided. Isoflurane probably safe. Regional and inhalation techniques are recommended, but regional block may not produce relaxation. Prolonged apnoea may follow the injection of normal doses of thiopentone. Dystrophia in babies (*see* Bray R. J. and Inkster J. S. *Anaesthesia* 1984, **39**, 1007). Dystrophia in obstetrics (*see* Blumgaret C. H., Hughes D. G. and Redfern N. *Anaesthesia* 1990, **45**, 26). *See* Chapter 3.1.

Ebstein's abnormality (tricuspid valve disease) Supraventricular tachycardia during induction. W. E. Ebstein (1836–1912), Gottingen physician.

Edward's syndrome (trisomy 18) VSD, patent ductus, pulmonary stenosis, micrognathia, short sternum, renal failure, clenched hands, low-set ears.

Ehlers–Danlos syndrome (collagen abnormality) Hypermobility of joints, fragile skin, veins, arteries and tracheal mucosa occur. Intubation may cause severe tracheal bruising. Spontaneous rupture of cerebral and other vessels. Associated aneurysmal thromboses occur. Spontaneous pneumothorax is a risk (even during anaesthesia). Mitral regurgitation occurs. (Wooley M. W. et al. *J. Ped. Surg.* 1967, **2**, 325; Dolan P et al. *Anesthesiology* 1980, **52**, 266; Ehlers E. *Derm. Zeit.* 1901, **8**, 173; Danlos H. *Bull. Soc. Franc. Dermatol. Syph.* 1908, **19**, 70.) *See also* Pseudoxanthoma elasticum.

Eisenmengers complex (pulmonary hypertension, VSD, right ventricular failure) Decreases of systemic vascular resistance (e.g. enflurane, isoflurane) cause problems by increasing the right to left shunt, but vasoactive agents (and hypercapnia and further hypoxia) also cause pulmonary vasoconstriction and require great caution. Strong tendency to right ventricular failure and asystole during anaesthesia. Very slow equilibration with inhaled gases.

Nitrous oxide, by producing mild arteriolar constriction, is a safe agent in this dangerous condition. Ketamine also has advantages. (Bird T. M. and Strunin L. *Anaesthesia* 1984, **39**, 48; Lumley J. et al. *Anesth. Analg. (Cleve.)* 1977, **56**, 543; and Foster J. M. G. and Jones R. M. *Ann. R. Coll. Surg.* 1984, **66**, 153; Pollack K. L., Chestnut D. H. and Wenstrom K. D. *Anesth. Analg.* 1990, **70**, 212.)

Ellis–Van-Creveld disease (chondro-ectodermal dysplasia)   Respiratory failure, congenital cardiac septal lesions.

Epidermolysis bullosa   Skin and mucous membranes of airway easily blistered with scarring. The no-touch technique is called for! May be on steroids; may be associated with porphyria. Sticky tape may damage skin. Ketamine has been recommended. Steroid cover often required. (Fox W. T. *Lancet* 1979, **1**, 766; Kubota Y. et al. *Anesth. Analg. Curr. Res.* 1961, **40**, 244; Reddy A. R. R. and Wong D. H. W. *Can. Anaesth. Soc. J.* 1972, **19**, 536; Frost P. M. *Anaesthesia* 1980, **35**, 918; James I. G. and Wark R. *Anesthesiology* 1982, **56**, 323; Tomlinson A. A. *Anaesthesia* 1983, **38**, 495; James I. G. *Anaesthesia* 1983, **38**, 1106.)

Epilepsy   Convulsions due to perioperative drug withdrawal. Loose teeth due to phenytoin therapy.

Erythema multiforme   Postintubation laryngeal oedema. (Cucchiara R. C. and Dawson B. *Anesthesiology* 1971, **35**, 537.)

Exomphalos and gastroschisis   Postcorrection respiratory failure is a major problem.

Fabry's syndrome (lipidosis)   Myocardial ischaemia in early adult life, renal failure.

Factor V Leiden mutation   High risk of pulmonary embolus, requiring carefully controlled anticoagulation in pregnancy, trauma and surgery. (Price D. T. and Ridker P. M. *Ann. Intern. Med.* 1997, **127**, 895–903; Sarasin F. P. and Bounameaux H. *Br. Med. J.* 1998, **316**, 95–99.) There is resistance to the anticoagulant effect of protein C. Similar risk in protein C, S, or antithrombin deficiency.

Familial dysautonomia (Riley–Day syndrome)   Described in 1949. It is an inherited disease showing abnormally active parasympathetic system with sporadic storms of sympathetic activity. It is mainly confined to Ashkenazi Jews. The child cries without tears, is highly emotional with bouts of sweating and unexplained fluctuations of blood pressure. Reduced autonomic stability, hypersalivation, regurgitation, poor temperature control, sensitive to respiratory depressants. Intrinsic pulmonary disease may give postoperative problems. Volatile anaesthetics can cause bradycardia and hypotension and thus must be used carefully. Nitrous oxide and O_2 are usually sufficient. Intermittent positive-pressure ventilation often required while anaesthetized, due to CO_2 insensitivity. Dopamine hydroxylase is deficient, with hypersensitivity to dopamine and other adrenergic and cholinergic drugs. Reduced sensitivity to pain. (Meridy A. W. and Greighton R. E. *Can. Anaesth. Soc. J.* 1971, **18**,

563; Cox R. G. and Sumner E. *Anaesthesia* 1983, **38**, 293; Foster J. M. G. *Anaesthesia* 1983, **38**, 391; Stenquist O. and Sigurdsson J. *Anaesthesia* 1982, **37**, 929; Sweeney B. F. et al. *Anaesthesia* 1985, **40**, 783; Axelrod F. B. et al. *Anesthesiology* 1988, **68**, 631–635.) Conrad M. Riley (1913–), Denver paediatrician; R. L. Day (1905–), Pittsburg physician.

Familial periodic paralysis The hyperkalaemic type is associated with paralysis after general anaesthesia, especially thiopentone and relaxants. (Streeten D. J. In Stanbury J. B. (ed.) *Metabolic Basis of Inherited Disease.* McGraw-Hill, New York, 1972.) (For anaesthesia, *see* Fozard J. R. *Anaesthesia* 1983, **38, 294.**)

Fanconi syndrome (renal tubular acidosis) Acidosis, dehydration, hypokalaemia, renal failure all require correction. (Morris R. C. *N. Engl. J. Med.* 1969, **281**, 1405.) Guido F. Fanconi (1903–), Zurich paediatrician.

Fanconi's anaemia Defect in DNA regeneration with sensitivity to X-rays which should be restricted, e.g. in ITU.

Farber's disease (lipogranulomatosis) Cardiomyopathy and renal failure. Granulomas may exist in the larynx, making intubation difficult. (Gilbertson A. A. and Boulton T. B. *Anaesthesia* 1967, **22**, 607.)

Farmer's lung Pulmonary fibrosis. May be on steroids.

Fat embolism Sudden, severe respiratory and renal failure, mental confusion with disseminated intravascular coagulation (DIC), classically 1–2 days after fracture. May require full intensive care support. *See* Orthopaedic anaesthesia Chapter 4.1.

Favism (glucose-6-phosphate-dehydrogenase deficiency) Anaemia; haemolysis may result from sulphonamides and aspirin. (Gilbertson A. A. and Boulton T. B. *Anaesthesia* 1967, **22**, 607.)

Felty's syndrome (a form of idiopathic thrombocytopenic purpura) Anaemia, haemmorrhage, neutropenia, infections. May be on steroids. Augustus R. Felty (1895–), US physician.

Femoral hypoplasia syndrome Difficult intubation (micrognathia).

Fetal surgery Anaesthesia is necessary after 26 weeks. *See* Glover V. and Nicholas F. *Br. Med. J.* 1996, **313**, 796; Wise J. *Br. Med. J.* 1997, **315**, 1112.

Fibrodysplasia ossificans (myositis ossificans) May be difficult to intubate, with reduced thoracopulmonary compliance. (Newton M. C., Allen P. W. and Ryan D. C. *Br. J. Anaesth.* 1990, **64**, 246.)

Fibromatosis (including juvenile and hyaline forms) *See* Vaughn G. C. et al. *Anesthesiology* 1990, **72**, 201.

Fibrosing alveolitis (Hamman–Rich syndrome) Cyanosis, left heart failure. May be on steroids.

Fluid retention syndrome Risk of associated obesity, diabetes, hypo- and hyperthyroidism, depression. Worsened by steroids, carbenoxolone, non-steroidal anti-inflammatory drugs (NSAIDs), guanethidine, hydralazine, prazosin and calcium channel antagonists. Increased capillary permeability may cause problems during operation. (Dunnigan M. G. *Hospital Update* 1990, **16**, 653–664.)

Freeman–Sheldon syndrome Difficult intubation due to micrognathia.

Friedreich's ataxia Myocardial degeneration with failure and dysrhythmias, Hypertrophic cardiomyopathy may coexist. respiratory failure, diabetes, and peripheral neuropathy. Cases may be treated like those with amyotrophic lateral sclerosis. Very sensitive to non-depolarizing relaxants. Atracurium can be used (Bell C. F. et al. *Anaesthesia* 1986, **41**, 296 and *see* Bird T. M. and Strunin L. *Anesthesiology* 1984, **60**, 377). An autosomal recessive inherited disease causing progressive ataxia and usually additional myopathy. (Bell C. F., Kelly J. M. et al. *Anaesthesia* 1986, **41**, 296). Nicolas Friedreich (1825–1882). Heidelberg physician.

Gardner's syndrome (multiple polyposis) No specific difficulties except from laryngeal polyps.

Gargoylism Respiratory obstruction after induction, very difficult intubation, cardiomyopathy and valve lesions occur.

Gaucher's disease Thrombocytopenia, neutropenia, anaemia. Pulmonary aspiration may be a problem during anaesthesia.

Gilbert's disease (familial unconjugated hyperbilirubinaemia) Jaundice (for which the anaesthetist may be blamed!) precipitated by minor upsets, including starvation. Nicholas A. Gilbert (1858–1927), Paris physician.

Glanzmann's disease (thrombasthenia) Abnormal haemorrhage, platelet infusion rarely effective. May be on steroids.

Glomus jugulare tumours There is a risk to cerebral blood flow and intense stimulation of baroreceptors is a major nuisance during excision. *See* Mather S. P. and Webster N. R. *Anaesthesia* 1986, **41**, 856; Braude B. M. et al. *Anaesthesia* 1986, **41**, 861.

Glucagonoma For anaesthetic management of glucagonoma, *see* Nicoll J. M. V. and Catling S. J. *Anaesthesia* 1985, **40**, 152.

Glue-sniffing At resuscitation, there may be unstable circulation due to grossly increased catecholamines.

Glycogenoses

Type I (Von Gierke's disease) Perioperative acidosis and hypoglycaemia. Diazoxide has been recommended.

Type II (Pompe's disease) heart failure and neuromuscular weakness, macroglossia. Rarely survive infancy (McFarlane H. J. and Soni N. *Anaesthesia* 1986, **41**, 1219).

Type III perioperative hypoglycaemia.

Type IV perioperative hypoglycaemia.

Type V (McArdle's disease) muscle weakness, cardiac failure. (*See* Cox J. M. *Anesthesiology* 1968, **29**, 1221.)

Goldenhar syndrome (oculoauriculovertebral syndrome, hemifacial microsomia) Difficult intubation and airway (small mandible, micrognathia with unilateral cleft defect, unilateral maxillary hypoplasia, cervical vertebral defects). Associated congenital heart disease (Fallot and VSD). *See* Madan R., Trikha A., Ventakaraman R. K., Batra R.and Kalia P. *Anaesthesia* 1990, **45**, 49. Atropine-resistant bradycardia may be a problem (Khan F. M. *Anaesthesia* 1991, **45**, 1102).

Golz–Gorlin syndrome (focal dermal hypoplasia) Difficult airway due to frequent dental and facial asymmetry, and stiff neck (Gorlin R. J. and Golz R. W. *N. Engl. J. Med.* 1960, **262**, 908–912). Hypertension due to prorenin/renin production has been a problem (Yoshizumi J. et al. *Anaesthesia* 1991, **45**, 1046–1048).

Goodpasture's syndrome Severe repeated intrapulmonary haemorrhage with fibrosis. Hypertension, anaemia, renal failure. May be on steroids. E. W. Goodpasture (1886–1960), Boston pathologist. Preoperative plasmapheresis may be required. *See* Urbaniak S. J. and Robinson E. A. *Br. Med. J.* 1990, **300**, 662–665.

Gorlin syndrome (*see* Golz–Gorlin)

Gout Avoid dehydration. Uricaemia may be worsened by methoxyflurane, ethanol and lactate.

Groenblad–Strandberg disease (*See* Pseudoxanthoma elasticum)

Guillain–Barré disease (acute idiopathic polyneuritis, with ventilation problems due to rising muscle weakness; autonomic storms and severe pain) May require IPPV in intensive care, circulation sometimes unstable due to autonomic dysfunction. Usually self-limiting in up to 6 weeks, but much moral support needed while on IPPV. Suxamethonium may cause dangerous hyperkalaemia for up to 3 months after onset. (Smith R. B. *Can. Anaesth. Soc. J.* 1971, **18**, 199; Perel A. et al. *Anaesthesia* 1977, **32**, 257.) G. C. Guillain (1876–1961), Paris neurologist. J. A. Barré (1880–), Strasbourg neurologist.

Haemochromatosis (bronze diabetes and haemosiderosis) Iron deposits in liver (cirrhosis); pancreas (diabetes); joints (arthritis); skin (bronzing) and heart valves (late cardiac failure). The patient may be having weekly venesections.

Haemolytic uraemic syndrome See Johnson G. D. and Rosales J. K. *Can. J. Anaesth.* 1987, **34**, 196–199.

Haemophilia Preoperative plasmapheresis may be required (Urbaniak S. J. and Robinson E. A. *Br. Med. J.* 1990, **300**, 662–665), with factor VIIIc and VIIIAg replacement. Perioperative DDAVP cover (4 μg/day) may be needed.

Haemorrhagic telangiectasia (Osler–Weber–Rendu syndrome) Postintubation laryngeal bruising and obstruction. Risk of epistaxis.

Hallermann–Streiff syndrome Difficult intubation, due to micrognathia, brittle teeth, hypoplastic nares.

Hallervorden–Spatz disease (Elejalde B. R. and de Elejalde M. M. *J. Clin Genet*. 1979, **16**, 1.) A rare progressive disorder of the basal ganglia which occurs in late childhood and leads to death. The patients are demented and show various types of myotonia and muscular rigidity, with trismus which would make intubation difficult. Volatile induction and maintenance relieve the dystonic posturing which returns after operation, as with other basal ganglion disorders. (Roy R. C. et al. *Anesthesiology* 1983, **58**, 382.)

Hamman–Rich syndrome Acute diffuse interstitial lung fibrosis.

Hand–Schuller–Christian disease (histiocytic granulomata) Diabetes insipidus with electrolyte problems, hepatic failure, pancytopenia, respiratory failure, laryngeal involvement. May be on steroids. Intubation difficulties due to small larynx. (Lieberman P. H. et al. *Medicine (Baltimore)* 1969, **48**, 375.)

Hare lip *See* Chapter 4.2 Cleft palate and paediatric anaesthesia.

Hay–Wells syndrome Difficult intubation (maxillary hypoplasia)

Henoch–Schonlein purpura Bruising tendency with haemmorrhage risk.

Hepatolenticular degeneration (Kinnier–Wilson disease) Defect in copper metabolism, hepatic failure, epilepsy, trismus, weakness and sensitivity to relaxants.

Hermansky syndrome (thrombasthenia, albinism) Bruising, platelet infusion may be required.

Holt–Oram syndrome (hand–heart syndrome) Congenital cardiac septal defects. (Lewis M. et al. *J. Am. Med. Assoc.* 1965, **193**, 1080.)

Homocystinuria A recessive inborn error of metabolism due to deficiency of cystothionine synthetase. Thromboses, pulmonary embolism (requiring heparinization), lens dislocation, osteoporosis, mental handicap, hypoglycaemia, urinary calculi and renal failure occur. (Carson N. A. J. *Br. J. Hosp. Med.* 1969, **2**, 439.)

Hunter syndrome (mucopolysaccharidosis II) Thoracic skeletal abnormalities with respiratory failure, cardiomyopathy, stiff joints, laryngeal and pharyngeal involvement with obstruction, macroglossia and increased secretions, all making intubation difficult. (Gilbertson A. A. and Boulton T. B. *Anaesthesia* 1967, **22**, 607.) C. H. Hunter (1872–1965), English paediatrician.

Huntington's chorea *See* Chapter 3.1. G. H. Huntington (1850–1916), New York neurologist.

Hurler syndrome (gargoylism, mucopolysaccharidosis I) Death before puberty from cardiac involvement, with aortic and mitral incompetence. Difficult intubation due to macroglossia and increased secretions; chest infections, heart failure. (Wilder R. T. and Belani K. G. *Anesthesiology* 1990, **72**, 205.)

Hydatid disease Pulmonary, hepatic, cardiac, renal and cerebral cysts may cause local problems.

Hydrocephalus If there is a ventriculo-atrial valve in place antibiotic cover is often advised before operation. The large occiput may make intubation difficult so that the body should be raised on a pillow or mattress. Great care needed in supporting head while unconscious.

Hyperparathyroidism May be associated with hypercalcaemia with danger of cardiac arrest. Risk temporarily diminished by potassium infusion. For anaesthesia *see* The experts opine. *Surv. Anesthesiol. 1985,* **29,** 72.

Hyperpituitarism *See* 'Medical diseases' Chapter 3.1.

Hyperviscosity syndrome (Waldenstom's macroglobulinaemia, multiple myeloma) Thrombosis risk. Preoperative plasmapheresis may be required. (Urbaniak S. J. and Robinson E. A. *Br. Med. J.* 1990, **300,** 662–665.)

Hyperthermia syndrome *See* 'Malignant hyperpyrexia' Chapter 3.1.

Hypokalaemic familial periodic paralysis Sensitivity to relaxants and risk of arrythmias. *See* Chapter 3.1.

Hypoparathyroidism (*see also* Albright's osteodystrophy) Hypersensitivity to sedatives and anaesthetics; hypocalcaemia with muscular weakness and tetany. Perioperative CaC_{12} or Ca gluconate may be needed.

I-cell disease (mucopolysaccharidosis VII) Hernias; pulmonary problems due to thick secretions, with airway obstruction, and chest-wall deformities. Difficult to intubate because of stiff neck. Cardiac valvular lesions coexist.

Ichthyosis A congenital condition in which there may be difficulty in fixing an extradural catheter to the skin, if adhesives are used. (Smart G. and Bradshaw E. G. *Anaesthesia* 1984, **39,** 161.)

Idiopathic myoglobinuria *See* Chapter 3.1.

Idiopathic thrombocytopenic purpura Bruising, haemorrhage. Heparin and aspirin are avoided. May be on steroids. Platelet infusions for surgery, rebound thromboses after splenectomy.

Infective mononucleosis Airway obstruction due to enlarged tonsils may prove fatal. (Catling S. J. et al. *Anaesthesia* 1984, **39,** 699; Carrington P. and Hall J. I. *Br. Med. J.* 1986, **292,** 195.)

Insulinoma For removal of, see Muir J. J. et al. *Anesthesiology* 1983, **59,** 371.

Ivemask syndrome Asplenia, situs inversus, dextrocardia, cyanotic heart disease.

Jaw, congenital fusion of in a neonate (Seraj M. A. et al. *Anaesthesia* 1984, **39,** 695.)

Jehovah's Witnesses Blood transfusion refused. These patients sign a special consent absolving doctors from problems arising from failure to transfuse blood or blood products. Extracorporeal circuits are usually acceptable.

For anaesthesia, *see* Harris T. J. B. et al. *Anaesthesia* 1983, **38,** 989, and in heart surgery, Henderson A. M., Maryniak J. K. et al. *Anaesthesia* 1986, **41,** 748; Wong D. H. W. and Jenkins L. C. *Can. J. Anaesth.* 1989, **36,** 578–585, *Management of Anaesthesia for Jehovah's Witnesses.* Association of Anaesthetists, London, 1999.

Jervell–Lange–Nielsen syndrome Deafness with cardiac dysrhythmias, long QT interval and enlarged T wave. Risk of cardiac arrest. Pacemaker insertion may help. (Jervell A. et al. *Am. Heart J.* 1957, **54,** 59). For anaesthesia, see Medak R. and Benumof J. L. *Br. J. Anaesth.* 1983, **55,** 361; Freshwater J. V. *Br. J. Anaesth.* 1984, **56,** 655; Ryan H. *Can. J. Anaesth.* 1988, **35,** 422–424.

Jeune's syndrome Lung problems due to chest-wall deformity.

Kaposi's sarcoma Pigmented sarcoma of the skin. M.K. Kaposi (1837–1902), Austrian dermatologist. May be associated with AIDS.

Kartagener's syndrome Dextrocardia, sinusitis, bronchiectasis (due to defective ciliary function), immunoincompetence.

Kasabach–Merritt syndrome Rarely survive more than a few weeks from birth, enlarging haemangioma with haemorrhage and thrombocytopenia. May be on steroids.

Kawasaki disease Children who have had this disease, and not been treated with gamma-globulin in the first 10 days, may have coronary and other aneurysms and are at risk of cardiac infarction even during operations.

Kearns–Sayer syndrome The reaction to muscle relaxants is normal, but complete and sudden heart block may develop during anaesthesia. (D'Ambra M. N. et al. *Anesthesiology* 1979, **51,** 343.)

Kelly–Paterson syndrome (Plummer–Vinson syndrome, sideropenic dysphagia) In the very advanced case, regurgitation on induction.

King Denborough disease Malignant hyperpyrexia association.

Klinefelter syndrome Crush fractures of osteoporotic vertebrae. May be very large in adult life. H. K. Klinefelter (1912–), Baltimore physician.

Klippel–Feil syndrome (congenital fusion of cervical vertebrae) Difficult intubation; cleft palate; neurological defects, scoliosis and VSD may coexist (Klippel M. and Feil A. *Soc. Anat. Paris Bull. et Memb.* 1912, **14,** 185). For anaesthesia *see* Naguib M. et al. *Can. Anaesth. Soc. J.* 1986, **33,** 60.

Klippel–Trenaunay syndrome (angio-osteohypertrophy) High output failure, thrombocytopenia, cleft palate, short wide neck and inability to extend neck.

Kneist's syndrome Difficult intubation due to stiff neck.

Kugelberg Welander syndrome (spinal muscular atrophy) Respiratory problem due to muscle weakness. Caution needed with relaxants.

Kwashiorkor Difficult to intubate due to pterygoid fibrosis. Low serum electrolytes and serum cholinesterase.

Larsen's syndrome (multiple joint dislocations) Difficult intubation due to unstable neck, pulmonary infections. (Wooley M. W. et al. *J. Ped. Surg.* 1967, **2,** 325.)

Laryngomalacia Upper airway obstruction with snoring, not relieved by an airway, especially in the paediatric patient.

Laryngotracheoesophageal cleft See Armitage E. N. *Anaesthesia* 1984, **39,** 706.

Laurence–Moon–Biedl syndrome Obesity, polydactyly, mental retardation; associated congenital heart disease, renal failure with diabetes insipidus.

Leber's disease Congenital optic atrophy. There may be idiopathic hypoventilation with sensitivity to diazepam and mild analgesics. *See* Hunter A. R. *Anaesthesia* 1984, **39,** 781.

Leiden factor V mutation See Factor V (Chapter 3.2).

Lentiginosis Hypertrophic cardiomyopathy may coexist.

Leopard syndrome Multiple leopard skin spots, hypertelorism, severe pulmonary stenosis. (*Scott. Med. J.* 1983, **28,** 300; Rodrigo M. R. C., Cheng C. H., Tai Y. T. and O'Donnell D. *Anaesthesia* 1990, **45,** 30).

Leprechaunism Abnormal endocrine state, mentally defective; hyperinsulinism, hypoglycaemia, renal failure. Maintenance of blood glucose during starvation is a priority.

Leprosy Leprosy patients are often on steroids. Some parts of the body may be analgesic.

Lesch–Nyhan syndrome (hyperuricaemia) Renal failure before puberty.

Letterer–Siwe disease (histiocytosis) As for leukaemia; gingivitis with very loose teeth, intrinsic lung disease.

Leukaemia Anaemia, thrombocytopenia, veins may be difficult. May be on steroids.

Lingual vein thrombosis Severe upper airways obstruction, mouth breathing impossible, nose breathing difficult, laying down may be impossible. Helium/oxygen mixture useful until fibreoptic intubation is achieved. (Approaching the patient in the sitting position from the front, the fibreoptic 'picture' is reversed.)

Lipodystrophy Liver failure, renal failure, diabetes, with anaemia. Halothane is to be avoided.

Lowe syndrome (oculocerebrorenal syndrome) Renal failure, hypocalcaemia, acidosis.

Ludwig's angina Acute airway obstruction. Difficult intubation due to infection. Woody swelling of floor of mouth, with trismus, unrelieved by suxamethonium or other relaxants. A gas induction or fibreoptic intubation is usually performed for anaesthesia.

Lyme disease Spirochaetal disease named after the town of origin. Intense pain requiring opioids, myocarditis occurs 6 weeks after initial attack, with atrioventricular block. Treated by penicillin, tetracycline, Ceftriaxone. Anaesthesia is postponed until remission. *See* Bateman D. E. *Hospital Update* 1990, **16,** 677–682.

McArdle's disease Glycogenosis V. A hereditary myopathy causing glycogen to accumulate in muscle, with weakness and respiratory problems, and cardiomyopathy. Atracurium appears to be a safe agent for the production of muscle relaxation in short procedures. Suxamethonium is to be avoided. *See* Rajah A. and Bell C. F. *Anaesthesia* 1986, **41,** 93.

Macroglossia Intubation and airway problem. Often a feature of congenital syndromes, e.g. Down's.

Mafucci syndrome (enchondromas and haemangiomas) Anaemia, sensitivity to vasodilator drugs, fragile bones, labile blood pressure.

Mandibulofacial dysostosis (Treacher–Collins syndrome) Micrognathia, difficult intubation; fibreoptic intubation is usually required. Coexistent congenital heart disease sometimes. Tracheal ventilation via a 16-G needle has proved useful. (Smith R. B. et al. *Br. J. Anaesth.* 1974, **46,** 313; Collins E. and Treacher J. *Trans. Ophthal. Soc. UK.* 1900, **20,** 190.)

Maple syrup urine disease (branched chain ketonuria with neuropathy) A metabolic disease of children involving an accumulation of ketoacids and amino-acids in the blood and urine, with abnormalities of blood sugar and electrolytes. *See* Delaney A. and Gal T. J. *Anesthesiology* 1976, **44,** 83.

Marchiafava–Michaeli syndrome Auto-immune haemolytic anaemia with paroxysmal nocturnal dyspnoea and venous thromboembolism. May be on steroids.

Marfan's syndrome (arachnodactyly, congenital connective tissue disorder) Emphysema, cataracts, high arched palate, pneumothorax, coronary thrombosis, dissecting aneurysms, easily dislocated joints, aortic and mitral regurgitation, kyphoscoliosis. (Wooley M. W. et al. *J. Ped. Surg.* 1967, **2,** 325.) Young patients with this syndrome are a high anaesthetic risk group (Verghese C. *Anaesthesia* 1984, **39,** 917). *See also* Annotation, *Br. Med. J.* 1982, **285,** 464. For maternal outcome of pregnancy in Marfan's syndrome *see* Lipscomb K. J., Smith J. C., Clarke B., Donnai P. and Harris R. *Br. J. Obstet. Gynecol.* 1997, **104,** 201–206. B. J. A. Marfan (1858–1943), Paris paediatrician (1896).

Maroteaux–Lamy syndrome (mucopolysaccharidosis IV) Cardiomyopathy, respiratory failure (partly due to chest-wall deformity), anaemia, thrombocytopenia. (Gilbertson A. A. and Boulton T. B. *Anaesthesia* 1967, **22,** 607.)

Myalgia encephalitis ('ME') Postviral weakness. Caution with dosage of non-depolarizing relaxants due to debility and reduction of muscle mass. Short-acting agents desirable (e.g. propofol, alfentanil, remifentanil), especially for day-cases. In the extreme case, reduction of myocardial muscle may pose a risk.

Meckel's syndrome (Mekel–Gruber Syndrome) (microcephaly, micrognathia, congenital cardiac disease, and polycystic kidneys) Difficult intubation, renal failure. Encephalocele and cleft palate may be present. J. F. Meckel (1781–1833), anatomist from Halle.

Median cleft face Difficult intubation due to micrognathia.

Meig's syndrome (ovarian cyst with embarrassing pleural effusion) The effusion should be tapped before anaesthesia to relieve respiratory failure. J. V. Meig (1892–1963), Boston gynaecologist.

Methaemoglobinaemia Exacerbated by prilocaine (*see* Chapter 3.1).

Mikulicz's syndrome (salivary and lachrymal gland enlargement) Difficult airway and intubation sometimes, due to glandular enlargement. It has been suggested that atropine and hyoscine are best avoided. J. von Mikulicz Radecki (1850–1905), Breslau surgeon.

Moebius' syndrome A rare congenital abnormality of the cranial nerves. Difficult intubation due to micrognathia. *See* Krajcirik W. J. et al. *Anesth. Analg. (Cleve.)* 1985, **64**, 371.

Mongolism See Down's syndrome.

Morquio's syndrome (mucopolysaccharidosis IV) Kyphoscoliotic dwarfs with atlanto-axial instability, making intubation difficult. Respiratory and cardiac failure by early adult life. Aortic incompetence. (Gilbertson A. A. and Boulton T. B. *Anaesthesia* 1967, **22,** 607; Birkinshaw K. J. *Anaesthesia* 1975, **30**, 46.)

Moschkowitz disease (a form of thrombocytopenic purpura) Renal damage. May be on steroids.

Motor neurone disease A progressive disease with muscle fasciculation and weakness. Hypersensitivity to all muscle relaxants. Laryngeal incompetence. Lung cancer may be present. *See also* Amyotrophic lateral sclerosis.

Moya-moya disease A rare and dangerous abnormality of the cerebral circulation with narrowing or occlusion of the anterior and middle cerebral arteries, first described in Japan in 1961. For anaesthesia *see* Bingham R. M. and Wilkinson D. J. *Anaesthesia* 1985, **40**, 1198. Brown S. C., Lam A. M. *Can. J. Anaesth.* 1987, **34**, 71–75. Straining, e.g. in labour, must be avoided. If general anaesthesia is unavoidable, a neuroanaesthetic is least open to criticism.

Mucopolysaccharidosis A hereditary connective-tissue disorder with deposition of abnormal amounts of mucopolysaccharides in body tissues. May be difficulties with airways and intubation because of secretions. Preoperative tracheostomy may occasionally be required. Other problems very slow recovery; with breath holding, bronchospasm and frequent cyanosis, postoperative dehydration and chest infection. A light premedication with oral diazepam and glycopyrronium, and antibiotics for those with valvular lesions has been described. (Baines D. and Keneally J. P. *Anaesth. Intensive Care* 1983, **11**, 198; Kempthorne P. M. and Brown T. C. K. *Anaesth. Intensive Care* 1983, **11**, 203; King D. H. et al. *Anaesthesia* 1984, **39**, 126; Brown T. C. K. *Anaesth. Intensive Care* 1984, **12**, 178; Herrick I. A., Rhine E. J. *Can. J. Anaesth.* 1988, **35**, 67–73.)

Multiple endocrine adenomatosis type IIb React as phaeochromocytoma.

Multiple mucosal neuroma syndrome May make intubation difficult.

Multiple myelomatosis Pathological fractures, especially of vertebrae, care needed in positioning. Hypercalcaemia, anaemia, hyperviscosity, renal failure, coagulopathies.

Multiple sclerosis *See* Disseminated sclerosis.

Muscular dystrophy Weak flaccid skeletal and eventually cardiac muscles. Sensitivity to atropine, opiates, thiopentone and non-depolarizing relaxants, which may not reverse after anticholinesterase drugs. May be confined to ocular muscles (Robertson, J. A. *Anaesthesia* 1984, **39**, 251). May be associated with a hyperpyrexial reaction. *See* Duchenne muscular dystrophy. Various other syndromes occur, usually with cardiomyopathy, e.g. Dreyfuss (limb girdle affected).

Myasthenia gravis and myasthenia congenita *See* Medical diseases (Chapter 3.1). There is weakness and extreme sensitivity to relaxants. Preoperative plasmapheresis may be required (Urbaniak S. J. and Robinson E. A. *Br. Med. J.* 1990, **300**, 662–665). May be on steroids and azathioprine. Isoflurane is useful (Nilsson E. and Muller K. *Acta Anaesth. Scand.* 1990, **34**, 126), as are regional blocks. Postoperative intensive care, with IPPV, is often needed.

Myasthenic syndrome Often due to carcinomatous myopathy, more commonly seen in older men. For anaesthesia during treatment with 3, 4-diaminopyridine, *see* Telford R. J. and Hollway T. E. *Br. J. Anaesth.* 1990, **64**, 363.

Myositis ossificans Difficult intubation sometimes due to stiff neck. In severe cases, reduction of thoracic compliance with respiratory failure. May be on steroids.

Myotonia congenita (Thomsen's disease) *See* Dystrophia myotonica. (Ravin M. et al. *Anaesth. Analg.* 1975, **54**, 216.) A. J. T. Thomsen (1815–1896), Danish physician.

Nemaline myopathy Inadequate ventilation due to muscle weakness. Sensitivity to non-depolarizing relaxants. Malignant hyperpyrexia association.

Neurofibromatosis Fibromas may occur in larynx or heart, excessive response to relaxants; rarely associated with phaeochromocytomas. (*See* von

Recklinghausen's disease.) F. D. von Recklinghausen (1833–1910), German pathologist.

Neuromuscular syndromes Associated with malignant disease, e.g. Eaton–Lambert syndrome.

Niemann–Pick disease (sphingomyelin infiltration, xanthomatosis) Anaemia, thrombocytopenia, respiratory failure.

Noack's syndrome (craniosynostosis) Sometimes difficult to intubate due to micrognathia.

Noonan syndrome Micrognathia, short, webbed neck, pectus excavatus, heart disease (pulmonary stenosis, VSD, hypertrophic cardiomyopathy), renal failure.

Ollier disease Great care required with joints.

Opitz–Frias syndrome The hypospadias dysphagia syndrome; the G syndrome. Rare congenital condition with genital and craniofacial abnormalities. (Opitz J. M. et al. *Birth Defects* 1969, **5**, 95.) For anaesthesia *see* Bolsin S. N. and Gillbe C. *Anaesthesia* 1985, **30**, 1189.

Orofacial–digital syndrome Cleft palate may coexist. Renal failure occurs.

Osler–Weber–Rendu syndrome See Haemorrhagic telangiectasia. W. Osler (1849–1919), physician, Baltimore and Oxford; F. Parkes Weber (1863–1962), London physician; H. J. Rendu (1844–1902), French physician.

Osteogenesis imperfecta (fragilitas ossium) Fragile bones, teeth easily damaged, excessive haemorrhage during surgery. Occasional respiratory problem due to chest-wall deformity. Malignant hyperpyrexia association. (Robinson C. and Wright D. J. *Today's Anaesthetist* 1986,**1**, 22; Cunningham A. J. et al. *Anesthesiology* 1984, **61**, 91.)

Osteopetrosis Similar to Osteogenesis imperfecta.

Ovarian hyperstimulation syndrome A self-limiting condition where excess vasoactive and endothelial peptides are secreted causing ARDS and systemic inflammatory response syndrome (SIRS), often requiring intensive care. Ascites is common.

Pancreatitis, acute High serum amylase levels. Severe toxaemia and shock, hypocalcaemia, relaxant reversal difficulties. Intensive care is indicated. ARDS may follow surgery. Surgery and anaesthesia are better avoided if possible.

Paramyotonia congenita Weakness and myotonia induced by exposure to cold. Sensitivity to relaxants, electrolyte abnormalities. Halothane and suxamethonium are better avoided.

Paraplegia Autonomic instability, liability to bedsores. Hyperkalaemia may follow suxamethonium. (For neuromuscular monitoring in tetraparesis *see* Fiacchine F., Bricchi M. and Lasio G. *Anaesthesia* 1990, **45**, 128.)

Parkinson's disease Restriction of movement of chest wall may give postoperative chest problems. (Severn A. *Br. J. Anaesth.* 1988, **61**, 761–770, ibid 1989, **62**, 580–581; Marsden C. D. *Lancet* 1990, **335**, 948.)

Patau syndrome (trisomy 13) Micrognathia, difficult to intubate due to micrognathia and cleft palate. VSD and dextroversion; microcephaly with skin defects.

Pellagra Neuropathy and difficult intubation.

Pemphigus vulgaris May be septic, and on steroids and immunosuppressives.

Pendred's disease Goitre may be found.

Pfeiffer's syndrome Craniostenosis, (may be very haemorrhagic operation, with difficult airway afterwards), syndactyly.

Pharyngeal pouch Regurgitation of contents, not controlled by cricoid pressure, rapid sequence intubation, intubation under local analgesia, etc. The pouch should be emptied manually by the patient before anaesthesia, or by carefully directed large bore nasogastric tube.

Phenylketonuria Sensitivity to opioids and barbiturates, so inhalation induction is recommended. Epileptic fits, hypoglycaemia.

Pierre–Robin syndrome Micrognathia, posterior displacement of the tongue, a hypoplastic mandible with glossoptosis, small epiglottis, high arched or cleft palate. Respiratory obstruction occurs, which tends to disappear after the age of 2 years. It may be necessary to suture the tongue to the alveolar ridge of the mandible to relieve respiratory obstruction. Such cases may be very difficult to intubate. The child should be nursed in the prone position both before and after operation.

Plummer–Vinson syndrome *See* Kelly–Paterson syndrome. H. S. Plummer (1874–1936), Mayo Clinic physician; P. P. Vinson (1890–1959), US surgeon.

Pneumatosis cystoides intestinalis Nitrous oxide is contraindicated. *See* Sutton D. N. and Ooskitt K. R. *Anaesthesia* 1984, **39**, 776.

Pneumoconiosis Pulmonary fibrosis and emphysema, excessive sputum, reduced compliance, cyanosis. May be on steroids.

Polyarteritis nodosa *See* Chapter 3.1.

Polycystic kidneys Renal failure, pulmonary cysts may coexist with danger of pneumothorax; 1 in 7 have cerebral aneurysms. Polycystic liver may coexist.

Polycythaemia May be associated with cardiorespiratory failure, congenital shunts, etc. Hyperviscosity thromboses are a risk. Isovolaemic predonation of blood may be helpful in the severe case. Haemmorrhage may be a problem in polycythaemia rubra vera.

Polymyositis *See* dermatomyositis.

Polysplenia Associated congenital heart disease.

Pompe's disease *See* Glycogenoses. Difficult to intubate because of macroglossia. Respiratory problems due to muscle weakness, and cardiomyopathy.

Porphyrias Paralytic crises precipitated by barbiturates, hydroxydione, diazepoxide, anticonvulsants, nikethamide and other non-anaesthetic drugs. Regional anaesthesia is possible. (McNiell M. J. and Bennet A. *Br. J. Anaesth.* 1990, **64**, 371.)

Potter's syndrome (Potter E. L. *Am. J. Obstet. Gynecol.* 1946, **51**, 855 and 559; Potter E. L. *Obstet. Gynecol.* 1965, **25**, 3.) Oligohydramnios in the mother and renal agenesis, typical facies and pulmonary hypoplasia in the baby. In spite of intubation, ventilation may be impossible (Van der Weyden, E. *Anaesth. Intensive Care* 1982, **10**, 90).

Prader–Willi syndrome Patients have (after the neonatal phase) extreme obesity, polyphagia, dental caries, congenital muscle hypotonia (with respiratory problems), mental retardation, hypogonadism and sometimes cardiovascular abnormalities. Blood glucose should be maintained intravenously during fasting. May be very large in adult life. (Mayhew J. F. and Taylor B. *Can. Anaesth. Soc. J.* 1983, **30**, 565; Yamashita M. et al. *Can. Anaesth. Soc. J.* 1983, **30**, 179.) A. Prader, H. Willi (1900–1971), Zurich paediatricians. (Prader A. et al. *Schweiz. Med. Wochenschr.* 1956, **86**, 1260; Ward O. C. *J. R. Soc. Med.* 1997, **90**, 694–696.)

Progeria (premature ageing) Myocardial ischaemia, hypertension, cardiomegaly. The patient, though small, looks old.

Progressive external ophthalmoplegia (PEO) All induction agents used intravenously should be given slowly and in small dosage (James R. H. *Anaesthesia* 1986, **41**, 216).

Progressive muscular dystrophy *See* 'Medical diseases' (Chapter 3.1).

Prolonged QT syndrome An inherited condition causing attacks of dysrhythmia leading to syncope. Has been treated with beta-blockers. *See* O'Callaghan A. C. et al. *Anaesth. Intensive Care* 1982, **10**, 50.

Prune belly syndrome (pseudoxanthoma elasticum, congenital absence of abdominal muscles) Inability to cough due to muscle weakness, causes postoperative respiratory problems. Renal failure may coexist. (Henderson A. M. et al. *Anaesthesia* 1987, **42**, 54.)

Pseudoxanthoma elasticum (Groenblad–Strandberg disease) Fragility of all connective tissue including upper airways, the heart, (with high incidence of coronary artery disease, hypertension, valve disease and dysrhythmias) and the retina. Thromboses are a problem. Fixation of intravenous lines may be difficult. *See* Ehlers–Danlos syndrome.

Pulmonary cysts Increase in size (especially with N_2O) with possible rupture during anaesthesia.

Pulmonary hypertension (primary) For extradural analgesia in, *see* Davies M. J. and Beavis R. *Anaesth. Intensive Care* 1984, **12**, 165.

Reiger's syndrome As for Dystrophia myotonica. The teeth are abnormal.

Rett syndrome Females with dementia, autism, movement disorders and abnormal respiratory control. Maquire D. and Bachman C. *Can. J. Anaesth.* 1989, **36**, 478–481.

Rheumatoid arthritis and Still's disease Difficult intubation, with risk of atlanto-axial subluxation, difficult veins, poor spontaneous respiration. May be on steroids. Great care is needed with padding and support on the operating table. *See* Chapter 3.1.

Rickets Kyphoscoliotic respiratory limitation, difficult spinal analgesia, hypocalcaemia.

Riley–Day syndrome *See* Dysautonomia and Familial dysautonomia.

Ritter disease Fragile skin, difficult veins.

Romano–Ward syndrome (Romano C. et al. *Clin. Pediatr.* 1963, **45**, 656; Ward O. C. *J. Irish Med. Assoc.* 1964, **54**, 103.) Congenital delay of cardiac depolarization and prolonged QT interval. May cause sudden death at any age during induction of anaesthesia; Transvenous pacing and stellate ganglion block have been used to prevent this (Callaghan M. L. et al. *Anesthesiology* 1977, **47**, 67–69; Ponte J. and Lund J. *Br. J. Anaesth.* 1981, **53**, 1347).

Rubinstein syndrome (microcephaly, chronic lung disease) Associated congenital heart disease.

Russel–Silver syndrome Short stature, facial asymmetry, micrognathia, macroglossia, cafe-au-lait spots, sweating, fasting hypoglycaemia and mental deficiency. Difficult airway and intubation, blood-glucose monitoring required.

Saethre–Chotzen syndrome *See* Chotzen syndrome.

San Filippo syndrome (mucopolysaccharidosis III) No specific problems. (Gilbertson A. A. and Boulton T. B. *Anaesthesia* 1967, **22**, 607.)

Sarcoidosis Pulmonary and laryngeal fibrosis, cardiac failure, dysrhythmias, hypercalcaemia. May be on steroids.

Scleroderma (diffuse thickening of skin, fibrosis leading to muscle degeneration in the diaphragm which may contribute to respiratory problems. Blood pressure is difficult to measure, poor lung compliance) Difficult intubation due to restricted mouth opening, difficult veins, regurgitation, respiratory failure, hypovolaemia, hypotension, renal failure, prolonged action of local analgesics. May be on steroids. (Birkhan J. et al. *Anaesthesia* 1972, **27**, 89; Sweeney B. *Anaesthesia* 1984, **39**, 1145; Iliffe G. D. and Pettigrew N. M. *Br. Med. J.* 1985, **286**, 337.)

Scurvy Anaemia, bruising, loose teeth. Surgical haemorrhage is severe.

Sebaceous naevus disease Congenital cardiac disease may coexist.

Senile hypertrophic cardiomyopathy Often unrecognized and dangerously asymptomatic; severe cardiac failure or arrest is a risk.

Sheie disease (mucopolysaccharidosis V) Hernias, joint stiffness, aortic incompetence in adult life.

Shprintzen syndrome Difficult to intubate (micrognathia). Deafness and congenital cardiac abnormalities occur.

Shy–Drager syndrome (central nervous and autonomic degeneration) (Shy G. M. and Drager G. A. *Arch. Neurol.* 1960, **2**, 51; King D. H. et al. *Br. J. Anaesth.* 1984, **39**, 126.) Highly labile blood pressure, ephedrine suitable for hypotensive crises. Cardiac dysrhythmias occur. It has been suggested that methoxyflurane, cyclopropane and ether be avoided. *See* Hutchinson R. C. and Sugden J. C. *Anaesthesia* 1984, **39**, 1229.

Siamese twins *See* Conjoined twins.

Sick sinus syndrome Uncoordinated atrial activity; dissociation of atrial from ventricular rhythm, with tendency to ventricular fibrillation. Usually in elderly men. (Reid D. S. *Br. J. Hosp. Med.* 1984, **31**, 341). *See also* Chapter 3.1.

Sickle-cell disease *See* Chapter 3.1.

Silver syndrome (dwarfism, micrognathia) Difficult intubation sometimes. (*See* Russel–Silver syndrome.)

Simmonds' syndrome and Sheehan's syndrome (post-partum pituitary necrosis) As for Addison's disease. M. S. Simmonds (1855–1925), Hamburg pathologist; Sheehan H. L., British pathologist.

Sipple syndrome (multiple endocrine adenomatosis) As for phaeochromocytoma (*see* Chapter 3.1).

Sjögren's syndrome (keratoconjunctivitis sicca) Worsened by atropine and hyoscine, improved by humidification. H.S. Sjögren (1899–), Stockholm ophthalmologist.

Smith–Lemli–Opitz syndrome (micrognathia, mentally defective, hypoplasia of thymus) Difficult intubation, infection problems and intrinsic lung disease.

Spinal muscular atrophy type I (Seddon S. J. *Anaesthesia* 1985, **40**, 821.) *See* Kugelberg–Welander disease.

Sponylometaphyseal dysplasia Difficult to intubate due to neck.

Sporadic cardiomyopathy Often unrecognized and dangerously asymptomatic; severe cardiac failure or arrest is a risk.

Sprengel's syndrome Difficult intubation due to neck.

Stevens–Johnson syndrome *See* Erythema multiforme. Fragile skin, difficult veins. A. M. Stevens (1844–1945), US paediatrician; F. C. Johnson (1897–1934), US paediatrician. Cardiomyopathy is a risk factor.

Stickler's syndrome (progressive arthro-ophthalmopathy) Progressive myopia, retinal detachment, secondary glaucoma, pain and stiffness of joints with hypotonia, kyphoscoliosis, maxillary hypoplasia, occasional cleft palate, deafness, possible intubation problems.

Still's disease (juvenile chronic polyarthritis) Airway maintenance may be difficult because of limited movement of the jaws and of the cervical spine. Atlanto-axial subluxation due to erosion of the odontoid process may be present. Blind nasal intubation, or the use of the fibreoptic laryngoscope may be necessary. Ketamine is a useful drug here. G. F. Still (1868–1941), London paediatrician.

Sturge–Weber syndrome (cavernous angioma of face with intracranial involvement) Epilepsy and hemiparesis may occur. the facial or cervical angioma is a warning sign for the anaesthetist. W. A. Sturge (1850–1919), F. Parkes Weber (1863–1962), English physicians.

Syringomyelia Occasional respiratory failure. Fingers may be anaesthetic.

Systemic lupus erythematosus Anaemia, bruising, renal and respiratory failure, nasal skin involvement. May be on steroids.

Takayasu's disease see Thorburn J. R. and James M. F. M. *Anaesthesia* 1986, **41,** 734, Necrotising vasculitis of systemic and pulmonary arteries.

Tangier disease (analphalipoproteinaemia) Sensitivity to muscle relaxants, ischaemic heart disease, anaemia, thrombocytopenia.

TAR syndrome (thrombocytopenia, absent radius) Concomitant Fallot's tetralogy occurs.

Tetraparesis See Paraplegia.

Thalassaemia Haemolytic anaemia with jaundice and cyanosis, intubation difficulties have been described. Homozygous form has fetal haemoglobin (Hb), heterozygous forms HbC, HbE, HbS with sickling problems (*see* Chapter 3.1). SC disease may have a Hb of 10–12 g/dl; AS disease may have normal Hb. In crisis, O_2, analgesics, intravenous fluids 3 $l/m^2/h$, and antibiotics are required.

Total body irradiation In children, with high dosage, there is poor response to infections. *See* Lo J. N. and Buckley J. J. *Anesthesiology* 1984, **61,** 101.

Thrombocytopenic purpura Bruising, haemorrhage; preoperative plasmapheresis and platelet transfusion may be required if the count is < 80 000. Platelet numbers may rebound following splenectomy. (Urbaniak S. J. and Robinson E. A. *Br. Med. J.* 1990, **300,** 662–665.)

Tourette syndrome For anaesthetic implications *see* Morrison J. E. and Lockhart C. H. *Anesth. Analg. (Cleve.)* 1986, **65,** 200.

Tracheo-oesophageal-fistula Milk aspiration into lungs, stomach full of air, causing respiratory embarrassment. Intermittent positive-pressure ventilation difficult with low fistula. For anaesthesia in adults, *see* Chan C. S. *Anaesthesia* 1984, **39**, 158. (*See* 'Paediatrics', Chapter 4.2.)

Treacher-Collins syndrome *See* Mandibulofacial dysostosis. E. Treacher-Collins, British ophthalmologist. Difficult intubation (micrognathia, maxillary and mandibular hypoplasia), ear deformities occur.

Tricuspid incompetence Antibiotic cover is usual. Afterload reduction and preload increases have proved helpful. (Stone J. G. et al. *Anesth. Analg. (Cleve.)* 1980, **59**, 737.)

Trisomy 13 *See* Patau syndrome.

Trisomy 18 *See* Edwards' syndrome.

Trisomy 21 *See* Down's syndrome.

Trisomy 22 Severe hypoglycaemia during perioperative starvation requires intravenous glucose.

Tuberous sclerosis Renal failure, cardiac rhabdomyomas with dysrhythmias, lung cysts, which may rupture. Ash-leaf and cafe-au-lait spots.

Turner's syndrome (X0 chromosome with micrognathia, short webbed neck, aortic coarctation and stenosis; and renal anomalies) Difficult intubation, prolonged effects from renally excreted drugs.

Urbach–Wiethe disease (mucocutaneous hyalinosis) Difficult intubation due to small laryngeal opening.

Urine drinking in psychiatric patients Produces moderate to severe hyponatraemia, which requires correction before anaesthesia.

Down's syndrome anaesthesia problems

1 Resistance to sedatives, and possible dislike of doctors and injections; need for appropriate strong premedication.

2 Large size.

3 Difficult veins, possibly managed by gas induction with sevoflurane.

4 Excess salivation and large tongue.

5 Associated ASD and VSD, with risk of intracardiac shunting, sudden cardiac failure and endocarditis (need for antibiotics).

6 Immune deficiency with risk of infection.

7 Communication problems resulting in fear and failure to comply with instructions (e.g. not starved; eating EMLA and dressing; rapport with parents is essential).

8 Postoperative problems: restraint, pain, airway obstruction, hypoxia.

VATER syndrome   Ventricular septal defect and intrinsic pulmonary disease. Renal failure occurs.

Ventricular septal defect (VSD)   'The louder the murmur, the smaller the defect'. Antibiotic cover is usual. Volume loading and mild reduction of pulmonary vascular resistance is desirable (without hypotension) to keep the shunt left-to-right. If the shunt reverses, sudden cyanosis occurs. Carefully titrated doses of ephedrine will usually restore left-to-right shunt. Hypovolaemia is to be avoided.

Von Gierke's disease (glycogen storage problems with hepatic and renal failure)   Perioperative starvation gives severe hypoglycaemia and acidosis, requiring correction.

Von Hippel–Lindau syndrome (haemangioblastomas)   Associated with phaeochromocytoma; hepatic and renal failure. (Steiner A. C. et al. *Medicine* 1968, **47,** 371.)

Von Recklinghausen's disease (neurofibromatosis)   May have fibromas of pharynx, larynx (making intubation difficult); and heart; may have phaeochromocytoma, kyphoscoliosis, multiple lung cysts and renal failure. There is an excessive response, sometimes, to non-depolarizing relaxants and suxamethonium.

Von Willebrand's disease (pseudohaemophilia)   Defective platelet adhesiveness with factor VIII deficiency. Controlled by tranexamic acid, 1 g, and desmopressin (DDAVP), 4 μg, given slowly, intravenously, 1 h before operation, 4 h after operation, and 24 h after operation. Tranexamic acid is then continued, 1 g orally, 8-hourly, for a week. Cryoprecipitate is considered if this treatment fails to correct coagulopathy (Miller B. E, Mochizuki T. and Levy J. H. *Anesth. Analg.* 1997, **85,** 1196–1202). Salicylates are avoided. E. A. von Willebrand (1870–1949), physician, Finland.

Weaver's syndrome   Rare developmental condition with unusual craniofacial appearance and micrognathia with airway and intubation problems. May be very large in adult life. (Weaver D. D. et al. *J. Pediatr.* 1974, **84,** 547.) *See* Turner D. R. and Downing J. W. *Br. J. Anaesth.* 1985, **57,** 1260.

Weber–Christian disease (global fat necrosis)   Adrenal failure, occasional constrictive pericarditis. Subcutaneous fat must be carefully protected at operation. (Spirak J. L. et al. *Johns Hopkins Med. J.* 1970, **126,** 344.)

Wegener's granuloma (ulceration of midline structures of face)   Possible airway involvement causes difficulties, also renal failure. May be on steroids. F. Wegener (1907–), Berlin pathologist.

Welander's muscular atrophy (peripheral muscular atrophy)   Very sensitive to thiopentone, relaxants and opiates.

Werdnig–Hoffman disease (infantile muscular atrophy)   Respiratory failure, worsened by relaxants and opioids. G. W. Werdnig, Graz neurologist; J. Hoffman (1857–1919), Heidelberg neurologist.

Wermer syndrome (type I endocrine adenomatosis) Renal failure, severe hypoglycaemia, bronchial carcinoid tumours, hypercalcaemia.

Werner syndrome (premature ageing) (cf. Hutchinson Gilford syndrome; progeria) Myocardial ischaemia, diabetes, hypercalcaemia.

William's syndrome Congenital stenosis of aortic and pulmonary valves may coexist. Hypercalcaemia occurs in infancy (20%). Stellate blue eyes.

Wilm's tumour Anaemia (7 g/dl is the lower acceptable limit), IVC obstruction may occur due to the size of the tumour.

Wilson's disease (hepatolenticular degeneration from copper deposits) Hepatic and renal failure, with ventilatory problems and difficulty reversing relaxants. S. A. Kinnear Wilson (1877–1937), London neurologist.

Wiskott–Aldrich disease Anaemia and coagulopathy problems.

Wolf–Hirschorn syndrome A rare chromosomal abnormality. Patients have poor intrauterine growth, severe psychomotor retardation, characteristic facies, and various midline fusion abnormalities (Lazuk G. I. et al. *Clin. Genet.* 1980, **18**, 6). Malignant hyperpyrexia may occur. For anaesthetic management, *see* Ginsburg R. and Purcell-Jones G. *Anaesthesia* 1988, **43**, 386.

Wolff–Parkinson–White syndrome Electrocardiogram shows prolonged QRS and short PR interval due to various cardiac disorders; worsened by neostigmine. Tachycardia produces ST depression. Paroxysmal supraventricular tachycardia may accompany induction of anaesthesia, and progress to ventricular fibrillation. Prevention by transvenous pacing. Termination of paroxysmal supraventricular tachycardia by carotid sinus massage or with phenylephrine (Jacobson L. et al. *Anaesthesia* 1985, **40**, 657), propranolol 0.01 mg/kg i.v., or verapamil 0.1 mg/kg slowly i.v. DC cardioversion should be immediately available.

Wolman's disease Anaemia and clotting problems.

ANAESTHESIA FOR VARIOUS SURGICAL OPERATIONS AND SITUATIONS

Surgical operations and choice of anaesthetic

INTRODUCTION, SIMULATORS AND GENERAL CONDUCT OF ANAESTHESIA

This chapter of the *Synopsis of Anaesthesia* does not attempt to provide 'cook-book' techniques for each situation. Nor should it. Every patient is different from every other, and every anaesthetist is different from every other. However, the problems to be expected in common situations are outlined, together with general guidance and things to avoid.

THE CONDUCT OF SIMPLE ANAESTHETIC TECHNIQUES

Intravenous cannulation is performed (Nitescu P. et al. *Acta Anaesth. Scand.* 1990, **34,** 120; Gunawardene R. D. and Davenport H. T. *Anaesthesia* 1990, **45,** 52) and appropriate monitoring instituted.

1 The intravenous induction agent is given until loss of the eyelash reflex. This is still one of the best signs of adequate induction of anaesthesia. Nitrous oxide/air and O_2 is given and a volatile agent is increased steadily (pausing or giving more intravenous agent if breath-holding occurs). Anaesthesia is deepened until respiration is quiet and regular. An opioid may be given. An airway can be inserted if necessary, provided that there is no tongue movement on opening the mouth or foot movement on depressing the chin (Ballantine's sign (Ballantine R. I. W. *Anaesthesia* 1982, **37,** 214)). Surgery may then begin.

2 Where intubation and relaxation are required, e.g. for abdominal surgery, the intravenous induction agent is followed by an opioid and a relaxant and the patient intubated after an appropriate interval. Intermittent

positive-pressure ventilation (IPPV) is maintained with N_2O/O_2 and volatile (or other) agent at about 50% minimum alveolar concentration (MAC_{50}) as long as the relaxant (or any subsequent relaxant) is acting.

3 Total intravenous anaesthesia (TIVA) may be substituted for volatile agents.

There are of course multitudes of variations on these themes, but the aim is to find a balance between the four principles of an anaesthetic, i.e. absence of awareness, analgesia, relaxation and attenuation of the stress response (the 'quadrant of anaesthesia'). The emphasis on any one of these will depend on which operation is being performed and the needs of the patient.

Anaesthesia (or analgesia) may be regarded as a process of modification of the normal physiological reflex response to the stimuli provided by surgery and anaesthesia, i.e.

1 inhibition of the afferent part of the reflex system;
2 depression of the central synaptic mechanisms of coordination;
3 block of the efferent part of the reflex arc.

ATTENUATION OF THE STRESS RESPONSE TO SURGERY

This is a hormone-mediated response to the noxious effects of surgery, a reaction designed to preserve life in trauma. However, in the anaesthetic situation, while these responses are often helpful, they may have disadvantages, e.g. the accelerated clotting cascade may lead to venous thrombosis. The stress response includes the 'fear, fight and flight' activity of adrenaline, resistance to the effects of insulin and the secretion of endogenous steroids and growth hormone.

Attenuation of the stress response is achieved with short-acting opioids in doses in excess of those required for simple analgesia, and also by the use of regional blockade during and after surgery. The disadvantages of attenuation of the stress response is that protective reflexes, e.g. vascular reflexes during epidural analgesia, are also attenuated.

ANAESTHESIA SIMULATORS

These may be used for training purposes in knowledge and skills in general anaesthesia for surgical situations.

Benefits of simulators

1 Focus on early recognition of critical incidents.
2 No patient risk: even patient death can be simulated safely!

3 Can easily repeat otherwise rare critical events of all types, with improved performance of trainees in second attempts (reaction times, diagnostic strategies, upgrade of professional practice, and detection of crises).
4 Individual or group teaching can be given.
5 Errors and mistakes are allowed. Hypotheses may be tested.
6 The simulation may be stopped at any time, for discussion, relaxation of tension in the trainee, or analysis of mid-crisis.
7 Trainee is debriefed at the end using a video record.
8 Equally good for experienced or novice anaesthetists.
9 Used to assess behavioural skills and psychological strengths of trainees.
10 Useful in revalidation.

Types of scenario

Monitoring artifacts; airway problems; difficult intubation; oesophageal intubation; aspiration; hypovolaemia; O_2 failure; anaphylactic shock; hyperpyrexia; arrythmias; use of inotropes; cardiac infarction and tamponade.

Note: a poor performer must be allowed to regain confidence *before they leave the simulation session*.

ABDOMINAL AND GENERAL SURGERY

Requirements for general anaesthesia

1 Unconsciousness (unless regional analgesia is employed), with complete absence of awareness.
2 Prevention of gastric contents entering the glottis.
3 Suppression of reflex responses to surgical stimuli.
4 Good relaxation of the anterior abdominal wall.
5 Reasonably rapid return of consciousness and of the upper respiratory tract reflexes.

A technique of general anaesthesia for abdominal surgery

1 Preoxygenation/denitrogenation; intravenous induction, using 2.5% thiopentone or alternative agent and opioid.
2 Injection of a non-depolarizing relaxant in a dose sufficient to allow easy intubation, giving time for maximal neuromuscular block to occur, during which the lungs are gently inflated with a N_2O/O_2 mixture (if there is a risk of vomiting or regurgitation and consequent aspiration of stomach contents, suxamethonium may be preferred, to allow more rapid intubation).

3 Tracheal intubation after optional spraying of the larynx with no more than 3 ml of 4% lignocaine solution, followed by careful inflation of the tracheal cuff and testing for oesophageal intubation.

4 Maintenance with a (N_2/O_2) mixture and IPPV, with opioid and volatile agent, to ensure complete unconsciousness. More relaxant is given as required, monitored by clinical response or a nerve stimulator.

5 At the termination of the operation, an anticholinesterase is injected to overcome neuromuscular block, preceded by atropine or glycopyrronium to counteract its muscarine-like effects. The nerve stimulator may be used to gauge the adequacy of reversal.

6 When spontaneous respiration is established, suction and pharyngeal toilet, deflation of the cuff and removal of the tracheal tube can be effected. The patient is then transferred back to bed to receive O_2 by catheter or mask, in the lateral position to facilitate nursing and a clear airway.

7 Monitoring throughout the perioperative period may include arterial blood pressure, electrocardiogram (ECG), capnography, temperature, oximetry, etc.

Alternative techniques

1 Use of volatile agent as the main drug to provide anaesthesia and relaxation of the abdominal wall,

2 Regional block (with or without general anaesthesia to provide unconsciousness), e.g. extra- or intradural, abdominal field block.

Preparation for emergency operations

Fluid and electrolyte balance must be corrected when possible.

The problem of regurgitation and vomiting is not confined to obstetric and emergency abdominal operations, and if there is suspicion that the stomach is not empty a nasogastric tube (6–12 G, 4–7 mm diameter) should be passed through the nose or an oesophageal tube (12 G) passed through either the nose or mouth. The stomach should then be aspirated with the patient supine and on each side in turn. When there is retroperistalsis, e.g. in acute intestinal obstruction, the stomach may refill from the duodenum between the time of emptying and the introduction of the tracheal tube with the risk of the inhalation of intestinal contents.

Rapid-sequence induction and intubation

The technique to induce anaesthesia followed almost immediately by tracheal intubation (so-called 'crash induction') is designed to forestall the dangers of vomiting, regurgitation and aspiration of stomach contents. Following pre-oxygenation, the induction dose of intravenous agent is immediately followed by suxamethonium or another fast relaxant. An assistant, who must be properly trained, applies cricoid pressure as the patient loses consciousness, while the anaesthetist proceeds to tracheal intubation and inflation of the cuff. Cricoid pressure is released and the tube tested for correct positioning. When suxamethonium is contraindicated, rocuronium has been used. This gives reasonable intubating conditions earlier than when any other nondepolarizing agent is used.

Acute intestinal obstruction

Factors to be considered are as follows.

1 *The degree of circulatory collapse.*
2 *The presence or absence of regurgitation or vomiting.* The former is a passive process requiring no muscular force: the latter is a muscular reflex act. The former is aided by a head-down tilt and rendered less likely if the head is tilted upwards 45 degrees.
3 *The degree of distention of the abdomen.*
4 *The degree of electrolyte and fluid imbalance.* This must be controlled with infusion of Hartmann's or other appropriate solution. The moderately dehydrated patient has lost 6% of total body fluids. The severely dehydrated patient has lost 10% of total body fluids, and shows loss of skin elasticity, sunken eyes, dry tongue and oliguria.
5 In all bowel operations except those of the shortest duration, N_2O inhaled into the lungs may be partially excreted into the gut, causing distention. In both normal people and those with intestinal obstruction, much fluid is excreted by the proximal small intestine, only to be reabsorbed lower down. In high obstruction, this subsequent reabsorption is prevented. Low obstruction gives rise to distention. Vomiting causes loss of chlorides and alkalosis, and consequently great fluid loss and dehydration. Distention causes interference with circulation of the bowel wall, and pressure on the great veins results in reduced venous return to the heart, hypotension and interference with cardiac action due to increased intra-abdominal pressure.

Biochemical changes in intestinal obstruction include:

1 haemoconcentration;
2 metabolic acidosis (but alkalosis if vomiting is prominent);
3 diminution of serum chlorides;
4 increased blood urea and non-protein nitrogen;
5 acid urine, with perhaps ketone bodies and low urinary chloride;
6 hypokalaemia.

The stomach should be emptied by either a nasogastric or a wider bore oesophageal tube, preferably the latter. Grave illness does not make this any less necessary. The tube should be taken out before induction of anaesthesia but may be reintroduced after induction and retained until the return of the reflexes. A patient with increasing cyanosis, tightly clenched jaws and faeculent material issuing from the nose is a truly terrifying sight, and one which carries a bad prognosis. That which cannot be easily treated had better be prevented.

General anaesthesia is safer in shocked subjects. The actual agents and techniques used to produce general anaesthesia vary with different workers.

Intra- and extradural analgesia (with or without a light general anaesthetic) produce good relaxation, contract the bowel and do not interfere with the cough reflex (when used alone). They produce hypotension and are questionable in shocked, hypotensive and debilitated patients.

Elective operations on the colon and rectum

Maximal relaxation of the abdominal wall is necessary and contracted intestines an advantage. Extra- or intradural analgesia with light general anaesthesia, or light general anaesthesia with a muscle relaxant are suitable. Adequate intraoperative fluid replacement must be maintained during colon resection and anastomosis which is a prerequisite for successful healing.

Biliary tract surgery

Anaesthetic technique is similar to that used for gastric operations. Morphine may, by stimulating the sphincter of Oddi to contract, increase the intrabiliary pressure up to 20 cmH_2O and thus produce pain. Fentanyl raises intrabiliary pressure but the effect wanes within 25 min. Pethidine is probably the safest in this respect.

The following drugs lower intrabiliary pressure by relaxing the sphincter:

1 amyl nitrate;
2 nitroglycerin 1 mg;
3 papaverine 30 mg.

If an intraoperative choledochogram is required, apnoea for up to 30 s may be necessary.

Cases of *acute haemorrhagic pancreatitis* have a terrible operative prognosis; thus, obscure abdominal emergencies should have serum amylase tests done so that operation can be avoided. Hypocalcaemia may complicate pancreatitis and may result in difficult reversal of non-depolarizing relaxants.[1] Intravenous aprotinin (Trasylol), an inhibitor of kallikrein, has been recommended. For description of anaesthesia for *excision of islet cell tumour* of pancreas (*see* Insulinoma, Chapter 3.1).

Portal hypertension

Endoscopic injection of oesophageal varices is used. Problems: severe haemorrhage; anaemia; coma; extreme sensitivity to most anaesthetic drugs; cardiovascular instability; respiratory failure; alcoholic history; blood flooding the airway, full stomach, ammonia intoxication; cross-infection risk for personnel; etc. General anaesthesia is to be avoided if possible, and conducted with great caution if necessary.

Liver transplantation

This presents complex problems. Atracurium is the relaxant of choice. Large and fast blood transfusions require special pressurized warmed infusors and huge cannulae. Metabolic acidosis is likely to occur. Wisconsin cardioplege solution gives up to 12 h of preservation for the donor liver and rises in serum potassium are common during operation (but hypokalaemia may be a feature later on). In the *anhepatic phase*, citrate is not metabolized, drug disposition is highly abnormal, and transplantation of an ice-cold liver produces a fall in body temperature. Coagulation is monitored by thromboelastography.

Haemorrhoidectomy

Surgical assault on the anal region results in severe pain, reflex response, e.g. movement of body muscles, and reflex laryngeal spasm (Brewer–Luckhardt reflex).

Light general anaesthesia alone has no place here. Some surgeons request maximal relaxation of the anal sphincter while others prefer a certain amount of tone to be retained. Strong short-acting analgesics, e.g. remifentanil, alfentanil are helpful, but bradycardia may need correction. Intubation may be required.

Local infiltration with lignocaine or bupivacaine gives excellent postoperative pain relief. From a point 2.5 cm (1 in) posterior to the anus, with the index finger of the left hand in the rectum, 1.5% lignocaine–adrenaline solution is injected: total amount, 25 ml. Only one site of injection used, and anus and anal canal are ensheathed by a cylinder of solution.

REFERENCE

1 Mallett S. V. *Lancet* 1990, **336,** 886.

CARDIOTHORACIC ANAESTHESIA

THORACIC ANAESTHESIA

Preoperative considerations

Any underlying lung disease is usually obvious clinically and assessed by lung function tests. Smoking and the cardiac disease that often coexist pose added problems. It is not always easy to advise on the extent of any proposed lung resection, and predict outcome, especially if postoperative lung collapse or infection occurs.

Preoperative assessment will establish the extent of pulmonary disease and whether or not the patient is in the best state of preparation for surgery.

Assessment of pulmonary function

Formal measurement of pulmonary function should be performed routinely on all patients, although patients with a localized lesion or with no history of significant pulmonary disease may be exempt. Baseline function is most easily assessed using spirometry.

SPIROMETRY

The forced vital capacity (FVC), forced expired volume in 1 s (FEV_1), the ratio FEV_1/FVC and the peak expiratory flow rate (PEFR) can easily be measured at the bedside. If the flow rate is plotted against volume, a flow–volume loop can be obtained. Defects of spirometry are basically of two types: obstructive or restrictive.

An obstructive pattern is characterized by a reduction in FEV_1 and in the FEV_1/FVC ratio; the FVC is normal or slightly reduced.

A restrictive defect is characterized by a reduction in FVC but normal FEV_1/FVC ratio. Measurement of lung volume and gas transfer provide additional information.

ARTERIAL BLOOD GASES

Patients with chronic lung disease may have a low arterial O_2 tension and/or elevated CO_2 tension. Baseline measurement is routine.

Predictive value of pulmonary function tests[1]

No specific test can be used to predict morbidity and mortality. However, from the accumulated published data it would appear that a FVC or FEV_1 of less than 50% predicted and FEV_1/FVC ratio of less than 35% predicted are associated with an increased risk. Dyspnoea at rest and arterial hypoxaemia on room air also has predictive value.

Anaesthetic considerations

Open pneumothorax and lung collapse

Important features of IPPV are:

1 prevention of lung collapse;
2 the extent of lung movement in the operating field can be adjusted to suit the surgery;
3 deep anaesthesia is not needed;
4 it allows control of secretions;
5 it provides respiratory support for a patient with lung disease.

The lungs normally are kept inflated by the difference between atmospheric pressure in the alveoli and the negative pressure (about $-5\,cmH_2O$) in the potential space between the two layers of pleura. This balances the elastic recoil of the lung, and the tendency of the chest wall to spring outwards.

When the chest is opened, the negative pressure is lost and the elastic recoil causes collapse of the lung on that side. The mediastinum, unless fixed by adhesions, shifts towards the other side, compresses the healthy lung and interferes with cardiac function. If the lung is adherent to the chest wall, these effects may not be marked. The lung collapse causes $\dot{V}/\dot{Q}$ mismatch, shunting, hypoxia and a high pulmonary vascular resistance. If breathing spontaneously, the healthy lung breathes in and out partly from the trachea and partly from the other lung. This transfer of gas from one lung to the other is 'pendelluft', effectively increases dead space and can be lethal. These problems are overcome with IPPV, perhaps with the addition of positive end-expiratory pressure (PEEP).

The major disadvantage of IPPV is air leak from the lung if there is a bronchopleural fistula, or the creation of an air leak by rupture of emphysematous bullae.

Pulmonary secretions

Excessive secretions are uncommon, but occur in lung abscess, bronchiectasis, bronchopleural fistula and tumours, when infected secretions lie distal to an obstructed bronchus. Improvement may be obtained by preoperative postural drainage and antibiotics.

Methods for preventing the spread of secretions into healthy parts of the lungs during surgery include the following.

1 *Regional analgesia* and preserving the cough reflex, e.g. for drainage of empyema.
3 *Regular tracheal suction*, especially after the position is changed or the lungs manipulated.
3 *Surgical clamping of a bronchus*, as soon as the chest is open.
4 *Posture:* a drainage or an antidrainage posture may be employed. The patient can be positioned so that secretions from the diseased lung will flow into the trachea for suction and not contaminate the healthy lung. Alternatively, secretions can be retained in the diseased lobe, e.g. sitting

for lower lobectomy in bronchiectasis. An empyema is often drained with the patient sitting, especially if there is any chance of bronchopleural fistula.

5 *Endobronchial intubation* and blocking with inflatable cuffs.

Endobronchial instrumentation/intubation[2]

Isolation of one lung or major lobe has the following advantages:

1 secretions and blood are confined to the diseased area;
2 any bronchopleural fistula is isolated;
3 the lung to be operated upon is collapsed and still.

Methods include the use of a double-lumen (commonest) or single-lumen endobronchial tube. The former are not designed for use in children, but single-lumen bronchial tubes may be used. Bronchial blockers are now used very seldom.

DOUBLE-LUMEN ENDOBRONCIAL TUBES

One lumen ends just above the carina, the other extends into one main bronchus. There are versions to intubate left or right main bronchi, the right-sided tube having a slotted opening to allow inflation of the right upper lobe. The two tubes separate proximally for connection to two catheter mounts. The longer bronchial tube has a cuff which seals it in the main bronchus; a second cuff seals the whole tube in the trachea. Both cuffs have pilot balloons. The *Carlens* double-lumen tube was the first (originally used for differential bronchospirometry). The *Robertshaw* red rubber tube (three sizes: small, medium, large) was popular, now largely superseded by *disposable PVC double-lumen tubes*. These are easier to insert, and may cause less damage and be more economical.[3] Coaxial double-lumen tubes have been used.[4]

The double-lumen tube is passed into the trachea using an ordinary laryngoscope, and then advanced blindly until it reaches the natural end-point of resistance. The tracheal and bronchial cuffs are then inflated in turn, and checks made for leaks and correct positioning by inflating down each tube and auscultating the lung. Either lung can be ventilated, isolated or collapsed at will. Accurate placement may be difficult owing to alterations in anatomy or as a result of pathology, and may be checked further by fibreoptic bronchoscopy, and ultimately by the surgeon palpating the tube.

SINGLE-LUMEN ENDOBRONCHIAL TUBES

Normally left-sided, but if right-sided, the bronchial cuff is slotted to allow ventilation of the upper lobe. A tracheal cuff allows ventilation of both lungs and helps anchor the tube.

Macintosh and Leatherdale[5] described two tubes for right-lung surgery: a left-sided endobronchial tube with bronchial and tracheal cuffs and a small right-sided channel used to aspirate secretions or distend the right lung; an endotracheal tube combined with a left endobronchial cuffed suction blocker.

The *Green–Gordon* tube is right-sided, has a tracheal cuff and carinal hook, and is used for surgery on the left lung.

Magill endobronchial tubes are very long Magill tracheal tubes. The *Machray modification* has a short cuff.

The *Pallister* left endobronchial tube has a tracheal cuff and two bronchial cuffs, in case one is ruptured, as may happen during sleeve resection of the right upper lobe bronchus.[6] These last three are best inserted over a rigid or fibreoptic bronchoscope.[7] An intubating bronchoscope is the same diameter for its entire length, and has no lip at its tip, unlike a diagnostic bronchoscope.

The *Univent* is an endotracheal tube incorporating a movable bronchial blocker with a lumen for suction, giving O_2 or high-frequency ventilation.

ENDOBRONCHIAL INTUBATION IN INFANTS

An uncuffed tube, 1 cm longer than the distance from mouth to carina measured on the lateral chest radiograph, will tend to enter the bronchus on the opposite side to the bevel. The bevel is cut for the desired side, the tube passed into the bronchus and rotated through 180 degrees so that the upper lobe orifice is not obstructed. The bevel needs an extension on the right side to allow for the more proximal position of the right upper lobe orifice.

ENDOBRONCHIAL BLOCKERS

Passed through a rigid bronchoscope now seldom used. Fogarty or even Swan–Ganz catheters have been used in children.

PROBLEMS WITH ENDOBRONCHIAL TUBES

1 *Difficulty with insertion*, especially if anatomy is abnormal or distorted.
2 *Dislodgement*, during positioning the patient, and movement of the head and neck.
3 *Trauma*, to larynx and airways.
4 *Kinking*, of thin-walled single-lumen endobronchial tubes.
5 *Arterial hypoxaemia* during one-lung anaesthesia. Collapse of the upper lung and hypoxic pulmonary vasoconstriction increase its vascular resistance.

Nonetheless, blood does flow through this collapsed lung and the shunt causes hypoxaemia which is little improved by ventilation with 100% O_2. The lower lung will be at a disadvantage too, as its FRC will be reduced with some atelectasis.

These problems can be helped by:
(a) using a tidal volume large enough (about 12 ml/kg, but titrated against airway pressure) to reduce lower lung atelectasis, but not so large as to divert blood flow to the upper lung;
(b) cautious application of PEEP which can improve oxygenation in severe hypoxaemia[8] (but may divert blood to the upper lung and reduce cardiac output so worsening hypoxaemia);

   (c) insufflating, intermittently inflating, applying continuous positive airway pressure (CPAP) or using high-frequency jet ventilation in the collapsed lung with 100% O_2 – careful monitoring of arterial saturation is needed;
   (d) clamping the pulmonary artery when a pneumonectomy is performed.
6 *Hypercapnia*, which is seldom a problem in practice.

Principles of anaesthesia for thoracotomy[9]

Median sternotomy is used for access to the thymus, retrosternal goitres and anterior mediastinum; lateral thoracotomy is used for all other thoracic operations. For the problems posed by mediastinal masses, *see* Pullerits J. and Holzman R. *Can. J. Anaesth.* 1989, **36**, 681. Oat-cell bronchial carcinoma may be associated with *myasthenic syndrome* where there is marked sensitivity to all relaxants, *see* Chapter 3.1. Bleomycin therapy can cause pulmonary fibrosis, aggravated by a high F_1O_2.

Premedication should include a vagolytic drug and, depending on the patient's condition, a sedative agent. Atrial fibrillation may occur during or after thoracotomy (especially pneumonectomy), and the patient is often digitalized preoperatively.[10]

Invasive arterial and central venous pressure (CVP) monitoring are advisable and have the additional advantage of allowing assessment of arterial blood gases.

Most anaesthetic techniques including TIVA, have been used with success. Volatile anaesthetic agents have no significant adverse effect on the hypoxic pulmonary vasoconstrictor response at the concentrations used.[11]

Endobronchial techniques should be employed, although many lung resections can be carried out with ordinary endotracheal tubes. Intermittent positive-pressure ventilation is essential with an open chest (*see* above 'Open pneumothorax and lung collapse'). High-frequency jet ventilation during routine thoracotomy probably offers no advantage over conventional one or two-lung IPPV.[12,13]

Good analgesia is particularly important after thoracotomy to allow adequate respiration and coughing, and can be instituted preoperatively. Systemic opioids (i.v. infusion or PCA) are effective and are the cornerstone of analgesic therapy.[14,15] The following are also effective in reducing pain and analgesic consumption: intercostal and interpleural catheters for local analgesics; thoracic epidural opioids, low-dose ketamine and non-steroidal anti-inflammatory drugs (NSAIDs) (as adjunctive therapy). There is little evidence that lumbar epidural opioids or cryoanalgesia of the intercostal nerves are effective. There is insufficient information on the effectiveness of paravertebral block of the intercostal nerves (which is attractive because it provides unilateral analgesia over several segments). Transcutaneous nerve stimulation[14] may help. (*See also* Kavanagh B. P. et al. *Anesthesiology* 1994, **81**, 737.)

If sputum retention is troublesome postoperatively, minitracheostomy may be needed.[16]

Other considerations

1 *Positioning*. Care must be taken to avoid injuries due to pressure or to the brachial plexus by traction on the upper arm.
2 *Bronchial stapling/suturing* is usually performed with the bronchus clamped. Use of a double-lumen tube gives control of the opposite lung, and helps the anaesthetist test the bronchial stump for leaks.
3 *Blood loss*. May be extensive. At least one large-bore cannula is essential. A central venous catheter is important.
4 *Closure of the chest*. The lungs should be fully expanded before closure. Residual air in the pleural cavity can be removed by an intrapleural drain connected to an underwater seal or a Heimlich disposable flutter valve.[17]
5 *Accidental pneumothorax*. May occur on the contralateral side during thoracotomy with mediastinal dissection. Also during any operation near the pleura and during local blocks (brachial plexus block, intercostal nerves). Suspected if the pattern of spontaneous respiration is altered and breath sounds are absent. Diagnosed by radiography. The hole in the pleura should be closed if possible and the lung fully inflated. Puncture of the lung itself will usually close spontaneously but chest drains may be required as a safety precaution.
6 *Postoperative hypoxaemia*. Atelectasis, sputum retention, poor pain relief and fluid overload may all contribute. Patients who have undergone a thoracotomy will require O_2 in the immediate postoperative period for up to 24 h and chest physiotherapy.

Specific operations

Diagnostic procedures

BRONCHOSCOPY

Rigid bronchoscopy
For topical analgesia, *see* Chapter 5.2. Very rarely employed. For general anaesthesia, premedicate according to general condition. Commonly vagolytic drug only. An intravenous anaesthetic technique is employed; small doses of intermittent suxamethonium (but repeat dosing may induce bradycardia), atracurium or infusion of mivacurium are necessary to relax the larynx for insertion of the bronchoscope and prevent coughing. The haemodynamic effects of rigid bronchoscopy are similar to those of laryngoscopy (*see* Chapter 2.6), but greater and of longer duration.[18]

Respiration is maintained by *the Sanders injector*. Intermittent flow of O_2 via a small tube in the mouth of the bronchoscope entrains air by the Venturi effect to inflate the lungs despite the open proximal end. The injector can be permanently fixed to the bronchoscope, and pipeline O_2 used (410 kPa) with three different injector sizes (SWG 16 for adults and small adult, 18 for adolescent and 19 for child, infant and neonate). This technique is the most satisfactory, and can also be used for laryngeal microsurgery. Modifications include: transtracheal ventilation through a 14-G cannula; use of the O_2 side-arm of the bronchoscope to increase F_1O_2; use of Entonox as the driving gas to prevent awareness, but the air entrainment will make this of little use; high-frequency jet ventilation. Very little air entrainment occurs at rates over 1 Hz. May reduce coughing.

The ventilating bronchoscope allows IPPV at the same time as the operator visualizes the bronchial tree through a window.

Intermittent ventilation, using a tracheal tube pushed into the mouth of the bronchoscope. Useful in the occasional case when the Venturi injector is inadequate.

Deep inhalational anaesthesia, performing bronchoscopy as anaesthesia lightens. Gives a limited time.

Massive haemorrhage may occur after biopsy; treatment consists of topical adrenaline and/or sucking under direct vision through the bronchoscope until the bleeding subsides.

Drugs and instruments should always be available for endobronchial intubation. After the procedure, reflexes must return rapidly, and the patient placed in the lateral position on the same side as the biopsy to prevent soiling normal lung and to allow drainage of blood etc.

Fibreoptic bronchoscopy
This instrument allows most extensive visualization of the larynx and bronchial tree. The segmental divisions of the lung can be inspected and trans-bronchial lung biopsy performed. It is much more comfortable (under local analgesia) than the rigid instrument. Anaesthetic techniques include: *topical analgesia* with sedation and analgesia e.g. midazolam and alfentanil; *general anaesthesia*, passed down a rigid bronchoscope (when the Sanders injector functions normally), a standard tracheal tube or a laryngeal mask. Intermittent positive-pressure ventilation is also possible using a rubber diaphragm to provide an airtight seal, although the fibreoptic instrument (diameter up to 6.5 mm) will partially obstruct the lumen. For lengthy examinations, high-frequency jet ventilator may be used; Mallinckrodt 'Hi-Lo' tracheal tube will allow the PEEP generated by the expiratory obstruction to be monitored.

Removal of an inhaled foreign body
Most common in children and in the right lung, and is removed via a rigid bronchoscope under inhalation anaesthesia. Respiratory obstruction may be present and can act as a valve so that a segment of lung becomes hyper-inflated. These cases can be dangerous and need experience.

OESOPHAGOSCOPY

Relaxation of the postcricoid sphincter is needed for rigid oesophagoscopy; achieved using muscle relaxants or deep anaesthesia. In obstructive lesions, regurgitation may occur from a dilated oesophagus above the lesion. A tracheal tube should be passed and suction should always be available. The technique should allow rapid return of reflexes. At the end of the procedure the pharynx must be sucked clear of blood etc. and the patient turned on the side. Oesophagoscopy may cause trauma, perforation and bleeding after biopsy or with oesophageal varices. Intermittent propofol and suxamethonium, using IPPV with O_2 and N_2O, or spontaneous respiration using a volatile agent are both satisfactory techniques.

The flexible fibreoptic instrument usually requires light sedation only.

MEDIASTINOSCOPY

These patients may have obstruction of the superior vena cava and the trachea. An armoured endotracheal tube may be considered. The anaesthetist should be prepared for haemorrhage.

Intrathoracic surgery

PNEUMONECTOMY

A right pneumonectomy removes 55% of the patient's lung tissue, and if the function of the remaining lung is compromised the patient is in a precarious position postoperatively. The major problems are pulmonary hypertension worsened by hypoxia, and oedema of the remaining lung from mechanical damage, reduced lymph drainage and left ventricular failure.

The lateral or prone position may be used. A double-lumen tube is preferred but can be performed under ordinary endotracheal anaesthesia. If problems are encountered inserting a right-sided double-lumen tube, a left-sided tube may be used for a left pneumonectomy, by withdrawing it slightly for the bronchial suture.

Suction should not be applied postoperatively to pleural drains which should be clamped. Intermittent transient release of the clamp (e.g. 1 min every 1 h) will prevent mediastinal shift.

BILATERAL PNEUMONECTOMY

Lung volume reduction surgery or reduction pneumoplasty; either 'open' through a median sternotomy or bilateral thoracoscopy. The principle is to reduce lung volume by resecting the worst functioning lung tissue, allowing better function from remaining lung tissue and improved pulmonary and diaphragmatic mechanics. Any degree of sedation postoperatively is undesirable and interpleural or epidural analgesia is preferable to opioid analgesia.

LOBECTOMY

One or (in the case of the right lung) two lobes may be resected. Upper lobectomy is sometimes carried out for carcinoma along with a segment of the main bronchus (sleeve resection). There will be a large air leak and difficulty with ventilation unless one-lung anaesthesia is used. Lower lobectomy is usually for tumour, but may be for bronchiectasis in children, and the volume of sputum may be large. In older children a Magill blocker may be useful. In young children with copious sputum the sitting position should be considered.

There may be considerable alveolar air leak afterwards, which decreases when IPPV is stopped. Low-pressure suction (-5 cmH$_2$O) should be applied postoperatively to pleural drains to keep the lungs expanded.

LUNG CYSTS AND BULLAE

Large cysts compress surrounding lung tissue, and may have a valvular communication with a bronchus allowing gas to pass in more easily than out. Intermittent positive-pressure ventilation and coughing may therefore cause further distension or even a tension pneumothorax. Isolate cyst with a double-lumen tube or bronchial clamp. If the cysts are bilateral, high-frequency jet ventilation (HFJV) should be considered in order to minimize barotrauma.[19] Nitrous oxide may distend lung cysts because of its much greater solubility than nitrogen. If a tension pneumothorax occurs, it should be aspirated through a large needle or drain through the second intercostal space anteriorly.

Pulmonary hydatid cysts are common in the Middle East and in sheep-rearing communities within the UK. They can be bilateral and multiple, and need excision if they become large. They may erode the bronchial wall and become infected. Accidental rupture of the cyst into the bronchi during surgery risks dissemination of the disease. Endobronchial intubation is indicated.

BRONCHOPLEURAL FISTULA

An abnormal communication between the intrathoracic respiratory system and the pleural cavity. Aetiology: traumatic, neoplastic, infective and congenital (bullae, tracheo-oesophageal fistula, etc). Most commonly presents after pneumonectomy, especially if right-sided. This produces two complications: a gas leak from the lung which may make ventilation impossible, but usually is small; a collection of fluid in the pleural cavity or post-pneumonectomy space may flood the bronchial tree. A bronchial blocker in the bronchial stump may easily be pushed through the weakened suture line. Ideally a double-lumen tube is used to isolate the opposite lung, maintaining spontaneous respiration until this is achieved. This has been done using only a propofol infusion.[20] The experienced anaesthetist, however, may simply use suxamethonium to perform a bronchoscopy and then pass an endobronchial tube. Awake endobronchial intubation may also be considered. High-frequency jet ventilation may be valuable in diminishing any gas leak. For the radiological characteristics of bronchopleural fistula following pneumonectomy, *see* Lauckner M. E. et al. *Anaesthesia* 1983, **38,** 452.

LUNG ABSCESS AND DRAINAGE OF EMPYEMA

Lung abscesses may be caused by aspiration, obstruction by tumour or spread from elsewhere. Preoperative postural drainage, physiotherapy and antibiotics are the mainstays of treatment, but lung resection may be needed. Endobronchial instrumentation protects against contamination of the bronchial tree.

Rib resection for empyema and operations more extensive than simple drainage, and in children require general anaesthesia. The presence of a possible bronchopleural fistula will normally require a double-lumen tube. Awake intubation under local analgesia in the sitting position should be considered with a large fistula or empyema.

OTHER INTRATHORACIC OPERATIONS

Mediastinotomy, segmental lung resection, open lung biopsy, pleuradhesis
The pleural cavity is opened; endobronchial intubation will assist by collapsing lung.

Pleurectomy, decortication
Haemorrhage may be a problem. For decortication keeping the lung inflated can aid surgery.

Thoracoscopy
Minimal access thoracic surgery has undergone a resurgence of interest. Video-assisted thoracoscopic surgery (VATS) can be used for many of the above operations; VATS is particularly useful for treatment of spontaneous pneumothorax and pleurectomy. It is associated with less postoperative respiratory dysfunction than open thoracotomy.

The conversion rate of VATS to open thoracotomy is 10%, indications being:

1 continuing air leak;
2 adhesions;
3 inability to collapse lung;
4 technical problems with surgery.

Retrosternal goitre
Performed through an upper median sternotomy. Postoperative tracheal collapse with respiratory embarassment is treated with CPAP, helium–oxygen or, if severe, tracheal intubation.

Tracheal, oesophageal and chest-wall surgery

TRACHEAL STENOSIS

Preoperative dilatation may allow passage of a tracheal tube with inflation of the cuff beyond the operation site. Difficulties are more likely in children. Insertion of tracheal stents has been managed with HFJV, or venturi ventilation and partial cardiopulmonary bypass.[21] A bronchoscope can be used to place catheters for HFJV beyond an obstruction, although a free outflow for the gas must be provided to prevent lung distension.[22] Resection of central airway tumours with the Nd-YAG laser may need HFJV with air to avoid the risk of fires, together with TIVA.[23]

OESOPHAGECTOMY

The patient's general condition is often poor due to lack of nutrition. Assessment and treatment to correct nutritional and electrolyte deficiencies are therefore important. A short period of enteral nutrition (or parenteral if needed) preoperatively may be of great benefit (*see* Chapter 1.4). The operation may be long and bloody, and may involve opening the abdomen as well as the thorax.

THYMECTOMY

Thymectomy for myasthenia gravis
The approach is transcervical, or by splitting the sternum when one or both pleural cavities may be opened. For preoperative and anaesthetic management of myasthenia, *see* Chapter 3.1.

PECTUS CORRECTION

A relatively small proportion of patients with pectus excavatum undergo surgical correction. Surgery is undertaken towards the end of the pubertal growth spurt. Lung function should be assessed preoperatively. Intraoperative blood loss may be dramatic. Postoperative pain control may be difficult. The metal bar is removed after 6 months or so.

Transplantation

LUNG TRANSPLANTATION[24]

Lung transplantation encompasses a range of operations: single lobe, single lung, double lung, bilateral sequential single lung and heart–lung.

Indications
Emphysema and pulmonary fibrosis account for 60% of transplants, the remainder include sarcoid, α_1-antitrypsin, primary pulmonary hypertension. The best results are in patients with fibrotic lung disease, although the sepsis associated with cystic fibrosis may be a problem when immunosuppressed.

Anaesthetic technique
Conventional one-lung anaesthesia is used for single lung transplants. Use IPPV with slow inspiration, small tidal volume and high rate. Aim to keep $PaCO_2$ as low as possible to prevent pulmonary artery pressure rising. In patients with emphysema undergoing single lung transplantation, the remaining diseased lung is very compliant and tends to be ventilated at the expense of the transplanted lung. Continuous cardiac output and mixed venous O_2 monitoring is useful. All efforts are made to avoid cardiopulmonary bypass (CPB) (but some centres routinely employ CPB).

Respiratory support with extracorporeal gas exchange may be needed as a bridge to transplantation.

Problems

These include haemorrhage as adhesions are separated, pulmonary hypertension when the pulmonary artery is clamped in which case CPB will be needed. Postoperative accumulation of lung water (due to ischaemia before implantation, denervation and section of lymphatic drainage in new lung), hence restricted fluid regimen postoperatively.

Obliterative bronchiolitis is a late complication.

(*See* Bracken C. A. et al. *J. Cardiothor. Vasc. Anesth.* 1997, **11**, 220.)

Pneumothorax

Spontaneous pneumothorax

Spontaneous pneumothorax is common in two age groups: young adults and elderly patients with emphysema.[25]

Spontaneous pneumothorax indications for surgery are:[26]

1 persistent air leak;
2 recurrent pneumothorax;
3 contralateral spontaneous pneumothorax;
4 first pneumothorax in high-risk patient.

Tension pneumothorax

Thoracic trauma (*see* below), rib fractures, ruptured bullae and CVP insertion may all cause a tension pneumothorax. Signs suggestive of a tension pneumothorax include:

1 cyanosis;
2 rapid deterioration in vital signs;
3 decreased or absent breath sounds;
4 tracheal deviation;
5 decreased pulmonary compliance during anaesthesia.

Tension pneumothorax is treated with urgent thoracocentesis.

Thoracic trauma

Chest trauma is often associated with multiple other injuries (head injury, abdominal injury, bony injury, etc.). The mortality from chest trauma is 30% when associated with a head injury. Flail chest is associated with 10–30% mortality.[27]

Thoracic injuries can be classified as:

1 penetrating – stab, gunshot, etc.;
2 non-penetrating – blunt chest trauma, deceleration injury, barotrauma and blast injury.

Non-penetrating injuries may be associated with contusions of myocardium, rupture of thoracic aorta, tracheal and bronchial rupture, pulmonary contusions, oseophageal injury (rare) and diaphragmatic rupture (loops of bowel in the chest on X-ray).

Haemothorax

Diagnosis is based on history and clinical examination. The origin of the bleeding includes punctured lung, tears of the internal mammary artery, injury to the great vessels and injury to the intercostal vessels. Initial treatment is chest drain, this may be only surgical treatment in > 80% of patients presenting with haemothorax. The decision to proceed to thoracotomy is based on an assessment of rate and total volume of bleeding associated with injury as follows:

1 persistent hypotension despite aggressive volume replacement;
2 bleeding > 300 ml/h for 4 h;
3 massive continuing haemorrhage > 2000 ml;
4 left haemothorax in presence of a widened mediastinum.

Cardiac tamponade

Cardiac tamponade is suggested by the following.

1 Site of the wound: neck, praecordium, upper abdomen (but may also be seen in non-penetrating injury).
2 Beck's triad: distension of neck veins, hypotension and muffled heart sounds.
3 Pulsus paradoxus.
4 A rising CVP and falling blood pressure (BP).
5 Electrical alternans on the ECG is diagnostic but the ECG is not always helpful. The chest X-ray is also of limited value.
   Pericardiocentesis is necessary to relieve tamponade in the rapidly deteriorating patient, but surgery is the definitive treatment (*see* below).

Rupture of descending thoracic aorta

Traumatic rupture of the descending thoracic aorta usually occurs at the level of the ligamentum arteriosum. The adventitia holds the aorta in place, consequently control of arterial pressure is critical. Computed tomography (CT) scan or an arch aortogram is necessary to define the extent of the injury. The left lung will need to be collapsed to allow surgical access. Urinary output should be monitored as the renal arteries may be involved.

CARDIAC ANAESTHESIA[28]

Anaesthetic problems in cardiac surgery

1 Effects of the disease process, e.g. poor ventricular function which may be further depressed by anaesthetic drugs and hypoxia, pulmonary oedema, valvular stenosis restricting cardiac output which cannot increase to compensate for a fall in vascular resistance. Anaesthetic agents must therefore be given with particular care. The function of other organs, especially lungs, liver and kidney may be impaired.
2 Blood loss and replacement. Haemorrhage can be sudden and rapid. It is easy to overload the circulation in the presence of a failing left ventricle.
3 Surgical manipulations of the heart may cause ectopic beats, asystole, other dysrhythmias or hypotension, especially in the presence of acid–base or electrolyte disturbances.
4 The problems of CPB (and perhaps hypothermia), which allows surgery on a heart that is isolated from the circulation without damage to vital organs. See below.

Closed-heart surgery without bypass

Premedication with morphine is well tolerated. Hyoscine is preferred to atropine which may produce excessive tachycardia. An intravenous infusion is started before induction, and arterial cannulation under local analgesia so that changes in arterial pressure during induction and tracheal intubation may be monitored continuously. The ECG and saturation are monitored as usual. After preoxygenation, minimal intravenous anaesthetic provides a smooth induction without undue cardiovascular depression. A slow circulation time delays the response. A small dose of benzodiazepine before giving thiopentone or methohexitone allows smaller doses and less disturbance of the circulation. Intubation is performed using either suxamethonium or a non-depolarizing muscle relaxant, and IPPV continued with N_2O, O_2 and opiate or volatile supplements if needed.

Blood must be immediately available. Additional monitoring includes CVP, body temperature and urine output. During manipulation of the heart, a close watch should be kept of the heart's rhythm and function along with direct observation of the heart. If manipulation causes bradycardia with hypotension, a short period of rest may be required. The lungs must be fully expanded before the chest is closed. Oxygen therapy is important in the immediate postoperative period.

Closed mitral valvotomy

Performed in some cases of pure mitral stenosis with an uncalcified valve. Other closed valvotomies are very unusual.

Ligation of patent ductus arteriosus

If closure does not occur after birth, blood flows from the aorta to the pulmonary artery, the reverse of flow in intra-uterine life. The left side of the heart dilates to cope with the increased flow through it. Less blood flows down the aorta and the diastolic blood pressure is low. Cyanosis only occurs if pulmonary vascular disease has developed, or if other congenital abnormalities exist. There is a continuous murmur, and there may also be pulmonary regurgitation. Endocarditis is a hazard. The ductus is easily torn when it is ligated, especially in an adult, with major bleeding.

Coarctation of aorta

Surgery is more risky in an adult because of associated hypertension, coronary artery disease and cerebral aneurysms. Enlarged collaterals in the chest wall prevent a severe rise in pressure when the aorta is clamped. Induced hypotension has a place to reduce blood loss from these collaterals and make the actual suturing of the aorta easier. The blood pressure should be rising again when the clamps are removed. If the collaterals are poorly developed (as in children) and the pressure distal to the coarctation is therefore low, the blood supply to the spinal cord may be at risk. Hypothermia or an assisted circulation in the descending aorta has been used.[29]

Pericardectomy

Constrictive pericarditis limits diastolic expansion of the heart. The rise in atrial pressure leads to venous congestion, ascites, peripheral oedema and sometimes atrial fibrillation. The blood pressure may almost vanish on inspiration (pulsus paradoxus). These patients present considerable risks. Cardiac output may not be able to increase if there is a sudden fall in peripheral resistance, and intravenous induction needs great care. An inhalational induction can also be used. The surgical procedure is lengthy and involves considerable manipulation of the heart. Blood loss should be replaced precisely, as the circulation is easily overloaded.

Drainage of cardiac tamponade

The patient depends on a tachycardia and vasoconstriction to maintain the blood pressure. Treatment of medical cases is normally by aspiration, but in the postoperative case open drainage is needed. Pulsus paradoxus is not a useful sign in these latter patients. Intermittent positive-pressure ventilation may cause severe hypotension before the pericardium is opened, and adrenaline 10–20 μg may be useful, repeated if necessary.

Coronary revascularization

Single vessel coronary vein grafting without cardiopulmonary bypass avoids the adverse effects of bypass.

Open-heart surgery with cardiopulmonary bypass

Used when the surgery needs a circulatory arrest longer than the 7 min which is normally considered safe under conventional hypothermia, e.g. surgery of the coronary arteries[30] (the commonest operation), heart valves, septal defects and other more complex congenital abnormalities. Extracorporeal circulation (bypass) is made possible by anticoagulation with heparin and its reversal with protamine.

Assessment

Ventricular function is assessed from the history, examination and data at cardiac catheterization. A high left ventricular end-diastolic pressure (LVEDP) of over 10 mmHg, a low ejection fraction of under 50% and abnormalities of ventricular wall motion indicate poor function. Left main stem coronary stenosis presents a high risk. Any pressure gradients across valves and calculated valve areas should be noted. Pulmonary arterial pressure and vascular resistance are important in patients with mitral stenosis or congenital disorders. Dental assessment should have been carried out. Cardiac drugs are usually continued until surgery. Relatively heavy premedication with opiates and/or benzodiazepines is usually well-tolerated, unless the patient is needing inotropic support.

Anaesthesia

Similar considerations apply as for surgery without CPB. Before bypass is instituted the anaesthetist must be prepared to control arterial pressure, dysrhythmias and any left ventricular dysfunction. If the latter is severe, inotropic support (adrenaline 5–20 μg/min) and rapid progression to bypass is needed. Tracheal intubation, skin incision and sternal splitting are the most stimulating events. Intermittent positive-pressure ventilation with N_2O and O_2 is used perhaps with opiate or volatile supplements. Halothane and enflurane are myocardial depressants. Isoflurane is a systemic and coronary vasodilator, and so may cause coronary steal. Most feel that this is unlikely to be significant at the low concentrations used and without severe hypotension, and there is even evidence that isoflurane may protect the myocardium against ischaemia.[31]

Alternatives include propofol infusion; large doses of opiates given slowly as the sole anaesthetic agent, e.g. morphine (1–5 mg/kg), fentanyl (up to 100 μg/kg) or equivalent doses of alfentanil, sufentanil; or remifentanil as an infusion. Such doses usually give good cardiovascular stability and suppress the endocrine response to stress. Disadvantages include the need for longer postoperative respiratory support, possible awareness and chest-wall rigidity.

Monitoring (see also Chapter 2.2)

1 *Myocardial ischaemia.* The ECG warns of ischaemia and dysrhythmias. An endocardial pacemaker wire may be inserted preoperatively, and an

epicardial wire used intra- and postoperatively. Transoesophageal echo-cardiography will detect abnormalities of wall motion usually due to ischaemia.

2 *Pulse oximetry.*

3 *Arterial pressure.* Usually by cannulation of the non-dominant radial artery. Flow is non-pulsatile during bypass. Rapid changes may occur.

4 *Central venous pressure.* Indicates right ventricular filling pressure. During bypass, a rise in CVP suggests obstruction or malposition of the venous lines. At the end of operation high pressure may be caused by overtransfusion or myocardial insufficiency; low pressure by inadequate transfusion. Two or more catheters, or a multilumen catheter, may be inserted into the internal jugular vein. One is then used for pressure measurement and another for drug administration.

5 *Left atrial pressure* can be measured directly via a catheter inserted by the surgeon, but risks embolization. Otherwise a Swan–Ganz pulmonary arterial catheter may be used to measure wedge pressure.

6 *Cardiac output.* Special Swan–Ganz catheters may be used for thermal dilution measurements, and for mixed venous O_2 saturation.

7 *Capnography.* Hyperventilation may be harmful if the cerebral perfusion is compromised.

8 *Cerebral perfusion.* An electroencephalogram (EEG) may indicate the adequacy of cerebral perfusion. Pupil sizes will warn of gross differences between the hemispheres.

9 *Temperature.* In the nasopharynx for core (or brain) temperature. Toe or bladder temperature may be used for peripheral temperature and gives an index of peripheral vasodilatation.

10 *Urine flow.* A simple index of adequate renal perfusion and thus cardiac output. Urine output should be recorded every half hour, and should exceed 0.5 ml/kg/h. Initially during bypass output is very small, but becomes high as rewarming occurs and the priming solution is excreted.

11 *Biochemistry.* Especially serum potassium and glucose. The latter is of particular interest as there is evidence that cerebral ischaemia causes more damage if there is hyperglycaemia. Some avoid giving dextrose solutions.[32]

12 *Arterial blood gases. See below.*

Cardiopulmonary bypass[33]

The extracorporeal circulation incorporates a pump(s), a heat exchanger and an oxygenator for gaseous exchange. Damage to blood must be minimal at the flows chosen; the apparatus must be capable of sterilization or be disposable.

Blood flow

Perfusion flows used in adults vary from 1.0 to 2.4 l/min/m² body surface area. Venous blood is taken from the right atrium or both venae cavae separately, and returned via an arterial cannula inserted into the aorta or femoral artery. Lower flows help keep the heart cold if cardioplegic arrest is used, and may cause less damage to the blood. Flow is usually non-pulsatile (but can be pulsatile) and generates a mean arterial pressure of about 30–50 mmHg. This pressure can be adjusted with small doses of vasoconstrictor or vasodilator drugs. It must be remembered that during rewarming and suturing of the proximal anastomoses during coronary artery grafting, the myocardium is still dependent on the diseased coronaries for its supply.

Acid–base balance

Most operations are performed under moderate hypothermia at 28°–32°C. Carbon dioxide is more soluble at low temperatures and so the PCO_2 drops and the pH rises, if the values measured in the blood-gas machine at 37°C are corrected to body temperature. Carbon dioxide may be added to the oxygenator gas mixture to avoid this apparent respiratory alkalosis. This is the 'pH-stat' approach.[34]

Allowing PCO_2 to fall (and pH to rise) as body temperature falls maintains electrochemical neutrality or the ratio of H^+ to OH^- constant. This means that the fraction of the histidine imidazoles in proteins which are unprotonated is constant. This is the 'α-stat' approach, as this fraction is called α. It keeps the major buffer systems, and perhaps enzyme function, at their most effective.[35] In practice it means that PCO_2 and pH should not be corrected for temperature when considering acid–base status, and that the apparent respiratory alkalosis should be accepted despite the possibility of cerebral vasoconstriction. The evidence that α-stat is the better policy is far from proven.[36]

Anticoagulation[37]

A control activated clotting time (ACT; 90–130 s) is measured before giving heparin, 2–3 mg/kg or 90 mg/m^2 body surface area, prior to arterial cannulation. A long control value may indicate rare antithrombin III deficiency, which requires greatly increased heparin dosage. The ACT should exceed 400 s before starting bypass. Additional heparin during bypass is given according to the ACT. Thromboelastography may be of use (*see* Mallett S. V. and Cox D. J. A. *Br. J. Anaesth.* 1992, **69**, 307).

Heparin is reversed with protamine 3–4 mg/kg after bypass, given over several minutes. If given too fast hypotension may occur as a result of systemic vasodilatation, or sometimes intense pulmonary arterial constriction perhaps after the release of thromboxane A_2 in the lung.[38] Patients who are allergic to fish, have been on isophane insulin, or who have had a vasectomy may be allergic to protamine.

For cardiopulmonary bypass in patients with cold agglutinins, *see* Park J. V. and Weiss C. I. *Anesth. Analg.* 1988, **67**, 75.

Haemodilution

The pump is primed with crystalloid, colloid (which may include blood) or a mixture of both so that the calculated haematocrit will drop to about 20–25% on bypass. Heparin and usually mannitol are added. Haemodilution may cause less lung damage and improve tissue capillary perfusion. Currently there is interest in pre-bypass plasmapheresis with reinfusion of platelet-rich plasma post bypass, but this is a time-consuming technique.

Oxygenators
Bubble oxygenators are now rarely used because they damage all types of blood cell. The polypropylene or silicone used in membrane oxygenators is less damaging to blood.

Blood loss
Although there is no venous return to the heart during bypass, blood reaches the heart from: (i) the coronary circulation; (ii) bronchial arteries via pulmonary veins (may be considerable in conditions such as Fallot's tetralogy); (iii) incompetent aortic valve. This heparinized blood is returned via suckers to the bypass reservoir.

Suction causes blood cell damage, and may be reduced by: (i) arrest of coronary circulation by a clamp across the aortic root. The heart is arrested and the myocardium protected against ischaemic damage by an ice-cold potassium-containing cardioplegic solution injected into the coronary circulation. For short periods ventricular fibrillation may be induced. (ii) Hypothermia to 15–20°C, *see* below.

Blood replacement
Via a cannula in an arm vein used solely for this purpose. It may also be added to the pump during bypass, when the proportion of blood in the patient and in the pump varies somewhat with vascular tone. After bypass blood is given according to the clinical state, the CVP, the appearance of the atria and the apparent blood loss. Target packed cell volume (PCV) is 24–30%. It may be given from the pump reservoir as long as the arterial cannula is still in place.

Hypothermia
Ventricular fibrillation occurs when body temperature falls below about 28°C, and asystole at even lower temperatures. Under deep hypothermia (15°C) cell metabolism is so low that total circulatory and ventilatory arrest is safe. The period for which this is true was taken to be 1 h, but may be shorter. The operating field is still and dry, and this is used for repair of the aortic arch and of some congenital defects. On rewarming, the heart can be defibrillated above 30–32°C.

COMPLICATIONS OF CARDIOPULMONARY BYPASS

Excessive bleeding
Occurs especially with repeat surgery. The problems arise after bypass and may be due to:

1 preoperative bleeding diathesis, especially treatment with anticoagulant, antiplatelet or thrombolytic drugs, aspirin;

2 inadequate neutralization of heparin;
3 fibrinolysis and fibrinogen depletion (< 1 g/l);
4 platelet sequestration and dysfunction;
5 failure of surgical haemostasis;
6 hypothermia.

Bleeding usually responds to careful surgical technique, more protamine (if indicated by the ACT) and FFP. Platelets are not usually needed. Antifibrinolytic therapy (tranexamic acid 1 g) reduces loss.[39] Reduction in Von Willebrand factor may occur (and so a failure of platelet adhesion) and is treated with cryoprecipitate or desmopressin 0.3 mg/kg over 15 min.[40] The plasmin and kallikrein inhibitor, aprotonin, has been used with success,[41] although it probably acts on platelets.

Gas embolism
From an empty venous reservoir, faulty oxygenator, leaks and faults in the bypass circuit, or ejected from the heart before air has been completely removed. Retrograde cerebral perfusion can minimize brain damage after massive gas embolism. Bubble detectors and filters in the arterial line are used. Even with meticulous technique small bubbles can be introduced, so N_2O should be avoided for up to 20 min after bypass to prevent their expansion.

Brain damage[42]
May be global or focal, and caused by ischaemia, embolism of gas bubbles, blood clot, calcific fragments from a stenosed aortic valve or fat droplets. More subtle neuropsychiatric sequelae and personality changes also occur. Dysfunction may be worsened by hypocapnia before bypass, low perfusion pressure and hyperglycaemia. Cerebral autoregulation may be better preserved with the α-stat approach to acid–base balance.[43] The contribution that drugs can make to the lessening of brain damage is slight. However, doses of thiopentone large enough to make the EEG flat (about 40 mg/kg) have been shown to reduce cerebral complications after surgery involving an open left ventricle, although this study was at normothermia.[44] Also the calcium-channel blocker nimodipine 0.5 mg/kg/min during surgery has resulted in a minor improvement in some neuropsychological tests after CPB.[45]

Awareness
The need to avoid both myocardial depressant drugs just before discontinuing bypass, and N_2O because of possible bubble emboli, can leave the patient with very little anaesthetic. The risk of awareness is inherent in the technique of bypass. Sweating at this stage can be striking, but probably because warm blood is perfusing the hypothalamus.

Lung changes
Due to poor left ventricular function, high pulmonary venous pressure and pulmonary oedema; postperfusion lung syndrome. Activation of the

complement and kallikrein cascades causes neutrophils to aggregate in the pulmonary circulation. These affect vascular tone and capillary permeability. Gas and particulate emboli also contribute to the development of an inflammatory response which can progress to full-blown adult respiratory distress syndrome: perivascular oedema and haemorrhage, congestion and thickening of interalveolar walls, patchy collapse, intra-alveolar haemorrhage, disturbance of ventilation/perfusion relationships; fentanyl sequestered in the lungs during bypass and released again afterwards; phrenic nerve damage due to cold solutions applied to the heart.

Cardiac tamponade
Clots may block drainage of the pericardium and tamponade results.

Hypertension after coronary artery surgery
Controlled by vasodilators, e.g. sodium nitroprusside, but this may increase pulmonary shunting.

Postoperative hypothermia
Rewarming on bypass may leave some vascular beds still cold. As these are gradually reopened postoperatively, body temperature falls. Vasodilatation during bypass and monitoring of peripheral temperature helps avoid this problem.

Kidney and liver dysfunction
Although haemolysis and haemoglobinuria occur during bypass, the condition usually clears spontaneously. Development of renal failure is more related to the cardiovascular state before and after the operation. The same is true of jaundice and liver dysfunction.

Postoperative care

Patients are nursed in an intensive care area with full monitoring continued as needed. Artificial ventilation is often maintained until cardiovascular stability and rewarming is complete, although patients who have had uneventful coronary artery surgery are extubated immediately in some centres. Postoperative pain from a median sternotomy is not severe and is treated by conventional analgesics.

CARDIOVASCULAR SUPPORT

Inotropic drugs and/or vasodilators are often needed after discontinuing bypass and are usually continued for a while. The following is a suggested approach when information from a Swann–Ganz catheter is available (*see* Table 4.1.1):

Table 4.1.1

PCWP	Cardiac	Index
	< 2.2	> 2.2
< 18	Volume loading	No treatment necessary
> 18	Inotropes	Vasodilators
	Vasodilators	Diuretic
	Volume loading	

If drug therapy fails to maintain cardiac output, the intra-aortic balloon pump should be considered. This is inserted percutaneously into the femoral artery and advanced to the descending aorta. The balloon is inflated in diastole (to help coronary perfusion) and deflated in systole (to reduce afterload). It can increase the output of a failing heart by 10–20%, is relatively simple and provides useful but limited assistance.

If the patient's condition is not improved (such a situation is also seen after massive infarction or particularly in those awaiting transplantation), various other mechanical devices have been used to assist the failing ventricles. They include the haemopump, a spinning turbine placed in the left ventricle after surgery; extracorporeal centrifugal pumps; either implanted or external ventricular assist devices and a totally artificial heart.

SURGERY FOR DYSRHYTHMIAS

Accessory conducting pathways that are causing intractable dysrhythmias may be ablated by an electric shock delivered down a special cardiac catheter. Alternatively subendocardial resection is carried out under CPB. Either method requires extensive electrophysiological mapping of the conducting tissues. Apart from the dysrhythmias themselves, these patients do not present any unusual anaesthetic problems.

ANAESTHESIA FOR CARDIAC TRANSPLANTS

The main indications for the operation are ischaemic cardiomyopathy or dilated cardiomyopathy. Most patients are warfarinized. Phosphodiesterase inhibitors have been useful in patients awaiting heart transplantation. Anaesthetic problems do not differ from those of any open-heart operation in a seriously ill patient. Active infection or malignant disease are contra-indications.

Elevated pulmonary vascular resistance is a relative contraindication. The specific immunosuppressive action of cyclosporin has greatly improved results but may result in postoperative impairment of renal function.

Heart-lung transplants are technically easier than heart-only transplants and are performed for primary pulmonary hypertension, primary lung disease and cardiomyopathies. The tracheal anastomosis heals better than a bronchial anastomosis. If the recipient's heart is normal it may be used for transplantation into a third patient. Long-term results are improving.[46]

CARDIAC CATHETERIZATION

Usually performed under local analgesia and sedation, except in small children and when accessory pathway ablation is intended.

INSERTION OF INDWELLING PACEMAKERS

Patients should seldom present for anaesthesia without adequate pacing. The apparatus itself is now usually implanted in the chest wall under local analgesia. For patients with pacemakers who require other surgery, *see* Chapter 3.1.

IMPLANTABLE DEFIBRILLATORS

Used for patients with drug refractory dysrrythmias. Consist of a pulse generator located in a pocket in the abdominal wall connected to two epicardial sensing leads and two defibrillator patches. Can deliver shocks of up to 20 J.[47]

CARDIOVERSION

Anaesthesia is necessary as the shock is painful, more so at higher strengths. Although barbiturates may be used, some have noted fewer dysrhythmias using benzodiazepines. Propofol is an alternative.

FURTHER READING

Gothard J. W. W. (ed.) *Clinical Anaesthesiology*. Vol. 1. Baillière, London, 1987.

Benumof J. L. *Anesthesia for Thoracic Surgery*. W. B. Saunders, Philadelphia, 1987.

Kaplan J. A. (ed.) *Thoracic Anesthesia*, 2nd edn. Churchill Livingstone, New York, 1991.

Kaplan J. A. (ed.) *Cardiac Anesthesia*. W. B. Saunders, Philadelphia, 1993.

Hensley F. A. (ed.) *The Practice of Cardiac Anesthesia*. Little Brown, Boston, 1995.

REFERENCES

1 Boysen P. G. In Kaplan J. A. (ed.) *Thoracic Anesthesia*, 2nd edn. Churchill Livingstone, New York, 1991.

2 Dunne N. M. and Gillbe C. E. In Gothard J. W. W. (ed.) *Thoracic Anaesthesia. Clin. Anaesthesiol.* 1987, **1,** 79.

3 Linter S. P. K. *Anaesthesia* 1985, **40,** 191.

4 Conacher I. D. *Anaesthesia* 1991, **46,** 400.

5 Macintosh R. R. and Leatherdale R. A. L. *Br. J. Anaesth.* 1955, **27,** 556.
6 Pallister W. K. *Thorax* 1959, **14,** 55.
7 Aps C. and Towey R. M. *Anaesthesia* 1981, **36,** 415; Watson C. B. In Gothard J. W. W. (ed.) *Thoracic Anaesthesia. Clin. Anaesthesiol.* 1987, **1,** 33.
8 Klingstedt C. et al. *Acta Anaesth. Scand.* 1990, **34,** 421.
9 Benumof J. L. *Anesthesia for Thoracic Surgery.* W. B. Saunders, Philadelphia, 1987.
10 Ritchie A. J. et al. *Ann. Thorac. Surg.* 1990, **50,** 86.
11 Eisenkraft J. B. In Atkinson R. S. and Adams A. P. (eds) *Recent Advances in Anaesthesia and Analgesia – 18.* Churchill Livingstone, Edinburgh, 1994.
12 Lunkenheimer P. P., Whimster W. F. and Sykes M. K. (eds) *Acta Anaesth. Scand.* 1989, **33** (Suppl. 90).
13 Jenkins J. et al. *Anaesthesia* 1987, **42,** 938; Howland W. S. et al. *Anesthesiology* 1987, **67,** 1009.
14 Kavanagh B. P. et al. *Anesthesiology* 1994, **81,** 737.
15 Conacher I. D. *Br. J. Anaesth.* 1990, **65,** 806.
16 Wain J. C. et al. *Ann. Thorac. Surg.* 1990, **49,** 881.
17 Harriss D. R. and Graham T. R. *Br. J. Hosp. Med.* 1991, **45,** 383.
18 Hill A. J. et al. *Anaesthesia* 1991, **46,** 266.
19 McCarthy G. et al. *Anaesthesia* 1987, **42,** 411.
20 Donnelly J. A. and Webster R. E. *Anaesthesia* 1991, **46,** 383.
21 Sherry K. M. et al. *Anaesthesia* 1987, **42,** 61.
22 Larsson S. and Nordberg G. *Anesth. Analg.* 1987, **66,** 471.
23 Blomquist S. et al. *Acta Anaesth. Scand.* 1990, **34,** 506.
24 Conacher I. D. *Br. J. Anaesth.* 1988, **61,** 468; Smyth R. L. et al. *Respir. Med.* 1989, **83,** 459; Dark J. and Corris P. *Thorax* 1989, **44,** 689; Conacher I. D. et al. *Anaesthesia* 1990, **45,** 971.
25 Miller A. C. and Harvey J. E. *Br. Med. J.* 1993, **307,** 114.
26 Waller D. A. *Ann. Thorac. Surg.* 1994, **58,** 372.
27 Webb A. K. *Br. J. Hosp. Med.* 1978, **20,** 406, 411.
28 Kaplan J. A. (ed.) *Cardiac Anesthesia.* W. B. Saunders, Philadelphia, 1987; Hensley F. A. and Martin D. E. *The Practice of Cardiac Anesthesia.* Little Brown, Boston, 1990.
29 Buckels N. J. et al. *Thorax* 1988, **43,** 1003.
30 Streisand J. B. and Wong K. C. *Br. J. Anaesth.* 1988, **61,** 97.
31 Priebe H.-J. *Anesthesiology* 1989, **71,** 960.
32 Lanier W. L. *Anesth. Analg.* 1991, **72,** 423.
33 Tinker J. H. (ed.) *Cardiopulmonary Bypass: Current Concepts and Controversies.* W. B. Saunders, Philadelphia, 1989.
34 Tinker J. H. and Campos J. H. J. *Cardiothorac. Anesth.* 1988, **2,** 701.
35 Murkin J. M. J. *Cardiothorac. Anesth.* 1988, **2,** 705.
36 Bashein G. et al. *Anesthesiology* 1989, **71,** 7.
37 Stow P. J. and Burrows F. A. *Can. J. Anaesth.* 1987, **34,** 632.
38 Lowenstein E. and Zapol W. M. *Anesthesiology* 1990, **73,** 373.
39 Horrow J. C. et al. *J. Thorac. Cardiovasc. Surg.* 1990, **99,** 70.
40 Editorial. *Lancet* 1988, **i,** 155.

41 Royston D. et al. *Lancet* 1987, **ii,** 1289; Van Oevren W. et al. *J. Thorac. Cardiovasc. Surg.* 1990, **99,** 788.

42 Hilberman M. (ed.) *Brain Injury and Protection during Heart Surgery.* Martinus Nijhoff, Boston, 1988; Shaw P. J. et al. *Q. J. Med.* 1989, **267,** 633.

43 Murkin J. M. et al. *Anesth. Analg.* 1987, **66,** 825.

44 Nussmeier N. A. et al. *Anesthesiology* 1986, **64,** 165.

45 Forsman M. et al. *Br. J. Anaesth.* 1990, **65,** 514.

46 Glanville A. R. et al. *J. R. Soc. Med.* 1990, **83,** 208.

47 Manolis A. S. et al. *Clin. Cardiol.* 1989, **262,** 1362; Shapira N. et al. *Ann Thorac. Surg.* 1989, **48,** 371.

DAY-STAY (DAY-CASE) ANAESTHESIA

INDICATIONS

An operation lasting up to 30 min is not likely to be associated with severe postoperative pain, the use of drains or catheters, or complicated by postoperative haemorrhage. Patients should be generally fit and the social and domestic arrangements should be suitable. Particular indications include surgery in children. Another advantage is the reduced incidence of hospital-acquired infections. Parents of children being driven home are advised to have an accompanying person in addition to the driver.

Adult patients must be accompanied home and not travel alone on public transport. They should be supported for 24 h. The mental attitude towards illness and pain must be constructive.

Postponement should occur if medical disease is found on the day of admission. Provision should be made for admission overnight if postoperative sequelae or unexpected complications occur.

SELECTION OF PATIENTS

Often done by surgeons, who may need guidelines from the anaesthetist. There is often a wide difference between the ideal and the actual in this area.

ASA grades 1 or 2 and age under 70 years are acceptable. In practice this means no interference with lifestyle by medical conditions. Obesity is a problem. Under 0.5 kg/cm or 35 lb/ft of height, body mass index (BMI) 30, is quite acceptable.

Patients should not be presented for day-case general anaesthesia with the following conditions: ischaemic heart disease; insulin-dependent diabetes; those on steroid medication; those living more than one hour's journey from the hospital; those living alone; and those with acute respiratory infection or chronic respiratory failure.

A preoperative history and general examination in the surgical clinic, anaesthetic clinic or at domiciliary visit is performed. Cooperation with the family doctor is important. Preoperative standardized checklists, which the patient or relatives fill in, are useful.

Patients and relatives have an absolute obligation to disclose all medical, therapeutic and relevant social facts. *See* Chapter 1.1.

THE DAY OF OPERATION

Preoperative and postoperative instructions (e.g. fasting or inability to drive), should be in writing and easy to understand. Patients and relatives are responsible for obeying these exactly. Regional analgesia may be considered. Oral temazepam, triazolam, or antacids are suitable for premedication if required (but *see below*).

TECHNIQUE

Ideally the day-stay theatre should be adjacent to the day-stay ward and the postoperative observation room. Operations should be performed early in the day. Premedication should be minimal or avoided completely. Small children should be first on the list to prevent hypoglycaemia from starvation. The anaesthetic is only started when the surgeon and operating team are ready and the anaesthetic should be the lightest compatible with safety. Only agents which are rapidly eliminated are used, e.g. propofol for induction of anaesthesia, alfentanil, remifentanil, N_2O, isoflurane, sevoflurane or desflurane. Suxamethonium may cause muscle pains the following day unless precautions are taken. Tracheal intubation is not contraindicated. Diazepam and fentanyl have a rebound effect 4–8 h after administration which although not greater than the initial effect, may be dangerous. Midazolam may be the benzodiazepine of choice when full general anaesthesia is not required. Local analgesia on its own or combined with light general anaesthesia has the advantage of excellent postoperative pain relief. In suitable patients both intra- and extradural block may be employed, taking care to avoid residual postoperative muscle paralysis.

RECOVERY FROM ANAESTHESIA

Assessment of recovery and fitness to go home is usually undertaken by an experienced nurse. It is more important for the patient to be escorted home and public transport avoided than for any particular test to be carried out.

Someone should stay with the patient until the next day. Factors to be taken into account in assessing recovery include:

1 awakening, ability to answer questions and obey commands;
2 stable arterial pressure and pulse;
3 can swallow and cough;
4 fitness to walk to the bathroom without feeling faint – Romberg's test and stabilometry;
5 has eaten and drunk without nausea, has passed urine;
6 fitness to return home – have their (un)written postoperative instructions and medications, if any; reaction time tests may be performed;
7 fitness to go out alone – usually allowed the day after anaesthesia; research tools to assess this include the electroencephalogram (EEG), the track tracer, psychomotor tests, choice reaction tests;
8 fitness to go to work – usually the following day (depending on the surgery).

ASSESSMENT OF FITNESS TO DRIVE

Views differ. The drugs used, their amounts and timing are important in assessment. An interval of 48 h has been suggested whereas others think a shorter time is safe. Perhaps a median time is 24 h.

Following the injection of local analgesics, 1 h after the return of normal function.

FURTHER READING

Commission on the Provision of Surgical Services. Guidelines for Day-Stay Surgery. *Royal College of Surgeons England*, London, 1985.

Bradshaw E. G. and Davenport H. T (eds) *Day Case Surgery, Anaesthesia and Management*. Arnold, London, 1989.

White P.F. (ed.) *Outpatient Anesthesia*. Churchill Livingstone, Edinburgh, 1990.

Klepper I. D., Sanders L. D. and Rosen M. (eds) *Ambulatory Anaesthesia and Sedation*. Blackwell, London, 1991.

DENTAL ANAESTHESIA[1]

UPTAKE AND ELIMINATION OF NITROUS OXIDE

During dental anaesthesia peak inspiratory flow rates may be between 30 and 200 l/min, tidal volumes between 300 and 3000 ml, and respiratory minute volume between 11 and 50 l/min. The arterial blood concentration of N_2O reaches an initial plateau within 10 min. In this time, depending upon factors such as inhaled concentration, alveolar ventilation and cardiac output, the arterial tension will be over 90% of the inhaled tension. On discontinuing, blood levels fall rapidly over 10 min.

Four 'zones' of N_2O anaesthesia have been described:

1 Moderate analgesia (6–25% N_2O inhaled); 25% N_2O is more potent than 10 mg morphine.
2 Dissociation analgesia (26–45%); 30% gives rise to psychological symptoms and lack of ability to concentrate. This is more severe at 45%.
3 Analgesic anaesthesia (46–65%). Near complete amnesia. Patient may respond to commands.
4 Light anaesthesia (66–70%). Complete analgesia and amnesia. Not possible to communicate with patient.

There is considerable variation between patients.

POSTURE DURING 'DENTAL CHAIR' ANAESTHESIA

The supine position for dental anaesthesia is favoured because of the dangers of hypotension (due to vasodilatation and bradycardia) and inadequate

---

Apparatus for dental surgery anaesthesia

1 Anaesthetic machine with spare gas supply and volatile agents.
2 Full intubation set.
3 Full resuscitation set.
4 Intravenous infusions with crystalloids, colloids and range of cannulae.
5 Intravenous agents, atropine and suxamethonium.
6 Emergency drugs.
7 Monitors – electrocardiogram (ECG), arterial pressure, pulse oximetry, capnography, nerve stimulator.
8 Defibrillator.

Indications for general anaesthesia in dentistry

1 Anxiety.

2 Infection (localized or spreading).

3 Disability – mental, physical or medical.

4 Age, e.g. childhood.

5 Allergy to local analgesics.

6 Following failed local analgesia, for any reason.

7 Larger or more prolonged operations.

---

cerebral perfusion (fainting). The dependent position of the legs is always to be avoided since blood may pool in them. A faint is vasovagal syncope, requiring immediate diagnosis, treatment with 100% O_2, and intravenous atropine.

MONITORING IN THE DENTAL CHAIR

1 'Finger on the pulse'.
2 Electrocardiogram. Adhesive electrodes may be placed on arms and leg. Ventricular ectopic beats are common during extractions.
3 Arterial pressure – an automated monitor with good artifact rejection is best. The cuff may also be placed on leg (ankle).
4 Pulse oximetry and capnography.

COMMON DIFFICULTIES

1 Patients who are frightened and have a poor command of themselves ('dentophobia'). These are difficult to control and may need premedication. Intravenous induction is usually indicated.
2 Patients who resist all anaesthetics, e.g. alcoholics; vigorous young men. In addition to larger doses of induction agents, short-acting opioids and even muscle relaxants may be needed.
3 Children under 4 years. Premedication may be helpful. A sympathetic but firm approach, using N_2O/O_2 and sevoflurane, via face mask for induction. At the age of about 4–7, intravenous induction is often easier. Above the age of 12, most children can be treated as adults.
4 Obesity. Difficult veins; difficult airway.

5 Patients who have missed periods and may be pregnant. Elective general anaesthesia is undesirable during pregnancy.
6 Patients who are anaemic.
7 Patients with decompensated heart disease. These are best managed in hospital.
8 Patients with hypertension. The risk is sudden severe hypotension. These risk cases are better managed in hospital. Volume loading with 70–150 ml/kg of a plasma expander is a good prophylactic in the untreated case.
9 Diabetics.
10 Patients on steroid therapy. Hydrocortisone 100 mg may be given intravenously just prior to anaesthesia.
11 Patients taking monoamine oxidase inhibitors (MAOIs). These drugs are contraindications to the use of pethidine, related compounds and pressor drugs. Pressor drugs may be needed at any time during dental anaesthesia.
12 The physically or mentally disabled require careful management. Even for conservation, it may be necessary to administer general anaesthesia with tracheal intubation. Premedication is important and combinations such as temazepam 20 mg and droperidol 2–5 mg (in adults) orally 2 h before induction have been recommended. Sedation by diazepam before local analgesia or general anaesthesia is also useful. Initial dose in children up to the age of 10 years is 1 mg/year of age. In older patients 5–20 mg. Down's syndrome patients are usually very resistant to sedatives and large doses may be required.

A SUGGESTED PREOPERATIVE QUESTIONNAIRE

1 Are you reasonably physically fit?
2 What drugs or medicines do you take?
3 Have you taken aspirin in the last week?
4 Have you ever received a general anaesthetic before? If so, how did it affect you?
5 How old are you?
6 What do you weigh?
7 Could you be pregnant?
8 Have you ever had a heart attack, 'stroke' or angina?
9 What diseases do you suffer from (if any)?
10 Have you any allergies? If so, to what are you allergic?
11 Do you faint easily?

CONTRAINDICATIONS TO GENERAL ANAESTHESIA IN THE DENTAL CHAIR

1 Patients who have not fasted before surgery.
2 Patients with acute infections or tumours in the region of the upper airways which cause or may cause obstruction.
3 Sickle-cell disease.
4 Severe coronary disease.
5 Cerebral vascular disease.
6 Extreme obesity.
7 Severe chronic bronchitis and obstructive airways disease.
8 Spastic states.
9 Haemophilia.
10 Patients on medication with certain drugs, e.g. MAOIs, anticoagulants.

It is unwise to allow patients who have received intravenous anaesthetics to return home alone, to drive a car or to cook or go shopping on the day of the anaesthetic.

Anaesthesia administration in the dental chair is now usually by sevoflurane/N_2O/O_2 or intravenous induction and laryngeal mask.

The stomach and bladder should be empty, the nose should be blown and dentures removed. The anaesthetist must be sure that the patient is fit for the proposed operation and tight garments must be loosened. Premedication may or may not be given, but the patient should be treated sympathetically and the procedure explained sympathetically. Dental forceps and other instruments should be prepared unobtrusively and an atmosphere of calm confidence adopted.

COMPLICATIONS OF DENTAL CHAIR ANAESTHESIA

1 *Hypoxia.*
2 *Respiratory arrest.* This may be due to:
   (a) respiratory obstruction and is treated accordingly;
   (b) breath-holding in light anaesthesia treatment – careful deepening of anaesthesia;
   (c) apnoea due to severe hypoxia – treatment is by inflation of the lungs with oxygen;
   (d) grave cardiovascular depression – full resuscitation required;
   (e) apnoea due to deep anaesthesia – treatment is by inflation of the lungs with O_2. In practice it may be difficult to make the diagnosis between over-light and over-deep anaesthesia.
3 *Cardiac arrhythmias*, due to increased sympathetic activity during dental operations.
4 *Fainting and hypotension.* Blood pressure, SpO_2 and pulse are continuously monitored. Should the patient even become pale, immediate restoration of

normal pulse, BP and SpO_2 are essential to prevent cerebral ischaemia. If this is neglected, delayed recovery from anaesthesia, permanent cerebral damage from hypoxia or even death may result. (Note that collapse and death has also followed local analgesia). *Causes of faint and collapse during dental anaesthesia may include:*

(a) emotional factors;

(b) hypoxia.

(c) pressure on the carotid sinus area when supporting the jaw;

(d) bradycardia and hypotension due to surgical stimulation of vagal reflexes; the patient is pale (cyanosis is a late feature) with a weak, slow, feeble pulse – immediate elevation of feet, intravenous atropine and possible vasopressor is needed;

(e) cardiac arrest diagnosied by the ECG – O_2 is given, cardiopulmonary resuscitation is started;

(f) anaphylactic reaction;

(g) convulsions due to epilepsy (or cerebral hypoxia) – usually self-limiting – the patient is placed in the recovery position and protected from injury;

(h) intravenous injection of local analgesic with vasopressor, especially when a patient is on tricyclic drugs;

(i) cessation of anaesthesia – anaesthesia may protect against syncopal reactions, which become manifest at the end of the procedure.

5 *Nausea and vomiting.* The risk is greater in those who have had it in the past, and where opioids are used. Prophylaxis is by ondansetron, metoclopramide, or cyclizine or droperidol.

6 *Minor morbidity.* Following extraction under local or general anaesthesia there is a high incidence of sore lips, trismus, drowsiness, nausea, vomiting, giddiness and headache.

7 *Pain.* Short-acting opioids, non-steroidal anti-inflammatory drugs (NSAIDs) and dexamethasone may be given during the procedure. The cyclo-oxygenase 2 (COX-2) inhibitors do not have the gastric and cardiovascular side-effects of other NSAIDs and may be given as an oral premedication.

8 *Death.* It is often difficult to determine the true cause of death, but hypoxia and pulmonary oedema feature in a number of reports. Cardiomyopathy presents a special and often undetectable risk in patients of any age. Diabetic autonomic neuropathy is an important risk factor, calling for hospital treatment (*see* Medical diseases Chapter 3.1).

IN-PATIENT DENTAL ANAESTHESIA

Preoperative assessment and premedication are as usual. The anaesthetic technique usually involves nasotracheal intubation and a throat pack to prevent aspiration of blood and debris.

Complications and hazards

1 Epistaxis and nasal trauma due to passage of a nasal tube. Can be minimized by prior spraying of the nasal mucosa with a vasoconstrictor (e.g. cocaine 4%, Sudafed or ephedrine).
2 Sore throat. Due to the insertion of a throat pack, when bruising and abrasion of the mucus membrane of the palate and fauces can readily occur.
3 Muscle pains due to suxamethonium.
4 Ventricular dysrhythmias resulting from dental extractions. Premedication with a beta-blocker reduces the incidence. Less common if halothane avoided.

Medical conditions indicating in-patient care for any dental surgery

1 Patients with congenital mental defects, Down's syndrome and spasticity.
2 Significant cardiac disease, requiring special anaesthetic management. In valvular disease, antibiotic cover is given to prevent subacute bacterial endocarditis. Low-risk cases – amoxycillin; high-risk cases (previous SBE and prosthetic valves) – augmentin plus gentamycin, injected very slowly. In penicillin allergy, vancomycin, clindamycin or teicoplanin may be used.
3 Cases of chronic respiratory disease, particularly where there is gross derangement of ventilation/perfusion relationships. (*see* Chapter 3.1).
4 Coagulopathy, e.g. haemophilia, Christmas disease thrombocytopenia, or where there is a history of severe postextraction haemorrhage. Preoperative correction is performed.

FACIOMAXILLARY OPERATIONS[2]

Fractured jaws

Preassessment

This may be part of a major trauma with intraoral haemorrhage, obstructed airway, head injury and loss of consciousness. In these very severe cases the protective laryngeal reflexes may be obtunded with danger of aspiration of blood, teeth and other debris and cerebral hypoxia. Airway, breathing and circulation are the first priority, preventing secondary brain damage and correcting shock. It may be wise to pass a tracheal tube, usually via the nose. Rarely a tracheostomy may be required; however, most mandibular fractures are unilateral and do not require urgent treatment. In others trismus may be a feature. The operative treatment of jaw fractures is usually carried out as an elective procedure. Fractures of the maxillae can be classified according to the Le Fort scheme. Respiratory and intubation problems may arise if the mobile maxilla approximates to the posterior pharyngeal wall or the dorsum of the tongue.

The anaesthetist who is asked to help with a fractured mandible and/or maxilla should look out for the following:

1 Associated injuries, especially:
   (a) head injuries – loss of consciousness, depressed fractures, raised intra-cranial tension;
   (b) chest injuries – pneumothorax or haemothorax;
   (c) abdominal injuries – ruptured viscera;
   (d) major bone fractures.
2 Presence of blood and debris in the pharynx, larynx and trachea, with respiratory obstruction. Occasionally bronchoscopy is necessary.
3 Possibility of swallowed blood, food and drink in the stomach which may be regurgitated.

Premedication

None.

Induction

The following should be available: two or more good laryngoscopes; experienced dedicated, and adequate help, an operating table or trolley that can be instantly tipped; suction, instantly available and switched on; equipment for emergency cricothyroid puncture. Rarely bronchoscopy may be indicated, but this is not usually a situation for fibreoptic intubation.

Atropine and an antiemetic are given.

Rapid-sequence induction is usually carried out unless trismus is present. Visualization of the larynx may be rendered difficult if blood and debris are present, but the shattered tissues do not often resist introduction of the laryngoscope. A mobile maxilla makes this more difficult!

A cuffed nasotracheal tube is usually preferred. A pharyngeal pack can also be inserted, but must be removed and pharyngeal toilet performed immediately before the jaws are wired together.

Criteria for extubation after wiring of the jaws

1 Fully awake.

2 Adequate respiration.

3 Well oxygenated.

4 No nausea or vomiting.

5 Wire clippers present.

Maintenance

By inhalation anaesthesia. Smooth anaesthetic technique is desirable, with rapid return of reflexes at the end of operation and absence of vomiting, coughing and straining. Remifentanil has a place here. Antiemetic drugs are very important.

Postoperatively

If the jaws have been wired together the patient should leave theatre with a nasopharyngeal airway in situ and be extubated awake. A pair of wire cutters should remain near the patient, so that they can be used in an emergency to free the jaws, and the mouth and pharynx can be sucked out. The nursing attendants should know how to use the instrument and which wires to cut. In fact on occasion it may be life-saving, in the presence of severe respiratory obstruction.

In cases of elective rewiring, fibreoptic intubation via the nose is an easy and safe technique.

REFERENCES

1 Meechan J., Robb N. and Seymour R. *Pain and Anxiety Control for the Conscious Dental Patient*. Oxford University Press, Oxford, 1998.
2 Jones N. *Craniofacial Trauma*. Oxford University Press, Oxford, 1997.

ANAESTHESIA FOR ENDOCRINE SURGERY

THYROID GLAND

Thyroid function

Clinical assessment can be supplemented by the following.

1 Radioactive iodine uptake after 20 min and 48 h.
2 Thyroid scan.
3 Measurement of total plasma levels of T_3 (tri-iodothyronine) and T_4 (thyroxine). These are normally about 1–3 and 50–150 nmol/l respectively.
4 Measurement of free (unbound) T_3 and T_4 levels. These distinguish thyroid disease from abnormalities of the carrier proteins (which are raised in pregnancy, for example).

5 Thyroid-stimulating hormone (TSH) level, before and after giving thyrotrophin-releasing hormone (TRH). The serum cholesterol is high in myxoedema.

Preoperative preparation

Hyperthyroidism is almost always caused by primary thyroid disease. The commonest form is Graves' disease, in which there are IgG autoantibodies that mimic TSH. Toxic patients can be treated medically (with antithyroid drugs such as carbimazole, or with radioactive iodine) or surgically. When surgery is advised the patient should first be rendered euthyroid by medical treatment, although beta-blockade is also used as it inhibits the cardiovascular actions of the thyroid hormones, as well as slowing the conversion of T_4 to T_3. Carbimazole increases the vascularity of the gland, and iodine is used to reduce it in the 7–10 days immediately before surgery, as Lugol's iodine (iodine 5% in 10% potassium iodide) or potassium iodide (60 mg three times daily). Radiography and computed tomography (CT) scan are important to check the possibility of respiratory obstruction from retrosternal goitre, compression or deviation of the trachea. Indirect laryngoscopy should be performed to assess vocal cord movement and the function of the laryngeal nerves.

Anaesthetic technique

All the commonly used agents have their advocates, and respiration may be spontaneous or controlled. Coughing must be prevented by a volatile agent, topical analgesia or by muscular paralysis. A tracheal tube is usually employed to maintain the airway in thyroid surgery, and is essential when the trachea is deviated or compressed, if there is stridor or if the vocal cords move abnormally. Intubation should also be used if the goitre is retrosternal (the sternum may have to be split) or if malignancy is suspected (when surgery will be more extensive).

Stimulation of the recurrent laryngeal nerve causes spasm of the corresponding cord, with inspiratory stridor if patient is not intubated. If nerve is divided, the cord first becomes abducted and flaccid; later it assumes the cadaveric position between abduction and adduction. Later still, some voluntary control is gained.

The eyes should be protected from the towels, etc. Hyperextension of the neck is unnecessary and should be avoided. A head-up tilt reduces venous oozing. Infiltration of the skin and subcutaneous tissues with 1 : 200 000 to 1 : 400 000 adrenaline in the zone of the incision reduces oozing in the skin flaps. The incidence of arrhythmias is reduced by beta-blockers and by avoiding acid–base disturbances. The pharynx should be suctioned before extubation, but coughing immediately after operation is to be avoided as it may contribute to reactionary haemorrhage. The cords can be examined when respiration returns, to *see* that they move normally.

Respiratory obstruction after thyroidectomy

The causes may be as follows.

1 *Reactionary haemorrhage.* This may cause pressure on the trachea and requires immediate intubation, evacuation of the haematoma, often deep in the tissues of the neck, unrelieved by merely removing skin sutures; and restoration of the airway. The diagnosis may be obvious, but if the patient has a subjective sensation of being 'unable to breathe properly' this is usually very significant. Reintubation is usually very difficult because of swollen and distorted tissues.

2 *Oedema of the larynx.* Usually seen on the second or third day after operation. Diagnosis is by indirect laryngoscopy and if stridor becomes troublesome a tracheal tube or tracheostomy will be required. Oedema of the pharynx may also be a cause of obstruction.

3 *Recurrent laryngeal nerve injury.* Injury to the recurrent laryngeal nerve may be transient or permanent. The former is not uncommon and even if bilateral need not be serious unless there is, in addition, oedema causing obstruction. Permanent injury to one nerve may be symptomless and is not serious unless the patient earns his living with his voice as the opposite cord compensates for the immobile cord. Permanent injury to both cords is very serious because both voice and airway are impaired owing to the narrow glottis. Either a permanent tracheostomy or an operation to widen the glottis is required. Even slight obstruction may prove fatal in patients with cardiorespiratory disease, and tracheostomy is always better done early than late. Routine examination of the larynx before and after thyroidectomy has shown that one-third of cases of unilateral paralysis resulting from trauma to the recurrent nerve are symptomless and in nearly all of these a normal voice is re-established. Treatment is unnecessary.

4 *Collapse of trachea.* This can occur due to erosion of the tracheal cartilages by a large goitre, but is rare unless the actual tracheal cartilage is removed in malignant cases. The unsupported walls of the trachea may collapse inwardly, causing partial or even total obstruction when the tube is removed. Reintubation must be performed at once.

5 *Injury to the superior laryngeal nerve.* This is rare but can be suspected if there is a voice change, or difficulty in swallowing. The former is due to cricothyroid paralysis, the latter to sensory paralysis. The condition soon improves. In a series of over 300 thyroidectomy operations, the operation carried a hazard to the voice in 5% of patients, with permanent damage, measured by sophisticated methods, in 3%. There is as great a need for

the surgeon to take care of the external laryngeal nerve as for the recurrent branches.[1]

6 *Mucus or blood in the airway.*

Other complications after thyroidectomy

1 *Thyroid crisis.* Rarely seen. The patient may complain of abdominal pain, fever, diarrhoea, gross nervousness and restlessness, or even mild mania, with tachycardia and dysrhythmias. An acute abdomen may be suspected. A sudden crisis in an unsuspected thyrotoxic patient after operation requires administration of a beta-blocker, together with potassium iodide and hydrocortisone. Mild tachycardia or pyrexia during the first few post-operative days may indicate a lesser degree of thyroid overactivity and may be abolished or prevented by oral potassium iodide.

2 *Hypoparathyroidism.* A low serum calcium requiring calcium gluconate 10%, up to 20 ml i.v. slowly. There may be tetany, with positive Chvostek's and Trousseau's signs.

HYPERPARATHYROIDISM

Primary hyperparathyroidism results from excessive secretion, usually due to an adenoma, occasionally to diffuse hypertrophy of the glands. It may be associated with renal stones, bone pain and cysts progressing perhaps to osteitis fibrosa, loss of appetite, nausea and thirst. Very high calcium levels cause a short QT interval, and severe and intractable cardiac arrhythmias, which in an emergency may respond to cautious intravenous administration of potassium chloride. After parathyroidectomy the serum calcium falls and there may be tetany, requiring intravenous calcium gluconate. In advanced cases of hyperparathyroidism there may be dehydration, sodium depletion from polyuria and renal failure. Full hydration and oral (or intravenous) phosphates may be required.

PRIMARY ALDOSTERONISM (CONN'S SYNDROME)

Described by Conn in 1955.[2] Tumours of the adrenal cortex occur in two-thirds of cases, secrete excessive amounts of aldosterone and require surgical removal. Clinical features include hypertension, hypokalaemic alkalosis and hypokalaemic nephropathy. Preoperative management includes correction of metabolic disturbances and potassium depletion (spironolactone and potassium supplements). Anaesthetic management is likely to be complicated by difficulty in controlling large swings of blood pressure. Temporary hypo-aldosteronism can occur after operation and may require fludrocortisone 0.1–0.5 mg daily.

PHAEOCHROMOCYTOMA

First reported by Frankel in 1886 and named by Ludwig Pick (1868–1935), of Berlin.[3] A tumour of the adrenal medullary cells of chromaffin origin, which, although it may be histologically benign, may be dangerous because of excessive secretion of adrenaline and noradrenaline. Ten per cent are bilateral and 10% are malignant. Ten per cent are found outside the adrenal in other chromaffin tissue, e.g. in the paravertebral space, in the organ of Zuckerkandl near the aortic bifurcation, and in the coeliac plexus. The patient exhibits hypertension, either paroxysmal or continuous, hyperhidrosis and elevated basal metabolic rate with some fever and reduced blood volume. Some cases of hypotension have also been described. The catecholamines cause a cardiomyopathy. Diagnosed by estimation of urinary catecholamines which may be 100–300 μg daily (normal 20–40 μg) and their metabolites, by CT or magnetic resonance imaging (MRI), or by imaging with ^{131}I-meta-iodobenzylguanidine.

Preoperative preparation

1 *Alpha-adrenergic blockade* prevents dangerous elevation of blood pressure during surgery and restores blood volume. Usually phenoxybenzamine 10 mg orally 8-hourly, increased by 10-mg increments until the recumbent diastolic pressure is 90–100 mmHg without postural hypotension. Therapy should continue for 1 week preoperatively. In an emergency, phentolamine i.v. in 1-mg increments is rapidly effective.
2 *Beta-adrenergic blockade* is indicated in the presence of tachycardia or dys-rhythmia, e.g. propranolol 40 mg orally, 8-hourly. It should not be started before alpha-blockade, or the blood pressure may rise dangerously.
3 *Tyrosine hydroxylase inhibitors* prevent the synthesis of catecholamines, e.g. metirosine 250–1000 mg, four times daily for at least a week before surgery.

Anaesthetic technique[4]

The effects of excess adrenaline or noradrenaline during operation when the tumour is manipulated may cause a problem. Full invasive vascular monitoring is usual. Premedication should include sedatives to reduce anxiety. General anaesthesia is usually employed, but agents which cause sympathetic stimulation are to be avoided. Drugs that release histamine should also be scrupulously avoided as this stimulates the release of catecholamines. Intravenous agents with N_2O, O_2 and relaxants are recommended. Short-acting beta-blockade with esmolol 20 mg i.v. helps avoid tachycardia at intubation. Excessive hypertension may be controlled by the use of sodium nitroprusside; further rise when the infusion is discontinued may indicate the presence of more chromaffin tissue. The blood sugar should be checked, as hypoglycaemia may occur, especially with beta-blockade.

NEUROBLASTOMA

This is a catecholamine-secreting malignant tumour arising from the sympathetic nervous system in infants and children, situated in the retroperitoneal or retropleural region. It may secrete catecholamines during surgery and should be managed like a phaeochromocytoma with alpha-adrenergic blocking agents, e.g. phentolamine, and blood volume expansion.

REFERENCES

1 Kark A. E. et al. *Br. Med. J.* 1984, **289**, 1412.
2 Conn J. W. *J. Lab. Clin. Med.* 1955, **45**, 6.
3 Frankel F. *Virchow Arch. Path. Anat.* 1886, **103**, 244; Pick L. *Berl. Klin. Wochenschr.* 1912, **19**, 16.
4 Russell W. I. et al. *Anaesth. Intensive Care* 1998, **26**, 196.

ANAESTHESIA FOR OTORHINOLARYNGOLOGY

In throat and nose surgery, the problems of anaesthesia are related to the fact that the operations are carried out on the upper respiratory tract. The anaesthetist preserves a clear airway, uses a circuit optimizing surgical access, uses reliable monitoring at all times, and takes steps to prevent soiling of the trachea and bronchial tree with blood and debris. There should be a protocol for dealing with failure of any of these. The problems are most evident during operations on the larynx itself.

The following factors should be considered when surgery is to be carried out on the upper respiratory tract

1 Premedication must be adequate, but not heavy enough to prevent postoperative airway control.

2 Smooth induction will reduce the incidence and degree of haemorrhage.

3 In operations producing blood and debris, entrance into the lungs is prevented by cuffed tracheal tube and/or efficient pharyngeal packing.

4 The use of a slight reversed Trendelenburg position minimizes venous oozing, but precautions are taken to prevent air embolism. A degree of tilt not quite enough to empty the external jugular veins is ideal.

INTRANASAL OPERATIONS

For example polypectomy, septoplasty, rhinoplasty, fibre-endoscopic sinus surgery.

General anaesthesia is maintained via a preformed orotracheal tube sealed off with a cuff, and pharyngeal pack to prevent blood going down the oesophagus. These packs must be removed before extubation. Forgetfulness to remove a pharyngeal pack is one of the easiest mistakes for an anaesthetist to make and it can readily prove fatal. To reduce bleeding, topical intranasal cocaine 1–10%, injection into the nasal septum of octopressin and prilocaine (or adrenaline), or block of the sphenopalatine ganglion which carries the vasodilator fibres to the nasal blood vessels may be used.

MANIPULATION OF FRACTURED NASAL BONES

The safe technique involves tracheal intubation with cuff and/or pack to prevent aspiration of blood should haemorrhage occur. The anaesthetic agents should permit rapid return of protective reflexes, e.g. propofol, suxamethonium, remifentanil, alfentanil. If plaster of Paris is applied, the closed eyes may be protected with adhesive tape. Minor manipulation can sometimes be carried out under intravenous anaesthesia in the head-down position.

TONSILLECTOMY IN CHILDREN

Risks of tonsillectomy during a genuine cold

1 Risk of laryngeal spasm/bronchospasm, poor oxygenation/ cyanosis during operation.

2 Risk of cardiac arrest in children – up to 4–6 weeks after infection.

3 Surgical profuse haemorrhage.

4 Postoperative laryngeal spasm.

5 Postoperative chest infection.

Provision of the right psychological atmosphere is of the greatest value in obtaining smooth induction of anaesthesia without tears, requiring rapport with the child, the parent and even the child's toys.

Both preoperative crying and tachycardia increase bleeding in these operations.

Temazepam (0.5 mg/kg) or midazolam (0.1 mg/kg) syrup are suitable premedicants, especially for fractious children.

Amethocaine gel or EMLA cream are used for painless venepuncture. Marking the area of the best veins helps nurses locate the patch correctly. Sevoflurane may be used for induction in the sizeable minority of children who have needle phobia, and the parents are warned that either approach may be needed for induction.

A preformed oral tube may be kept clear of the operative field if a Doughty blade on the Boyle–Davis gag is used.

Intermittent positive-pressure ventilation (IPPV) or spontaneous respiration are both acceptable. Some workers use a reinforced laryngeal mask.

The aim should be to have the patient fully oxygenated, comfortable and able to cough within a minute or two of the completion of the operation. (A nasal tube is very satisfactory for teenagers or adults.)

The patient enters the recovery ward in the 'tonsil position' (semi-prone, prevented from rolling on to his face by a pillow beneath the chest, and by flexed knees and hips) and remains in this position until full consciousness is regained.

Topical application to the tonsillar fossae of 10% lignocaine, used carefully in a spray, is reported to reduce postoperative pain, without interfering with protective reflexes.[1]

ANAESTHESIA FOR POST-TONSILLECTOMY HAEMORRHAGE

This can be a grave responsibility.

Assessment for 'post-tonsillectomy haemorrhage' anaesthesia

1 Blood loss (often underestimated).

2 Resuscitation (transfusion is used earlier in children).

3 Amount of cross-matched blood available.

4 Adequacy of analgesia.

5 Adequacy of airway and oxygenation.

The patient is likely to have a stomach full of blood clot and to be shocked. Visible blood loss is only a fraction of total haemorrhage. Anaesthesia may be induced by rapid-sequence induction ('crash') technique. Some workers prefer induction with an inhalation agent with the patient in the lateral position, initially. In either case, cricoid pressure is used.

Small doses of anaesthetics are all that is needed.

Gastric aspiration before leaving theatre is advisable. It reduces the risk of postoperative regurgitation.

ANAESTHESIA IN UPPER RESPIRATORY TRACT OBSTRUCTION

This may occur:

1 at the lips;
2 in the mouth;
3 in the nose;
4 in the pharynx;
5 in the larynx;
6 in the trachea.

Signs: stridor; dilating alae nasi; rib and intercostal retraction; use of accessory muscles, e.g. scalenes and sternomastoids; indrawing over clavicles; perhaps cyanosis.

Symptoms: dyspnoea; anxiety, restlessness; inability to sleep.

Diagnosis: inspiratory stridor suggests obstruction at or above cords; expiratory stridor suggests obstruction in bronchial tree; inspiratory with expiratory stridor suggests tracheal obstruction. X-rays and CT scan of the neck are useful.

Some causes of stridor

1 Croup.

2 Inhalation of foreign body.

3 Diphtheria.

4 Retropharyngeal abscess/haematoma.

5 Inhalation injury (burn or chemical).

6 Trauma of upper airways.

7 Angio–neurotic oedema.

8 Epiglottitis (stridor and cough are not common in this condition).

9 Airway tumours.

These cases present life-threatening difficulties because of possible:

1 trismus, e.g. in Ludwig's angina which may not relax with suxamethonium;

2 loss of accessory muscle tone in unconsciousness results in complete airway obstruction. Thus, tracheostomy or minitracheostomy under local analgesia may be necessary, or awake fibreoptic intubation before the induction of general anaesthesia. Awake blind nasal intubation after spraying the nares and larynx with local analgesic solution (cocaine 4% in the nares) has been used in some cases. The inhalation of a mixture of helium 79% and O_2 21 % has a density of 330 as against 1000 for air.

Premedication must not depress respiration. (e.g. atropine only)

When inducing general anaesthesia in a patient with an acute infection of the neck or chronic laryngeal obstruction, apnoea must not be produced until it is certain that the lungs can be inflated. One hundred per cent O_2 should be given for 10 min, followed by a smooth 'gas' induction.

In trismus, early passage of a nasal airway will overcome obstruction due to a bulky or oedematous tongue or pharynx. The volatile agent will release the trismus, enabling intubation. A rather small tube, e.g. size 6.5 or 7 mm, is easier to insert than a larger one, and is permissible for short operations.

LARYNGECTOMY

Anaesthetic management

Compromised airway: it is important to assess the likelihood of narrowing of the laryngeal aperture clinically (stridor = aperture 6 mm or less; indirect laryngoscopy), by peak flowmeter and from soft-tissue X-rays and CT and MRI scans of the neck.

Anaesthetic problems during laryngectomy

1 Laryngeal obstruction.

2 Haemorrhage.

3 Air embolism.

4 Interrupted airway during operation.

5 Vascular reflexes from retraction of carotid sinus, giving unstable arterial pressure and bradycardias.

6 Prolonged surgery, risk of hypothermia, bedsores, etc.

7 Postoperative care of the tracheostome; humidification, aseptic suction.

8 Parenteral nutrition or jejunostomy feeding required while the wound heals.

A tracheostomy may be performed at the beginning. In significant respiratory obstruction, fibreoptic intubation or preliminary tracheostomy under local analgesia is performed. Atropine premedication is important.

Even where there is no obvious obstruction, after careful induction, relaxant is not given until the anaesthetist can ventilate the lungs manually.

In an emergency, cricothyroid puncture and cannulation may be needed.

PHARYNGOLARYNGECTOMY

Cancer of the hypopharynx treated by simple pharyngolaryngectomy to be followed by multistage plastic repair causes similar anaesthetic problems to laryngectomy. But the one-stage operations using colon or stomach as replacement are very lengthy and pose additional problems:

1 Space around the patient is restricted, and it is important that the anaesthetist has adequate access.
2 Bradycardia, hypotension and cardiac arrhythmias can occur during mobilization of the oesophagus and transference of stomach or colon to the neck.
3 Damage to the contents of the mediastinum. Rupture of the trachea has occurred, requiring immediate endobronchial intubation.
4 Total thyroidectomy is also performed. Thyroxine will be required as replacement therapy. Parathyroidectomy may cause postoperative hypocalcaemia with tetany.
5 Postoperative intravenous feeding will be necessary.

LARYNGOSCOPY AND MICROSURGERY OF THE LARYNX

Problems include:

1 need for relaxation of the jaw and cords;
2 facility to observe cord movement in some cases;
3 vascular reflexes with hypertension and tachycardia;
4 the possible presence of lesions which cause obstruction to the airway;
5 requirement to keep the patient oxygenated and ventilated;
6 rapid postoperative recovery of airway control without spasm.

General anaesthesia is used with a volatile agent to prevent awareness. A long plastic 5- or 6-mm cuffed tracheal tube is inserted through the nose (an oral tube is more likely to be dislodged by the surgeon) so that the tube lies between the arytenoids, enabling the full length of the cords to be seen. The relaxant is chosen depending on the expected length of the operation. A ventilating laryngoscope, employing Sanders injector can be used for children, with total intravenous anaesthesia (TIVA). A tracheal injector is available for insertion through the cords but there is a risk of hyperinflation of the lung and surgical emphysema if upper airway obstruction prevents free exhalation. In combined laryngoscopy/bronchoscopy, the anaesthetist is advised to use a tracheal tube during the laryngoscopy to avoid long hypoxic delays while changing scopes.

LASER SURGERY TO THE LARYNX

The surgeon, using the operating microscope, guides the laser beam to excise lesions of the larynx. Anaesthesia is as for laryngoscopy. Ignition of the tube by the laser is prevented by the following.

1 Use of a metal tube which will not ignite.
2 Protection of the tube by wrapping it in aluminium tape.
3 Avoidance of a tube, ventilation being maintained by a Sanders injector attached to the surgeon's laryngoscope.
4 Air/oxygen/volatile agent mixtures are preferable, as nitrous oxide also supports combustion.
5 Patients with a pre-existing tracheostomy are well managed by retaining the silver tracheostomy tube in position.

TRACHEOSTOMY

1 Extreme emergency: cricothyroid puncture and cannulation.
2 Emergency: Minitrach type of device – much more difficult to insert than in the elective situation.

Anaesthesia problems of injuries to larynx and trachea

1 Airway obstruction, requiring emergency intubation, often difficult, especially if due to damaged epiglottis.

2 Massive carotid haemorrhage with cerebral ischaemia.

3 Pneumothorax.

4 Concomitant cervical spine injury and spinal cord lesions.

5 Air embolism. The patient should be nursed in head-down position to prevent air being sucked into an open vein.

6 Concomitant head injury or drug overdose.

7 Full stomach.

---

3 Elective:
   (a) percutaneous dilation tracheostomy device, often used in intensive care;
   (b) formal surgical tracheostomy under general anaesthesia.

Patients in the intensive therapy unit may well have a tracheal tube in place already. If not, after assessment of the airway (*see* above), an orotracheal tube is inserted after induction of light general anaesthesia with muscle relaxants if necessary. The cuff of the tracheal tube should not be deflated before the trachea is opened and the tube is withdrawn above the incision but not through the cords until the tracheostomy tube is satisfactorily in place. This allows ready replacement of the original tube should difficulties arise. There is a rapid and smooth transfer of anaesthetic connections from one tube to the other.

EXCISION OF PHARYNGEAL POUCH

Pharyngeal pouch first described by Ludlow of Bristol in 1764. Considerable contents of a full pouch may spill into the pharynx during induction of anaesthesia, not controllable by cricoid pressure, making awake fibreoptic intubation a safer proposition. The anaesthetist may pack the pouch with gauze, after induction, to help with its identification. Sometimes operative treatment may be carried out endoscopically when the 'carina' between pouch and oesophagus is removed by diathermy.

The patient may have recurrent chest infections due to aspiration of pouch contents.

OPERATIONS ON THE MIDDLE AND INNER EAR

The main problems are as follows.

1 The theatre is often relatively darkened (the anaesthetist is advised to refuse to work in total darkness). The patient's skin must be clearly visible at all times.
2 Nitrous oxide diffusion may raise the pressure in the obstructed middle ear.
3 Strong tendency to postoperative vomiting.

Myringotomy

General anaesthesia, e.g. via laryngeal mask, is suitable. Vagal cardiac arrest may occur if the 'vagal' area of the tympanic membrane (supplied by the auricular branch) is incised (prevented by atropine).

Mastoid operations

Some surgeons like to be able to observe facial twitching should the facial nerve be stimulated by manipulations in the vicinity. Immediate steps can then be taken for decompression should injury be demonstrated. This involves anaesthesia with spontaneous respiration. The operations of myringoplasty, tympanoplasty and stapedectomy are greatly facilitated by the provision of a relatively ischaemic field. This may be provided by the use of standard techniques (*see* Chapter 2.7, production of ischaemia).

In operations with obstructed middle ears, N_2O can cause increased pressure within the middle ear with bulging of the intact drum. With spontaneous respiration, middle ear pressure can increase by 39 mmH_2O per minute; with IPPV it may increase by 63 mmH_2O per minute, and these pressures can be reached within 5 min.[2] This may be important during operations such as myringoplasty. The problem is avoided if N_2O is discontinued 30 min before anticipated placement of the graft. Anaesthesia may be maintained with intravenous agents and air or O_2, volatile agents, sedatives and opioids until surgery is completed. Withdrawal of N_2O has caused subatmospheric pressures.

SLEEP APNOEA SYNDROME

This is far from being a benign condition, and may present for palatoplasty, or be an associated condition in any other situation. Difficult intubation, pre- and postoperative hypoxia, CO_2 narcosis, and excessive respiratory sensitivity to opioids are major risks, requiring at least postoperative high-dependency unit (HDU) care, and at worst IPPV in the intensive therapy unit (ITU). It also occurs in children.[3]

REFERENCES

1 Williams A. and Hamilton A. *Anaesthesia* 1986, **41,** 222.
2 Casey W. F. and Drake-Lee A. B. *Anaesthesia* 1982, **37,** 896.
3 Warwick J. P. and Mason D. G. *Anaesthesia* 1998, **53,** 571–579.

NEUROANAESTHESIA

SPECIAL PROBLEMS IN NEUROSURGERY

1 Control of intracranial pressure (ICP) and cerebral blood flow (CBF) by control of ventilation and $PaCO_2$.
2 Maintenance of the airway. The tracheal tube and connections are often inaccessible.
3 Control of venous pressure by absence of straining or coughing at any stage of the operation. Even a short period of straining may cause cerebral oedema persisting for hours.
4 Length of surgery.
5 Positioning in the sitting, lateral or prone positions requires special care.
6 Air embolism in head-up positions.
7 Induced hypotension may be needed.
8 Brain retraction or surgical trauma may affect vital structures.
9 Postoperative care of airway and respiration.
10 Fits.

CEREBRAL HAEMODYNAMICS

Intracranial contents are: brain 80% (which is one-seventh extracellular fluid (ECF), and three-quarters water), cerebral blood volume 12% and cerebrospinal fluid 8%. All are incompressible and restricted within the rigid skull, although some venous blood and cerebrospinal fluid (CSF) may be squeezed out into the jugular veins and the spinal canal respectively.

The brain weighs about 1.5 kg (but only 50 g when suspended in CSF) and its total blood flow is 750 ml/min (15% of cardiac output). Grey matter has a higher blood flow than white matter (70 and 20 ml/min/100 g respectively). Over two-thirds comes from the carotid arteries, the rest from the vertebrals. Its O_2 consumption is about 50 ml/min (20% of that for the whole body). Different regions of the brain have differing functions and patterns of blood flow. The status of important areas may not be reflected in global measurements, e.g. of jugular venous O_2 saturation.

Cerebral blood flows below about 20 ml/min/100 g cause electrencephalogram (EEG) changes. Values below 10 ml/min/100 g cause impaired ionic homeostasis and histological changes of ischaemia.

Factors affecting cerebral blood flow

Regional blood flow is closely related to local brain metabolism. Global CBF is affected by the following (in approximate order of importance):

1 *Arterial PCO_2*. Linear response between a PCO_2 of 2.7 kPa (20 mmHg) when CBF is halved, and 10.7 kPa (80 mmHg) when CBF is doubled.[1] Little change outside these values. Mediated through the associated changes in H^+ concentration. Cerebral blood flow returns to normal over about 24 h if the change in PCO_2 is maintained, as CSF bicarbonate is adjusted. This limits the period that hyperventilation is of value in reducing ICP. Reactivity to CO_2 indicates healthy cerebral (and spinal) vessels, is increased by volatile agents and may not be seen in abnormal areas of brain.

2 *Cerebral perfusion pressure*. Mean arterial blood pressure (MAP) minus ICP (or cerebral venous pressure if this is higher). *Autoregulation* maintains a steady CBF as perfusion pressure varies between 50 and 150 mmHg. Both these pressure limits are higher with sympathetic stimulation and in hypertensives. Vasodilators or cervical sympathectomy allows a lower blood pressure to be tolerated than when sympathetic tone is high (e.g. in haemorrhage). As with CO_2 reactivity, autoregulation is a sign of healthy brain, and is impaired by volatile agents.

3 *Venous and intracranial pressures*. A rise in venous pressure will raise the ICP which tends to lower CBF because:
   (a) cerebral perfusion pressure is lowered;
   (b) a high ICP compresses the cerebral vessels.
   The normal brain compensates to some extent. Abrupt rises in venous pressure during straining or coughing may cause serious falls in CBF, especially if arterial pressure also falls (e.g. during induction).

4 *Arterial PO_2*. Inhalation of 100% O_2 only reduces CBF by 10%. The PO_2 must be reduced below 6.7 kPa (50 mmHg) before CBF starts to rise.

5 *Autonomic system*. Extensive sympathetic supply, mainly from the superior cervical ganglion, but relatively little effect. Alpha-2 stimulation causes vasoconstriction, β_1 stimulation causes dilatation. A vasodilator parasympathetic supply derives from the facial nerve.

6 *Temperature*. CBF falls by 20–50% if body temperature is dropped 10°C. Hyperthermia increases CBF.

7 *Blood viscosity*. CBF rises as viscosity falls and vice versa.

8 *Age*. Cerebral blood flow falls by about 0.5% per year in later life, and this fall is confined to the grey matter.

9 *Drugs*. All inhalation agents are cerebral vasodilators but this effect can be modified by hyperventilation. Any resultant rise in ICP is greater in patients with a space-occupying lesion, and 'shift' may occur at the level of the

tentorium or foramen magnum. Ketamine is also a cerebral vasodilator and increases CBF. Other intravenous anaesthetics (e.g. barbiturates, propofol, etomidate, benzodiazepines) reduce CBF together with a drop in cerebral metabolism. *See below.*

Cerebral steal and inverse steal

Brain pathology may produce maximal local vasodilatation or a loss of normal regulation. In these circumstances, a rise of $PaCO_2$ may dilate vessels in surrounding normal brain and 'steal' blood from the abnormal area. The converse may happen if $PaCO_2$ falls, and blood be diverted to the abnormal part ('inverse steal' or Robin Hood effect). The clinical importance of these possibilities is uncertain.

Intracranial pressure

Normal ICP is 10–15 mmHg, and varies slightly with both the heartbeat and respiration. The zero level is taken to be the base of the skull or the external auditory meatus. Measured by an intraventricular catheter, a subdural or extradural transducer. All can be inserted via a burr-hole. An approximate value of ICP can be obtained from a CT scan.

Raised ICP occurs with coughing, sneezing, straining, etc. Raised pathologically with:

1 pressure from outside, e.g. bony tumour or craniostenosis;
2 space-occupying lesions, e.g. neoplasm, abscess or haematoma;
3 hydrocephalus;
4 venous obstruction and positive end-expiratory pressure (PEEP);
5 arterial dilatation, e.g. high $PaCO_2$;
6 cerebral oedema;
7 head-down position.

Raised ICP causes headache, vomiting, papilloedema, drowsiness, bradycardia and hypertension (Cushing reflex). Neurogenic pulmonary oedema may occur. If ICP equals arterial blood pressure, CBF cannot occur.

Decreased ICP occurs after: (i) dehydration or loss of blood or CSF; (ii) removal of a space-occupying lesion. It is of little significance.

As a space-occupying lesion grows, ICP rises little at first as (by the Monroe–Kellie hypothesis) there is a corresponding decrease in volume of cerebral venous blood and CSF. The pressure–volume curve is still flat. Later, however, this compensatory mechanism fails, and then a small rise in intracranial volume (e.g. hypercapnia or volatile agents causing arterial dilatation; coughing or turning the neck causing venous distension) causes a big rise in ICP. Measurement of intracranial compliance may indicate how nearly this danger point has been reached.

TECHNIQUES OF ANAESTHESIA FOR NEUROSURGERY

Many patients are generally fit, but those having surgery for cerebrovascular or cervical spine disorders or for secondary tumours may have important associated disease.

Local analgesia

May be considered where facilities for skilled administration of general anaesthesia are not available. Since most of the brain is insensitive to surgical stimuli, local analgesia is useful for e.g. decompression of a haematoma when ICP may be rising rapidly, burr-hole biopsy or cortical mapping. Sometimes the patient's cooperation is required during the operation, e.g. localization of subjective phenomena.

The skin and scalp may be infiltrated with 0.5% lignocaine with adrenaline 1 : 200 000 to cut down oozing. The bone is only slightly sensitive and drilling is usually tolerable. The only sensitive parts of the brain are the dura mater at the base of the skull, the dural sheath around arteries, especially in the region of the middle meningeal artery, and the dura on cranial nerves in the posterior fossa and at the base of the brain, especially the trigeminal ganglion.

Unsuitable for children and uncooperative adults, and for long operations. Alterations in level of consciousness, fits or vomiting may occur, sometimes needing respiratory support. The patient may need restraint. Oxygen blown under the towels near the mouth prevents a feeling of suffocation. Full monitoring is used.

General anaesthesia

The brain should be soft, the veins uncongested, ICP low and CBF adequate for the cerebral metabolic rate.

Premedication

Sedative drugs, particularly narcotic analgesics, should be avoided with:

1 raised ICP;
2 head injury;
3 the prone, sitting or steep head-up position with spontaneous respiration.

A modest dose of temazepam will calm an anxious patient without leading to confusing postoperative drowsiness. Glycopyrrolium is a useful anti-sialogogue if needed.

Induction

Coughing and straining can raise the venous pressure for up to half an hour, and must be avoided. Thiopentone or propofol and a short-acting opioid (fentanyl 0.2–0.3 mg) are commonly used.

The airway

Any rise in ICP on intubation may be obtunded by the opioid and perhaps an extra dose of thiopentone. Some workers give lignocaine 1–1.5 mg/kg i.v. 4 min before laryngoscopy. Topical analgesic spray to the larynx may be used, which does little to prevent the rise in ICP, but helps avoid coughing and straining on the tube. A generous dose of relaxant is better in this regard and gives best conditions for laryngoscopy. Jugular venous obstruction can be caused by laryngoscopy.

Care should be taken to prevent disconnections and kinking. Reinforced tubes may be used. The tube is *securely* fixed with strapping rather than tapes which can cause venous obstruction. Intermittent positive-pressure ventilation is almost universal for neurosurgery, but spontaneous respiration may be used for some infra-tentorial operations if it is felt that the pattern of breathing may indicate the proximity of the surgeon to vital structures. In either case there should be no obstruction, especially to expiration. Adequate muscle relaxation means that airway pressures are kept to a minimum.

Choice of anaesthetic agents

INTRAVENOUS BARBITURATES

Cerebral metabolism and blood flow are reduced by similar amounts. This may amount to 30% in light (burst suppression on the electroencephalogram (EEG)) and 50% in deep thiopentone anaesthesia (isoelectric EEG). The latter requires repeated administrations. There is no added advantage in giving doses higher than those needed to cause an isoelectric EEG, as metabolic activity to maintain neuronal integrity persists. Evoked potentials are unaffected. Intracranial pressure is reduced. However, in head injuries other agents (e.g. mannitol) are probably as good, and outcome is not improved. Thiopentone may protect the brain from incomplete ischaemia (e.g. as may occur during cerebral vascular surgery) if given in burst suppression dosage (3–7 mg/kg) before the ischaemia occurs, or by infusion shortly afterwards to equilibrate throughout the brain. Inverse steal may contribute to this protection. Haemodynamic and respiratory support are likely to be needed. Barbiturates are of no value after cardiac arrest because the EEG will be flat anyway.

PROPOFOL

This causes a similar reduction in cerebral metabolism and blood flow to thiopentone, although less effective as protection against cerebral ischaemia.[2] The pressor response to laryngoscopy is less pronounced with propofol. Fits have been reported after its use in other types of surgery. Since postoperative fits are a complication of intracranial surgery, some prefer to avoid propofol in these patients. Widely used for sedation in patients being ventilated in neurological intensive care.

OTHER INDUCTION AGENTS

Ketamine raises CBF with little change in metabolic rate. It retains a place for children undergoing diagnostic radiological procedures. Midazolam suppresses cerebral metabolism to only a limited extent. Etomidate has similar effects to thiopentone, but myoclonus after etomidate may increase ICP.

NARCOTIC ANALGESICS

Little effect on CBF, and CO_2 reactivity is preserved. The rapid onset and offset of remifentanil is particularly appropriate to treat the few painful stimuli that occur in intracranial surgery.[3]

MUSCLE RELAXANTS

These do not penetrate the blood–brain barrier and have no direct effects on the brain. Suxamethonium increases muscle afferent discharge, which can raise CBF and ICP unless the patient is adequately anaesthetized or has been pretreated with a non-depolarizing agent. Atracurium may release histamine, and its metabolite laudanosine is a cerebral stimulant, but not at the levels seen in clinical practice. Vecuronium has no effect on the brain, but phenytoin therapy may increase requirements.

NITROUS OXIDE

Fifteen per cent N_2O was used by Kety and Schmidt as the diffusible indicator in their classic measurement of CBF.[4] Little effect on cerebral metabolism, probably increases blood flow and so may increase ICP in susceptible patients. These effects are of little significance as they are readily modified by barbiturates, opiates and hyperventilation. Nitrous oxide diffuses into air-filled spaces, e.g. air embolism and perhaps the subarachnoid space after dural closure. The latter is not a problem clinically. Should be turned off if air embolism occurs. Commonly used in neurosurgery.

ISOFLURANE

Only a mild cerebral vasodilator with little impairment of autoregulation. No increase in CBF below 1–1.5 minimum alveolar concentration (MAC) (1.15–1.7%). May increase ICP in susceptible patients, but this can be controlled by hyperventilation. No evidence that it is harmful to introduce isoflurane before lowering the $Pa CO_2$. Reactivity of the cerebral circulation to CO_2 is preserved or enhanced by all volatile agents.

All the volatile agents tend to decrease the amplitude and increase the latency of evoked potentials. Isoflurane decreases cerebral metabolism and the EEG becomes isoelectric at the relatively low concentration of about 2 MAC. This is similar to thiopentone, and isoflurane offers some protection against incomplete global or regional ischaemia, although some steal may occur in the latter case. Useful for carotid artery surgery, and for all intracranial surgery.

SEVOFLURANE

Similar to isoflurane in its effects on the central nervous system (CNS). There is no increase in CBF below about 1 MAC with preservation of autoregulation and CO_2 reactivity. There are no excitatory phenomena.

HALOTHANE

Most potent cerebral vasodilator of the volatile agents, but decreases metabolism to a moderate degree. Cerebral blood flow is tripled and autoregulation abolished at 1 MAC (0.75%). The associated rise in ICP is prevented by prior reduction of $PaCO_2$ to about 3.3 kPa (25 mmHg) by hyperventilation, even in patients with tumours. May worsen regional ischaemia by cerebral steal.

ENFLURANE

Cerebral vasodilator (less than halothane, more than isoflurane). Cerebral blood flow doubled at 1 MAC (1.68%). May increase ICP in susceptible patients, but this causes little problem in normal doses and with prior hyperventilation. Tends to cause EEG discharges and sometimes convulsions over about 1.5 MAC (2.5%), especially if the $PaCO_2$ is low. This can be used to identify the focus in surgery for epilepsy. Little used otherwise in neurosurgery.

Thiopentone or propofol, fentanyl, vecuronium or atracurium, and 70% N_2O plus isoflurane is a widely used combination.

Hyperventilation

The $PaCO_2$ should be lowered before introducing a volatile agent, although this is not essential with isoflurane or sevoflurane. Many workers aim for a $PaCO_2$ of about 3.5 kPa (26 mmHg). This gives near-maximal cerebral vasoconstriction, lowered ICP and an excellent surgical field. Some prefer less hyperventilation if possible. Below 2.7 kPa (20 mmHg) there is no improvement in ICP and EEG and metabolic signs of cerebral ischaemia occur, mainly because of the left-shifted dissociation curve.

Monitoring

In addition to the normal monitoring, invasive intra-arterial pressure measurement is used for intracranial and high spinal cord surgery. Changes in ICP and surgical manipulation, particularly in the posterior fossa can cause profound changes in pulse and blood pressure which should be reported to the surgeon. Any difference in height between the arterial pressure transducer and the brain must be considered for the calculation of cerebral perfusion pressure. If much bleeding is expected, e.g. cerebral vascular surgery, or if air embolism is a possibility, a central venous line is useful.

Electrophysiological monitoring

1 *Electroencephalogram.* Usually a 16-channel record on huge amounts of paper, but computer processing of the signals enables them to be presented in form useful for monitoring purposes, e.g. the cerebral function analysing monitor. Normal rhythms are: α (8–12 Hz, the dominant rhythm), β (18–30 Hz), θ (4–7 Hz), δ (less than 4 Hz). As CBF drops the fast rhythms disappear, slow rhythms predominate and the voltage drops. The EEG can detect cerebral ischaemia during carotid artery surgery.

2 *Sensory evoked potentials.* Unlike EEGs, these test specific neural pathways and are less influenced by anaesthetics, but the voltages measured are smaller and so computer averaging techniques are needed. They are difficult to record in the electrically hostile environment of an operating theatre, and are influenced by other factors such as body temperature and $PaCO_2$.

Somatosensory (SSEP) and brainstem auditory (AEP) evoked potentials are the most useful intraoperatively. (Visual evoked potentials show too much variation.) Used to detect: (i) awareness or depth of anaesthesia; (ii) damage to the nervous system during surgery. Characteristic positive (P) and negative (N) voltage peaks occur, e.g. N2O, a negative peak in SSEPs occurring 20 msec after the stimulus (i.e. with a *latency* of 20 msec). Ischaemia, injury and inhalational anaesthetics tend to decrease SSEP amplitude and increase latency. Intravenous agents have less effect. AEPs test brainstem pathways, e.g. during surgery for acoustic neuroma, and are short latency. SSEPs are used (especially with extradural sensors) to help check spinal cord integrity during, for example, operations to stabilize the spine.[5] This is more reliable than the 'wake-up' test. Descending motor pathways also may be assessed by cortical stimulation.[6]

Control of intracranial pressure

A raised ICP produces a tight dura and brain and makes retraction more hazardous. Methods of reducing ICP are as follows.

1 *Hyperventilation*, which is of value for at least 24 h, until the CSF pH returns towards normal (*see above*).

2 *Diuretics*. Hyperosmotic agents: mannitol ($C_6H_{12}O_6$). A hexahydric alcohol related to the hexose sugars. An isomer of sorbitol. Solutions (e.g. 20%) can be sterilized by autoclaving. Dose 0.5–1.5 g/kg i.v. over 10–20 min, which starts to lower ICP in 5 min, is maximal at 45 min, and lasts up to 4–6 h. The larger doses are no more effective, but last longer. Shrinks brain ECF, but may also produce cerebral vasoconstriction and reduce CSF production. Lowers blood viscosity which augments CBF for a given perfusion pressure. Some do not give it before a bone flap is raised, to avoid tearing of bridging veins. Disadvantages: initial transient rise in blood volume and so ICP if given too fast; excessive fluid depletion; small rebound rise in ICP later; may increase ICP if blood–brain barrier is disrupted; may precipitate heart failure. Often combined with a loop diuretic, e.g. frusemide 0.5–1 mg/kg. A urinary catheter is needed.

3 *Removal of CSF*. (Up to 150 ml.) Via a needle or catheter in the lateral ventricle. Catheters are less likely to block if drained against a pressure of about 15 mmHg. Spinal drainage is useful for aneurysm surgery, but can cause tonsillar herniation if there is a space-occupying lesion.

4 *Control of arterial and venous pressures*. Hypotensive agents and head-up tilt.

5 *Steroids*. Dexamethasone 4 mg 6-hourly gives a rapid, if temporary, clinical improvement in patients with oedema around tumours, but the reduction of ICP is often delayed. Of no value in head injuries.[7]

6 *Intravenous anaesthetics and lignocaine* cause cerebral vasoconstriction. The latter (1–1.5 mg/kg) is used to prevent coughing and ICP rises at intubation and extubation.

7 *Hypothermia*. Reduces ICP and provides some protection against brain ischaemia, as the ischaemic time is doubled to about 8 min at 30°C. This is achieved by surface cooling, but is rarely used now. Profound hypothermia (15°C) with cardiopulmonary bypass is still occasionally used for surgery on giant aneurysms.[8]

Postoperative care

Intermittent positive-pressure ventilation is not usually necessary, unless control of ICP is likely to be difficult. Neurological deterioration may result from haematoma or oedema formation. Localizing signs are eagerly sought. Postoperative ICP monitoring is not used routinely, rather clinical assessment and CT scanning when indicated. The need for analgesia after intracranial surgery is slight. Codeine phosphate is effective and causes little sedation. Antiemetics are often needed. Phenytoin is often given after supratentorial surgery to reduce incidence of fits, although its efficacy is uncertain.[9] Hyponatraemia due to inappropriate secretion of antidiuretic hormone may follow trauma or some tumours.

PARTICULAR NEUROSURGICAL PROCEDURES

Intracranial aneurysms and subarachnoid haemorrhage[10]

Operation is performed to prevent rebleeding, which is most likely early after the first bleed. The desire for early surgery is tempered by the danger of vasospasm in the first few days, and by the poor prognosis of patients with significant neurological deficit. The sympathetic outflow after subarachnoid haemorrhage can cause asymptomatic widespread ST and T-wave changes on the ECG, which do not necessarily mean coronary artery disease and need not contraindicate surgery. Although the CT scan may indicate the site of the aneurysm, angiography is needed to define it more precisely. Its exact site will determine the surgical approach and be important in assessing risk. Surgery is normally performed on relatively fit patients. If the aneurysm neck cannot be clipped, wrapping it with a reinforcement material or perhaps embolization or ligation of a feeding artery may be performed. Giant aneurysms can need cardiopulmonary bypass and profound hypothermia (15°C).[11] Rupture of the aneurysm as the dissection proceeds is not uncommon, and blood loss may be severe. Deliberate hypotension is much less used now. Subarachnoid haemorrhage impairs autoregulation, and hypotension will therefore worsen cerebral ischaemia.[12] Postoperative recovery can be complicated by cerebral vasospasm, hydrocephalus and hyponatraemia. Spasm can be treated by keeping the blood pressure high with fluid loading and inotropes, or with nimodipine 1–2 mg/h i.v. or 60 mg 4-hourly orally. Prostaglandins and polypeptides from platelets may be factors causing vasospasm.

Controlled hypotension

Still may be occasionally used during the removal of vascular tumours (e.g. meningioma) or malformations. Nitroprusside is easily controllable, but is a cerebral vasodilator and may increase ICP slightly. Some therefore use trimetaphan before the dura is opened, which is not a cerebral vasodilator, but this gives fixed and dilated pupils for some hours after operation. Autoregulation is impaired after induced hypotension, especially if volatile agents have been used too, and postoperative IPPV may be needed. For the techniques of controlling arterial pressure *see* Chapter 2.7.

Posterior fossa craniotomy

Performed in the prone, semi-prone (park-bench) or sitting position, and needs careful attention to positioning. Cerebral venous pressure is harder to keep low in the prone position or if the head is flexed. Particular hazards are as follows.

1 Air embolism in the sitting position (*see below*).
2 Hypotension in the sitting position. Prevented by bandaging and elevating the legs, and by pressor drugs.

3 Surgical damage to vital brainstem structures. The pattern of spontaneous respiration has been used to indicate brainstem integrity, but the improved surgical field obtained by IPPV is striking. In the paralysed patient proximity to these vital structures is indicated by dramatic changes in pulse, cardiac rhythm and blood pressure.
4 Hydrocephalus, due to CSF obstruction in the fourth ventricle.
5 Cranial nerve damage. Stimulation of the trigeminal nerve during excision of an acoustic neuroma may cause hypertension. Vagal stimulation may also occur, with bradycardia and hypotension. Damage may cause postoperative laryngeal obstruction. Glossopharyngeal damage will predispose to postoperative aspiration.
6 Massive swelling of the face and tongue may occur up to 36 h postoperatively and obstruct the airway.[13]

Air embolism in neurosurgery

Venous air embolism is common if the patient is in the sitting position, which is also sometimes used for surgery of the cervical spine. Many veins in the occipital muscles and other tissues of the back of the neck do not collapse readily after they have been divided, but are held open, allowing air to be sucked in. The mastoid emissary vein is a particularly common site for air entry, as are the major dural sinuses. Portals of entry within the dura are relatively uncommon.

An oesophageal or precordial stethoscope may pick up the typical murmur of air in the heart, end-tidal CO_2 falls rapidly, and a Doppler ultrasonic probe over the precordium or in the oesophagus will detect small amounts of air. Diathermy interferes with the latter, so in practice it is of least value when it is most needed. Although significant amounts of air may be aspirated through a correctly placed right atrial catheter, serious air embolism is best prevented by good surgical technique and prompt flooding of the surgical site with saline if air is suspected. Nitrous oxide should be discontinued. The cerebral venous pressure is quickly raised by compressing the jugular veins, either manually or by a special cuff around the neck.

A patent foramen ovale is a common (25–35%) incidental finding at postmortem,[14] but can be readily detected preoperatively by contrast Doppler echocardiography.[15] Paradoxical air embolism can occur through a patent foramen ovale (PFO), as the atrial pressure gradient can reverse transiently at certain phases of the cardiac cycle, even if the mean LA pressure exceeds mean RA pressure. A small bubble of air entering the left side of the heart in the sitting position is likely to enter a cerebral or coronary artery.

Many surgeons have abandoned the sitting position in neurosurgery, believing the risks of air embolism outweigh the excellence of the surgical conditions that it gave.

Craniofacial surgery

The main problems are airway difficulties and heavy blood loss.

Trans-sphenoidal surgery

Usually for pituitary tumours. Not suitable for suprasellar extensions. Although operating through an unsterile part of the body, meningitis is surprisingly rare. The operation is well-tolerated, with minimal trauma and blood loss. Diabetes insipidus is uncommon. Vasoconstrictors should be applied to the nasal mucosa. The patient should be warned that the nose will be packed when he or she awakes. Full steroid cover is needed, and thyroid hormone replacement.

Operation for intractable epilepsy

Electrophysiological mapping of the cortex during craniotomy may be done in specialized centres under intravenous sedation and local analgesia.

Operations on the spinal cord and vertebral column

Usually performed for degenerative and disc disease, tumours or extradural haematoma. Tumours of the spinal cord may interfere with intercostal or even the phrenic nerve roots. Operations are usually carried out in the lateral or prone position, but supine for anterior cervical fusion. *See above* for electrophysiological monitoring of spinal cord function.[16]

Bleeding from extradural veins is the chief problem. Any increase in abdominal pressure, from coughing, straining or incorrect positioning, forces blood through the vertebral veins and distends them. For lumbar surgery, if the patient is supported prone with his or her weight on the upper chest and the pelvis so that the abdomen is free, and the lumbar spine flexed, then the extradural veins collapse. This also prevents hypotension due to vena caval obstruction. Special padded frames with an adjustable angle of flexion are available. Full relaxation helps. The arms may be placed above the head, giving excellent venous access.

Intermittent positive-pressure ventilation is usual. Induced hypotension should not be necessary, especially if extradural block is combined with general anaesthesia. Damage to the bowel, IVC and aorta may occur if the surgeon pierces the anterior longitudinal ligament. During high spinal surgery, cardiac dysrhythmias may occur. Cervical cord surgery may be followed by sleep apnoea (Ondine's curse).[17] The surgeon may stimulate the carotid sinus during an anterior approach to the cervical spine.

Excision of the odontoid peg and spinal fusion may be needed in patients with rheumatoid arthritis. It is approached through the mouth. Atlanto-axial instability is also common in Down's syndrome, often asymptomatic and so a trap for the unwary anaesthetist.[18] Lateral radiographs of the cervical spine should be performed in neck flexion and extension.

Anaesthesia for diagnostic procedures

The same considerations for monitoring and control of ICP and CBF are needed as for major neurosurgery. Conditions for the anaesthetist are never easy in a radiology department. Angiographic techniques are also used in the occlusion or embolization of cerebral aneurysms or arteriovenous malformations.

Ketamine (2 mg/kg i.v. or 10 mg/kg i.m.) may be used for diagnostic procedures in children such as CT/MRI scanning or lumbar puncture. The airway should be maintained without the need for tracheal intubation.

Computed tomography scanning

First described in 1973.[19] The head must be completely still for the several seconds taken for imaging each slice. General anaesthesia may be required in uncooperative adults and young children. Ketamine is useful, or tracheal intubation and the use of a very long Bain system, allowing machine and monitors to be outside the room, with the patient in sight through a window or camera. Contrast is often given intravenously to improve scan quality.

Magnetic resonance imaging

First used in 1973.[20] Immobility is vital for good images. The patient is placed in a strong magnetic field (above 0.5 Tesla) and exposed to radiofrequency pulses. Protons in certain atoms, especially hydrogen, realign themselves with the magnetic field, emitting an RF signal that induces microvoltages in the detector coils. The decay of this RF signal is described by two time constants T_1 and T_2, directed with and transverse to the magnetic field respectively. Imaging is achieved by varying the field strength across the body.

X-rays are avoided, but the magnetic field can:

1 attract ferromagnetic materials inside or outside the body, e.g. older vascular clips, laryngoscope batteries, gas cylinders, anaesthetic equipment; also such materials distort the image;
2 cause malfunction of pacemaker circuits, analogue and digital watches, magnetic storage media;
3 cause T-wave changes on the ECG of no clinical significance;
4 induce tiny currents inside the body which seem to be harmless.

The scanners are claustrophobic and noisy.

The anaesthetic machine and ventilator are best placed remotely, and a long circuit used with a suitably low expiratory resistance. A coaxial circuit may need modifying to achieve this. Monitoring is difficult as even non-ferromagnetic wire connections to the patient may degrade the image, but equipment compatible with high magnetic fields is available. The patient has to be removed from the body of the scanner in an emergency.

ELECTROCONVULSIVE THERAPY

Relative contraindications

1 Recent myocardial infarct or stroke.
2 Severe osteoporosis or a major fracture.
3 Raised ICP.

Pulse rate, blood pressure, cardiac output and catecholamine levels rise during the fit. Ventricular arrhythmias may be seen, although severe bradycardia or even asystole can occur just after the passage of the electric current. These circulatory changes are usually well tolerated, and the procedure is remarkably safe.[21]

Technique

Methohexitone (1 mg/kg) is given intravenously with a small dose of atropine, followed by suxamethonium 25–40 mg. Propofol (1.5 mg/kg) can be used, but shortens the duration of the fit. It is not clear whether this reduces the efficacy of treatment, but in any case, propofol and methohexitone have much the same recovery characteristics after electroconvulsive therapy (ECT).[22] The lungs are inflated with O_2 during the apnoeic period, and the electric current applied. There is usually a pilomotor reaction and unreactive pupils even if limb movements are absent. The current directly stimulates the muscles of mastication, and this can cause damage to teeth and lips. A rubber bite block should be used. Prolapsed disc and long bone fracture can occur.

BRAIN PROTECTION

Various measures have been put forward to 'protect' the brain from ischaemic insults. Hypothermia is the only established intervention that does so. Cerebral O_2 consumption falls progressively with temperature, and the EEG becomes isoelectric below about 21°C. Enough barbiturate will produce a flat EEG, but cerebral O_2 consumption can only be reduced by about 50%. Isoflurane behaves similarly. Both barbiturates and isoflurane may offer some protection against incomplete ischaemia. None of these agents has been useful given after an ischaemic insult. Intracranial pressure and blood glucose should be carefully controlled.

MANAGEMENT OF ACUTE HEAD INJURIES

The brain may be damaged by contusion, haemorrhage, oedema and microscopic diffuse axonal injury. The latter is important for long-term prognosis.

Initial treatment

First aid – airway management (lateral position as vomiting is likely), control of haemorrhage, speedy hospitalization. The first few minutes after the injury are crucial in determining the ultimate outcome. Subsequent treatment is then directed towards prevention of further brain injury.

Ventilation and adequacy of the airway are assessed

Oxygenation of the brain must be maintained. If tracheal intubation is needed it should be performed as a rapid sequence induction, after preoxygenation, thiopentone and suxamethonium, and with cricoid pressure. Ensuring the best conditions for intubation is more important than any transient rise in ICP after suxamethonium. Nasal tubes should be avoided if CSF drainage from the mouth, nose or ears suggests a base of skull fracture, as they can be passed into the cranial cavity by mistake. Precautions should be taken in case of instability of the cervical spine (radiography if there is time; immobilization of the neck if there is not). The chest should be examined for injury; a chest drain may be indicated to prevent a tension pneumothorax. If sedation is needed for a ventilated patient, a propofol infusion up to 4 mg/kg/h is satisfactory.

Circulation

Arrest any serious haemorrhage and maintain an adequate blood pressure. Blood loss from scalp wounds may require transfusion. It may not be wise to insert a central venous pressure (CVP) line from the neck if this is also injured. Disturbances of body temperature, fluid balance and fat embolism may occur.

Blood gases

Hypoxia, hypercapnia and acidosis must be avoided. Intermittent positive-pressure ventilation should be used early to correct any deterioration in blood gases. Neurogenic pulmonary oedema (NPO) is a rare complication of head injury, and is treated by IPPV, control of ICP and vasodilators to counteract the intense sympathetic outflow which causes NPO.

Neurology

Assess level of consciousness by the Glasgow Coma Scale, which uses the best verbal and motor responses on scales of 1 to 5 (or 6), and eye opening on a scale of 1 to 4.[23] The total score can thus range from 3 to 14 (or 15). Look for lateralizing signs (limb movements, pupil sizes and reflexes). Computed tomography or MRI scans if available. IPPV may be needed to control decerebrate spasms. Hypothermia, barbiturates and steroids[24] have no place in head injuries.

Associated injuries

Associated injuries should be sought. The patient may have taken drugs or alcohol. Uncomplicated head injury should not prevent the urgent treatment of abdominal injuries, compound limb fractures or haemothorax, though treatment of faciomaxillary fractures can usually be delayed.

Control of intracranial pressure

Many centres insert an ICP monitor (*see* above) if the Glasgow coma score is 8 or less. It also allows assessment of ICP waveform,[25] cranial compliance and the importance of a small haematoma. It cannot reflect regional variations in ICP, however, and the extent to which measurement of ICP improves outcome is contentious. Intermittent positive-pressure ventilation to a $PaCO_2$ of 4–4.5 kPa (30–34 mmHg) is recommended. Further reduction in $PaCO_2$ may reduce ICP, but at the expense of ischaemia caused by the cerebral vasoconstriction, and is of no benefit. Mannitol 0.5–1.0 g/kg is effective, but for a limited time.

Fits

These may be overt, or seen on the EEG of a paralysed patient. Voltage on the cerebral function monitor should be 5–15 μV. (Less may indicate ischaemia.) Fits markedly increase the brain's need for O_2 and must be controlled with barbiturates or benzodiazepines. Intermittent positive-pressure ventilation may well be needed if large doses are used.

Blood sugar

The dangers of hypoglycaemia are well-known, but hyperglycaemia may increase the brain damage after ischaemic episodes.

Anaesthesia for acute head injury surgery

Anaesthesia may be required for diagnostic procedures, evacuation of haematoma, elevation of a depressed fracture or for other associated injuries. There may be considerable blood loss. Pain relief may also be required after non-cranial surgery in the presence of a head injury.

Each case needs individual assessment. Special care will be needed over the ICP, airway (there may be bleeding into the airway with a fractured base of skull), ventilation, full stomach, aspiration, hypovolaemia and associated injuries. An antacid regimen is used if the patient is conscious. A rapid sequence induction and tracheal intubation is usually indicated. Fractures through the base of the skull or the sinuses may allow pneumoencephalus if face-mask ventilation is used, which may worsen with N_2O.[26]

Intracranial haematoma

May be extradural, often from the middle meningeal artery, subdural or intra-cerebral. Urgent operation is especially needed for the former. The results can be dramatic. Physical signs are a progressive:

1 increase in coma score;
2 dilatation of a pupil;
3 bradycardia and hypertension;
4 hemiparesis opposite to the side of the injury.

Confirmed by CT scan. If the clinical picture progresses to apnoea, the prognosis is poor, even when instantly remedied by IPPV. Burr-holes under local analgesia may be performed with success, but formal craniotomy is often needed immediately after CT scanning.

Transportation of patients with head injuries[27]

The airway must be secure. It is safer to sedate the patient, intubate the trachea and start IPPV *before transfer* if there has been any change in level of consciousness, if bleeding threatens the airway, or if there have been fits. Intubation will be much more difficult if it has to be performed during the journey. Facilities must be carried for intubation and IPPV with O_2 in all cases (tubes can fall out). Suction equipment must be available.

The cardiovascular system should be stable, and haemorrhage excluded as a cause of hypotension, *before transfer*. Intravenous and intra-arterial cannulae will be *in situ*, and a CVP line will often be useful. Electrocardiogram, O_2 saturation, body temperature, blood pressure and end-tidal CO_2 should be monitored during transfer. Normal drugs for resuscitation should be available, as well as sedatives, thiopentone, suxamethonium, a non-depolarizing relaxant, vasoactive agents such as ephedrine, dobutamine, etc., steroids and diuretics.

Prognosis

The long-term effects of head injury can seldom be assessed at the time of admission to the ITU. In general, younger patients have a better prognosis. Of those patients in coma for 6 h or more, mortality is around 50%. Permanent disability may result. Even if physical recovery is good, social and personality problems may arise.

Brainstem death

First described clinically in 1959,[28] but has been challenged.[29] For this diagnosis *all* the following signs must be present, in addition to a clear diagnosis of the underlying condition, for at least 12 h. Pupils have no response to light. Caloric and oculovestibular reflex absent. (There should be no wax in the ear.) The 'doll's-eye reflex' does not mean that there is brainstem death. Absent corneal, gag and carinal reflexes. No response to pain inflicted on head. No spontaneous respiration for 4 min in the absence of hypothermia and hypoxia, with a $PaCO_2$ of 6.7 kPa (50 mmHg) or more, provided that no drugs which affect these reflexes persist in the body. If blood-gas analysis is not available, ventilate with 100% O_2 for 10 min and then 5% CO_2 in O_2 for 5 min before disconnection.

In the UK the diagnosis is made by two senior doctors independently, the interval between such examinations depending on the clinical situation. The time of death is at completion of the last test. Other countries differ, e.g. in France the two examinations must be performed at least 24 h apart. Spinal reflexes may persist after brainstem death. Electroencephalography or cerebral angiography can confirm brainstem death. This is not necessary in the UK, but is more often used in the US.

Brainstem death and organ donation

Problems in the management of the brain dead for organ donation are hypotension, arrhythmias, oliguria, diabetes insipidus and coagulopathy. The 'rule of 100s' is useful:[30] keep systolic blood pressure over 100 mmHg using volume loading and, if needed, dopamine up to 5–10 μg/kg/min; keep urine output over 100 ml/h by maintaining the cardiac output, dopamine infusion and frusemide 20–40 mg; keep PaO_2 over 13.3 kPa (100 mmHg), and haemoglobin over 100 g/l. Some details vary with the organ(s) to be retrieved. For the lung, any tracheal suction should be performed in a sterile manner, O_2 toxicity avoided and 5 cmH$_2$O PEEP used to prevent atelectasis. For the kidney, give mannitol 0.5 g/kg before excision to ensure good urine flow.

Spinal cord injury

See 'Paraplegia' in Chapter 3.1. See also Hambly P. R. and Martin B. *Anaesthesia For Chronic Spinal Cord Lesions.* (Review) *Anaesthesia* 1998, **53,** 273.

REFERENCES

1 Brian J. E. *Anesthesiology* 1998, **88,** 1365.
2 Todd M. M. and Warner D. S. *Anesthesiology* 1992, **76,** 161.
3 Warner D. S. et al. *Anesth. Analg.* 1996, **83,** 348.
4 Kety S. S. and Schmidt C. F. *J. Clin. Invest.* 1948, **27,** 476.

5 McTaggart Cowan R. A. *Can. J. Anaesth.* 1998, **45,** 387; Manninen P. H. *Can. J. Anaesth.* 1998, **45,** 460.
6 Kawaguchi et al. *Anesth. Analg.* 1996, **82,** 593.
7 Dearden N. M. et al. *J. Neurosurg.* 1986, **64,** 81.
8 Thomas A. N. et al. *Anaesthesia* 1990, **45,** 383.
9 Shaw M. D. M. and Foy P. M. *J. R. Soc. Med.* 1991, **84,** 221.
10 Guy J. et al. *Anesth. Analg.* 1995, **81,** 1060; McGrath B. J. et al. *Anesth. Analg.* 1995, **81,** 1295.
11 Thomas A. N. et al. *Anaesthesia* 1990, **45,** 383.
12 Miller J. D. *Br. J. Anaesth.* 1995, **75,** 518.
13 Howard R. et al. *Anaesthesia* 1990, **45,** 222.
14 Thompson T. and Evans D. C. *Q. J. Med.* 1930, **23,** 135.
15 Konstadt S. N. et al. *Anesthesiology* 1991, **74,** 212.
16 Kawaguchi et al. *Anesth. Analg.* 1996, **82,** 593; McTaggart Cowan R. A. *Can. J. Anaesth.* 1998, **45,** 387; Manninen P. H. *Can. J. Anaesth.* 1998, **45,** 460.
17 Vella L. M. et al. *Anaesthesia* 1984, **39,** 108.
18 Powell J. F. et al. *Anaesthesia* 1990, **45,** 1049.
19 Hounsfield G. N. *Br. J. Radiol.* 1973, **46,** 1016 and Ambrose J. p. 1023; New P. F. J. et al. *Radiology* 1974, **110,** 109.
20 Lauterbur P. *Nature* 1973, **242,** 190.
21 Simpson K. H. and Lynch L. *Anaesthesia* 1998, **53,** 615.
22 Boey W. K. and Lai F. O. *Anaesthesia* 1990, **45,** 623; Matters R. M. et al. *Br. J. Anaesth.* 1995, **75,** 297.
23 Teasdale G. and Jennett W. B. *Lancet* 1974, **2,** 81.
24 Dearden N. M. et al. *J. Neurosurg.* 1986, **64,** 81.
25 Lin E. S. et al. *Br. J. Anaesth.* 1991, **66,** 476.
26 Finch M. D. and Morgan G. A. R. *Anaesthesia* 1991, **46,** 385.
27 Association of Anaesthetists. *Recommendations for the Transfer of Patients with Acute Head Injuries to Neurosurgical Units.* Association of Anaesthetists, London, 1996.
28 Mollaret P. and Goulon M. *Rev. Neurol.* 1959, **101,** 3.
29 Hill D. J. In Dobb G. J. (ed.) *Intensive Care: Developments and Controversies. Clin. Anesthesiol.* 1990, **4(2),** 601.
30 Gelb A. W. and Robertson K. M. *Can. J. Anaesth.* 1990, **37,** 806.

ANAESTHESIA FOR OPHTHALMIC SURGERY

In anaesthesia for intraocular surgery, a sudden rise in intraocular tension from the normal 10–20 mmHg following coughing, vomiting, contraction of the orbicularis oculi or straining may cause displacement of iris or vitreous into the wound.

ANATOMY OF THE EYE

1 Sclera – the leathery outer coat of the globe. The cornea, the transparent front part, has a very delicate posterior membrane which must not be damaged during operations. The cornea is oxygenated from air and aqueous humour.
2 The inner coat – the vascular choroid continuous anteriorly with the ciliary body and iris (which divides the anterior segment into anterior chamber in front and posterior chamber behind. These contain aqueous humour (secreted at about 0.1 ml/h), the controller of intraocular pressure).
3 Retina – the innermost, sensory layer, with focus on the cone-rich macula. Contains retinal blood vessels, and optic nerve.
4 Lens, held to the ciliary body by the suspensory ligament, separating vitreous from anterior segment.
5 Extraocular muscles controlling direction (exquisitely sensitive to relaxants).

INNERVATION OF THE EYE

1 Motor. Superior oblique muscle from fourth cranial nerve. Lateral rectus from sixth. All other extraocular muscles from the third nerve. Orbicularis oculis from the seventh.
2 Sensory. Optic nerve conveys vision. Other sensation from ophthalmic division of the fifth nerve.
3 Parasympathetic. Fibres arise from the Edinger–Westphal nucleus and run with the third nerve to synapse in the ciliary ganglion, then via the short ciliary nerves. Stimulation of the parasympathetic causes constriction of the pupil and of the ciliary muscle.
4 Sympathetic. Fibres from T1 synapse in the superior cervical ganglion and travel via the carotid plexus to join the long and short ciliary nerves. Stimulation produces dilatation of the pupil.

LOCAL ANALGESIA

This avoids complications of general anaesthesia, postoperative sedation, nausea and vomiting, and risks in cardiac and respiratory disease, but some patients do not like it and some are too restless or uncoordinated.

Loss of memory function in the elderly after cataract extraction under general anaesthesia is no different than after regional analgesia plus sedation, but regional analgesia is often preferred. The advent of phacoemulsification has transformed local analgesia for cataract surgery. Amethocaine drops are quite adequate for this. Lid retractors or facial nerve block may be used to prevent blinking.

Retrobulbar (retro-ocular) block

After topical analgesia of the cornea and conjunctival sac, the long and short posterior ciliary nerves and ciliary ganglion are blocked within the muscle cone. These supply the uveal tract and cornea and reduce the tone of the extraocular muscles. Retro-ocular block dilates the pupil, causes exophthalmos, reduces intraocular pressure and makes prolapse of the vitreous less likely. Two per cent lignocaine or prilocaine is a suitable solution, 2 ml (4 ml for enucleation).

1 Superior approach, through the superior rectus, with the patient looking downwards, from a weal just above the middle of the tarsal plate. A fine 5-cm needle is used and is inserted 3–4 cm backwards, slightly inwards and downwards. During movement of the needle, injection is continuous as a safeguard against injuring veins.
2 Inferolateral, from a weal at the inferolateral margin of the orbit. A fine 5-cm needle is inserted backwards along the floor of the orbit, until its tip is posterior to the eye at the apex of the orbit: 1–2 ml of solution are injected. A transconjunctival approach may also be employed. Deposition of a little solution is also necessary in superior rectus.

Retrobulbar haemorrhage

This is likely to follow puncture of a vessel by the needle used for retrobulbar block. It results in a rise in intraorbital pressure with proptosis and requires postponement of the operation.

Retrobulbar block using bupivacaine has been reported as resulting in brainstem anaesthesia with apnoea, needing IPPV and intubation.[1]

Periocular (peribulbar) block[2]

The block is advocated as simple to perform with a low incidence of complications.

Solution used: 2% lignocaine or 0.5% bupivacaine, or equal mixture of the two, or with added vecuronium 0.5 mg.[3] Total volume used 12–15 ml, occasionally 20 ml (especially in the elderly when fluid is likely to leak out from the space). Caution is needed if the axial length of the eye is < 26 mm.

Technique

1 Lower block. Skin weal in lower lid, just superior to inferior orbital rim, 1.5 cm medial to lateral canthus. Needle advanced through weal with bevel towards orbit. 'Pop' felt as passes through lower orbital septum. Needle point advanced towards equator of eye, angled supero-medially, 4 ml injected at depth of about 2.5 cm. Tension within orbital tissues monitored by testing eyeball movement by means of lid palpation. Often

there is a temporary proptosis and conjunctival oedema. On needle withdrawal 1 ml is delivered to the orbicularis oculi muscle.

2 Upper block. Skin weal to upper lid 1–2 mm medial and inferior to the supraorbital notch. Needle advanced through weal aimed at roof of orbit, parallel to nose. Advanced posteriorly over eyeball to depth of about 2 cm. Then it is directed medially and advanced 0.5–1.0 cm. Two to three millilitres are injected and eyeball tension checked. One millilitre injected into substance of orbicularis oculi on withdrawal. A pressure cuff is applied to the eye for 10–20 min. Degree of blockade checked 5 min after application. If there is mobility still present a further 3–4 ml is injected (lower injection for infero-lateral and upper injection for supero-medial movement).

Mechanism

Thought to be by diffusion of solution to branches of cranial nerves 3, 4, 5, 6 and 7 and to ciliary ganglion.

GENERAL ANAESTHESIA

The main priority is to avoid rises of intraocular pressure (normal 10–20 mmHg), because of risk of iris or vitreous prolapse during operation. Ideally the eye should be soft before the anterior chamber is opened, as a sudden decompression may produce stresses which can in turn result in choroid haemorrhage. Choroidal blood flow is affected by $PaCO_2$ (similar to the cerebral circulation).

Intraocular pressure may be lowered by:

1 mechanical methods, preoperative use of a pressure pad, or manual milking of fluid from the anterior chamber immediately prior to start of the operation;
2 hypocapnia;

The ancillary problems often faced in the eye case

1 Diabetes, with the problems of control (*see* Chapter 3.1).

2 Old age, with severe respiratory disease and recognized or asymptomatic cardiac disease.

3 Other medical diseases, e.g. rheumatoid arthritis, Down's syndrome and rare congenital disorders (*see* Chapter 3.2).

4 Associated trauma in cases of perforating eye injury.

3 hypotension;
4 reduction of CVP;
5 acetazolamide;
6 intravenous anaesthetics, narcotic analgesics and volatile anaesthetic agents (provided $PaCO_2$ not allowed to rise).

It is raised by:

1 hypercapnia;
2 coughing, sneezing, straining, intubation and other causes of raised CVP;
3 suxamethonium;
4 locally administered atropine (in narrow-angle glaucoma);
5 local steroids.

ANAESTHETIC DRUGS IN OPHTHALMIC SURGERY

Premedication. Drugs used must not contribute to postoperative vomiting. *Benzodiazepines* are often employed.

Short-acting *opioids* are a useful adjunct in the anaesthetic sequence and do not overcome the local midriatics used. Antiemetics may be given routinely.

Non-steroidal antinflammatory drugs are excellent for postoperative analgesia, as are other simple analgesics.

Suxamethonium. This increases intraocular tension but the rise is probably confined to the period of apnoea and so is no reason for banning this useful aid to intubation. The average rise is 7–8 mmHg. It comes on in 30 s, is maximal at 2 min and has disappeared in 6 min after injection. It is normally avoided in open eye operations.

The mechanism of the rise in intraocular pressure is not fully understood. It may be that contraction of the extraocular muscles is important, but there is evidence that pressure rises even when these muscles have been detached from their insertions.

These effects can be minimized by the injection of a small dose of a non-depolarizing relaxant or acetazolamide, 500 mg immediately before induction of anaesthesia.

Non-depolarizing relaxants reduce the tone of extraocular muscles, enable intubation and produce apnoea. Intermittent positive-pressure ventilation has the advantage that $PaCO_2$ can be controlled. Relaxants also allow light planes of anaesthesia to be maintained with rapid recovery on completion of surgery.

Intravenous agents. Thiopentone, propofol and etomidate reduce the tension in normal and glaucomatous eyes.

Inhalation agents. The volatile agents offer good conditions, facilitating IPPV or spontaneous breathing (with quiet respiration and minimal postoperative nausea and vomiting). Intraocular pressure falls.

Nitrous oxide is avoided when SF_6 is used in vitrectomies to prevent a rise of pressure due to diffusion.

Ecothiopate iodide (phospholine iodide, an organophosphate derivative of choline). Low levels of serum cholinesterase amounting to a twofold reduction in one-third of patients can occur within a few days of commencing the use of drops of this agent in the treatment of glaucoma. Although a 50% reduction in enzyme activity should not prolong apnoea with suxamethonium for more than 10–15 min a non-depolarizing agent may be preferred. The effects of these drops on the enzyme level lasts 2–4 weeks after the cessation of treatment.

SOME SUITABLE GENERAL ANAESTHETIC TECHNIQUES

Intraocular operations

For example phacoemulsification, and intraocular lens implant for cataract, or corneal grafts.

Standard techniques are satisfactory with use of a tracheal tube to ensure the airway. Coughing on the tube is prevented by relaxants, If the eye is open this complication may be disastrous as vitreous can be extruded.

Advantages of general anaesthesia

1 Cooperation of patient ceases to become a problem.

2 No risk of retrobulbar haematoma from injection of local analgesic drug.

3 Less of an ordeal for the patient.

4 Quiet atmosphere in theatre facilitates delicate surgery.

An alternative to the use of a tracheal tube is the laryngeal mask.

Coughing may be prevented by codeine 1 mg/kg i.m.

Ventilation laryngeal masks, with a better seal around the larynx, are being developed.

Particular care is taken when inflating the cuff of the endotracheal tube, so that it just seals the airway. A higher pressure in the cuff than this may damage the tracheal mucosa, causing serious postoperative coughing and rise of intraocular pressure.

Two suitable techniques are:

1 propofol, muscle relaxant, N_2O and O_2, supplementation with a volatile or intravenous agent and IPPV;

2 spontaneous respiration can be allowed, via laryngeal mask. Volatile agents must be given in sufficient concentration to ensure that coughing does not occur. Eye cases have an extraordinary tendency to cough. It may be worth suppressing this by codeine 1 mg/kg i.m.

Cataracts in young adults may be associated with dystrophia myotonica or with diabetes.

Vitrectomy

This raises the following problems for the anaesthetist:

1 Avoiding a rise of intraocular pressure due to suxamethonium, intubation, (esmolol may be used prophylactically).
2 Avoiding hypertension due to intubation (may cause choroid haemorrhage). Esmolol may be used prophylactically.
3 Relaxant wearing off during a prolonged procedure (neuromuscular monitoring required, with appropriate top-ups of relaxant).
4 Nitrous oxide diffusion into CF_6 (gas used in the vitreous space), causing rise of volume and pressure, with local pressure effects. (Nitrous oxide is discontinued 10 min before SF_6 is instilled.)
5 Postoperative vomiting and coughing, with risk of iris herniation. (Prophylactic antiemetics and intramuscular codeine are very helpful.)

Repeated operations at short intervals may be required. Non-depolarizing relaxants, IPPV and full monitoring techniques are recommended.[4]

Retinal detachment

This is often an extraocular operation; a smooth and quiet induction, emergence and postoperative period are required in order to reduce the likelihood of further detachment. The oculocardiac reflex may be a problem.

Perforating eye injuries

Other injuries should be considered. Smooth anaesthesia is the order of the day. Induction of anaesthesia must avoid coughing and straining as these are associated with an acute rise in intraocular pressure with the danger of loss of vitreous fluid. Surgery is rarely urgent and the optimal time of operation must be discussed with the surgeon. Each case must be judged on its merits, attention being paid to:

1 urgency of surgery;
2 likelihood of full stomach;
3 possible difficulty of tracheal intubation.

Few anaesthetists have personal experience of a large series of cases. A suitable technique for many cases includes preoxygenation, thiopentone induction, generous dose of non-depolarizing relaxant, e.g. rocuronium. Intubation as soon as possible, use of cricoid pressure and maintenance along the usual lines. There are workers of experience who have used suxamethonium for intubation without vitreous loss, especially when there is judged to be a risk of aspiration of stomach contents.

Squint correction

Intravenous propofol, opioid and N_2O/O_2, volatile agent with spontaneous respiration via a laryngeal mask is usually suitable. As the patient is usually a child, gas induction may be appropriate.

The oculocardiac reflex: a variety of stimuli arising in or near the eye (especially following traction on the internal rectus, or pressure on the eyeball), may cause bradycardia and arrythmias, especially in the young, with (sometimes almost immediate) cardiac arrest. Prophylactic use of atropine is recommended. Adequate cardiac monitoring must accompany these interventions. Immediate action may be required. The surgeon is asked to relax the eye muscles, more atropine is injected intravenously.

The oculocardiac reflex may also be seen during operations for the correction of facial fractures, in patients with the Marcus Gunn syndrome and in operations on the empty orbit.

Examination of the eyes or tonometry

In small children. Spontaneous breathing using a small laryngeal mask for volatile agent with N_2O and O_2 is satisfactory.

REFERENCES

1 Chang J. L. et al. *Anesthesiology* 1984, **63**, 789.
2 Fry R. A. and Henderson J. *Anaesthesia* 1990, **45**, 14.
3 Reah G., Bodenham A. R., Braithwaite P., Esmond J. and Menage M. J. *Anaesthesia* 1998, **53**, 551–554
4 Mirakhur R. K. *Ann. R. Coll. Surg. Engl.* 1985, **67**, 34.

ANAESTHESIA FOR ORTHOPAEDIC OPERATIONS

INTRODUCTION

Orthopaedic operations lend themselves to the use of regional anaesthesia – a particularly gratifying form of the art of anaesthesia producing high-quality postoperative pain relief. The Synopsis of Anaesthesia has been an enthusiastic proponent of these regional techniques for over half a century. It is therefore appropriate, in a discussion of orthopaedic anaesthesia to include some gentle warnings about the use of regional blockade.

1 Many patients do not like large areas of the body being numb and paralysed postoperatively. Blocks should cover as small an area as relevant.
2 Day-case patients may not be able to go home if their limbs are paralysed for several hours after operation. Sensory blocks are preferred to motor block. Ropivacaine 1–2 mg/ml or bupivacaine are suitable.
3 Anaesthetists are advised not to offer to conduct caudal epidurals in place of the surgeon.
4 When compartment syndrome is a risk (e.g. in tibial nailing), the cardinal sign of this (pain) would be obscured by a regional block, leading to a dangerous delay in diagnosis.
5 Orthopaedic regional blocks may be performed to avoid instability in patients with serious cardiovascular disease. However, spinal blockade may cause hypotension, or the conscious patient may have uncontrollable hypertension due to fear. Both are dangerous to the safety of the patient.
6 The old orthopaedic aphorism is also relevant to the anaesthetist: 'bones are not filled with marrow, they are filled with dark ingratitude'.

A high proportion of orthopaedic operations are conducted in very old and ill patients with major medical and anaesthetic problems. Tourniquets are the responsibility of the operating surgeon. However, their use affects the anaesthetic: exsanguination of the lower limb causes a rise in CVP and arterial pressure, which may be serious in patients, with actual or potential congestive

---

Prevention of venous thromboembolism:
Mechanical methods

Graduated compression stockings (TED), intermittent pneumatic compression, foot pumps.

Pharmacological methods

1 Heparin and low-molecular-weight heparins.

2 Dextran 70.

3 Aspirin and non-steroidal anti-inflammatory drugs (NSAIDs).

4 Oral anticoagulants, e.g. warfarin.

Use of regional blocks

They have a lower incidence of deep venous thrombosis (DVT) than under general anaesthesia.

cardiac failure. The pressure in a pneumatic tourniquet should be the arterial pressure plus 30–50 mmHg in the arm and plus 50–70 mmHg in the leg; duration of inflation in the arm should not exceed 1 h and in the leg, 1.5 h, and should be used with the greatest care in patients with ischaemic vascular disease and if sickle-cell trait is present. Application of an Esmarch bandage or Rhys–Davies exsanguinator may cause the release of a blood clot causing pulmonary embolism. The acidosis resulting from ischaemia in the limb may precipitate a crisis in a patient with sickle-cell disease (*see* Chapter 3.1). A tourniquet may also be associated with postoperative DVT, and with changes of blood levels of drugs[1] and CO_2.[2]

The pressure gauges of tourniquets used for surgery and anaesthesia, especially if intravenous regional analgesia (IVRA) is used (Chapter 5.2), should be tested regularly to ensure that their measurements are reasonably accurate. An Esmarch bandage should not be used as a tourniquet.

MANIPULATIONS

Require good relaxation for a short time; are conveniently done under intravenous agents, a relatively large dose being given just before the surgeon is ready to produce the trauma. A short-acting opioid, e.g. remifentanil may be added if required. Preoxygenation is beneficial.

LEG AMPUTATIONS

These patients are often elderly, ill, with a high incidence of vascular disease, sepsis, diabetes and atrial fibrillation. Rheumatoid arthritis, obesity and severe respiratory disease are also common.

Because of the possibility of phantom limb pain, unilateral intradural spinal analgesia is useful. Care must be taken, hopefully to keep a spinal block unilateral, by maintaining the lateral position for 20–30 min after subarachnoid injection with the diseased side down, to limit the degree of sympathetic block. A good alternative is lumbar plexus blockade which does not block the sympathetic nerves. Otherwise light general anaesthesia or ketamine (especially s-ketamine) is suitable.

In the emergency situation, with an unprepared patient, local infiltration by the surgeon ('squirt-and-cut'; Schleich technique) is a very safe technique.

Meticulous preoperative preparation and postoperative care together with low-dose heparin can improve the prognosis of this potentially dangerous operation.

Anaesthetic problems of the elderly

Cardiovascular system

Ischaemic heart disease, poor cardiac function and perfusion of vital organs, atherosclerosis and hypertension.

Respiratory system

Increased closing capacity, with airway collapse and hypoxia; poor respiratory response to hypoxia, increased incidence of atelectasis, pulmonary embolus and postoperative chest infection.

Nervous system

Cerebrovascular impairment, hearing and sensory impairment; confusion.

Pharmacology

Increased sensitivity to central nervous system (CNS) depressants and other drugs. Impaired drug distribution, metabolism and elimination. altered plasma protein and drug binding.

Metabolism

Slower metabolic rate; impaired renal blood flow and function; impaired fluid balance, especially dehydration; and malnutrition.

Other problems

Physically frail with impaired temperature control; increased likelihood of gastro-oesophageal reflux; cervical spondylosis and arthritis with limitation of movement; thin vulnerable skin. Diabetes more common.

INTERNAL FIXATION OF HIP FRACTURES

Main problem[3]

The patient is usually elderly and often handicapped by heart failure, hypertension and respiratory failure, stroke, diabetes, anaemia, osteoporosis, dehydration, mental deterioration and sometimes hypothermia. Many will be suffering from hypoxia, perhaps due to fat embolism, and this will be made worse by operation. These conditions are dangerous and must be treated before surgery; postponement of the fixation for a few days after injury will not increase morbidity or mortality. A femoral nerve block will ease the pain during movement of the patient. Rehydration by intravenous infusion is commenced on arrival in hospital.

Anaesthesia

Any reasonable method of anaesthesia, if carefully applied and if dosage is kept low, is usually safe on the operating table, but postoperative mortality is influenced by:

1 depressed mental function preoperatively;
2 age greater than 85 years;
3 neoplasia;
4 postoperative chest infection;
5 deep wound infection.[4]

There are arguments for and against most of the commonly employed techniques. The usual choice is between general anaesthesia and spinal block (which gives good results and reduces postoperative hypoxaemia and even early mortality). Spinal block tends to be avoided in patients with low cardiac reserves, who will not compensate for sympathetic blockade. General anaesthesia tends to be avoided in patients with respiratory failure. The patient may have a preference for one or the other.

Hypocapnia is avoided because of its cerebral vasoconstriction. The target is to keep all monitored parameters normal. Intraoperative short-acting opioids, e.g. fentanyl are used in small dosage, as they last much longer in the elderly.

Patients in poor condition may be managed by a combination of nerve block, intravenous ketamine (and benzodiazepine).[5] Intermittent ketamine, with or without diazepam, has given better results than IPPV with relaxant.[6] S-ketamine could be used if available. Postoperative analgesia has been obtained by lateral cutaneous nerve block.[7]

Oxygen may need to be given for 1–2 nights postoperatively.

Sequelae and complications

Mortality is high in the elderly and is chiefly due to patient problems rather than anaesthesia problems. Oxygen therapy and plasma volume expanders are usually continued in the postoperative period. Postoperative cognitive deficit (POCD) is common. Its lack of response to advances in anaesthesia over the last 50 years implies a non-anaesthetic cause.[8]

TOTAL REPLACEMENT OF THE HIP OR KNEE JOINTS

Problems

Old age, obesity; severe cardiac and respiratory disease; haemorrhage; possible lateral position of the patient. The use of *polymethyl methacrylate cement*, is often followed by systemic absorption of the monomer causing hypotension and even by cardiac arrest, probably due to vasodilatation and cardiac depression. The prior infusion of 500 ml of a suitable plasma volume expander usually counteracts this, and a head-down tilt of the table may be helpful. Femoral marrow embolism also occurs, mediated by prostacyclin, thromboxane and other mediators.[9] A vent tube should be placed in the marrow cavity when cement is forced in, to prevent absorption and embolism.

When cement is used in knee replacement, the tourniquet delays absorption and hypotension. The patient collapses just as the surgeon removes the cuff and walks away.

The surgical contortions may cause injury to leg veins leading to thrombosis and embolism. Cardiovascular collapse during this operation may also be due to air embolism.

Full cardiac and respiratory work-up are advised. Dyspnoea is an unreliable symptom in these cases, because of immobility of the joints.

Anaesthesia

Bleeding is usually a problem. Availability of transfusion is double-checked. Normovolaemic haemodilution[10] has been employed.

The choices lie between general anaesthesia, spinal block and lumbar plexus block. The latter has the advantage that there is no sympathetic blockade, and is suitable for patients with both cardiac and respiratory failure, giving postoperative analgesia. It may be combined with light general anaesthesia.

Central neural blockade by lowering the blood pressure reduces bleeding and may reduce the incidence of thrombosis. Maintenance of usual blood pressure by ephedrine, is important. Intradural and extradural blocks have their advocates. Hypothermia must be prevented. A small catheter is inserted into the femoral shaft before cement is forced in, to prevent fat, monomer and air embolism.

Whatever the anaesthetic technique, all monitored parameters are kept as normal as possible.

COMPLICATIONS AND SEQUELAE OF MAJOR LOWER LIMB JOINT SURGERY

Detectable vein-wall plaque thrombosis occurs in the majority of patients after operation. This may lead to pulmonary embolism, and the therapeutic

---

Key features of fat embolism

1 Cerebral – severe confusion.

2 Pulmonary – hypoxia needing IPPV.

3 Ophthalmic – blocked vessels visible.

4 Renal – acute renal failure.

5 Other – disseminated intravascular coagulation (DIC).

---

target is the prevention of this.[11] With extradural block there is normal fibrinolysis during and after surgery and so less tendency for clot formation than if a general anaesthetic is given.[12] Fat embolism occasionally accounts for postoperative hypoxaemia and adverse cerebral effects. Air embolism may occur. Blood loss is monitored and carefully replaced, including postoperative loss.

SPINAL OPERATIONS

Lumbar laminectomies and fusions are performed in the lateral or prone position, which interferes with respiration and inferior vena caval flow, unless special frames are used. However, air embolism has been reported in patients on these frames.[13] General anesthesia is commonly used.

Surgery of the thoracolumbar spine demands scrupulous anaesthetic technique and careful positioning to avoid an increase in pressure in the extradural veins; the main problem is to produce an ischaemic field. Some surgeons infiltrate the skin incision and interspinal region with adrenaline saline solution to aid haemostasis. Extradural lumbar block has also been used, e.g. for the grossly obese; with the warning to the surgeon that there will be clear fluid in the extradural space (as well as within the dura).

Anterior cervical fusion may result in vocal cord paralysis.

FRACTURES OF THE CERVICAL SPINE

The patient should be intubated and placed on the operating table with the cervical collar and traction still in place so that the position is not altered. This may be difficult, but the patient usually adopts the position providing the clearest airway. Intubation may be difficult and may require fibreoptic intubation. Cervical fusion itself makes intubation more difficult.

OPERATIONS FOR KYPHOSCOLIOSIS

Assessment: is there interference with respiratory function (with cardiac failure)? Lung and cardiac function tests are needed. Are there other congenital problems? Will the (teenage) patients be anxious, needing premedication?

The main problems are prolonged surgery, heat loss, blood loss (haemorrhage may be profuse – cross-match 5–10 units), invasive monitoring is often needed; poor access to the patient who will be on a Toronto frame, pneumothorax (requiring chest drains) may occur.

The patient may be woken up in the middle of the operation and asked to move his or her toes, to exclude possible cord damage. Light sedation is useful for this phase. The alternative is spinal cord evoked potential monitoring.[14]

At the end of the operation, during which a narcotic, relaxant, N_2O and O_2 technique, with **IPPV** is usually satisfactory, the muscle relaxant is reversed after the patient is placed supine, to prevent coughing while being moved. A rapid wake-up allows early testing of spinal cord damage.

For severe postoperative pain, a morphine infusion has proved useful (large doses are required), or extradural differential block including opioids. The catheter is placed by the surgeon towards the end of the operation. Postoperative respiratory failure, metabolic acidosis, and ileus are problems requiring routine ITU or HDU care. *See also* Chapter 4.2.

LONG BONE FRACTURES

Existing patient problems: pain, fat embolism (with adverse cerebral effects), other injuries (e.g. head, chest, abdomen), potential full stomach (delayed emptying in trauma).

Operative problems: blood loss may be severe in femoral fractures.

ARTHROSCOPY

General anaesthesia, e.g. via a laryngeal mask, avoids damage to the instrument from movement (which is not always prevented by regional block). Some strange positions are adopted for arthroscopy of shoulder and hip joints, and require care in supporting the patient. Air embolism has been reported.

Local anaesthetic in the joint cavity is effective for postoperative analgesia (e.g. 20 ml 0.25% bupivacaine in the knee). Intrajoint morphine has also been tried but is without effect.[15]

Anaesthesia for bone-marrow harvest, for transplantation, *see* Filshie J. and Pollock A. N. *Anaesthesia* 1984, **39**, 480.

REPEATED JOINT AND BONE MANIPULATIONS IN CHILDREN

Ketamine has a place in the management of small children who require repeated manipulation and application of plaster of Paris. Some multifactorial congenital diseases may coexist.[16] *See* 'Rare diseases', Chapter 3.2.

Pain after finger and toe operations can be relieved by simple metacarpal and metatarsal blocks with plain bupivacaine.

REFERENCES

1 Schmitt H., Batz G., Knoll R., Danner U. and Brandl M. *Acta Anaesth. Scand.* 1990, **34**, 104.
2 Bourke D. L., Silberberg M. S., Ortega R. and Willcock M. M. *Anesth. Analg.* 1989, **69**, 541–544.
3 Sinclair S., James S. and Singer M. *Br. Med. J.* 1997, **315**, 909–912.
4 Wood D. K. et al. *J. Bone Joint Surg.* 1992, **74**, 199–202.
5 Howard C. B. et al. *Anaesthesia* 1983, **38**, 993.
6 Spreadbury T. H. *Anaesthesia* 1980, **35**, 208.
7 Jones S. F. and White A. *Anaesthesia* 1985, **40**, 682.
8 Moller J. T. et al. *Lancet* 1998, **1**, 857–861.
9 Byrick R. J., Wong P. Y., Mullen J. B. and Wigglesworth D. F. *Anesh. Analg.* 1992, **75**, 515–522.
10 Thorburn J. *Br. J. Anaesth.* 1985, **57**, 290.
11 Palmer A. J. et al. *Haemostasis* 1997, **27**, 75–84.
12 Rosenfield BA, et al. *Anesthesiology* 1993,**79**, 435–443.
13 Albin M. S., Ritter R. R., Pruin C. E. and Kalff K. *Anesth. Analg.* 1991, **73**, 346–349.
14 Shimogi K., Kurokawa T., Tamaki T. and Willis W. D. *Spinal Cord Monitoring and Electrodiagnosis.* Springer-Verlag, Berlin, 1990.
15 Kalso E. et al., *Pain* 1997, **71**, 127–134; Picard PR et al. *Pain* 1997, **72**, 309–318.
16 Rochoff M. A. and Hall S. C. *Anesth Analg.* 1997, **85**, 1185–1190.

ANAESTHESIA FOR PLASTIC SURGERY AND BURNS

PLASTIC SURGERY

Anaesthesia

Skin grafts can often be removed painlessly from the thigh after block of the lateral femoral cutaneous and, if necessary, femoral nerves, or by intradermal and subcutaneous infiltration of skin. An alternative approach is to apply EMLA cream to the donor site preoperatively.

The main problems in anaesthesia for plastic surgery are: access to the airway may be restricted because of facial injuries, scars, cleft palate (*see* Chapter 4.2), or because of bizarre positions requested by plastic surgeons; provision of hypotension to facilitate the work of the surgeon – this may conflict with the absolute priority for cerebral perfusion, e.g. during mammoplasty with the patient in the sitting position.

The anaesthetist must be firm in upholding safe practice.

For anaesthetic management of patients undergoing operations for free flap transfer it is important to ensure adequate skin blood flow with: vasodilator drugs, e.g. GTN; light general anaesthesia; maintenance of arterial blood pressure and CVP; maintenance of normal blood gases, circulating volume, cardiac output and body temperature; and good postoperative analgesia. Central neural blockade does not prevent arterial muscle spasm.[1]

Microvascular surgery has become increasingly ambitious, and these operations can take extreme lengths of time, even into a second day. The patient must be kept immobile under the operating microscope, protected from bedsores and warm. A nasogastric tube may be needed to keep the stomach empty, while anaesthetic agents chosen should not be cumulative nor toxic (e.g. N_2O) if used for such long periods. Isoflurane is an ideal agent. General anaesthesia is usual, although adequate pain relief may be a problem. Postoperative shivering can destroy many hours of the plastic surgeon's work. Pethidine and chlorpromazine may be useful. Regional block may be used, even as the sole technique, for operations exceeding 20 h.[2]

BURNS

Initial assessment and management

The anaesthetist is more concerned with the extent and location of the burn, which determine fluid and airway management, rather than the thickness which dictates the surgical care. Percentage of body surface burned assessed by 'rule of nines': front and back of trunk 18% each, each leg 18%, each arm 9%, head and neck 9%, genitalia 1%. For children the 'rule of tens' is used: front and back of trunk 20% each, each limb 10%, head and neck 20%. The size of the patient's hand and fingers is 1% of surface area. Nearly 80% of patients admitted have less than 20% burns. Adults with burns exceeding 20% (or children over 10%) will need fluid resuscitation and those over 30% need the care of a burns unit. If the burn is over 60%, or if the patient's age added to the percentage burn exceeds 100, he or she is unlikely to survive. Many patients may be burned in the same accident.[3]

Monitoring

SpO_2, respiration, arterial pressure, ECG, arterial blood gases, COHb, and perhaps cyanide levels.

Pain and analgesia

Cooling with water gives immediate pain relief, but only influences burn thickness if applied within 30 s. Subsequent analgesia may be Entonox, increments of intravenous opiate, volatile agent and ketamine (which has been given orally). Analgesia may require large doses and respiration must be monitored.

Respiratory injury

Nearly 20% of burns patients have a respiratory component to their injury. Dry heat or sometimes inhaled irritants may damage the lining of the upper airway. If this has occurred, evidenced by oral burns, singed nasal hairs, carbon-stained sputum or any sign of upper airways obstruction, then early intubation should be performed, preferably awake using a fibreoptic laryngoscope. A nasotracheal tube is preferred if the mouth is burnt. Complete obstruction can supervene rapidly; delay may make the identification of landmarks and intubation impossible. Tracheostomy in burned patients is associated with a high incidence of infections and of subsequent tracheal stenosis.[4]

Oxygen therapy

Carbon monoxide and cyanides are also inhaled. COHb over 15% is significant. COHb over 50–60% or a plasma cyanide over 130 mmol/l is likely to be fatal and may require hyperbaric O_2. Some pulse oximeters and co-oximeter blood gas machines can measure COHb. Blood gases and chest radiography should be performed, and humidified 100% O_2 given by mask with reservoir bag if PaO_2 is below 10 kPa, or to shorten the half-life of COHb from several hours, to less than 1 h. Ventilatory support may be needed. Regular steroids increase mortality, but a single large dose given early may benefit.[6]

Direct thermal damage is rare below the trachea, but pulmonary damage results from inhalation of irritants, e.g. aldehydes from wood smoke, oxides of nitrogen and sulphur and hydrochlorides, or from chemical burns, e.g. phosgene. Copious sputum, wheezing, pulmonary oedema, infection and an ARDS-like picture develop some 4–10 days after the burn. Escharotomies may be needed to allow adequate respiration in the presence of circumferential burns of the trunk.

Fluid therapy

Capillaries in the burnt tissue become leaky and large amounts of fluid and plasma proteins are lost into the extracellular space, mostly in the first 2–3 h.[7] Intravenous infusion will probably be needed and perhaps central venous or even pulmonary wedge pressure monitors. Venous access may be difficult because the usual sites are burnt. The patient should be weighed, and a urinary catheter may be needed with careful asepsis. Haemoglobin, packed cell volume (PCV), plasma and urine electrolytes should be measured.

There are many different formulae for calculating fluid requirements. A common one is that of Muir and Barclay:[8]

Fluid requirement (ml) = 0.5 × body weight (kg) × area of burn (%)

This volume is given (in addition to normal water and electrolyte needs) as colloid (human albumin), 4-hourly for the first 12 h, 6-hourly for the next 24 h, and then as needed to keep the PCV normal. However, it has been suggested that fluid resuscitation with human albumin may be associated with an increased mortality.[9]

In the US up to 4 ml/kg/% area of burn are given as lactated Ringer's solution in the first 24 h. Another regimen is hypertonic saline (Na 250 mmol/l) to keep the urine output greater than 1 ml/kg/h for the first 24 h, and 0.5 ml/kg/h after that.[10] This may be difficult because of the high secretion of vasopressin. A mixture of Hartmann's solution and gelatin solution has been used.[6] Blood may be needed to replace red cells damaged by deep burns, to keep PCV up to 35%.

Metabolic and immune effects

The hypercatabolism and rise in metabolic rate following burns is greater than after other forms of trauma. This compensates for the loss of heat by evaporation and impairment of vasoconstriction. The hypothalamic thermostat is reset at a higher temperature. There is a rise in plasma catecholamines, cortisol, glucagon, and particularly in vasopressin.[11] Hyperglycaemia is common. Energy requirement is 20 kcal/kg + 50 kcal/% burn, and may exceed 17 MJ/24 h (4000 kcal/day) with insulin infusion. Protein needed is 1 g/kg + 2 g/% burn. Palatable food is best but will often need to be supplemented by enteral tube feeding and sometimes parenteral nutrition. During anaesthesia, the increased metabolism requires a high alveolar ventilation. All aspects of the immune response are suppressed. Infections are a particular danger, and are treated energetically as they arise. Aminoglycosides, ticarcillin, azlocillin are commonly used.

Problems for the anaesthetist after the initial resuscitation

1 *The need for repeated procedures*, e.g. dressings. This may be done with neurolept analgesia or opiate analgesia supplemented by Entonox if needed. Ketamine, (2 mg/kg i.v. or 10 mg/kg i.m.) is useful particularly in children or where scarring of the neck makes airway maintenance difficult, but it does not always prevent aspiration.
2 *Further major operations* such as tangential excision of burnt tissue under general anaesthesia is associated with considerable haemorrhage. Intermittent positive-pressure ventilation with large tidal volumes is needed. Propofol and alfentanil infusions have been successful.[12] Controlled hypotension or the use of tourniquets if possible has been advocated to reduce blood loss.
3 *Practical difficulties of venous access*, applying a face mask, difficult airway if the neck is scarred, siting the blood pressure cuff, ECG electrodes or oximeter probe. An oesophageal stethoscope is useful. The patient may need to be placed in an unusual position on the operating table.
4 *Associated trauma to other organs*. Particularly if the patient has jumped out of an upstairs window.
5 *Deep venous thrombosis*.
6 *Suxamethonium* may cause a dangerous rise in serum potassium and cardiac arrest, especially if given between 3 and 8 weeks after the burns, due to increased number of extrajunctional receptors. Others recommend the avoidance of this drug at any time between 5 days and 4 months after.
7 *Resistance to the action of non-depolarizing relaxants*.[13] ED_{95} doubled (peak effect 2 weeks after burn) possibly for the same reason.
8 *Renal failure*, associated with either haemoglobinuria or myoglobinuria. Urine output should be watched closely. Alkalinization of the urine may be protective.
9 *Loss of drugs* into oedema fluid and because of decreased binding proteins. Aminoglycosides and cimetidine may need higher doses.

See also Martyn J. A. J. *Acute Management of the Burned Patient.* W. B. Saunders, Philadelphia, 1990; Robertson C. and Fenton O. *Br. Med. J.* 1990, **301,** 282.

REFERENCES

1 Aps C. et al. *Ann. R. Coll. Surg. Engl.* 1985, **67,**177.
2 Shanahan P. T. *Anesth. Analg.* 1984, **63,** 785.
3 Griffiths R. W. *Br. Med. J.* 1985, **291,** 917.
4 Lund T. et al. *Ann. Surg.* 1985, **201,** 374.
6 Williams J. G. et al. *Br. Med. J.* 1983, **286,** 775.
7 Arturson G. *Acta Anaesthesiol. Scand. Suppl.* 1985, **82,** 55.
8 Muir I. *Intensive Care Med.* 1981, **7,** 49.
9 Schierhout G. and Roberts I. *Br. Med. J.* 1998, **316,** 961; Cochrane
   Injuries Group Albumin Reviewers. *Br. Med. J.* 1998, **317,** 235.
10 Monafo W. W. et al. *Surgery* 1984, **95,** 129.
11 Crum R. L. *Arch. Surg.* 1990, **125,** 1065.
12 Reyneke C. J. et al. *Br. J. Anaesth.* 1989, **63,** 418.
13 Martyn J. A. J. et al. *Anesth. Analg.* 1982, **61,** 614.

ANAESTHESIA FOR UROLOGY

For anaesthesia in patients with impaired renal function, *see* Chapter 3.1.

CYSTOSCOPY AND BLADDER TUMOURS

If *general anaesthesia* is used, there must be:

1 complete loss of sensation;
2 relaxation of bladder sphincters and abdominal wall;
3 no straining, coughing or respiratory obstruction.

These can be difficult to accomplish smoothly, especially in the elderly with
heart and lung disease, and receiving many different drugs. It should never
be undertaken lightly, and may rarely even require tracheal intubation. Spontaneous respiration using O_2, N_2O and volatile agent with a small dose of
intravenous narcotic is a common technique.

A patient with bladder cancer may present for cystoscopy at regular intervals. Anaemia (sometimes severe) is common in these patients. If resection of
tumour is performed there is no significant absorption of the irrigation fluid.
Irrigation with normal saline is used postoperatively to prevent clot retention.
Bladder perforation may occur. Stimulation of the obturator nerve may cause
adduction of the patient's legs. Muscle relaxants or obturator nerve block will
prevent this.

Topical analgesia, e.g. lignocaine 1 or 2% gel may be satisfactory, especially
in women, or if a flexible fibreoptic cystoscope is used in men. Severe cystitis

makes local analgesia unsuitable as the distension of the bladder with irrigating fluid causes painful spasm. Extradural sacral block or intradural spinal analgesia is very satisfactory. Sympathetic supply to the bladder is from T11 to L2.

All instrumentation of the lower urinary tract is likely to cause significant bacteraemia. Prophylactic antibiotics are used (a single dose of gentamicin 120 mg). This must be combined with amoxycillin 1 g if the patient is at risk of endocarditis, and a further dose of amoxycillin 500 mg given orally 6 h afterwards.

TRANSURETHRAL RESECTION OF THE PROSTATE

General anaesthesia, either with spontaneous respiration or IPPV, may be supplemented by caudal extradural block to reduce bleeding and for postoperative pain. Intradural spinal block is also very satisfactory, e.g. 2–4 ml heavy or plain bupivacaine 0.5%. The block must reach at least T10.

Glycine 1.5%, at a pressure of less than 70 cmH$_2$O, is widely used for irrigation. Although slightly hypotonic (2.1% is isotonic) it has good optical properties, is non-electrolytic and prevents dissipation of diathermy current during resection. Glycine has a half-life of 85 min. Metabolic products include oxalate which may precipitate in the renal tubules if urine flow is low during the first 10 postoperative days, and ammonia which is a cerebral depressant. Glycine is an inhibitory neurotransmitter and may cause transient blindness. The amount which may be absorbed via the prostatic veins is typically around 700 ml or 20 ml/min, but can reach several litres, depending on the surgical skill, pressure of irrigant and duration of operation.

Glycine absorption can result in *TURP (transurethral resection of the prostate) syndrome*:[1] water intoxication, cerebral oedema, pulmonary oedema, hypoxia, nausea, vomiting, headache, fibrinolysis, bradycardia, hypertension, cardiac arrest, convulsions and coma. Burning sensations of the hands and face are early symptoms. The dilutional hyponatraemia may prolong the action of non-depolarizing relaxants, and cause QRS widening and T-wave inversion. Bacteraemia may confuse the clinical picture. Ideally the syndrome should be prevented by close observation of the patient and by monitoring the serum sodium. General anaesthesia will obscure the early symptoms. End-tidal ethanol levels after marking the irrigant with 1% ethanol have also been used as a measure of amount absorbed.[2] A sodium level below 120 mmol/l should be treated. The fully established syndrome is more difficult to manage. Treatment includes loop diuretics, e.g. frusemide 20–80 mg, water restriction, hypertonic saline (500 ml of 1.8%, 100 ml of 5%, 20 ml of 30%) with CVP monitoring, inotropic agents or even dialysis. Cold irrigating solutions may cause hypothermia.

Blood loss during this operation is difficult to measure, but is usually about 7–20 ml/g prostate resected. It will be increased by raising venous pressure (straining, overtransfusion, excessive absorption of irrigant), prolonged operation time and release of plasminogen activators from the prostate. Tranexamic acid 0.5–1 g may be useful. Blood loss is usually less with regional neural blockade than with general anaesthesia.

ABDOMINAL PROSTATECTOMY[3]

Better if the prostate is especially large. Relaxation is required and considerable haemorrhage may occur. General anaesthesia with IPPV is often used. Caudal or lumbar extradural analgesia (7–15 ml of plain bupivacaine 0.5% for the latter) is a useful supplement. Spinal intradural block to T10 with 2–4 ml heavy or plain bupivacaine 0.5%, is satisfactory. It provides relaxation and reduces bleeding. (*See also* Chapter 5.3). During transvesical prostatectomy there is considerable heat loss.

CIRCUMCISION

Babies and children may be given a normal intravenous or inhalational induction and spontaneous respiration maintained using O_2, N_2O and volatile agent. Laryngeal spasm may easily develop if anaesthesia is too light, and may need the surgery to be interrupted, the application of continuous positive airway pressure (CPAP) or even suxamethonium and intubation. Some prefer intubation and IPPV, using a volatile agent and a narcotic. In adults spontaneous respiration is generally used.

Extradural sacral block with bupivacaine 0.25%, 0.5 ml/kg, is an extremely useful adjunct, especially in children.[4] Penile block is a good alternative, blocking the dorsal nerves with 0.25% bupivacaine, 0.25 ml/kg in children, or 10 ml in adults. Postoperative sedation or beta-blocker for 3 days may help prevent painful erections after operation.

PRIAPISM

Erection may occur under anaesthesia when the penis is handled and can be difficult to treat. It may even preclude the insertion of a cystoscope. Deepening anaesthesia, topical local analgesics, dorsal nerve block,[5] nitroglycerin[6] or intracorporeal metaraminol 1 mg[7] may help. Terbutaline 0.25–0.5 mg or salbutamol 25 µg i.v. (in paraplegics)[8] have been used with success, as has ketamine in children.[9]

VASECTOMY

Innervation of the scrotum and its contents is derived from T10–L2 (splanchnic) and S2–3 (somatic). This operation is often done under local infiltration analgesia, but some surgeons prefer general anaesthesia as there is less likelihood of haematoma formation. This may be partly due to the postoperative sedation and the short bedrest required. Traction on the cord may result in bradycardia or even asystole. Atropine or glycopyrronium should be available and some give it preoperatively.

NEPHRECTOMY

First performed by Gustav Simon (1824–1913) of Heidelberg, in 1870.

Nerve supply to kidney and ureter arises from T10–L2. The pain of ureteric colic may be relieved by atropine, probanthine, hyoscine-n-methyl bromide (Buscopan), NSAIDs and narcotic analgesics. The bladder, lower ends of the ureters and the prostate are supplied by filaments of the inferior hypogastric plexus. This is formed from the sympathetic T11–L2, and parasympathetic S2–4.

Intermittent positive-pressure ventilation in the lateral position impairs respiratory efficiency, for although the lower lung has the higher blood flow, it receives less ventilation. Use of the kidney bridge further impairs lung function and predisposes to dependent atelectasis. When the patient is turned on the back at the end of the operation the lower lung should be fully inflated. Use of the kidney bridge in the lateral position may also cause inferior vena caval obstruction, leading to sudden severe hypotension. The patient may also be placed supine with a sandbag under the loin.

Renal tumours are extremely vascular. The anaesthetist should be prepared for torrential bleeding, and set up a wide-bore intravenous cannula. General anaesthesia with relaxant, IPPV, N_2O, volatile agent plus narcotic is usual, although spontaneous respiration may be employed. Both intradural and extradural analgesia up to T8 may be used, but is best combined with general anaesthesia. Ureteric tone is not greatly affected. Thoracic paravertebral block produces excellent unilateral analgesia without so much hypotension as an epidural. A paravertebral catheter may be inserted for postoperative analgesia.[10]

Rarely, the pleura is damaged during kidney operations; the resulting collapse of the upper lung may prove dangerous unless IPPV is employed. An underwater drain may be required. Tumour embolus causing collapse and cardiac arrest is an occasional complication of operations for carcinoma of the kidney.

TOTAL CYSTECTOMY

Much bleeding may occur, but there is an impressive reduction when employing extradural blockade. Circulatory monitoring is likely to include intra-arterial and central venous cannulae. A diuretic (e.g. frusemide 20 mg) is often requested at the end of the procedure.

HAEMODIALYSIS

Insertion of a Scribner shunt involves the insertion of an arterial and venous cannula with connecting link, in either the arm or leg. General anaesthesia and local infiltration with lignocaine have been used but are not always satisfactory. Regional analgesia has been advocated: axillary brachial plexus block with 10–20 ml 0.5% bupivacaine for the arm; sciatic (15–20-ml) and femoral (10-ml) blocks for the leg.

Anaemia is usually present; there may be impaired excretion of some of the drugs used; intravenous infusions must not be given into the arm with the fistula; suxamethonium should be avoided if the patient is hyperkalaemic. The further rise is likely to be less than 0.7 mmol/l with a single dose of 1 mg/kg but may be greater with repeated doses or in the presence of peripheral neuropathy.[11]

RENAL TRANSPLANTATION

First transplantation of a kidney by Richard H. Lawler (1935–1982) in 1950.[12] Immunological basis of tissue rejection described by Medawar in 1944.[13] Over 80% of first transplants function for more than a year, and the peripoerative mortality is less than 1%. Patients awaiting renal transplantation are in end-stage renal failure and have had repeated haemodialysis. Some will have already had nephrectomies. Hypertension, anaemia, pulmonary oedema, infections are common, and multiple drug therapy is likely. Neurological problems include mental changes, tremor, convulsions, coma, peripheral and autonomic neuropathy and myopathy. Problems during the operation include the maintenance of a stable cardiovascular system, and fluid and electrolyte balance.

Preoperative preparation

There is a limited time available for the correction of anaemia, acidosis and electrolyte imbalance. As there is an increased risk of aspiration, antacid, ranitidine or metoclopramide is given. Preoperative transfusion seems to confer no additional immunological advantage over cyclosporin.[14] Erythropoietin is very expensive but may be used in the most anaemic patients.

Technique[15]

Sedative premedication with an oral benzodiazepine may benefit the hypertensive, anxious patient. Some insert a multilumen internal jugular venous catheter before induction, which spares the arm veins and provides useful monitoring during and after the operation. Suxamethonium may be used for intubation despite the risk of hyperkalaemia if it is felt that the risk of aspiration warrants it. Intermittent positive-pressure ventilation is continued with N_2O, O_2, a volatile agent or fentanyl. Enflurane is best avoided because it is metabolized to fluoride. Atracurium is often the preferred relaxant as its elimination does not depend on renal function, but the need for relaxation in this extraperitoneal operation is slight. An automated oscillotonometer (on the opposite arm to any shunt) is used in preference to intra-arterial measurement to spare any trauma to the artery. There may be a rise in blood pressure on release of the vascular clamps. Regional techniques are not usually favoured. Fluid overload and potassium-containing fluids are to be avoided. Transfusions should not be used if possible as they may lead to haemosiderosis. Cryoprecipitate or desmopressin 0.3 μg/kg may counter any bleeding diathesis. Diuretics and low-dose dopamine are used to encourage urine output from the graft. Immunosuppression is usually with prednisolone, cyclosporin and azathioprine.

LITHOTRIPSY AND LITHOTOMY

Renal stones can now be treated without open operation in many cases. Bacteraemia is likely and should be covered by antibiotics.

PERCUTANEOUS NEPHROLITHOTOMY

This involves the passage of a telescope into the renal pelvis under radiological control, irrigation with saline, and electrohydraulic fragmentation until the stone can be extracted. Large volumes of saline may be absorbed if the pressure is allowed to rise above 75 cmH$_2$O in the pelvis.[16] The patient is semiprone, and IPPV is normally used, although neural blockade up to T8 may be satisfactory.

EXTRACORPOREAL SHOCK-WAVE LITHOTRIPSY (ESWL)

This fragments the stone by acoustic shock waves. It is non-invasive but painful. The patient is placed in a water bath to allow the shock to be focused on the stone. Arrhythmias are minimized by the shock wave being triggered 20 ms after the R wave. As many as 2500 shocks may be given at one treatment. Other problems include: variable length of procedure (up to 1–2 h); awkward positioning of the patient with poor access in an emergency; transfer of blood from the periphery into the thorax when immersed in water and back again at the end, with accompanying swings in blood pressure; use of image intensifier; noise of the shock waves. Lumbar extradural analgesia up to T4 using a catheter has been widely used.[17] Intradural analgesia is too inflexible, general anaesthesia technically difficult. Local infiltration alone (or even no analgesia at all) seems satisfactory for the newest generation.[18] Air used to identify the epidural space may be hazardous to the surrounding structures when the shock wave passes through.[19] Postoperative backache, nausea and vomiting are common. Extracorporeal shock-wave lithotripsy (ESWL) is contraindicated in pregnancy or with an uncorrectable bleeding disorder. Care must be taken if the spine is deformed, if the arteries in the abdomen are calcified or if the patient has a cardiac pacemaker.

REFERENCES

1 Gravenstein D. *Anesth. Analg.* 1997, **84**, 438.
2 Hahn R. G. *Anaesthesia* 1990, **45**, 577; Hultén J. et al. *Anaesthesia* 1991, **46**, 349.
3 Freyer P. *Lancet* 1900, **1**, 774.
4 Armitage E. N. *Clin. Anaesth.* 1985, **3(3)**, 535.
5 Papworth D. P. *Can. J. Anaesth.* 1987, **34**, 428.
6 Snyder A. R. and Ilko R. *Anesth. Analg.* 1987, **66**, 1022.
7 Block T. et al. *Urologe* 1988, **27**, 225.
8 Shantha T. R. *Anesthesiology* 1989, **70**, 707; Watt J. W. H. *Anaesthesia* 1998, **53**, 825.
9 Benson T. H. et al. *Anesth. Analg.* 1983, **62**, 457.
10 Richardson J. and Lönnqvist P. A. *Br. J. Anaesth.* 1998, **81**, 230.
11 Walton J. D. and Farman J. V. *Anaesthesia* 1973, **28**, 626.
12 Starzl T. E. *Surg. Clin. North Am.* 1978, **58**, 552.
13 Medawar P. B. *J. Anat.* 1944, **78**, 879.
14 Opelz G. *Transplant. Proc.* 1987, **19**, 149.
15 Cottam S. and Eason J. In Kaufman L. (ed.) *Anaesthesia Review 8*: Churchill Livingstone, Edinburgh, 1991, 159.
16 Sugai K. et al. *Br. J. Anaesth.* 1988, **61**, 516.
17 Richardson M. G. and Dooley J. W. *Anesth. Analg.* 1998, **86**, 1214.
18 Wilbert D. M. et al. *J. Urol.* 1987, **138**, 563.
19 Bromage P. R. and Bonsu A. K. *Anesth. Analg.* 1988, **67**, 484.

ANAESTHESIA FOR VASCULAR SURGERY

'Peripheral vascular surgery is surgery on ruins'

PREOPERATIVE EVALUATION[1]

This is a matter of risk assessment, optimization, timing of surgery, planning of anaesthesia, and arranging suitable postoperative intensive care.

Heart

Assessment of the degree of coronary disease and ventricular wall function, in addition to arrythmias. Known or silent myocardial infarctions may have occurred in 40–50% of these cases[2] (compared with 3–4% of all other preanaesthetic cases), and if recent, are a strong predictor of morbidity. The preoperative cardiovascular work-up is a controversial area and there is little consensus.

A scheme for preoperative cardiac risk assessment			
(*See* Davies J. M. et al. *Can. J.Anaesth.* 1994, **41**, 1156–1160)			
Disease history	Primary tests (if history positive)	Secondary tests (if primary tests positive)	Tertiary tests (if secondary tests positive)
Angina Previous myocardial infarction, etc. Diabetes High cholesterol Smoking Hypertension Age over 70 years Orthopnoea; dyspnoea (Heart failure)	ECG

Exercise ECG

Echo-cardiography

Dobutamine echo | Dipyridamole Thallium Scan | Coronary

Angiography |

Prophylactic coronary artery surgery may be indicated (but this surgery carries a significant mortality of its own). Control of hypertension (50–60% of these cases), while increasing peripheral perfusion, is also a difficult area, often requiring physician referral.[3] Routine use of serum troponin I and T in patients with chest pain would go some way to help identify those patients who have sustained myocardial damage.[4] A cardiac risk index is calculated.

Routine echocardiography, coronary angiography[5] and thallium scan with dipyridamole-induced maximum coronary vasodilatation have been used as important indicators of cardiac status. Myocardial ischaemia is a common (20%) operative complication, and causes over half the mortality of aortic surgery. Even 20 min of operative myocardial ischaemia gives hours of poor cardiac function ('stunning' effect, treated by adenosine modulation with acadesine[6]).

Class IV (HIGH RISK) patients with significant diabetes, previous stroke or previous myocardial infarction, may be better managed conservatively.

Cerebral perfusion

A history is sought (from a relative), of declining mental function, or of transient ischaemic attacks (TIAs) and the patient is tested for cognitive deficit, to assess likely operative risk. Angiography, MRI and positron-emission tomography (PET) scans may be required, especially for carotid endarterectomy.

Lung function

Is the patient a smoker or ex-smoker and has lung function been affected? Chronic obstructive pulmonary disease is common in these patients (25–50%). This will affect risk and duration of IPPV in the postoperative period.

Renal function

The incidence of postoperative acute renal failure is about 1%.

The existence of renal artery stenosis, preoperative mild renal failure (about 10%), age > 50, dehydration, hypotension, massive transfusion and warm ischaemia time > 30 min are predictors of perioperative acute renal failure.[7]

Blood

There may be high blood viscosity. The haemoglobin level and red-cell count are often high, and abnormal fibrinogens also contribute to this viscosity. Haemodilution with dextran 70 or other colloid is often beneficial.

> **Key points in preventing hypothermia**
> 1 Ambient temperature above 24°C.
> 2 Warm and humidify gases (100% at 37°C).
> 3 Airway heat exchangers.
> 4 Warm mattress.
> 5 Reflective blankets.
> 6 Intravenous fluid warmers.
> 7 Oesophageal thermal tubes.
> 8 Warm air convectors.

Concomitant disease

For example diabetes (in about 10%), puts the patient in a high-risk category.

Is the patient taking aspirin?

This is a common medication. If oozing haemorrhage is uncontrollable, platelet transfusion may be indicated.

MAIN PROBLEMS

This surgery is sometimes prolonged; the prognosis worsens after first hour; hypothermia is a major risk (active external warming is required) leading to peripheral vasoconstriction and coagulopathy in theatre.

Regular monitoring of coagulation status is required in every case, not only those where heparin is used. An IPPV technique with high-dose opiate supplements is usually used because of the poor general condition of these patients.

Cardiovascular stability

Cardiostable anaesthetic agents are used, with full invasive monitoring. The target is to maximize splanchnic, cerebral, coronary and peripheral perfusion; dopamine[8] and dopexamine[9] infusions (0.5–2 μg/kg/min) are frequently recommended. Levosimendan has been recommended to prolong cardiac systole without extra myocardial O_2 demand. Mesenteric artery ligation during aortic surgery may cause ischaemic colitis with all the postoperative intensive care problems that causes.

The compliance of the circulation is often very limited, with moderate blood loss causing major falls of CVP and MAP. Rapid response to this is required, and the CVP is often kept high, around 10–15 mmHg. Autoregulation of organ perfusion is reduced in arteriosclerosis. Therefore the arterial pressure is kept near the patient's normal, and normocapnia is maintained to optimize cardiac output and peripheral perfusion.

Cross-clamping the aorta (especially suprarenal) exerts maximum stress on the impaired myocardium, with 40–50% increased afterload resulting in failure. Nitroglycerin infusion 1–2 μg/kg/min may be used to prevent hypertension at this point. Inotropic support with dobutamine may be needed.

The magnitude of the effect of unclamping the aorta is critically dependent on the intravascular volume at the time. Central venous pressure and PCWP 10–15 mmHg is the target to prevent hypotension. Release of lactic acid from the limbs often requires bicarbonate 50–100 mmol i.v. to maintain cardiovascular stability and responsiveness to inotropes.

Haemorrhage

This may be massive (> 100ml/min). Transfusion is often needed and red-cell salvage autotransfusion an advantage. Intraoperative autotransfusion is deficient in platelets and clotting factors, and these should be given separately. All transfused blood must be warmed. There is still a great need for good synthetic O_2 carriers with better flow characteristics than blood.

Renal function

This may already be compromised by arteriosclerosis, diabetes and rarely, sepsis. Urine flow is monitored. good hydration is maintained throughout. Nephrotoxic antibiotics and NSAIDs are avoided. 'Renal dose' dopamine and dopexamine[9] can reverse intrarenal vasoconstriction and produce diuresis. Low-dose frusemide infusion may decrease renal O_2 consumption (in the absence of dehydration) and reverse oliguria. Care is needed to avoid a dehydrating polyuria with this drug. Mannitol may reduce renal medullary oxygenation.[10] Risk factors for renal failure include reduced renal perfusion,[11] due to aortic cross-clamping. Infrarenal cross-clamping reduces it; suprarenal cross-clamping abolishes it. Warm ischaemia time is critical in both situations.

Hypothermia

This causes coagulopathy, respiratory and cardiovascular problems and must be prevented. A high-efficiency patient warmer is positioned before surgery commences.

Pain control

Systemic opioids and regional analgesia are frequently employed. Sympathetic blockade from epidural analgesia, while helping lower limb vasodilatation, carries the risk of destabilizing the circulation. Therefore small incremental doses, with opioids, are used to achieve analgesia, without hypotension. The epidural catheter is sited at least 1 h before heparin is used. Myocardial ischaemia in the postoperative period is equally common (about 20%) whether epidural or patient-controlled analgesia (PCA) is used for analgesia,[12] although there is evidence that high thoracic block may be cardioprotective.[13] This has been disputed.[14]

Monitoring

Invasive monitoring of circulation as above, urine flow, coagulation status, arterial blood gases, acidosis, temperature, cerebral function during carotid endarterectomy. Pulmonary artery catheterization is especially useful in patients with ventricular dysfunction. An abnormal V wave on PCWP is a very early sign of myocardial ischaemia, as is wall motion changes seen on transoesophageal echocardiography.

Postoperative

1 After major vascular cases, the peripheral circulation may remain 'shut down' for 3–5 h, with hypertension (treated by nitroglycerin infusion). During this time some crystalloid infusions go into 'the third space', then, over a matter of $\frac{1}{2}$ h, the peripheral circulation 'opens up' with falls of peripheral resistance, and venous and arterial pressure. Lactate is washed in to the circulation from the peripheral tissues, causing cardiac failure. Intravenous colloids and inodilators are needed. Ileus, bowel ischaemia, restrictive respiratory failure and temporary renal failure[15] occur. Postoperative cardiac ischaemia is typically 'silent'. The α_2-agonist mivazerol has been used as a prophylactic.

2 Analgesia: epidural dilute local analgesic with added opioid, e.g. fentanyl 2–3 μg/kg is the gold standard for operations in the lower half of the body; in the emergency case insertion may have to wait for postoperative cardiovascular and coagulation stability: PCA; morphine or fentanyl infusions are also appropriate.

3 Intermittent positive-pressure ventilation with IMV or pressure support is frequently continued in ITU, except after the shorter operations. This maximizes O_2 supply and allows profound opiate analgesia, with time for normalization of the physiological insults of surgery.

Postoperative chest infection problems occur and are treated in the normal way. Extradural or other regional blockade is helpful in the postoperative period.

Reasons for perioperative stroke after carotid endarterectomy:

1 Clamping of carotid: emboli released by surgeon.

2 'Dissection' of arterial wall.

3 Cerebral haemorrhage resulting from anticoagulants

4 Emboli – thrombi develop on new raw surface of the artery.

5 Poor existing collateral vessels.

6 Recent preoperative strokes.

ANAESTHESIA FOR CAROTID ENDARTERECTOMY

Strong predictors of operative stroke are: preoperative stroke, female sex, age over 75, hypertension, peripheral vascular disease, occlusion of contralateral artery, stenosis of ipsilateral carotid siphon or external carotid artery. Weaker predictors are: TIAs, smoking. diabetes, angina, recent myocardial infarction (MI), or transient ocular ischaemia, plaque surface irregularity.

The patients are usually receiving aspirin, to which patients have very unpredictable responses.

The operation requires a good head position for the surgeon (poor for the anaesthetist – a preformed endotracheal tube is used). Warming blanket is usual, large-bore intravenous cannulae.

Anaesthesia

1 Total intravenous with propofol and remifentanil infusion.
2 Volatile anaesthesia.
3 Cervical plexus block with long-acting local analgesic; the mildest sedation is likely to be required in this situation, e.g. midazolam 1–2 mg i.v., possibly repeated every hour or two.

Monitoring

Intra-arterial pressure (kept as near usual as possible), CVP (may be inserted in jugular vein by surgeon), surgical angioscopy, doppler and stump pressure (by surgical finger or manometer), transcranial Doppler and EEG.

Heparin is often needed during the operation, and magnesium (4–10 mmol) may be considered. Nimodipine is widely used for cerebral protection and remacemide has been recommended.

The anaesthetist requires a quick response to reflex bradycardias (these may be prevented by carotid sinus nerve block).

The pressure ratio (MAP-stump pressure) is recorded. A shunt is not needed in all cases.

Postoperatively, rapid wake-up at the end to test cerebral function may be achieved by using TIVA with propofol and short-acting opioid for some or all of the operation. Hypertension may require control by GTN infusion (*see* Chapter 2.7).

ANAESTHESIA FOR RUPTURED AORTIC ANEURYSM

First resection of an aortic aneurysm performed in 1951. This condition carries a high mortality, and there is of course no opportunity for preoperative preparation as for elective cases. Patients are usually in poor general condition and are suffering from shock, ileus due to retroperitoneal haematoma, or haematemesis from leakage into the duodenum from the aneurysm. The patient may already have suffered irreversible brain and cardiac damage.

Resuscitation

Pain is relieved, O_2 is given, circulating blood volume is restored.

Induction of anaesthesia

Preoxygenation and rapid-sequence tracheal induction. Reduction of intra-abdominal pressure by anaesthesia may lead to renewed bleeding and should take place in the operating room, so that an aortic clamp can be applied very rapidly. Maintenance may be light general anaesthesia with non-depolarizing relaxants and opioids. The patient is in a critical shocked condition. Group-specific massive warmed blood transfusion is started as quickly as possible.

Large volumes of blood will be required with the usual risks which may follow massive transfusion, such as a failure of clotting mechanism (requiring intraoperative monitoring), accidental hypothermia, and calcium and potassium imbalance (requiring intravenous calcium). Blood filters and warmers are used. Autotransfusion is often useful, with care to avoid getting atheroma in the cell saver. Several large-bore drips are needed for high-speed massive transfusion until the clamps are on, and bleeding is controlled. Infrarenal cross clamping affects spinal haemodynamics.

Monitoring as above.

Metabolic acidosis is serious and requires regular blood gas analysis, with correction by bicarbonate as necessary.

Renal function is encouraged, e.g. by low-dose dopamine or frusemide infusion.

A high-efficiency warming blanket is applied before surgery begins.

If the ruptured aneurysm extends above the renal arteries the outlook is especially grave as this often causes renal and spinal cord ischaemia with irreversible damage.

REFERENCES

1 Pollard J. B., Garnerin P. and Dalman R. L. *Anesth. Analg.* 1996, **83,** 407–410; ibid. 1997, **85,** 1307–1311; Mangano D. T. and Goldman L. *N. Engl. J. Med.* 1995, **333,** 1750–1756.
2 Hollenberg M. and Mangano D. T. *Am. J. Cardiol.* 1994, **73,** 30B–33B.
3 American College of Physicians. *Guidelines For Assessment And Management Of Perioperative Coronary Disease Risk.* American College of Physicians, 1997.
4 Haft E. et al. *N. Engl. J. Med.* 1997, **337,** 1257.
5 Beven E. G. *J. Vasc. Surg.* 1986, **31,** 682–684.
6 Mangano D. T., McSPI Research Group. *J. Am. Med. Assoc.* 1997, **277,** 325–332.
7 Godet G., Fleron M.-H. and Vicaut E. *Anesth. Analg.* 1997, **85,** 1227–1232.
8 Thompson B. T. and Cockrill B. A. *Lancet* 1994, **344,** 7–8; Juste R. et al. *Intensive Care Med.* 1997, **23(suppl.2),** S80; Chertow G. M. *Am. J. Med.* 1996, **101,** 49–52
9 Berendes E. et.al. *Anesth. Analg.* 1997, **84,** 950–957; Rosseel P. M. J. et al. *Intensive Care Med.* 1997, **23,** 962–968.
10 Heyman S. N., Fuchs S. and Brezis M. *New Horizons* 1995, **3,** 597–607.
11 McHugh M. I. *Care Crit. Ill* 1997, **13,** 55–57.
12 Bois L. et.al. *Anesth. Analg.* 1997, **85,** 1233–1239.
13 Meibner A., Rolf N. and Van Aken H. *Anesth. Analg.* 1997, **85,** 517–528.
14 Bode R. H. et al. *Anesthesiology* 1996, **84,** 3–13.
15 McHugh M. I. *Care Crit. Ill.* 1997, **13,** 55–57.

Paediatric anaesthesia

It is almost impossible to generalize about 'paediatric anaesthesia' because this age group comprises several distinct age subgroups, whose physiology and pharmacology differ from one another. Special considerations include anatomical differences, differences of physiology, differences in pharmacology, and differences of psychology.

THE NEONATE

Anatomy

Defined as an infant during the first 28 days after birth or more than 44 weeks gestational age. The mature 3-kg infant is normally one-third the length, has one-ninth the body surface and one-twentieth the weight of the average adult. The head is large compared with the body, and the neck muscles are inadequately developed to maintain it in position without support. The anatomy of the upper airway predisposes to obstruction; the tongue is often pushed against the palate, causing respiratory obstruction under anaesthesia; the epiglottis is soft, large, patulous, 'U'-shaped and inclined at 45 degrees. Indeed the whole larynx is anteriorly inclined. The vocal cords are at the level of C4. The subglottic region rather than the rima glottidis is the narrowest portion of the airway. The trachea bifurcates at the level of T_2.

Physiology

The physiology of the neonate differs from that of the adult in many ways.

Respiratory system

In comparison with adults, neonates have a larger proportion of respiratory dead space. The ribs are nearly horizontal in the position of deep inspiration, while the large liver pushes up the diaphragm. The intercostal muscles are poorly developed and the diaphragm is the major muscle of ventilation.

The lungs are much less efficient, with a respiratory surface per unit weight one-third that of adults. To compensate for this, the respiratory rate is increased in infants. The laryngeal reflexes are very active.

The respiratory pattern of the neonate may be one of three types:

1 Regular: inspiration and expiration take equal time in the cycle with no expiratory pause.
2 Cogwheel: a definite, extended respiratory pause follows a lengthened expiratory phase.
3 Periodic: regular pattern, interrupted by apnoeic intervals or groups of shallow respirations. Periodic respiration may be seen in premature infants, or as a result of birth injury or hypoxia of the respiratory centre.

Pauses in breathing of up to 5 s occurring up to five times an hour are normal and have usually ceased by 6 weeks of age. Apnoeas of > 10 s are abnormal.

Because of the variations seen in respiratory patterns it is difficult to measure a 'normal' rate in the neonate, an average figure would seem to be 30–40/min. An average tidal volume (V_T) for the neonate is 7 ml/kg. The airway is narrow and this causes a high airway resistance with low compliance.

In infants, a negative pressure is sometimes created in the stomach during inspiration and gas may be sucked in. To relieve this a catheter should be used as a stomach tube if the abdomen is distended or if breathing is laboured.

Alveolar ventilation is 100–150 ml/kg/min (cf. 60 ml/kg/min in adult) and the minute volume (MV)/functional residual capacity (FRC) ratio is 5:1 (cf. 1.5:1 in adult).

Intubation may be difficult because of the relatively large head. A small amount of mucus secretion may cause considerable obstruction to respiration.

The cardiovascular system

In the fetus the left ventricle drives blood through the aorta to the body tissues and to the placenta in the proportion of one-third to two-thirds. Oxygenated blood from the placenta mixes with venous blood in its return to the heart. About half of this mixed blood passes through the foramen ovale to the left heart. The other half flows to the right heart for the pulmonary circulation, though a variable part of this passes through the ductus arteriosus to the aorta.

At birth, when the umbilical cord is tied, systemic arterial resistance rises because blood passing formerly to the placenta now has to pass through the arterial system to the body tissues. At the same time, as regular respiration is established, there is a profound reflex fall in pulmonary vascular resistance, and an increase in blood flow to the lungs. Pressure in the pulmonary artery falls and a reversal of flow occurs in the ductus arteriosus. The lumen of this vessel decreases in size over the next 7–10 days and is usually finally obliterated. The foramen ovale also closes (Fig. 4.2.1).

At birth the blood pressure (BP) averages 80/50 mmHg. Falls of systemic vascular resistance in neonates can cause serious right-to-left shunts. The

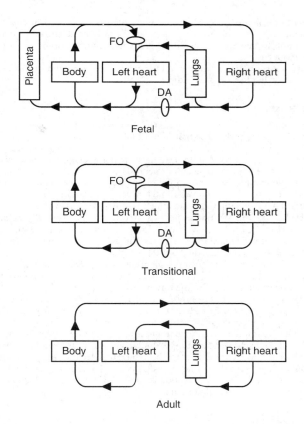

DA   Ductus arteriosus
FO   Foramen ovale

Figure 4.2.1 Alterations of circulation from fetal to adult type

pulmonary circulation is very labile and readily constricts in response to hypoxia, acidosis and hypercapnia.

The blood volume of the neonate is about 70–90 ml/kg, while haemoglobin is 17–21 g/dl. Cyanosis appears at high SpO_2s because of this haemoglobin concentration. (HbF persists for up to 3 months hence sickle-cell status cannot be reliably assessed before this time.) Average normal heart rates (bpm) are: birth 135; 1 month 160; 6 months 140; 1 year 120; 3 years 100.

Only 30% of the myocardium is contractile mass (cf. 60% in adult), and the neonate is less able to increase its stroke volume. Cardiac sympathetic innervation is incomplete, vagal tone is higher, and thus bradycardia occurs much more easily.

Body water is 75% of body weight (cf. 50% in adult), and of this, 45% is extracellular fluid (cf. 16% in adult).

Metabolism

Brown adipose fat is an important source of energy in the newborn and its metabolic rate is nearly twice that of the adult. It contains α-adrenergic receptors. Asphyxia at birth can result in exhaustion of carbohydrate reserves in muscles, liver and myocardium, leading to hypoglycaemia and acidosis. The normal neonate has a mild metabolic acidosis and respiratory alkalosis. Exposure to cold can also give rise to the same changes. Hyperventilation during anaesthesia is best avoided even though it will compensate for the metabolic acidosis. Hypoglycaemia and metabolic acidosis (ketosis) may be present if the child is starved for undue periods preoperatively, especially below the age of 4 years and below a weight of 15 kg. Blood-sugar estimations should be done in these circumstances. Figures below 1.5 mmol/l may be found, in which case administration of 0.5–1.0 g/kg glucose is indicated. In extreme cases it may be necessary to infuse concentrated glucose solutions, 20% or 25%, into central veins. To prevent hypoglycaemia, children should, if possible, be operated on early in the day or fed appropriately.

Oxygen consumption is 6–8 ml/kg/min (cf. 3 ml/kg/min in adult). Heat loss is of the order of 50% by radiation to cold walls of rooms or incubators, in addition to conduction, convection and evaporation. It has recently been appreciated that it may be unwise to nurse babies naked in an air temperature of 35°C, and it is more logical to use 'double-glazing' of the incubator or use a radiant heat shield. Draughts are to be avoided. Space blankets retain heat at first but are ineffective later when wet. Reduced renal function, especially urea concentrating capacity. Full function is reached by 2 years. Fetal albumin has a lower affinity for drugs than adult.

Stress response

Under light non-opioid anaesthesia, the stress response is even greater than the adult.[1] High-dose opioid anaesthesia is associated with a reduced morbidity and mortality.[2]

Pharmacology

Muscle relaxants in neonates

In babies, muscular relaxation requires neither deep anaesthesia nor large doses of relaxants. Protrusion of the intestines from the abdomen is due to diaphragmatic breathing and distention due to gas in the bowel, not to the muscular tone of the abdominal wall.

The neonate is more sensitive to non-depolarizing relaxants than the adult, though this sensitivity gradually decreases over the first 2 months of life.[3] Less acetylcholine is released in infants. Postoperative difficulties may be experienced if anticholinesterase drugs are not used, if hypothermia is allowed to occur, or when there is potentiation by volatile agent, hypokalaemia or antibiotics.

Atracurium should be preferred to suxamethonium in neonates even for short operations as suxamethonium may cause bradycardia in infants.

Opiates and postoperative analgesia in neonates

Neonates are very sensitive to opiates; these drugs have reduced clearances and prolonged durations of action. Neonates also have smaller respiratory reserves. Administration of opioids requires intensive monitoring and nursing in a high-dependency area.

Some suggested intraoperative intravenous doses:

1 morphine 25 μg/kg (60 μg/kg inhibits stress response); infusion rate 5–15 μg/kg/h;
2 fentanyl 1–3 μg/kg (spontaneously breathing); 5–10 μg/kg (intermittent positive-pressure ventilation (IPPV));[4]
3 alfentanil 10–20 μg/kg (50–120 μg/kg inhibits stress response); infusion rate 1 μg/kg/min;
4 sufentanil 1–3 μg/kg (5–20 μg/kg inhibits stress response);[5]
5 pethidine 0.5 mg/kg.

If other opioids have already been given, these doses are reduced. Postoperative analgesia, although desirable, has been associated with deaths.[6] The opiate-sparing effect of regional blockade is particularly beneficial in neonates and infants.[7]

Problems associated with neonates

The neonate may suffer from respiratory distress syndrome, haemorrhagic disease of the newborn with jaundice, birth trauma, hypoglycaemia, or infection. Congenital disease may be present. Venepuncture is difficult. There is sensitivity to non-depolarizing relaxants but resistance to suxamethonium. Hypothermia must be avoided.

Dehydration is recognized clinically by thirst, sunken eyes and fontanelle, oliguria, loss of skin turgor, empty veins, dry mouth, acute weight loss, slow (> 2 s) capillary return. Moderate dehydration represents a water deficit of about 75 ml/kg body weight. Biochemical estimation of electrolytes and glucose is required for calculated exact replacement of deficits. Special infant ventilators have been designed. The usual problems of infection exist.

Prematurity

Up to 6 months of age (longer if there are residual organ disorders) these children are more complex than usual. Their problems include: relative sensitivity to volatile anaesthetics with minimal alveolar concentration (MAC) equal to adult values, in turn due to:

1 high progesterone levels;
2 high endorphins;
3 immature central nervous system;
4 lower than usual body lipid content.

IMMATURE CARDIOVASCULAR SYSTEM

Nitrous oxide, associated with a small increase in cardiac output, is useful. Volatile anaesthetic agents cause dose-dependent depression of baroreceptor activity leading to hypotension with failure of heart-rate response to it, and of chemoreceptor activity, leaving the preterm child vulnerable to hypoxia without protective reflexes. For these reasons, most preterm babies should remain intubated after an anaesthetic until fully awake. Postoperatively they are monitored as if they were still anaesthetized.

IMMATURE RESPIRATORY SYSTEM

With smaller tidal volumes, greater respiratory rates, and high alveolar ventilation. The metabolic rate and O_2 consumption are high.

IMMATURE HEPATIC METABOLIC PROCESSES

For example paracetamol is excreted mainly as the sulphate in neonates rather than as the potentially more damaging glucuronide as in adults. The glucuronide/sulphate ratio only approaches adult level at 12 years of age. The average rate of drug metabolism is 2% of the adult value up to 2 months of age but by 3 years it is five times the adult rate.[8] Glucose, electrolytes and calcium balance are frequently abnormal.

FRAGILE INTRACEREBRAL BLOOD VESSELS

With greater risk of spontaneous intracerebral haemorrhage.
   Enflurane in particular depresses muscle. Nitrous oxide has minimal effect on muscle power. Minimum alveolar concentration values are related to post-conceptual age, they are often higher than expected, e.g. MAC halothane of preterm infants of 1–6 months is 1.2%, and isoflurane 1.8–1.9%.[9]

Anaesthesia in the neonate[10]

The choice lies between:

1 a 'volatile' technique;
2 balanced anaesthesia with relaxant and IPPV.

Ketamine has a longer elimination half-life than in older children.[11,12]

Inhalation induction and awakening, particularly with sevoflurane, is more rapid than in adults. A reliable intravenous infusion is an essential prerequisite in neonatal anaesthesia.

The presence of congenital abnormalities increases the risks of neonatal anaesthesia.

In premature infants, perioperative apnoea is a significant risk; operative ventilation to normocapnia is indicated. For the first postoperative 18–24 h, respiratory monitoring, with facilities for ventilation, should be available. Intraoperative ventilation may result in severe overventilation.

It has been suggested that, where possible, operation before the 44th week of conceptual age should be postponed. Vitamin K treatment should be given.

Causes of postoperative apnoea in the neonate are:

1 immaturity;
2 hypothermia, 34°C or below;
3 overdose of relaxant;
4 overdose with inhalation agent;
5 potentiation of non-depolarizing relaxant by volatile anaesthetic agent;
6 concurrent aminoglycoside antibiotics;
7 overdose of opioid analgesics;
8 a combination of the above.

Tracheal intubation in small babies

This is mandatory during anaesthesia. A straight laryngoscope blade, the tip of which is placed posterior to the epiglottis, is used. An endotracheal tube with internal diameter of 2.5–3 mm is suitable for neonates. An assistant, skilled in holding the baby, can prevent side-to-side movement by placing a hand either side of the head. The tube is inserted to about 10 cm from the lips, on average.

When intubated, there must be a leak of air between tube and trachea, to prevent pressure on the mucosa, with subsequent development of subglottic stenosis.

The risk of misplacement of the tube is always present.

Monitoring

See also Chapter 2.2. *As always, careful clinical observation of the condition of the patient throughout the operation is vital.*

CIRCULATION

A precordial or oesophageal stethoscope acts as a useful monitor of heart sounds, rate and rhythm. An electrocardiogram (ECG) should be routine. Lead III or CM3 give the best signal. The ECG monitor should show heart rate, since bradycardias are more frequent.

It is important that blood-pressure cuffs are of the correct size (*see* Chapter 2.1). Too narrow a cuff gives a reading which is too high and vice versa; the cuff should almost encircle the upper arm. The automated oscillotonometer is accurate. Monitors using ultrasonic detectors require protection from movement artifact. Finger arterial pressure monitors indicate non-invasive beat-to-beat pressure. For pulse oximetry *see* 'Metabolic status' below.

RESPIRATION

A stethoscope attached to the side-arm of a T-piece provides audible monitoring of respiration. Use of disposable oesophageal probes is now routine. Apnoea monitoring will be needed in the ward for 24 h postoperatively.

METABOLIC STATUS

Pulse oximetry (SpO_2) and transcutaneous oxygen tension (Tc PaO_2) monitoring makes continuous observation of the PaO_2 a realistic proposition. Pulse oximetry has some innaccuracies due to haemoglobin F, bilirubin and lag time, (*see* Chapter 2.2), but is very useful in the sudden-cyanosis situations of paediatric anaesthesia. Capnography is possible, but technically more difficult to obtain a proper alveolar sample, in small babies under 8 kg,[13] overcome by automatic fresh gas flow interruption during expiration,[14] and a capnograph with a rapid response time. Temperature monitoring is important. Urine flow may be useful in major operations.

Blood loss and replacement

The blood volume of a neonate is small, 85 ml/kg (about 300 ml in the newborn), and so blood replacement must be accurate. This can be done with the help of calibrated small suction bottles, swab weighing or colorimetric methods to estimate blood loss. Blood transfusion can be undertaken from small reservoirs coupled with an automated drip counter to transfuse an accurate volume in replacement. Replacement should be commenced when > 10% of the estimated blood volume has been lost. Blood should be warmed to prevent hypothermia.

Fluid balance

It is rare for preoperative fluid and electrolyte balance to require correction during the first 12 h of life but 0.45% normal saline with 4% dextrose is suitable in small babies. Haemoglobin, haematocrit electrolytes and blood glucose should be available before major surgery. In infants over 12 h of age correction of fluid and electrolyte abnormalities is of major importance. In the perioperative period, glucose-containing fluids are suitable until normal oral ingestion can be resumed.

Nutrition

The neonate requires energy in excess of 0.45 MJ/kg/day in order to grow. For enteral and parenteral nutrition, *see* Chapter 1.4. Aseptic technique must be scrupulous.

Temperature

The neonate loses 580 cal for every 1 g of water evaporated. This amount alone is enough to reduce the temperature of 580 g of the neonate's body water by 1°C.

The newborn rapidly loses heat if placed in a cold environment. The heat-regulating mechanisms are immature in the premature infant and in the mature newborn baby for some weeks. The newborn maintains its body heat through the metabolic activity of brown fat, which is to be found mainly around the kidneys and back. This fat has a rich blood and β-adrenergic nerve supply and the cells are profusely equipped with mitochondria. It may be deficient in small or premature babies. Care must be taken that undue heat loss does not occur on the operating table.

ROUTES OF HEAT LOSS

Conduction (e.g. to operating table), convection (e.g. due to draughts), radiation (worsened due to a baby's large surface area – especially the head, which should be covered) and evaporation (of perspiration, exhaled vapour and water from exposed viscera). Drapes provide an efficient insulation of the exposed surface of the infant. Cold blood transfusion may also produce hypothermia. It should be warmed. Cold stress and hypoxia lead to hypoglycaemia. For operations on babies below 10 kg, a warming mattress is important. Temperature is monitored at rectum, oesophagus, axilla or nasopharynx. The response to cold may be shivering, which increases O_2 consumption. (A 10°C fall of room temperature increases O_2 consumption by 50%). Neonatal environmental thermal neutrality is 33°C and 35°C for the premature. Hypothermia moves the oxyhaemoglobin dissociation curve to the left, reducing O_2 delivery to the tissues.

Common neonatal operations

Thoracic surgery

TRACHEO-OESOPHAGEAL FISTULA WITH OESOPHAGEAL ATRESIA

Incidence 1 in 3000 births, 50% weigh less than 2.5 kg and there is a greater than 50% incidence of other congenital abnormalities. Presents as maternal polyhydramnios and premature labour; with neonate dribbling at birth and inability to pass a nasogastric tube. Aspiration of food and secretions results in pneumonia within a few days of birth. Operation is no longer a hazardous procedure.

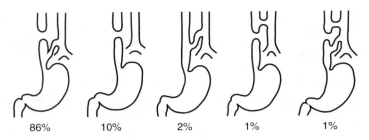

Figure 4.2.2 Anatomical classification of tracheo-oesophageal fistula

There are various anatomical variations. Much the commonest finding is the blind upper oesophageal pouch, with a fistula between the posterior trachea and lower oesophagus (Fig. 4.2.2).

Anaesthetic management may be difficult. Preoperative care includes transfer to a special unit. A Replogle tube should be passed into the blind upper end of the oesophagus for suction. Controlled ventilation via a tracheal tube is generally advocated. It is imperative that the anaesthetist be able to use effective suction in the airway at all times and a suitable fine catheter must be available. In a minority of cases artificial ventilation can result in gastric distention; gastrostomy is necessary for decompression. Good relaxation enables ventilation to be carried out at minimal pressures. Accurate replacement of blood is essential.

Recommended techniques
Premedication with atropine or hyoscine 0.05 mg/kg. An intravenous infusion is set up. Awake intubation is no longer recommended; asleep intubation in the premature child reduces the risk of intracerebral haemorrhage. Nitrous oxide/oxygen, volatile agent and muscle relaxant are suitable. The Replogle tube should remain in situ in the upper oesophageal pouch to allow removal of secretions. Care must be taken to avoid intubation of the fistula and inflation of the stomach. Intraoperative lung retraction may be associated with severe arterial desaturation. Elective postoperative ventilation is the routine.

DIAPHRAGMATIC HERNIA

Incidence 1 in 4000. Commoner in male infants (ratio 2:1). Seventy-five per cent occur in the left chest, 14% in the right chest the remainder in the anterior mediastinum. The commonest type is posterolateral defect on the left (foramen of Bochdalek) displacing the mediastinum to the right and compressing the right kidney. Diagnosed shortly after birth, the child may exhibit cyanosis resistant to O_2; dullness of the chest, absent breath sounds, scaphoid abdomen and later bowel sounds on the affected side of the chest. Chest X-ray shows gas-filled intestine in the chest with displacement of lung. The lung may be severely hypoplastic on the affected side, with mediastinal shift and compression of the opposite lung. Immediate decompression of hypoplastic lung does not result in a significant improvement in respiratory insufficiency. The current trend is therefore to delay surgery.

Initial management

1 Intubation of the trachea and gentle ventilation. The chest should not be inflated with a face mask, as this merely fills the stomach and intestines and worsens the degree of compression.
2 Insertion of a gastric tube to prevent aeration of the gut.
3 Measurement and correction of acidosis.
4 Prevention of hypothermia, dehydration and hypoglycaemia.

Perioperative management

Small defects are amenable to direct closure whilst large defects will require a mesh patch and as a result have a worse outcome. Some of these neonates revert to transitional circulation, with decreased pulmonary vascular bed, high pulmonary vascular resistance, and reopening of the ductus arteriosus and foramen ovale. Tolazoline, 2 mg/kg bolus, followed by the same dose infused over each hour, has been used to control these problems. Profound muscular relaxation may be required for short periods. Rapid infusion of colloids, e.g. plasma, may be required to counteract cardiovascular collapse during surgery. Elective ventilation is used postoperatively in severely ill cases. Pneumothorax is a constant danger which must be detected and treated immediately.

PATENT DUCTUS ARTERIOSUS

In a proportion of preterm neonates with severe respiratory distress syndrome (RDS) the ductus arteriosus remains patent. In cases where medical treatment such as indomethacin does not result in ductal closure it may be necessary to perform a thoracotomy and surgical ligation of the ductus. Intraoperatively the aorta can be mistaken for the ductus so most surgeons perform a trial clamping. An oximeter probe placed proximally (right arm) and another placed distally (either leg) will assist in confirming that the correct vessel has been clamped. Otherwise the anaesthetic management is similar to that for tracheo-oesophageal fistula (TOF). In particular intraoperative lung retraction may be associated with severe arterial desaturation.

Abdominal surgery

In neonates, muscular relaxation does not require deep anaesthesia or relaxants, except in special cases such as when a large volume of viscera has to be returned to the peritoneal cavity. The Jackson–Rees modification of Ayres T-piece is very convenient for IPPV. Bowel handling is associated with significant 'third space' fluid loss and necessitates intra- and post-operative colloid administration. (But *see* Cochrane Injuries Group Albumin Reviewers *Br. Med. J.* 1998, **317,** 235.)

INTESTINAL OBSTRUCTION

Pyloric stenosis

The commonest disease requiring surgery in the first 6 months of life. Incidence 1 in 300 births. Commoner in males than females (ratio 5 : 1) and in first born. Rarely presents before 2 weeks of age. The operation of pyloromyotomy is not an emergency procedure.

Preoperative preparation should be conducted in collaboration with paediatricians.[15]

Fluid and electrolyte replacement is the major consideration. Loss of gastric acid results in metabolic alkalosis and low serum chloride. There is marked loss of sodium and potassium in the urine in an effort to conserve hydrogen ions. Classic signs of dehydration occur: weight loss (0.5–1.0 kg); oliguria; dry mouth; sunken eyes; depressed fontanelles and loss of skin elasticity. The result is an ill, dehydrated, alkalotic, hypochloraemic, hyponatraemic, hypokalaemic infant.

Treatment is by intravenous drip infusion, initially normal saline with potassium chloride 20–40 mmol/l, until urine flow restarts, then 0.45% saline in 2.5% glucose with potassium chloride 20–40 mmol/l until urine flow is normal, then 0.18% saline in 4.0% glucose. A suitable drip flow rate is 2–3 ml/kg/h. The glucose is important to prevent hypoglycaemia. Surgery should not be undertaken until the chloride is at least 90 mmol/l and the bicarbonate 24–30 mmol/l. Intravenous feeding is rarely required.

Hourly gastric washouts are undertaken until the washout fluid is returned clear and odourless.

General anaesthetic technique: premedication with atropine 0.1 mg i.m. Perioperative body warming, precordial or oesophageal stethoscope and other routine monitoring. Suction on the gastric tube. Inhalation or intravenous induction and cricoid pressure. Intubation with 3-mm (or smaller) tracheal tube, facilitated by suxamethonium 1–2 mg/kg i.v. Maintenance with inhalational agents, supplemented by muscle relaxants and artificial ventilation. Extubation with the child awake, preferably lying on the side. Postoperative 0.18% saline in 4.0% glucose for 24 h when the child resumes partial or full feeds.

The local anaesthetic technique is obsolete since the operation is increasingly being performed in specialist paediatric surgical units where highly specialized anaesthetists are in charge. Ketamine as sole anaesthetic is not recommended.[16]

Duodenal atresia

Incidence 1 in 10 000 births, 30% also have Down's syndrome and 15% have cystic fibrosis. Other gastrointestinal and renal abnormalities are common.

Maternal polyhydramnios and failure to pass meconium in a neonate with aspiration, dehydration, shock and acidosis are all highly suggestive of the diagnosis. There are few specific anaesthetic problems. A nasogastric tube should be inserted as distention may result in diaphragmatic splinting.

Necrotizing entercolitis

Occurs in up to 5% of special care baby unit (SCBU) babies. Increased incidence with increasing prematurity especially if history of respiratory distress syndrome (RDS) and IPPV for hypoxia. Present with distended abdomen and classic radiological picture 'pneumatosis intestinalis'. Often require total parenteral nutrition (TPN). Remember to remove any umbilical artery catheter before surgery commences.

Exomphalos and gastroschisis

Incidence of exomphalos 1 in 5–10 000 births; incidence of gastroschisis 1 in 30 000 births. Requires emergency operation since rupture of the thin sac covering the intestines will result in peritonitis. The liver may be part of the eviscerated structure. Associated with multiple abnormalities including the Beckwith–Wiedemann syndrome (*see* Chapter 3.2). Anaesthetic management is similar to that for diaphragmatic hernia with protection against hypothermia. Prolonged ileus is a common complication and problems of fluid and electrolyte balance and parenteral nutrition may have to be solved. Plasma volume expanders will be needed and postoperative ventilation. Peritonitis is a common cause of death and intestinal obstruction due to adhesions may occur. The overall mortality is high.

Postoperative care

Neonates require special postoperative care after major surgery. Attention must be paid to the following.

1 *Environmental temperature:*
2 *Feeding:* a weight loss of 44 g/day/kg birth weight may occur in the first 2 days of life; it is possible for the blood sugar (normal level 3 mmol/l at birth) to fall to very low levels if early feeding is not commenced; oral feeding is preferable if possible.
3 *Acidaemia:* if present must be corrected.
4 *Oxygen therapy with pulse oximeter monitoring:* respiratory failure is a not uncommon complication and especially if opioids are administered. Assisted respiration may be necessary; rates of 60–80/min may be required using air enriched with O_2; estimation of PO_2 can be obtained using umbilical artery catheters.
5 *Cross-infection* is a particular hazard.
6 *Jaundice:* this may occur in any sick newborn baby; after surgery, haematomas provide an additional source of bile pigments.
7 *Postoperative analgesia:* opioid infusions are used, especially where IPPV is employed, e.g. morphine 5–15 μg/kg/h.

Day-case surgery in neonates

Many minor surgical procedures can be performed as a day-case in neonates older than 44 weeks postconceptual age so long as there have been no neonatal problems. Ex-premature neonates should remain in hospital overnight even after minor surgery especially if there is a history of apnoeic attacks. Spinal analgesia may be used in this latter group, especially if they are still O_2 dependent. (*See* Somri M. et al. *Anaesthesia* 1998, **53,** 762.)

INFANTS AND YOUNGER CHILDREN (UP TO 3 YEARS)

These children have better developed anatomy and metabolism but are still prone to hypothermia and shock due to blood loss and dehydration. The most risky cases are emergencies and those children with congenital disorders.

THE LARGER CHILD (3–10 YEARS)

In children up to 10 years of age the tidal volume (7 ml/kg), FRC (30 ml/kg) and dead space (2 ml/kg) are similar to adults. Resting respiratory rate decreases throughout childhood towards adult rate. Body lipid content rises up to 9 months of age, falls somewhat up to 6 years and then rises again towards puberty.

Preanaesthetic assessment

One should seek evidence of congenital or general medical disease especially recent upper respiratory tract infection (URTI). Elective anaesthesia should probably be postponed in the presence of a URTI. The children's experiences of previous general anaesthetic will influence how they react.

Preanaesthetic preparation

The traditional period of fasting (solids 6 h preoperatively; fluids 4 h preoperatively) has been challenged. Infants may have the last milk feed 4 h and the last clear fluid drink 2 h before anaesthesia, other considerations permitting.[17] Laboratory testing, as appropriate.[18]

Premedication

Morphine is much less widely used, as care is needed in infants (*see* 'Opioids in neonates' above). Some anaesthetists aim to give heavy premedication so that children arrive in the theatre suite asleep; they can then be anaesthetized using sevoflurane without the child regaining consciousness. Other anaesthetists prefer to establish rapport with the child and to provide an environment without fear; no premedication is given and the child 'talked' to sleep; anaesthesia being induced by inhalation or intravenous routes. Choice about premedication depends much on the state of the individual child. In the ideal world they would all be calm and relaxed, open to the charm of the kindly anaesthetist. In the real world they may be preconditioned to be otherwise.

However, sedative premedication is usually unnecessary when the weight is less than 10 kg.

'Complicated' children

The congenital or medical condition needs to be defined and optimized before anaesthesia. The presence of such conditions does make anaesthesia more difficult and adds risk of morbidity and mortality for the patient. They may have had many hospital visits and be highly cautious about anaesthetics.

Routes of sedative premedication[19]

Oral

There is a danger of vomiting and absorption of drugs may be uneven.

Benzodiazepines: temazepam syrup (2 mg/ml); dose 0.53 mg/kg (short-acting, 2–4 h).

Trimeprazine tartrate: a phenothiazine derivative, has central sedative, antihistaminic, antiemetic and spasmolytic action. It has none of chlorpromazine's antiadrenaline properties. Its side-effects include dryness of the mouth, vertigo, depression and fainting. Available in a palatable syrup as Vallergan Forte (6 mg/ml), 2 mg/kg 1.5 h before surgery. Associated with postoperative restlessness. The 'Liverpool regimen' is trimeprazine, 1.5 mg/kg orally 3 h preoperatively, then morphine 0.25 mg/kg 1 h preoperatively.

Analgesics: paracetamol 5–10 mg/kg.

Chloral and related compounds: chloral elixir, 35 mg/kg; dichloralphenazone, (contraindicated in porphyria), 35 mg/kg; triclofos, 70–100 mg/kg. All 1–2 h before anaesthesia. May also be given before an intramuscular opioid premedication.

Intranasal

Midazolam may be given intranasally in a dose of 0.2–0.3 mg/kg. Onset of sedation occurs within 10 min.

Rectal

The barbiturates methohexitone (20 mg/kg) and thiopentone (40 mg/kg) have been used but are unreliable; also diazepam 0.2 mg/kg.

Intramuscular

Generally intramuscular injections should be avoided, but are required when a fractious child refuses oral premedication. Pethidine: 1 mg/kg up to 5 years, 2 mg/kg over 5years (maximum 75 mg). Pethidine/promethazine mixture is available. Morphine, 0.1 mg/kg up to 5 years, 0.2 mg/kg over 5 years (maximum 10 mg).

Atropine 15 μg/kg and hyoscine 10 μg/kg can be useful in children, especially as salivation is often profuse; may also be given by mouth in double the dose. Hyoscine may be preferred because of its antiemetic action and sedative effect. Glycopyrronium 5 μg/kg (max. 400 μg) is satisfactory.

Anaesthesia

Informed consent in paediatric surgery is obtained from parent or guardian. In the ideal world the child should agree to the surgical procedure. There is often a gap between the real situation and the ideal situation here.

Paediatric resuscitation equipment should be available in every site where children are cared for.

The presence of parents in the anaesthetic room causes much debate. Some parents exert a helpful and calming influence on the child. Other parents generate tension and fear. This issue should be discussed at the preoperative visit, and not at the last minute. It helps to explain to the parent beforehand what will happen.

The classic method of anaesthesia, in infants and children with spontaneous respiration, of various mixtures of anaesthetic gases and vapours is widely used. Inhibition of the stress response with analgesics is important. Nitrous oxide and opioids are suitable but opioids carry the risk of respiratory depression, and require great care.

Intravenous induction of anaesthesia

For a nomogram to estimate drug dosage in children, *see* Wilson M. E. and McCleod K. R. *Anaesthesia* 1982, **37,** 951.

A 27-SWG needle is helpful. Topical analgesia of the skin e.g. using EMLA (eutectic mixture of local analgesics) cream,[20] or Ametop (amethocaine) cream applied an hour before, helps. Eutectic mixture of local analgesics cream does have complications.[21] More than two attempts at venepuncture should not be allowed in the conscious child, unless the skin analgesia has worked perfectly. (*See also* Whitelaw A. and Valman B. *Br. Med. J.* 1980, **2,** 602.) To facilitate intravenous puncture, a light shining from the side, casting a shadow is helpful. Suitable veins include those on the back of the hand, the dorsum of the foot, the internal saphenous vein, in front of the medial malleolus, and scalp veins in babies. Intravenous induction of anaesthesia with a sleep dose of thiopentone, is common, followed by a relaxant, intubation and IPPV with an N_2O/O_2 mixture, with or without volatile agent or opioid. There should be a small leak of air between tube and trachea.

INTRAVENOUS AGENTS

Thiopentone: dose 2.5 mg/kg in infants; 5 mg/kg in children. Laryngeal reflexes remain active.[22] The effects are similar to those seen in the adult. There is a progressive fall in the dose of thiopentone required for anaesthesia throughout childhood.

Methohexitone: dose 1.5 mg/kg of 1% solution; has triexponential decay, shorter $T\frac{1}{2}\alpha$ (2.4 min) and $T\frac{1}{2}\beta$ (23 min), than adults, with higher clearance, (18.9 ml/kg/min), giving faster postoperative psychomotor recovery than thiopentone.

Propofol: dose 2–2.5 mg/kg. Not licensed for use in children under 3 years of age. Hypotension (-24%) and apnoeas (< 30 s in 13%) are similar to adults.

Etomidate: dose 0.2–0.4 mg/kg.

Ketamine: dose 2 mg/kg i.v. or 5–10 mg/kg i.m. Elimination half-life 100 min in children.[23] Useful for diagnostic procedures and minor operations in small children and infants and to control restlessness before induction of general anaesthesia. Recommended when scarring of the neck as a result of burns produces an airway problem during induction of anaesthesia for plastic surgery. The agent may produce hallucinations even in children but this can be reduced if recovery is allowed to be quiet and if diazepam is given before and after. Infusion dose 40 μg/kg/min.

'Gas' induction of anaesthesia

Suxamethonium, syringes, needles and tracheal tubes should be immediately available in the anaesthetic room. Gas induction, e.g. using sevoflurane, is indicated if there is difficulty finding a vein, where the child has needle phobia, where EMLA cream has been unsuccessful or forgotten, or if the anaesthetist feels it is the best approach. Intravenous access should be gained at the earliest possible opportunity.

A suitable method is to administer O_2 with or without N_2O and either halothane or sevoflurane from a mask or tube held closely above the child's face. A flow of about 10 l/min may be required. The gas flow is subsequently reduced, and the percentage of volatile agent increased steadily. The child equilibrates with halothane 30% faster than the adult.[24] Halothane is well tolerated in children in whom the risk of halothane-associated hepatitis on repeated administration is very small.

Enflurane and isoflurane being more pungent, are not recommended. Reduced incidence of breath-holding, coughing and laryngospasm make halothane safer than enflurane and isoflurane. However, sevoflurane if available is the agent of choice. Cyclopropane is no longer used for gas induction.

It is quite acceptable to change the volatile agent to isoflurane or enflurane after induction as above.

MINIMAL ALVEOLAR CONCENTRATION VALUES AND PHYSIOLOGICAL EFFECTS

Minimal alveolar concentration is highest at 1 year of postconceptual age, being about 1.5 times the young adult value. At 32 weeks gestation (e.g. an

8-week preterm baby) it equals the adult figure. It falls steadily through child-hood and adolescence to reach adult levels by the mid-20s.

Nitrous oxide 70% or 2.5 mg/kg morphine reduces the MAC of halothane by 61–63%. High-dose sufentanil reduces it by 90%. However, opioids have a ceiling effect, and may not prevent awareness.

Hypotension (about 25% reduction at 1 MAC, about 50% reduction at 2 MAC of halothane enflurane and isoflurane) is largely heart rate-dependent and responds to atropine. Systemic vascular resistance is slightly increased with N_2O, unchanged with halothane, slightly reduced with enflurane, and halved at 2 MAC isoflurane. Isoflurane 1–2 MAC does not depress cardiac output.

Cerebral blood flow (at constant MAP and $PaCO_2$), is unaltered at 0.5 MAC of the volatile agents, but thereafter increased most by halothane (doubled at 1 MAC, quadrupled at 1.5 MAC), and least by isoflurane (unaltered at 1.2 MAC).

The volatile agents greatly potentiate non-depolarizing muscle relaxants in children.

Nitrous oxide is particularly useful because of the speed of induction, its absence of cardiovascular and respiratory depression, its rapid onset and offset, its dilution of over-high O_2 tensions, its reduction of volatile require-ment, its near-absence of metabolism and its powerful analgesic effect.

Monitoring in paediatric anaesthesia

See 'Neonatal monitoring' above, and Chapter 2.2.

Children require the same clinical and basic instrumental monitoring. Pulse oximetry is essential. Temperature monitoring is routine if a child is on a warming mattress (in case of hyperpyrexia). Capnography should also be routine. Indwelling arterial cannulae are likely to be required in cardiac, intra-cranial, and craniofacial operations, phaeochromocytomas, neuroblastomas, transplantations and complex spinal operations.

Central venous pressure monitoring, which has similar indications to the adult (*see* Chapter 2.2), is also used in neuroblastoma surgery and in children with unstable circulation due to congenital heart disease. The antecubital fossa approach is very difficult in small children. The subclavian approach has the problem that passage of a cannula from the right subclavian vein to the superior vena cava (SVC) is difficult unless aided by a guide-wire. Swan–Ganz catheters are likewise difficult to insert and maintain in infants, partly due to the reactivity of the pulmonary vasculature. In neonates, alter-native information about transitional circulation may be obtained indirectly from pre- and postductal PaO_2. Cardiac output measurements via Swan–Ganz catheters require great technical care if errors are to be avoided. Non-invasive Doppler ultrasound cardiac output measurement records velocity-flow and cross-sectional area of aorta for single beats, and is reason-ably accurate.[25] Aortovelography gives reasonable sequential estimates of changes in output.[26] Thoracic impedance techniques have proved difficult in children.[27]

Left atrial pressure monitoring lines for cardiac surgery can be inserted at operation via the right upper pulmonary vein. Coagulation monitoring (baseline and after each 50% of blood-volume loss) includes: platelet count (platelets needed if below 50 000/mm^3); prothrombin time and partial thromboplastin time (fresh frozen plasma needed if 25% prolonged); clotting time (can be performed at any time in the theatre itself); and fibrinolysins.

Neuromuscular monitors should deliver a 50-mA supramaximal stimulus. Positioning of stimulating and recording electrodes on the infant wrist is a problem. The median nerve has been used. Sensory-evoked potentials (SEPs) are used for testing neurone integrity during spinal, cardiac and carotid surgery. Transcutaneous SEPs require huge amplification of the signal and interference is always a problem.[28]

Blood glucose calcuim levels, bilirubin/kernicterus (unconjugated bilirubin, 300 μmol/l) especially dangerous in sick children with congenital intestinal malformations.

Malignant hyperpyrexia is uncommon in children but its occasional occurrence still calls for vigilance.[29]

Anaesthetic equipment for children

One or more 'paediatric trolleys' are organized containing all the special equipment required.

Dead-space and resistance to respiration must be minimal; weight and size of the equipment, with its tubing, must be suitable for small children. Valves must not cause undue obstruction; inhaled gases should be humidified; the reservoir bag should be smaller than in adults so that its movements with respiration can be seen easily. The closed system should not be used unless specially designed apparatus is available to minimize dead space.

Clear latex face masks which mould to the contours of the child's face should be preferred to the Rendall–Baker mask. Although care must be taken that dead space is not too high when small children and infants are anaesthetized, previous fears about mask dead space have proved ungrounded because of 'streaming' of gas within them.

The Magill attachment (Mapleson-A) or Bain coaxial circuit is suitable in older children, if the fresh gas flow exceeds the alveolar ventilation, during spontaneous respiration.

AYRE'S T-PIECE [30] AND JACKSON REES MODIFICATION[31]

This has a minimal resistance to respiration. *See* Chapter 2.1. Jackson Rees[31] modified the system by fitting a 500-ml bag with an open tail to the expiratory limb. This makes controlled ventilation and easy monitoring of respiration possible. During spontaneous respiration the fresh gas flow should be 150 ml/kg to eliminate rebreathing. During controlled ventilation the input need only be 100 ml/kg body weight with a minimum flow of 3 l/min. This is likely to produce a $PaCO_2$ of about 4 kPa. A flow of 3 l/min is recommended during neonatal anaesthesia.

Intubation

Indications: Difficult or obstructed airway; Children under 6 months or less than 5 kg; full stomach; hypoventilation requiring IPPV; use of relaxants requiring IPPV; operations limiting access to the airway; and operations over 1 h.

It may be performed under deep anaesthesia or relaxant. 'Awake intubation' causes rises of intracranial pressure.[32] It is similar to the adult, except that the larynx appears to be more anterior, and the epiglottis is doubly curved and more floppy. A straight-bladed laryngoscope is often helpful, especially in the smaller child, and this is inserted posteriorly to actively lift the epiglottis out of the way.

The smallest part of the trachea is the cricoid ring and the tracheal tube should be a loose fit in this indistensible ring evidenced by a small gas leak on IPPV, to avoid mucosal damage. The shoulder of the Cole tube was very prone to cause this damage. Preshaped RAE tubes with Murphy eyes are very convenient. Uncuffed tubes are used below the age of 10 years. For longer-term intubation, polyvinyl chloride (PVC) nasal tube may be considered. There is always the risk of misplacement of the tube in the oesophagus, and this must be checked for at every intubation.

$$\text{Tube internal diameter (mm)} = 4 + \frac{\text{age}}{4}$$

$$\text{Oral tube length to teeth in cm} = \text{internal diameter (mm)} \times 3$$

$$\text{Nasal tube length to nostril in cm} = [\text{internal diameter (mm)} \times 3] + 2$$

DIFFICULT INTUBATIONS IN CHILDREN

The Bullard laryngoscope has been developed for these situations. It has a long, thin, rigid blade (over which the tube is passed), and fibreoptics.[33] For those situations where intubation is sometimes difficult, *see* Chapter 2.6. Flexible fibreoptic intubation may be used.

Subglottic stenosis is a special case. It may be easy to intubate the larynx, only to find that the tube will not pass down the trachea. It should not be forced, but replaced with a smaller one.

It is still necessary to have a small leak between tube and trachea.

Complications of intubation in children

Disconnections; displacements (down – bronchial; up – oesophageal); obstruction by kinking and secretions; and after extubation, viz. sore throat (50%) hoarse voice, subglottic oedema. Highest incidence between 1 and 3 years, especially in Down's syndrome (3–10% of whom have been intubated in the past), epithelial damage (due to ischaemic pressure or chemical irritation).

INTUBATION AND THE ACUTE ABDOMEN IN CHILDREN

In acute appendicitis, for example, rapid-sequence induction is indicated. Because of the high gas flow rates it is exceptionally rare for the small leak between tube and trachea to allow soiling of the trachea by gastric contents.

Vomiting and acid regurgitation risk: trauma, anxiety and pain all delay emptying of the stomach. Although metoclopramide 0.1 mg/kg i.m. may be useful the incidence of side-effects is higher than in adults. Cimetidine 10 mg/kg orally, 2–3 h before induction of anaesthesia reduces the volume of gastric juice and increases the pH above 2.5.[34]

Artificial ventilation–IPPV

Controlled respiration has the advantage that it relieves the respiratory muscles of work and ensures adequate gas exchange. The Jackson Rees system or a paediatric ventilator[35] is suitable. Anaesthesia can be maintained at light levels with N_2O/O_2 and a muscle relaxant, and recovery is rapid. The risk to be avoided is severe hypocarbia (< 21 mmHg or 3 kPa). Capnography is therefore very important.

Small babies have a reduced FRC and airways closure may cause problems during spontaneous respiration.

Extubation and recovery from anaesthesia

Extubating a child in stage 2 anaesthesia is likely to cause coughing, straining and laryngospasm. Most infants can be extubated awake (i.e. stage 1 or lighter), except after intraocular surgery, where a cough on the tracheal tube as they pass through stage 2 should be avoided. In this case, and in older children, extubation may be done in stage 3 plane 1, and the child left (with extra O_2) to awaken very quietly under close supervision in the postoperative recovery room. The tracheal tube, laryngoscope and T-piece can be left close by in case reintubation is needed. Postoperative recovery staff monitor (and initiate correction of) breathing, colour, SpO_2, airway patency and peripheral pulse.

Intravenous infusions in children

Infusion sets should include a burette, so that small and measured volumes of fluid can be given. Infusion pumps and heaters may be required.

Perioperative hyperpyrexia

This is likely to occur: when the child is pyrexial; in hot climatic conditions; when there are too many coverings over the child; rare malignant hyperpyrexia (MH), and if there is inhibition of sweating following atropine premedication which may interfere with heat loss. A mattress with circulating water coils placed under the patient may be useful for cooling.

Paediatric pharmacology

Intraoperative opioids in children

See Table 4.2.1. Fentanyl 1–10 μg/kg (may cause significant muscle stiffness). Sufentanil 0.1–10 μg/kg has a place in cardiac anaesthesia because of its cardiostability, especially if bradycardia is prevented. *See also* Chapter 2.4.

Muscle relaxation in children

See Table 4.2.1. The volatile agents (especially isoflurane and enflurane) potentiate non-depolarizing muscle relaxants four- to fivefold in children. The usual relaxants and reversing drugs are satisfactory; infants require only half the dose of neostigmine.[36]

SUXAMETHONIUM

Infants are resistant to it (in spite of low cholinesterase levels) due to their greater extracellular volume (ECV) (40% of body weight cf. 18% in adults),

Table 4.2.1 Some suggested drug doses.

	Neonate		Child	
Drug	*Initial dose (mg/kg)*	*Repeat dose (mg/kg)*	*Initial dose (mg/kg)*	*Repeat dose (mg/kg)*
Atropine	0.01	–	0.02	–
Hyoscine	–	–	0.01	–
Ketamine i.v.	–	–	1–2	5–10
Ketamine i.m.	–	–	5–10	5–10
Methohexitone i.v.	–	–	2–4	1–2
Propofol i.v.	–	–	1–3	–
Thiopentone i.v.	–	–	4–8	2–4
Thiopentone rectal	–	–	40	–
Alfentanil i.v.	0.1	–	0.01	–
Fentanyl i.v.	0.01	–	0.001	–
Morphine i.m.	0.1	0.1	0.15	0.15
Pethidine i.m.	0.5	0.5	1.0	1.0
Atracurium	0.5	0.25	0.5	0.25
Doxacurium	0.03	0.01	0.03	0.01
Gallamine	1.0	0.25	2.0	0.5
Mivacurium	0.1	0.1	0.2	0.1
Pancuronium	0.06	0.01	0.1	0.02
Suxamethonium	2–3	1.0	1.0	1.0
Tubocurarine	0.25–0.8	0.1	0.25–0.8	0.1
Vecuronium	0.1	0.05	0.1	0.05

and may require 1–2 mg/kg i.v. Intramuscular dose 5 mg/kg for infants, 4 mg/kg for children. Phase II block occurs after 4 mg/kg. Suxamethonium in children (even in single doses) causes more bradyarrythmias than in adults.

Side-effects

Muscular fasciculation is not seen in infancy and there is no rise in intragastric pressure under 4 years of age while the rise in older children is less than in adults. Cricoid pressure is effective in preventing regurgitation. Suxamethonium should be preceded by atropine, 0.05 mg/kg to reduce the greater muscarinic effects seen in children. Hyperkalaemia is insignificant except after burns, paraplegia and tetanus. Post-suxamethonium/halothane myoglobinaemia is prevented by previous low-dose non-depolarizing relaxants. Successful use of suxamethonium in open-eye injuries in children has been reported. Suxamethonium is best avoided in children with Duchenne progressive muscular dystrophy because of cardiac effects and risk of MH. In children known to have MH, an N_2O/O_2/opioid/non-depolarizing relaxant technique is recommended.[37] Suxamethonium exacerbates congenital dystrophia myotonica with body rigidity preventing respiration and intubation. Such myotonia has also rarely followed the use of neostigmine in this condition.

INTERMEDIATE-ACTING RELAXANTS

Neonates and infants are slightly more sensitive to vecuronium and atracurium than older children. Compared with adults, vecuronium has slightly longer action in infants, and slightly shorter in children.

Infusion doses: atracurium 5–10 μg/kg/min (depending on concomitant 'volatiles');[38] vecuronium 1.4–2 μg/kg/min (depending on concomitant 'volatiles').[39]

Onset 2 min. Bradycardia during intubation is unusual. Histamine release from atracurium is less marked in children, but occasionally significant.

Mivacurium is short-acting, hydrolysed by plasma cholinesterase. Dose: 0.1–0.2 mg/kg, Onset 1.8 min, duration 10–20 min. There is some histamine release.[40]

LONGER-ACTING RELAXANTS

The vagolytic action of pancuronium is useful since infant cardiac output is very rate dependent, but the hypertension it generates may be undesirable in neonates and hypertensive heart disease. Most neonates and infants are slightly more sensitive to pancuronium and tubocurarine, but a few are markedly resistant.

Doxacurium is almost devoid of cardiovascular side-effects. Dose: 30 μg/kg. Onset 1 min, duration 45–60 min.

Children with Duchenne progressive muscular dystrophy or myasthenia gravis require reduced doses of non-depolarizing relaxants, or none at all (*see* Chapters 3.1 and 3.2).

Sedation techniques

The Toronto mixture is in common use for infants. (Pethidine 25 mg; promethazine 6.25 mg; chlorpromazine 6.25 mg; in 1 ml: the dose is 0.06–0.08 ml/kg up to 14 kg.)

Rectal pentobarbitone 2–4 mg/kg or diazepam (in propylene glycol for rapid and predictable absorption) 0.5 mg/kg. Ketamine remains useful.

Total intravenous anaesthesia in children

See Chapter 2.4 for general principles. Children require rather larger doses of propofol, e.g. induction 2–2.5 mg/kg, and minimum infusion rate (MIR) 15–20 mg/kg/h. Analgesics such as alfentanil (10–20 μg/kg bolus then 1 μg/kg/min, stopped 10 min before the end of surgery) are required. Remifentanil would be useful. Relaxants are infused as appropriate.

Regional analgesia

The whole panoply of regional techniques (extradural sacral, penile, ilio-inguinal nerve block, etc.), are commonly employed and give good results for pain relief in the perioperative period.

The safe dose of lignocaine is 4 mg/kg and bupivacaine is 2–3 mg/kg.

Anaesthesia for some common paediatric operations

Cleft palate and cleft lip in infants

Incidence 1 in 1000 births; can occur separately or together, unilaterally or bilaterally. May be associated with the Pierre Robin syndrome (*see below*) Treacher–Collins, Klippel–Feil, congenital heart disease, congenital endocrine disease (e.g. hypopituitarism) and congenital subglottic stenosis. Many surgeons prefer to operate when the child is about 10–16 weeks old for cleft lip and about 1 year old for the palate. (However, a current trend is to operate on cleft lip within days of delivery as this may give a better cosmetic result.) The child should be fit and healthy.

Atropine alone is suitable as premedication. Anaesthesia can be induced by any suitable method, but gas induction should be employed if there is any doubt about the ease of intubation or maintenance of the airway. An oro-tracheal tube, preferably a preformed RAE tube, is essential. Introduction may be hindered by an anteriorly displaced premaxilla obstructing the field of vision. To prevent the blade of the laryngoscope from sinking deeply into a wide cleft, gauze packing or adhesive tape can be used. Careful oropharyngeal toilet is necessary prior to removal of the tube. A tongue suture can be inserted to aid immediate postoperative control of the airway following cleft palate surgery. The infant should be nursed in a high-dependency unit (HDU) or paediatric intensive care unit (PICU) postoperatively, particularly if operated on as a neonate or if there are associated congenital abnormalities.

Tumours about the face and neck

Cystic hygromas and other tumours may occur in these regions and may make tracheal intubation difficult. Guided blind tracheal and fibreoptic intubation may be needed. Ketamine may have a place.

Anaesthesia in asthma

Avoid anaesthesia during an attack. For patients on long-standing steroid therapy, preoperative hydrocortisone will be required. Bronchospasm during the operation may be due to problems with a tracheal tube, e.g. irritation of the carina.

Anaesthesia for removal of inhaled foreign body

Should never be undertaken unless the services of an experienced bronchoscopist and anaesthetist are available. Intermittent positive-pressure ventilation can force the foreign body further down. (*See* Baraka A. *Br. J. Anaesth.* 1974, **46,** 124; Moussali H. *Br. J. Hosp. Med.* 1981, **25,** 300; Bush G. H. and Vivori E. *Br. J. Hosp. Med.* 1981, **26,** 102.)

Anaesthetic management of major spinal surgery in children (e.g. kyphoscoliosis)

The surgical approach to the spine is via vascular tissues and blood loss can be large. Good arterial and intravenous lines and monitoring are essential with major cross-match.

SCOLIOSIS

The timing of scoliosis surgery is a balance. Surgical correction tends to be delayed until after the growth spurt in the mid-teens. However, scoliosis, which is progressive, is likely to result in long-term cardiorespiratory deterioration.[41] Total lung capacity and vital capacity are both reduced. Forced expiratory volume (FEV) may be diminished as a result of mechanical inefficiency of the respiratory muscles. Airways closure encroaches on the FRC earlier than in normal subjects. Abnormal ventilation/perfusion ratios may result in relative arterial hypoxaemia. During operation, full cardiovascular and respiratory monitoring is usual. General anaesthesia with muscle relaxation and IPPV is the rule. Some surgeons require the patient to wake up so that the integrity of the cord, after distraction of the spine, can be tested;[42] others use evoked potentials.[43] The wake-up technique must be explained to the patient beforehand and the timing of supplementary doses of muscle relaxant and fentanyl must be carefully gauged. Blood loss at operation may be considerable and deliberate hypotension is often used. Elective IPPV may be employed postoperatively.

Neurosurgical operations

These require general anaesthesia via an orotracheal tube. Halothane is a useful agent in children, since respiration is usually quiet, but hypoventilation is to be avoided. Ketamine can be used for diagnostic procedures.

OPERATIONS FOR HYDROCEPHALUS

Intubation may be difficult due to the large head which makes visualization of the larynx awkward. A support placed under the body is useful.

MENINGOCELE

Careful anaesthetic technique is required. The operation is performed in the face-down position. Tracheal intubation is mandatory. Controlled ventilation is likely to be required as spontaneous respiration, mainly diaphragmatic, is embarrassed in this position.

POSTERIOR FOSSA EXPLORATION

In infants IPPV is recommended with close attention to replacement of blood loss, avoidance of heat loss, with wrapping of abdomen and legs in bandages and elevation of the legs. Central venous pressure measurement is helpful.

Circumcision

Standard techniques of general anaesthesia are suitable. Tracheal intubation is seldom necessary in children over 6 months of age but laryngeal spasm may occur; this requires temporary cessation of the surgical stimulus, then deepening of anaesthesia. Caudal block (0.25% plain bupivacaine, 0.5 ml/kg), performed while the child is anaesthetized, gives good postoperative analgesia as does penile block and dressings incorporating lignocaine ointment or EMLA cream. *See* Chapter 5.1.

Conjoined twins[44]

Operations for separation of conjoined twins are highly complicated and are carried out in specialist units only. (*See also* Harrison V. L. et al. *Anaesth. Intensive Care* 1985, **13,** 82; and Roy M. *Anaesthesia* 1984, **39,** 1225.)

Burns dressings

Problems arise when small children require frequent anaesthesia for burns dressings. Excessive starvation is to be avoided. Multiple halothane administrations are undesirable. Possible techniques include neurolept analgesia, ketamine and inhalation analgesia (e.g. N_2O).

Diabetic children

See also Chapter 3.1. The juvenile type of diabetes is very labile and demands particular care at the time of surgery. In the severely ill, frequent estimations of electrolytes and acid–base balance are required. The anaesthetist should aim for a rapid return of consciousness at the end of the operation with no vomiting. It is usually wise to seek the advice of a paediatrician regarding the insulin regimen. All but the most minor procedures will require intravenous dextrose and insulin.

Postoperative pain[45]

Regional analgesia should be used whenever and wherever possible (*see* Chapters 5.2 and 5.3). Great care is needed when giving opioids to infants, not only because of respiratory depression, but also because cardiac output is also very rate dependent, with serious results from opioid bradycardia (*see* 'Opioids in neonates' above). For infants over 10 kg in weight or 1 year of age, codeine phosphate, 1 mg/kg (to a maximum of 3 mg/kg/day) is satisfactory but should not be given intravenously as it causes a severe fall in cardiac output. Older children may be given intramuscular opiate analgesics on a weight basis via an indwelling deltoid cannula. Morphine has been used as a continuous infusion, 0.5 mg/kg in 50 ml of saline, at a rate of 5–15 μg/kg/h (neonates) or 5–40 μg/kg/h (older children) following major surgery. Aspirin is avoided because of risk of Reyes syndrome.

Nausea and vomiting in children after operations

Below the age of 3 there is a low incidence. Vomiting is more frequent after operations for hernia, tonsils and adenoids, squint and after cardiac catheterization.

Airway and respiratory emergencies in paediatrics

1 Asphyxia of the newborn.
2 Choanal atresia. Nearly always posterior. If bilateral, the infant will breathe through the mouth. The airway must be kept patent by opening the mouth, keeping the child crying, or insertion and taping down of an oropharyngeal airway until surgical correction can be performed.
3 The Pierre Robin syndrome. *See* Chapter 3.2.
4 Laryngomalacia. The commonest congenital cause of stridor. This is caused by incomplete development of the laryngeal cartilages. Inspiratory obstruction to respiration occurs as the flaccid structures are drawn in. Usually improves after the age of 18 months.
5 Common causes of stridor in children are (in order): laryngotracheitis, laryngotracheobronchitis, congenital stridor, acute epiglottitis and spasmodic laryngitis.

Resuscitation in paediatrics

The majority of paediatric cardiac arrests are respiratory in origin. A foreign body impacted in the pharynx or larynx (choking)is a common cause of arrest.

See Chapter 4.4 for the Resuscitation Council (UK) algorithms for basic and advanced life support.

There is a real risk of giving over-large doses of resuscitation drugs and fluids.

Children in the intensive therapy unit

These present the usual problems, compounded by different anatomy, physiology, pharmacology and psychology (*see above*).

REFERENCES

1 Anand K. J. S. and Hickey P. R. *N. Engl. J. Med.* 1987, **317,** 1321.
2 Anand K. J. S. and Hickey P. R. *N. Engl. J. Med.* 1992, **326,** 1.
3 Goudsouzian N. G. *Br. J. Anaesth.* 1980, **52,** 205.
4 Koehntop D. E. et al. *Anesth. Analg.* 1986, **65,** 227.
5 Moore R.A. et al. *Anesthesiology* 1985, **62,** 725.
6 Campling E. A., Devlin H. B. and Lunn J. N. (eds) *The National Confidential Enquiry into Perioperative Deaths*, 1989, 1990.
7 Lloyd-Thomas A. R. *Br. J. Anaesth.* 1990, **64,** 85.
8 Miller R. P. et al. *Clin. Pharmacol. Ther.* 1976, **19,** 971.
9 LeDez K.M. and Lerman J. *Anesthesiology* 1987, **67,** 301.
10 Waugh R. and Johnson G. G. *Can. Anaesth. Soc. J.* 1984, **31,** 700.
11 Friesen R. H. and Henry D. B. *Anesthesiology* 1986, **64,** 238.
12 Cook D. R. *Can. Anaesth. Soc. J.* 1986, **33 (Suppl.),** 38.
13 Sasse F. J. *J. Clin. Monitoring* 1985, **1,** 147.
14 Badgewell J. M. et al. *Anesthesiology* 1987, **66,** 405.
15 Connor M. E. and Drasner K. *Anesth. Analg.* 1990, **70,** 176.
16 *See* correspondence Bush G. H. *Anaesthesia* 1984, **39,** 381; Battersby E.F. et al. *Anaesthesia* 1984, **39,** 381.
17 Splinter W. M. et al. *Can. J. Anaesth.* 1990, **37,** 36.
18 Connor M. E. and Drasner K. *Anesth. Analg.* 1990, **70,** 176.
19 Laub M. et al. *Anaesthesia* 1990, **45,** 110.
20 Wahlstedt C. et al. *Lancet* 1984, **2,** 106; Hopkins C. S. et al. *Anaesthesia* 1988, **43,** 198; Gunawardene R. D. and Davenport H. T. *Anaesthesia* 1990, **45,** 52; Bjerring P. and Arendt-Nielsen L. *Br. J. Anaesth.* 1990, **64,** 173.
21 Norman J. and Jones P.L. *Br. J. Anaesth.* 1990, **64,** 403.
22 Jonmarker C. et al. *Anesthesiology* 1987, **67,** 104.
23 Grant I. S. et al. *Br. J. Anaesth.* 1983, **55,** 1107.
24 Brandom B. W. et al. *Anesth. Analg.* 1983, **62,** 404.
25 Schuster A. H. and Nanda N. C. *Am. J. Cardiol.* 1984, **53,** 257.

26 Haites N. E. et al. *Br. Heart J.* 1985, **53,** 123.
27 Donovan K. D. et al. *Crit. Care Med.* 1986, **14,** 1038.
28 Lam H. S. *Can. J. Anaesth.* 1987, **34,** S232.
29 Allen G. and Rosenberg H. *Anesth. Analg.* 1990, **70,** 115.
30 Ayre T. P. *Lancet* 1937, **1,** 561; Inkster J. S. *Br. J. Anaesth.* 1956, **28,** 512; Ayre T. P. *Br. J. Surg.* 1937, **25,** 131 (reprinted in 'Classical File,' *Surv. Anaesthesiol.* 1967, **11,** 400).
31 Rees G. J. *Br. Med. J.* 1950, **2,** 1419; *Br. J. Anaesth.* 1960, **32,** 132.
32 Friesen R. H. et al. *Anesth. Analg.* 1987, **66,** 874.
33 Borland L. M. and Casselbrant M. *Anesth. Analg.* 1990, **70,** 105.
34 Yildiz F. et al. *Anaesthesia* 1984, **39,** 314.
35 Hatch D. J. and Chakrabarti M. K. et al. *Br. J. Anaesth.* 1990, **65,** 262.
36 Fisher D. M. and Miller R. D. *Anesthesiology* 1983, **58,** 519.
37 Michel P. A. and Fronefield H. P. *Anesthesiology* 1985, **62,** 213.
38 Ridley S. A. and Hatch D. J. *Br. J. Anaesth.* 1988, **60,** 31.
39 Mirakhur R. K. et al. *Anesthesiology* 1984, **61,** A293.
40 Miler V. et al. *Anesth. Analg.* 1988, **67,** S149.
41 Loach A. *Current Topics in Anaesthesia. Anaesthesia in Orthopaedics.* Arnold, London, 1983.
42 Vauxelle J. et al. *Clin. Orthop.* 1973, **93,** 173; Abbott T. R. and Bentley G. *Anaesthesia* 1980, **35,** 298.
43 Brown R. H. and Nash C. L. *Spine* 1979, **4,** 466.
44 Ballantine R. I. W. and Jackson I. *Br. Med. J.* 1964, **1,** 1339; Furman E. B. *Anesthesiology* 1971, **34,** 95; Towey R. M. et al. *Anaesthesia* 1979, **34,** 178; Chi-Ching Cho et al. *Can. Anaesth. Soc. J.* 1980, **27,** 565.
45 Lloyd-Thomas A. R. *Br. J. Anaesth.* 1990, **64,** 85.

Obstetrics and gynaecology

OBSTETRIC ANAESTHESIA AND ANALGESIA[1]

Pregnancy

Pregnancy and labour produce remarkable physiological and psychological changes in the mother.

CIRCULATORY SYSTEM

The enlarged uterus pushes the diaphragm and heart upwards resulting in a large Q-wave and inverted T-waves in Lead III on the electrocardiogram (ECG). Heart rate peaks between 28 and 36 weeks at about 10–12 beats above normal. Cardiac output reaches a peak 30–50% above normal at term – difficult for a diseased heart. Peripheral resistance is reduced with lowest mean blood pressure at term. Venous pressure is normal, except when the gravid uterus compresses the inferior vena cava. Blood volume is increased, plasma volume more than red-cell volume, so that haematocrit falls, and uterine blood flow is markedly increased.

RESPIRATORY SYSTEM

Upward displacement of the diaphragm results in decrease of vertical depth of the thorax and increase in transverse diameter. increased lung vascular markings on X-ray. Minute ventilation rises by 50%. Functional residual capacity (FRC) is decreased from the 20th week. Closing volume is greater than functional residual capacity in about half of women in late pregnancy.

Peak expiratory flow rate (PEFR) remains normal.[2]

$PaCO_2$ falls by the 12th week of pregnancy to about 4 kPa (30 mmHg) and stays low until term. PaO_2 is sometimes reduced at term and may be higher in the sitting than in the supine position. Oxygen consumption rises during the last trimester due to the metabolic needs of the uterus, placenta and fetus. Basal metabolic rate is increased by about 15%.

FLUIDS AND ELECTROLYTES

Water and salt retention occur, probably related to placental steroid secretion.

ENDOCRINE GLANDS

There is hyperplasia of the anterior pituitary, thyroid and adrenal cortex, in addition to the effects on the organs of reproduction.

PSYCHOLOGY

The impact of pregnancy and parturition may have a considerable emotional effect, not least in the demand for a perfect outcome from every situation.

Supine hypotensive syndrome of late pregnancy

The gravid uterus presses on the inferior vena cava causing diminished venous return and perhaps hypotension. Most patients compensate by blood flowing through the azygos system via the paravertebral and extradural veins (not possible if an adrenaline-containing local analgesic solution has constricted them!). A right (or perhaps left) lateral wedge is used to move the uterus off the inferior vena cava.

ANALGESIA IN VAGINAL DELIVERY

Analgesia is not necessary in every case of labour and the different levels of treatment available are appropriate to different patients.

Non-pharmacological methods

Since drugs administered may cross the placenta to depress the fetus, any method which avoids or restricts their use deserves attention.

1 'Natural childbirth'. Patients are taught the art of relaxation and a measure of pain control through learned breathing patterns and concentration.
2 Transcutaneous electrical nerve stimulation (TENS) is beneficial in an important group of patients – those with moderate to severe contraction pains in an otherwise reasonably normal labour. This technique is easy to apply, totally non-toxic, and frequently effective. Commonly, four electrodes are placed, one either side of the spine in the lower thoracic region (T10) and one either side of the spine at the sacral area. The patient may control up to three levels of intensity of stimulus, and can switch off if she wishes. Some patients find mental concentration difficult while TENS is operating.

Analgesics

Nitrous oxide

Nitrous oxide does not interfere with uterine contractions, nor has it any effect on the fetus.

Premixed 50% N_2O/O_2 (Entonox) is very acceptable to patients. Inhalation begins at the onset of the contraction. A new variant of this is *isoxane* (Entonox with 0.2% isoflurane) to achieve improved analgesia.

Opioids

Pethidine can be used by midwives acting alone if certain rules are observed. It is an excellent strong analgesic, relaxes spasm of the cervix and has a wide margin of safety.

It is very useful in cases with a rigid, slowly dilating os.

It can, however, depress fetal respiration, which can be reversed by naloxone 3 μg/kg.i.v or i.m.

Morphine is also used. In small doses, it increases the intervals between pains; in larger doses it may depress contractions.

An acetylcholine receptor blocker: ABT 594

ABT 594 is as powerful an analgesic as morphine but acts on other receptors. It is currently being investigated.[3]

S-ketamine

This does not have the dysphoric effects of the racemic mixture and has proved useful in some centres. Memantine and dextromethorphan work in the same way.

REGIONAL BLOCK FOR OBSTETRIC ANALGESIA

This is not recommended in situations where there is no resident anaesthetist.

THE EFFECT OF EPIDURAL ON PROGRESS AND OUTCOME IN LABOUR:

Epidurals can modify the course of labour: early epidural placement is associated with longer labours compared with late epidural placement; stronger solutions of local anaesthetics (LAs) are associated with reduced uterine contractility and reduced pelvic floor tone compared with weaker solutions. Volume loading is routine, but generous fluid loading is associated with reduced uterine contractility possibly due to decreased endogenous oxytocin.[4]

There is a widespread search for spinal blocking drugs to eliminate the need for local anaesthetics.[5]

Perineal anaesthesia removes the bearing-down reflex but saddle block does not greatly delay normal labour if, when the cervix is fully dilated, the patient is encouraged to bear down during the pains.

The emphasis is therefore on a differential block giving only analgesia rather than motor blockade so that ambulant labour is possible.

With all forms of regional block, hypotension must be avoided because of the risk of fetal hypoxia. To prevent supine hypotension the patient is nursed in the lateral position or a wedge used to prevent caval compression. If it occurs the legs should be elevated, plasma-volume expander infused and O_2 administered. Systolic pressure should not be allowed to fall below 90 mmHg. Vasoconstrictors reduce uterine blood flow and are best avoided. Recommended are phenylephrine (in patients with cardiac disease),[6] ephedrine 12–25 mg i.v. or metaraminol infusion.

Spinal blocks last a shorter time in late labour compared with early labour, and somatic analgesia is shorter than visceral analgesia.[7]

Extradural (epidural) lumbar block

(*See also* Regional anaesthesia Chapter 5.3.)

Indications

The aim is to reduce labour pain, prevent exhaustion and preserve morale. Other indications are:

1 pre-eclamptic toxaemia;
2 slow, unbearably painful labour;
3 cardiac and respiratory distress;
4 premature or high-risk fetus;
5 multiple pregnancy;
6 breech delivery;
7 diabetes;
8 incoordinate action of uterus;
9 failure of conventional analgesia;
10 predicted difficult intubation;
11 operative delivery;
12 rare maternal diseases (cardiorespiratory, neuromuscular, orthopaedic).

Block should reach T10. Uterine muscle can function without neural control and may have its own intrinsic pacemakers.

Contraindications

The absolute contraindications are:

1 patient refusal (note: some mothers who were initially willing, are retro-spectively resentful of having received an epidural block);

2 local sepsis;
3 lack of experience of anaesthetist and inadequate supervision; no resident anaesthetist in hospital;
4 inadequate facilities (apparatus or personnel) for immediate resuscitation should untoward events occur;
5 shock, hypotension, hypovolaemia.

Relative contraindications for which risk–benefit has to be assessed and optimized are:

1 haemorrhagic disease or anticoagulant therapy;
2 systemic bacterial infection;
3 spinal cord or nerve disease;
4 back deformities, previous back problems, previous spinal surgery (the problem is technical difficulty and unpredictable spread of analgesic) or difficult anatomy (perhaps including obesity);
5 severe heart disease and hydramnios;
6 existing supine hypotension;
7 cardiac disease with fixed output; other significant medical diseases.

Technique

An intravenous infusion is an essential prerequisite. Volume loading with more than 10 ml/kg carries no advantage over 10 ml/kg.[8]

Identification of the epidural space is by saline – the complications of air include pneumocephalus, headache, nausea, hemiparesis, delayed awakening after N_2O, nerve root compression, subcutaneous emphysema, venous air embolism, all rare.[9]

Distinguishing cerebrospinal fluid (CSF) from saline – CSF has a higher temperature, presence of glucose higher pH and shows turbidity with thiopentone.[10] Catheter design may be important. One with a closed tip and three lateral holes may be preferable to one with a single end hole; multiport catheters have less unilateral analgesia and unblocked segments than single port catheters.[11]

The catheter may be introduced in the L2–3 or L3–4 interspace. It should not be advanced more than a short distance into the extradural space as it may take an undesired direction. The markings on Lee needle and catheter are useful here. Head-down tilt may aid spread to T10. Warming of the solution has been recommended.[12]

Test dosing for intravenous mis-siting of catheter with isoprenaline 5 mg has been advocated. This increased maternal heart rate and uterine blood flow, no effect of fetal heart rate or umbilical blood flow (intravenous adrenaline lowers uterine blood flow, but improves sensory and motor block).[13]

Combined spinal/extradural block is often used to speed onset.[14]

The analgesic is given by infusion via a syringe pump, throughout labour[15] or by bolus dose and top-ups using agreed protocol. Patient-controlled analgesia (PCA) is also used by this route.[16]

Drugs used include the following.

1 *Bupivacaine* 0.0625–0.25%. Block may be patchy, and the weaker solutions require support from added fentanyl 2–3 μg/ml.[17] Onset: $\frac{1}{2}$ h. Duration: 2–3 h. Infusions of 0.1% solution Infusion rate of bupivacaine (following an initial dose of 7–10 ml of 0.25%) is 10 ml/h using a syringe pump. Preterm parturients need a higher spinal dose of bupivacaine than term parturients.[18] *Levobupivacaine* has less motor block and about half the cardiotoxicity of bupivacaine.[19]

2 *Lignocaine* 0.5–1%. Onset in minutes, very reliable. Duration: 1–2 h. Maternal plasma concentration at delivery is directly related to total dose of lignocaine.

   Widely used in the US. With epidural infusions, the shorter action makes no difference to duration, and adds a safety factor in the event of an intradural misplacement. A common practice is to give the initial dose of lignocaine as 5 ml of 0.5% solution. (If the epidural catheter is in fact subarachnoid, an effective but safe spinal block will develop very rapidly.) If the epidural catheter tip is in the epidural space, a second, third and even fourth 5 ml are given at intervals to complete the epidural block.

   Carbonated lignocaine solutions have given better results in clinical practice. Administering the first dose of lignocaine slowly gives lower blood levels and no difference in speed of onset.[20]

3 *Ropivacaine*[21] 0.2–0.5% (initial dose 50 mg, top-ups 25 mg), with or without fentanyl 3 μg/ml. Ropivacaine may have less motor block than bupivacaine at these low concentrations.[22] Metabolized in liver by CYP1A enzymes by aromatic hydroxylation. Plasma clearance 440 ml/min; renal clearance 1 ml/min. Plasma half-life 1.8 h. Protein bound to α_1 acid glycoprotein.

4 *Opioids,* diluted in 5–10 ml of solution, e.g. fentanyl 10–25 μg (a single bolus with the first dose of local analgesic intensifies analgesia, speeds its onset, overcomes any 'patchiness', lasts up to 6 h and does not depress the fetus[23]). Other drugs used include: morphine 2 mg, diamorphine 1 mg, buprenorphine 0.15 mg (may last 24 h), methadone 10 mg (lasts up to 12 h), sufentanil 10 μg.[24] Solutions without preservatives should be used. Cardiovascular effects are minimal. Maternal respiratory depression, itching and nausea may occur if the above doses are exceeded.

5 *Other drugs:* etidocaine, 1% solution, is a good agent for Caesarean section, but not for normal delivery because of motor block. Alpha blockers clonidine, mivazerol[25] and dexmedetomidine.[26] Dexmedetomidine has less placental transfer than clonidine in spite of being more lipophilic. Neostigmine has been used for postoperative analgesia.[27] Extenders are being investigated – liposomes, microcrystals and microsomes. Chloroprocaine had a rapid onset of action but was of short duration. It antagonizes fentanyl (binds to μ and κ receptors).[28]

Maternal complications (1 in 400 cases) of epidural analgesia for labour

COMMON

1 Inadequate analgesia in up to 5% of cases. This should be openly explained to the patient beforehand.
2 Hypotension – must be differentiated for supine hypotensive syndrome by insertion of wedge. Extreme care must be used with catecholamine vasopressors because of great sensitivity of placental circulation.
3 Motor blockade, preventing ambulation. Extremely weak solutions of analgesic with opioid should give differential (only sensory) block.
4 Loss of heat, hypothermia – need warm room and warm intravenous fluids.
5 Inability to sense urge to push – requires regular monitoring of progress, and use of more dilute epidural solutions.
6 Longer second stage – when fetal head is on the perineum, mother can push.
7 Urinary retention – check bladder and catheterize.

MILDLY DISTURBING (1 IN 1600 CASES)

1 Sixth cranial nerve palsy.
2 Horner's syndrome.[29]
3 Catheter broken off in epidural space.
4 Injection of local analgesic into wrong catheter (e.g. intrauterine).

PROLONGED (1 IN 2000 CASES)

1 Leg pain.
2 Numbness and weakness.
3 Pressure sores.
4 Reactions to skin preparation material.

MODERATE (1 IN 2000 CASES)

1 Hyperalgesia.
2 Spinal headache if the dura has been punctured.

SERIOUS (1 IN 13 500 CASES)

1 Introduction of foreign material to extradural space.
2 Extradural haematoma.
3 Extradural infection.

LIFE-THREATENING (1 IN 30 000 CASES)

1 Intravenous injection of local analgesic, with convulsions and cardiovascular collapse.
2 Intrathecal injection, with total spinal: respiratory failure and cardiovascular collapse.

PSEUDOCOMPLICATIONS

Many unconnected symptoms are unjustly blamed on the epidural, e.g. headaches, backaches, leg aches, arm pains and numbness. Careful neurological examinations usually enable an accurate diagnosis to be made. For example, the incidence of pregnancy backache is 50%, with no difference between epidural and non-epidural groups.[30]

Peripartum stroke and cerebral thrombosis occur without epidurals.[31]

Obstetric paralysis due to pressure of the fetal head or the forceps on the lumbosacral trunk may occur even in the absence of intradural or extradural analgesia.

Neuropathy if due to epidural block is likely to be bilateral and to have a segmental (radicular) rather than a peripheral distribution.

Subarachnoid lumbar block (intradural, 'spinal')
(*see also* Regional anaesthesia Chapter 5.3)

For normal delivery or for outlet forceps with episiotomy.
  Advantages:

1 fast onset – about 5 min;
2 an easy end-point when inserting the needle;
3 no fetal respiratory depression;
4 fully awake patient.

  Disadvantages:

1 risk of post-dural puncture headache (PDPH);
2 prolonged use with a catheter is relatively difficult.

In both subarachnoid and extradural (epidural) block, a given dose of local analgesic solution may ascend higher in pregnant than in non-pregnant patients, so doses should be given with care.[32]

Managing an accidental dural puncture

1 Insert epidural in another space.

2 Explain risk of headache (including late onset) to patient.

3 If headache occurs consider other causes: ordinary headache, meningitis, tumour. (Abdominal pressure in upright posture from behind relieves PDPH).

   (a) Conservative measures: lie flat, generous fluids, analgesics, caffeine.
   (b) Possible epidural saline infusion.
   (c) Organize early blood patch.
   (d) Repeat patch if unsuccessful.

Post-dural puncture headache

Postdelivery headaches have always been a problem for a nursing mother, but the incidence of PDPH is minimized if fine needles, e.g. 26-G, 29-G, with pencil-points, e.g. Sprotte[33] or Whitacre are used. It has been suggested that the target should be an incidence of fewer than 1% severe headache and fewer than 4% failure.[34]

The orientation of the pencil-point needle aperture is not important for the spread of spinals.[35]

Extradural sacral (caudal) block

A single injection can be given for forceps delivery if lumbar approach is impossible. Sixteen to twenty millilitres of analgesic solution are recommended. A catheter may be used, with the precautions noted above. High spread can occur following sacral injection as evidenced by reports of meiosis and ptosis.[36] It is not without its disadvantages and is accompanied by a higher forceps rate and increased frequency of anomalies of rotation, e.g. persistent occipitoposterior position and mid-transverse arrest of the head. The third stage is short and post-partum blood loss minimal. The method is useful in uterine inertia, in cervical dystocia, and episiotomy.

The dangers are:

1 accidental subarachnoid block;
2 infection;
3 intrafetal injection.

Placental transfer of drugs

All drugs found in maternal blood cross the placenta to some extent unless they are altered or destroyed in passage, especially those with a high lipid solubility and low degree of ionization. Placental vascular activity and metabolism also play a part.

Maternal mortality

There is a small but inescapable maternal death rate which includes deaths from anaesthetic complications.[37] Commonest causes of death are hypertensive states including eclampsia, haemorrhage and pulmonary embolism.

Other deaths are associated with:

1 aspiration of stomach contents;
2 hypoxia associated with difficulty in tracheal intubation;
3 hypotension from any cause;
4 inadequate blood transfusion;
5 amniotic fluid embolus and existing maternal diseases, e.g. cardiac disease, sickle-cell anaemia;
6 complications of rare congenital abnormalities.

Anaesthetists are often asked to help rescue patients from these potentially lethal problems. Transfer to the intensive therapy unit (ITU) is likely to be indicated[38] in 0.265% of deliveries (3/4 obstetric related, 1/4 due to general medical causes).

Equipment for all locations where anaesthetics are administered

(In addition to anaesthetic machines, tubes, laryngoscopes, drips, suction, tilting table and the full selection of anaesthetic drugs.)

Oxygenation: O_2 failure warning device; O_2 analyser; pulse oximeter.

Ventilation: ventilator disconnection alarm; respirometer; end-tidal CO_2 analyser.

Circulation: precordial or oesophageal stethoscope; ECG monitor; automatic blood pressure recorder.

Temperature: thermometer.

Neuromuscular transmission: peripheral nerve stimulator; syringe driver or pump.

Algorithms for management of cardiac arrest, anaphylactic reaction; malignant hyperpyrexia.

Also available nearby when required: central venous pressure (CVP), pulmonary artery pressure (PAP) and direct arterial pressure monitoring.

Prevention of vomiting during anaesthesia in labour
(*see also* Chapter 2.8)

Vomiting is always a real danger during labour as the patient may not be suitably prepared, while the gastric emptying time is delayed. There may, too, be associated hiatus hernia.

Diet

A satisfactory regimen must be instituted to lessen the likelihood of acid stomach contents being present should general anaesthesia be required. Patients can be classified as 'normal' or 'high-risk' cases:

1 'Normal' cases. Unlikely to require general anaesthesia. The aim is to provide a light, easily digestible diet and to avoid meat, vegetables, fried food and milk. Sieved foods are allowed. Strong glucose drinks may delay gastric emptying.
2 'High-risk' cases. In these cases the obstetric, anaesthetic or medical history suggests risk to mother or baby, and that operative delivery may be required. In these patients, once active labour is established, they should be given nothing by mouth except for antacids. They should receive intravenous fluids, e.g. 500 ml 5% dextrose, 4-hourly. Both pethidine and diamorphine delay gastric emptying time, and so does maternal fatigue

---

Clinical features of acid aspiration syndrome

1 Respiratory: cyanosis, dyspnoea, bronchospasm.

2 Circulatory: tachycardia, hypotension.

3 Blood gas abnormalities: hypoxia, metabolic acidosis.

4 X-ray: a regular 'butterfly-shaped' hilar mottling, initially without evidence of atelectasis. ARDS may develop.

---

and exhaustion. Normal labour does not retard gastric emptying time. (Note that aspiration of vomitus can also occur during spinal analgesia for Caesarean section.)

Acid aspiration (Mendelson's) syndrome

This serious condition was thought by Mendelson to be due to acid irritation of material at a pH of 2.5 or below, but shown to occur with fluid of a neutral pH as well.[39] Aspiration of alkali may also be harmful. The normal pregnant fasting gastric secretion has a pH of 1.5.

An interval of some hours may separate the initial aspiration from the development of symptoms. Most commonly seen in obstetric patients.

Prophylaxis

Acid aspiration syndrome during general anaesthesia can be made less likely by the following:

1 Giving only fluids by mouth during labour, or managing hydration by intravenous infusion in the high-risk case (*see above*).
2 Antacids: anticholinergic drugs, antacids e.g. 0.3 mol/l sodium citrate 30 ml; H_2 antagonists, e.g. ranitidine 150 mg i.v. or i.m. 60–90 min before general anaesthesia results in a gastric juice of pH 5 on induction. It crosses the placental barrier. Famotidine 40 mg or nizatidine 150 mg may be considered. Prokinetic drugs, e.g. metoclopramide, 10 mg i.v. increases the lower oesophageal sphincter tone and so may reduce the incidence of regurgitation.
3 The insertion of a No. 10 oesophageal tube before induction of any general anaesthesia (not very pleasant but useful in the extreme situation).
4 Anaesthetic techniques: regional anaesthesia with full consciousness; general anaesthesia – awake intubation, or preoxygenation, rapid-sequence induction, with cricoid pressure.

The acid pulmonary aspiration syndrome can occur without definite vomiting or obvious regurgitation. Patients for anaesthesia in the immediate post-partum days may also be at risk.

> **Complications of labour which may be blamed on anaesthesia**
>
> 1 Peripartum stroke and cerebral thrombosis (1 in 5000 deliveries) (Lanska D. J. and Kryscio R. *J. Obstet. Gynecol.* 1997, **89**, 413–418).
>
> 2 Backache (Russell R., Dundas R. and Reynolds F. *Br. Med. J.* 1996, **312**, 1384–1388; Reynolds F. and Russell R. *Br. Med. J.* 1998, **316**, 69–70).
>
> 3 Fetal distress.
>
> 4 Instrumental/operative delivery.
>
> 5 HELLP (haemolysis, elevated liver enzymes, low platelets) syndrome.

Treatment

These cases may require, in addition to careful tracheobronchial toilet, aspiration and lavage with solution of 1% sodium bicarbonate, O_2 therapy and postoperative intermittent positive-pressure ventilation (IPPV). Hydrocortisone in large doses reduces the inflammatory reaction and aids bronchodilatation.

OPERATIVE OBSTETRIC PROCEDURES

Anaesthesia for Caesarean section

It needs to be remembered that fetal morbidity and mortality following elective section are greater than following normal delivery, for many reasons.

Premedication

1 Sodium citrate, 15 ml, 0.3 mol/l is given orally and/or H2 blockers, e.g. ranitidine to antagonize gastric acidity.
2 Metoclopramide 10 mg, to hasten gastric emptying, increase oesophageal sphincter tone and combat nausea.
3 Analgesics are not indicated until the delivery of the baby, but pethidine may have been given during earlier labour.

Extradural lumbar block

Extradural block for Caesarean section does not decrease placental blood flow. Previous Caesarean section is not necessarily a contraindication to extradural block in a subsequent labour, provided that careful monitoring for a ruptured scar is well maintained. (Scar pain and 'peritoneal pain' are uncommon signs of rupture. Sudden reduction or cessation of contractions are more usual signs of rupture.)

Management of epidural analgesia for Caesarean section

This is similar to that for obstetric epidural analgesia (above).

Lateral tilt or a wedge is used to avoid supine hypotensive syndrome. Oxygen is given from the outset. The systolic blood pressure should not be allowed to fall below 90 mmHg (mean arterial pressure (MAP) 70 mmHg).

1 Explanation of having to lie still for at least an hour; being draped; breathing O_2; the premedication antacids; the risks.
2 Consent.
3 Premedication (*see above*).
4 A drip is set up – volume loading with Ringer's solution.[40] The kinetics indicate that normally 500 ml is enough, more than this may cause oedema. Baseline arterial pressure, pulse, O_2 saturation, fetal heart rate and other parameters are noted.
5 A lumbar epidural catheter is inserted using saline to find the epidural space. Three to four millilitres of plain 0.5% bupivacaine or 1% lignocaine, as test dose to detect intradural placement is injected up the catheter. Adrenaline is usually avoided as it lowers uterine blood flow, if given intravenously,[41] although isoprenaline may be used to test intravascular placement. Adrenaline does, however, prolong the duration of analgesia in labour.[42]

   The patient is sat up for 5 min; testing for hypotension and paralysis. If there is none, a further 5 ml analgesic solution (e.g. 0.0625–0.1% bupivacaine), perhaps with added fentanyl 10–25 μg, is injected up the catheter to achieve block of the sacral roots. The target concentration of fentanyl is 3 μg/ml.[43] The patient is laid flat again and a further 5 ml analgesic solution injected up the catheter. Diamorphine 2–5 mg or sufentanil 2.5–5 μg can also be used to potentiate and prolong the block.[44] If the block has not extended to T6, after 10 min, a further 5 ml analgesic solution is injected. When the block has reached T6, a left lateral tilt is put on, and the surgeon may proceed gently. Monitoring continues as before. Local analgesic may be infused by syringe pump.

   A fully agreed protocol for monitoring, top-up and documentation is followed (*see Recommended Minimal Standards For Obstetric Anaesthesia Services*, The Obstetric Anaesthetists Association, UK, 1995).

   A combined spinal/epidural is frequently used. Post-dural puncture headache is reduced by use of a fine-gauge pencil-point spinal needle[45] (the strong indications for this during obstetric analgesia are extreme distress at the time the epidural is requested, uncontrolled pushing in labour, multiparous twin/breech delivery). There have been several case reports of bacterial and chemical meningitis using this technique.
6 At delivery, synthetic oxytocin is given intravenously, and diamorphine 5 mg in 10 ml saline given epidurally. (Diamorphine is one of the quicker-acting opioids.)

7 Mother and father are congratulated.
8 Epidural opioid analgesia may be continued in the postoperative phase, with antiemetics if necessary. Itching may be noticed.

The systolic pressure should be maintained at 90 mmHg or above by infusion of fluids intravenously, and if necessary by intravenous ephedrine or phenylephrine.

Vomiting is not uncommon. Oxygen may be given to the mother.

One of the advantages of extradural lumbar block for Caesarean section is that the mother may remain awake with active cough reflexes. Even very nervous patients can be managed in this way if they are treated sympathetically and the surgeon is gentle.

Block should reach to T6 (allowing for dermatomal overlap[46]), and the surgeon should not start until it does. In the event of a failure of the upper part of the block, due to some abnormality of the patient's anatomy, either the epidural catheter is topped up with a further volume of analgesic (e.g. lignocaine which has a faster onset), or if this fails, the anaesthetist (and patient) must be prepared to proceed to full general anaesthesia.

Epidural lignocaine, 1–2% solution given by extradural infusion for labour and Caesarean section, has the advantage of being more controllable than bupivacaine because it is shorter acting.

Intradural block (subarachnoid block)

Block should reach at least to the costal margin and can usually be obtained with 3 ml of analgesic solution.

Isobaric 0.5% bupivacaine in a dose of 1.5–4 ml is satisfactory. Addition of fentanyl 10–25 μg improves analgesia[47], with the patient in the lateral position for the injection, and immediately placed in the supine position with a wedge under the loin. Note that the dose of drug for spinal analgesia varies from place to place. The reasons for this are unclear. When an anaesthetist moves to a new location, it is wise to take local advice on the appropriate dosage in that region.

Local anaesthetic infiltration for Caesarean section

This is without serious effect on the mother or child, but is unsuitable for frightened or uncontrolled patients. The surgeon performs the injections.

Intradermal and subcutaneous infiltration is carried out in the line of the incision and solution should be deposited for about 2.5 cm on each side of the midline. Extra solution is injected into the pyramidales and into the retropubic space of Retzius. Solution injected into the rectus sheath will improve relaxation. The parietal peritoneum is infiltrated; likewise the tissue overlying the lower segment if the classic operation is not to be employed.

General anaesthesia for Caesarean section

Proper measures to prevent aspiration of stomach contents must be taken (*see* Chapter 2.8). The apparatus should be checked. A common induction technique is: preoxygenation for 3 min, atropine 0.3 mg to prevent salivation and bradycardia, thiopentone 3–4 mg/kg, suxamethonium 100 mg, cricoid pressure, tracheal intubation, N_2O/O_2 with a trace of volatile agent, e.g. 1% isoflurane, non-depolarizing relaxant.

Avoidance of oesophageal intubation is essential.

The self-inflating bulb oesophageal intubation detection device is 100% effective in normal individuals but may give false negatives in the morbidly obese and late pregnancy.[48]

SCOTI (sonomatic confirmation of tracheal intubation) is less efficient than Wee's oesophageal intubation detection device.[49]

Rocuronium 1 mg/kg with thiopentone has been used successfully in rapid-sequence induction for LSCS.[50]

Atracurium 0.25 mg/kg, cis-atracurium 0.05 mg/kg, mivacurium 0.05 mg/kg, rocuronium 0.25 mg/kg and vecuronium 0.05 mg/kg, are useful relaxants in Caesarean section because of their short duration of action, rapid clearance and minimal placental transfer. Oxygen concentrations up to 66% used to be advocated. The disadvantage is that the mother may become aware of events during the operation. Lateral tilt is employed to prevent caval compression. Tilt to the left is usual but tilt to the right also has advantages for the venous system of the left leg. Half doses of relaxant are all that is necessary in Caesarean section. The abdominal muscles are stretched during pregnancy and muscle tone is seldom a problem.

An intravenous opioid is given to the mother as soon as the baby is delivered, to deepen anaesthesia.

Predelivery hyperventilation is avoided because it reduces placental blood flow and O_2 transfer. A fall of maternal $PaCO_2$ below 2.85 kPa causes fetal acidosis as a result of reduction in placental blood flow. It is desirable to keep $PaCO_2$ at or above 4 kPa which is normal for the pregnant mother at term.

Ketamine has been used as the sole agent for forceps delivery, manual removal of the placenta and similar procedures, and as an induction agent prior to Caesarean section. Should be avoided in eclampsia or hypertension. In very large doses, it may cause fetal respiratory depression. Ketamine increases uterine tone in the first and second, but not in the third trimester of pregnancy. S-ketamine has the analgesic effects but not the dreams or hypertensive side-effects of the racemic mixture.

Synthetic oxytocin (Syntocinon, 10 units i.v.) is often used to contract the uterus. It may cause transient dilatation of vessels containing both α and β receptors with hypotension, especially disastrous in patients with aortic stenosis.[51] Not emetic.

Complications of anaesthesia for Caesarean section

ACID ASPIRATION SYNDROME

See above.

AWARENESS DURING GENERAL ANAESTHESIA FOR CAESAREAN SECTION[52]

This is a problem of light anaesthesia, employed to minimize sedation of the baby. The risk makes the use of adjuvants essential, e.g. isoflurane 1%, sevoflurane 2% or enflurane 1%. Even so, there may be an irreducible minimum incidence. The place of remifentanil in prevention remains to be elucidated. It is very common to deepen anaesthesia after delivery with opioids.

Monitoring is possible, e.g. by isolated arm technique or bispectral index. Following reversal of muscle relaxant at the end of operation, a patient's response to command within 15 s of N_2O cessation suggests that there has been a risk of awareness (which is by no means always unpleasant, and may merely be auditory).

Pseudo-awareness is when the patient thinks that what happens as she awakes postoperatively, is happening during the operation.

CAVAL COMPRESSION SYNDROME

In the supine position the inferior vena cava is compressed by the gravid uterus at term. In 6% of patients this results in bradycardia, fall of cardiac output and hypotension of significant degree. Caval compression syndrome may be latent or overt. In either case placental blood flow is reduced. This may result in fall of PaO_2 and metabolic acidosis in the fetus. These ill effects are less when the fetus descends during labour and when the patient is put in the lateral position or when a tilt to the left is used on the operating table. Tilt to the left is preferred, but if this is not effective tilt to the right can be tried.

FAILED INTUBATION

See Chapter 2.6.

VISCERAL PAIN

Visceral pain may occur during regional block for the operation;[53] incidence 5–10%.

HYPOTENSION

Great care is required, especially in control of arterial pressure and in adequate oxygenation of the mother and hence of the child. Hypotension can be treated by a lateral tilt, elevation of the legs, infusion of plasma-volume expander, ephedrine and O_2 administration. Methoxamine and phenylephrine may reduce the blood supply to the placenta, but phenylephrine has been recommended for patients with aortic stenosis.[54]

Caesarean section in patients with severe systemic disease

The approach taken must be dictated by the nature of the disease. Cardiac arrest has occurred before and during induction of anaesthesia.[55] Coagulopathy and thrombocytopenia would contraindicate regional block, e.g. in HELLP syndrome. Aortic stenosis remains controversial.[56] *See* Chapter 3.2.

Other obstetric operations

Anaesthesia for forceps delivery and breech delivery

1 Low spinal analgesia.
2 Extradural block.
3 Extradural sacral block is excellent, if time is available. The disadvantage of these regional techniques is the time they take to perform (in what is a semi-urgent situation).
4 General anaesthesia with thiopentone, suxamethonium and N_2O/O_2, given through a cuffed tracheal tube.
5 Pudendal block is fast and efficient if care is taken in accurate placement.

Anaesthesia for retained placenta

Frequently the demand for manual removal of the placenta comes for a patient who merely has a slow third stage of labour. There is no shock nor any hurry. Occasionally, however, the patient may be shocked and a retraction ring may form an obstruction.

The patient is resuscitated as far as possible with O_2, blood transfusion and colloids. Coagulation status is monitored. If satisfactory, a spinal or general anaesthetic may then be given. If intravenous resuscitation is incomplete, a general anaesthetic is a better choice, although the problem of acid regurgitation and the full stomach persist well into the puerperium.[57]

In the absence of facilities for general anaesthesia, intravenous opioids (e.g. subapnoeic doses of remifentanil or alfentanil) make the manoeuvre of manual removal tolerable. In an emergency and to save life in severe postpartum haemorrhage it may be justified to remove the placenta from a collapsed patient without any analgesia.

ASSISTANCE WITH SOME OBSTETRIC EMERGENCIES

Management is the responsibility of obstetricians; however, in practice, anaesthetists are often called in to advise, and to help with resuscitation.

Severe pre-eclampsia

It is due to failure of distension of the placental spiral arteries, causing release of fibronectin and exists when the following are present:

1 systolic pressure >160 or diastolic >110 mmHg; or >90mmHg on two occasions more than 4 h apart (hypertension alone is termed 'gestational hypertension' and affects 10% of pregnant women);

2 rapidly increasing proteinuria; >300 mg/24 h;

3 Oedema (not essential for diagnosis).

Eclampsia and pre-eclamptic toxaemia

Eclampsia and pre-eclamptic toxaemia (PET) (eclampsia = Gk, to shine forth[58]) may occur especially in primigravidae between the 20th week of pregnancy and 7 days post-partum. Incidence 1 in 2000 deliveries.

Mild pre-eclampsia is defined as a diastolic pressure above 90 mmHg with proteinuria <25 mg/l.

The following also occur in the serious case:

1 oliguria (<400 ml urine in 24 h);
2 cerebral or visual disturbance;
3 pulmonary oedema or cyanosis;
4 eclampsia is manifest if convulsions occur at any time.

There may be hypertension, reduced blood volume, reduced colloid oncotic pressure, thrombocytopenia, increased fluid in extravascular compartment, increased risk of premature placental separation, hyperreflexia, headache, clonus, photophobia, cerebral oedema, abnormal electroencephalogram (EEG) (diffuse slow activity with paroxysmal spikes), and convulsions. PCWP may be normal.

Death (about 10% of maternal mortality in UK), can occur from:

1 heart failure with pulmonary oedema;
2 inhalation of saliva or vomit;
3 cerebral haemorrhage;
4 hepatorenal failure – the so-called HELLP syndrome may occur; management guidelines have been suggested;[59]
5 disseminated intravascular coagulopathy (DIC).

Thrombocytopenia occurs in one-third of patients, but prolonged bleeding time is unlikely with counts above 80 000/cu mm.[60]

Hepatic rupture has been reported.[61]

Acute renal failure may be associated with haemoglobinuria and can require dialysis.

Laryngeal oedema has been reported[62] and can cause intubation problems.

Management

1 The anaesthetist should be informed at an early stage. The patient is kept well oxygenated.
2 Coagulopathy and thrombocytopenia are monitored and corrected continuously. The bleeding time is measured if platelets < 150 000.
3 Plasma volume is corrected, with CVP monitoring.
4 Vasodilatation: arterial pressure is controlled by epidural block, alpha- and beta-blockers or even sodium nitroprusside (SNP) (10 μg/kg/min). (Fetal/maternal SNP cyanide toxicity has been prevented by co-infusion of thiosulphate (1 g for every 100 mg SNP) in the ewe model.[63])
5 The health of the fetus is of paramount concern and is monitored continuously. *The baby is delivered as soon as possible* which usually brings the condition to an end, although convulsions can occur in the immediate post-delivery period.
6 Prophylaxis and control of convulsions may be by *magnesium sulphate*,[64] loading dose 40–80 mg/kg followed by infusion at 2 g/h. Side-effects include neuromuscular blockade directly related to serum magnesium levels,[65] and potentiation of relaxants, reduction of peripheral resistance, increase of cardiac output and antiadrenergic effects in animals.

The hazards of general anaesthesia are difficult intubation, exaggerated pressor response to intubation, and prolonged action of relaxants.

All this is much easier to write about than to successfully achieve in practice! In a severe case, every parameter is violently fluctuating, often exceeding the availability of laboratory results and therapeutic resources. There may be wild instability in the pathophysiological status of both patients. Transfer to a high-dependency unit (HDU) or ITU is often indicated[66] in this situation.

HELLP syndrome

Haemolysis, causing anaemia; elevated liver enzymes, LDH > 600, AST > 70 u/l; low platelets, < 100 × 10^9/l, due to increased consumption. This syndrome is different from pre-eclampsia but a variant of the same process. Patients are likely to be ill and require fluid resuscitation. There may be painful hepatic haemorrhage and rupture indicating emergency delivery and repair. Oedema is usual, hypertension is less common. Spinal block is usually contraindicated by thrombocytopenia, and coagulopathy due to hepatic dysfunction.

Amniotic fluid embolism

A sudden infusion of amniotic fluid into the maternal circulation, after rupture of the membranes, gives rise to an acute shock-like state characterized by:

1 respiratory distress;
2 cyanosis;

3 chest pain;
4 peripheral vascular collapse;
5 coma;
6 DIC with hypofibrinogenaemia and excessive bleeding; this may occur without collapse and be the first sign of the condition; effect on blood-clotting mechanism described in 1950;
7 convulsions which must be differentiated from those of eclampsia or toxicity of local analgesics.

Its signs and symptoms may wrongly be attributed to anaesthesia.

The mortality is high. Chest X-ray reveals bilateral perihilar mottling. Electrocardiogram shows right heart strain. Pulmonary artery and central venous pressures are raised. The pulmonary bed may be blocked by fibrin deposits. The diagnosis is definite when elements of amniotic fluid are found in maternal tissues, especially blood, urine, lungs and sputum. Treatment may include:

1 blood transfusion;
2 administration of fresh frozen plasma or fibrinogen to combat defibrination;
3 vasopressors (ephedrine or mephentermine are to be preferred as they cause less pulmonary vasoconstriction);
4 IPPV with O_2;
5 bronchodilators;
6 steroids;
7 digoxin.

Disseminated intravascular coagulopathy (DIC)

May follow haemorrhage, abortion, hydatidiform mole, intra-uterine fetal death, amniotic fluid embolism.

Effects:

1 continued bleeding;
2 destruction of fibrin and fibrinogen by plasma fibrinolysins;
3 conversion of prothrombin to thrombin may be inactivated by release of heparin-like substance in amniotic fluid.

Normal fibrinogen is 150–700 mg%. Less than 150 mg% is dangerous.

Diagnosis: clotting screen shows widespread abnormalities, often with fibrin degradation products (FDPs).

Treatment:

1 fresh frozen plasma;
2 ε-aminocaproic acid, 4–5 g initial dose i.v. over 1 h, then 1 g 8-hourly; or tranexamic acid to antagonize fibrinolysis;
3 when heparin-like factor diagnosed, give 20–50 mg i.v. protamine sulphate slowly; coagulation analysis is repeated frequently to assess effects of therapy;

4 fibrinogen infusion;
5 blood transfusion is usually required;
6 treatment of the cause of the DIC.

The prognosis is not good and relatives are informed accordingly. Intensive care is often needed.

Shock

Causes of shock in the obstetric patient include:

1 haemorrhage, e.g. antepartum or post-partum haemorrhage, lacerations of birth canal, retained placenta, uterine atony;
2 traumatic – acute inversion of the uterus; surgical trauma;
3 septic shock;
4 supine hypotensive syndrome (*see below*);
5 amniotic fluid embolism;
6 anaphylaxis.

Massive intrapartum haemorrhage

More than 1 ml/kg/min blood loss. The main aim is to initiate resuscitation, to enrol senior and ancillary help and transfer the patient to theatre as soon as possible.

If the patient is undelivered, put in left lateral position. Administer O_2. Ask for senior anaesthetic/obstetrician/midwife. Establish large intravenous access. Inform the blood bank, arrange immediate cross-matching, full blood count, coagulation screen. O-negative blood is brought to the patient and group-specific blood sent for. Colloid is infused fast. With every 4 units of transfused blood, platelets and fresh frozen plasma are given, also via a fluid warmer. The fetal heart rate, direct arterial pressure, oxygenation and CVP are monitored. The patient is catheterized and urine output measured.

Bleeding is controlled by immediate operation and delivery if not already delivered. Syntocinon is given. Emergency hysterectomy is occasionally required.

Monitoring of basic parameters continues, including coagulation status.

Admission to ITU is arranged.

Sickle-cell disease and pregnancy

(*See* Chapter 3.1.)

Myasthenia gravis in pregnancy

(*See* Chapter 3.1.)

Acute inversion of the uterus

Shock is out of proportion to blood loss. Correction of circulating volume and bradycardia, with cautious use of ephedrine to correct hypotension. General anaesthesia for surgical correction may be requested.

Resuscitation of the newborn[67]

One of the earliest papers on treatment was 'The Asphyxia of the Stillborn Infant and its Treatment', by Marshall Hall in 1856.[68] Intra-uterine respiration of the fetus, the rhythmical amniotic tide into and out of the air passages, was first demonstrated by J.F. Ahfelt (1843–1929), Leipzig obstetrician, in 1888 and then by the Italian, Ferroni, in 1899.

The fetal blood haemoglobin is 15–20 g/dl and when fully saturated carries 22 vol% of O_2. But because of the low PO_2 at which maternal blood gives up its O_2, fetal haemoglobin is only 50% saturated. There is also a mild acidosis with PaO_2 of 7 kPa and a pH fall to 7.25. To compensate for this the dissociation curve of the maternal haemoglobin is shifted to the left, while the dissociation curve of fetal haemoglobin is shifted to the right, making it give up O_2 more easily. Brown fat is important in heat regulation of the newborn.

In the newborn the amount of carbonic anhydrase is half that found in adult blood so that release of CO_2 in lungs is handicapped.

During the process of birth, anaerobic glycolysis may aid the survival of the infant, energy being released from glycogen, of which the stores are small.

Fluctuation in maternal CO_2 tension may contribute to respiratory difficulties in the newborn, especially in premature infants. Maternal $PaCO_2$ may fall as a result of hyperventilation towards the end of the first stage of labour, reducing placental blood flow, but may rise during the second stage as a result of breath-holding.

Intrapartum fetal monitoring

The signs of intra-uterine hypoxia are irregularity of the fetal heart rate going on to tachycardia or bradycardia. In a cephalic presentation, the presence of meconium indicates hypoxic relaxation of the fetal anal sphincter.

Estimation of the pH of fetal blood as an index of fetal hypoxia has proved most useful. A pH of 7.15 indicates critical hypoxia.

Causes of distress in fetus and newborn

1 Maternal hypoxia.
2 The presence of haemoglobinopathy.
3 Maternal hypotension, maternal cardiac failure.

4 Maternal hypoglycaemia may affect the neonate: a minimum maternal blood glucose of 7 mmol/l prevents fetal hypoglycaemia.[69]
5 The trauma of labour. Fetal distress form uterine hyperactivity has been relieved by nitroglycerin 60–180 μg doses repeated every 2–3 min.[70]
6 Placental infarction or premature separation; prolapse or knotting of cord.
7 Fetal respiratory failure.
  (a) *Central.* Due to: (i) immaturity of respiratory centre, perhaps associated with gross fetal abnormality; (ii) damage to respiratory centre from trauma or from cerebral oedema due to diabetes or hydrops fetalis; (iii) O_2 lack perhaps associated with intrapartum fetal asphyxia; (iv) narcotics and sedatives given to mother. The threshold of maternal respiratory centre differs from that of the fetal centre, as a level of narcosis harmless to the mother may be depressing to the fetus. All anaesthetics, except N_2O and O_2, and all analgesic agents, other than chloral in reasonable dosage, depress the fetal respiratory mechanism, an effect made worse by any hypoxia of the mother during labour. The placenta acts as no barrier to these agents. The danger is increased with premature infants.
  (b) *Peripheral.* Due to: (i) immaturity of lungs, e.g. in diaphragmatic hernia; (ii) respiratory obstruction; (iii) muscular weakness; (iv) fetal lungs full of liquor amnii or meconium; (v) intranatal pneumonia; (vi) respiratory distress syndrome; (vii) tracheo-oesophageal fistula.

The baby recovering from asphyxia first takes a series of gasps which give place to a series of single prolonged inspirations. Finally, rhythmic inspiration and expiration set in. Periodic breathing is not of bad prognostic significance in newborn babies and is common in premature infants.

Management of asphyxia of the newborn

Immediate oxygenation via mask or tracheal tube, with IPPV if necessary. The fetal circulation can withstand 10–15 min of hypoxia but deficient cerebral blood flow may cause permanent damage. The fetus in utero is cyanosed. The normally delivered child should breathe rhythmically from the beginning, air replacing liquor amnii. Alveoli are opened up by the negative pressure exerted by normal respiratory movements (-50 cmH_2O), as in crying. In respiratory depression respiration begins differently, in gasps – the most primitive respiratory movement, involving many more muscles.

Monitoring neonatal status

Virginia Apgar (1909–1975) of New York City described a system whereby the condition of a neonate can be assessed, one (or more) minutes after delivery.

Naloxone may be indicated for opioid depression.

Apgar scoring system					
	Heart rate	Respiratory effort	Muscle tone	Colour	Reflex irritability
0	Absent	Absent	Flaccid	Blue or white	No response
1	Slow, less than 100	Weak cry, hypoventilation	Some movement	Blue hands or feet	Some movement
2	100 or over	Crying lusty	Well flexed	Healthy pink	Active movement

Indications for oxygen and intermittent positive-pressure ventilation by mask in the newborn

1 Central cyanosis.
2 Bradycardia.
3 Failure to cry on stimulation.

Face-mask resuscitation may be successful if Head's reflex[71] stimulates spontaneous respiration; if it does not, intubation will be required. It requires skill and may cause damage.

Indications for intubation of the newborn and short-term intermittent positive-pressure ventilation

The following guidelines may be considered when the baby's condition deteriorates in the minutes following birth:

1 central cyanosis for more than 3 min;
2 bradycardia less than 100 bpm for more than 3 min;
3 apnoea for more than 3 min;
4 'white asphyxia', i.e. skin vasoconstriction;
5 cardiac arrest or depression;
6 Apgar score of 0–2.

The cyanosis will fail to respond to O_2 therapy in the presence of cyanotic heart disease, severe tracheo-oesophageal fistula, large diaphragmatic hernia and severe respiratory distress syndrome.

The upper air passages are cleared by suction, using a catheter (No. 6 FG). Skin stimulation, passive limb movements, slapping, etc. are also very valuable, while O_2 is given via a face mask and neonatal inflating bag 30–40 puffs per min. In feeble babies, a small stomach tube may be passed to evacuate the stomach of liquor amnii and prevent its aspiration into the lungs.

If no improvement takes place within 2 min the trachea is intubated using a straight-blade laryngoscope and the lungs inflated with O_2. Any baby born apnoeic, flaccid or with a slow heart beat may be intubated immediately.

A neonate is intubated with no pillow. The head is gently extended. The straight blade of the infant laryngoscope is gently inserted into the vallecula (not posterior to the epiglottis) from the right side of the mouth and then lifted vertically. The commonest mistake is to insert the blade too far, missing the glottis completely.

The tracheal tube used should have an internal diameter of 2.5–3.5 mm. Various designs are available.

The pressure needed to expand the newborn lung is usually about 2.94 kPa (30 cmH$_2$O), but may be double this for a few inflations.

Estimation of blood gases and electrolytes is desirable.

Care is taken to prevent hypothermia.

Closed chest massage, if required, can be carried out by pressure of two fingers over the mid-sternum 60 times/min. In a baby who is hypotonic and is not responding, continued resuscitation beyond 30 min is unlikely to result in a favourable outcome.

Hypoglycaemia is considered if resuscitation is not immediately successful.

Premature babies must not be given pure O_2 for any length of time. If they are cyanosed they may receive 40% O_2 for short periods only, thus reducing the danger of retrolental fibroplasia.

GYNAECOLOGY

First successful removal of an ovarian cyst in 1817 by Ephraim McDowell (1771–1830), of Kentucky,[72] and first successful closure of a vesicovaginal fistula in 1852 by James Marion Sims (1813–1883), of New York.[73] First successful surgical treatment of ruptured ectopic pregnancy by Lawson Tait of Birmingham (1845–1899).[74]

The main problems are haemorrhage, postoperative vomiting and deep venous thrombosis.[76] The high-dose oestrogen 'pill' produced resistance to the anticoagulant effect of protein C.

Abdominal operations call for profound relaxation to prevent damage to muscles and the upper abdominal peritoneum from abrasion by packs. They can be performed under spinal analgesia, either intradural or extradural, or under general anaesthesia.

For Wertheim's hysterectomy (Ernst Wertheim, 1864–1920, of Vienna) extradural block up to T5 is recommended and light general anaesthesia is a useful adjunct as there may still be some surgical stimulation outside the field of the block.

Grades of thromboembolism risk

Low risk
Minor, brief surgery.
Age <40 years.
No defined added risk.

Intermediate risk
Major surgery.
Over 60 min surgery.
Trauma.
Varicose veins.
Upper abdominal surgery.
Obesity.

High risk
Previous thromboembolism.
Pelvic/hip/major leg surgery: fibrinolysis is reduced following surgery (except prostate and lung).
Oral contraceptive pill, factor V Leiden mutation.
Abdominal malignancy.

The Trendelenburg position is unphysiological and should be maintained for as short a time as possible. It may lead to headache, regurgitation, atelectasis, nerve palsies and a steep rise in CVP. The less steep it is the better for the patient's respiratory and cardiovascular function. Levelling of the table should be gradual, with a watch on venous and arterial blood pressure.

Vaginal operations can be performed under extradural lumbar or sacral block (*see* Chapter 5.3) or general anaesthesia.

The lithotomy position is a source of potential problems to the patient. Stretching of the cervix or trauma to the perineum may produce laryngeal spasm, requiring a deeper plane of anaesthesia or a small dose of a muscle relaxant. Spinal analgesia combines afferent block, muscular relaxation and moderate hypotension and ischaemia. For dilatation and curettage, intravenous induction, with N_2O and O_2, with or without a volatile agent is satisfactory.

Anaesthesia for laparoscopy

Laparoscopy was first employed in 1910, using a cystoscope.[77] It is not a minor procedure and is accompanied by an increase in blood glucose, plasma cortisol, prolactin and growth hormone. In addition lethal haemorrhage may occur. The patient is often in a steep Trendelenburg position.

Problems of the lithotomy position

Trapped fingers, contact with metal, due to arm position.

Backache and lumbar disc pathology if pelvis is placed too low.

Nerve damage

Sciatic: stretched by knee extension, thigh flexion, and external hip rotation.

Femoral: kinked adduction and rotation of thigh.

Common peroneal: compressed between fibula and stirrup.

Posterior tibial: compressed by stirrups.

Saphenous: compressed between stirrups and medial condyle.

Shoulder retainers can cause injury to brachial plexus.

Pressure on calf muscles

Deep venous thrombosis, muscle necrosis and compartment syndrome (pressure on antero-lateral aspect of lower leg). Pressure from leaning surgical assistants.

Regurgitation and aspiration of stomach contents
Worse if head down.

Spontanous respiration impaired
Particularly in obese patients.

Severity of blood loss disguised by increased venous return
Intraocular pressure raised.

A distended stomach may be injured by the operator; it must be prevented, or if present, deflated. The injected gas, usually CO_2, may cause cardiovascular disturbances due to the raised intra-abdominal pressure. These include rise or fall of arterial pressure, CVP and heart rate. Hypercapnia causes increase in circulating catecholamines and peripheral vascular resistance. Peak levels of $PaCO_2$ may not arise until after completion of the operative procedure. Carbon dioxide embolus occurs. The gas may accidentally be injected into aorta, inferior vena cava, retroperitoneal tissues causing caval compression, hollow viscera or abdominal wall. The intra-abdominal pressure should probably not exceed 30 cmH_2O, a pressure adequate for good surgical exposure. The gas is absorbed but can be removed from the bloodstream by hyperventilation and IPPV. These changes would be less frequent if N_2O were substituted for CO_2, although the risk of explosion from diathermy is introduced especially if gas from an injured viscus enters the peritoneal cavity. Light general anaesthesia via a tracheal tube, with IPPV and relaxants, is a suitable combination and preferable to techniques of spontaneous respiration when the incidence of dysrhythmia is high, although N_2O, oxygen and enflurane, with spontaneous respiration is stated to give good results.[78] Gross obesity, marked anxiety and the presence of peritoneal adhesions are relative contraindications. The gas must be let out at the end of the operation or shoulder pain may result, lasting several days.

Pneumothorax has been reported, due to the passage of gas through surgical wounds in the diaphragm.[79] Other complications reported include brachial plexus palsy (poor positioning) and regurgitation of gastric contents.

Postoperative analgesia, instilling lignocaine through a catheter whose tip lies in the pouch of Douglas, has given good results.[80]

REFERENCES

1 Urquhart J., Plaat F. and Collis R. *Modern Obstetric Anaesthesia.* Oxford University Press, Oxford, 1998.
2 Brancazio L. R., Laifer S. A. and Schwartz T. *Obstet. Gynecol.* 1997, **89,** 383–386.
3 *Science* 1998, **279,** 32–33.
4 McGrady E. M. *Br. J. Anaesth.* 1997, **78,** 115–117.
5 Miller A. C. *Int. J. Obstet. Anal.* 1997, **1,** 2–18.
6 Yentis S. M. and Dob D. P. *Anaesthesia* 1998, **53,** 606–607.
7 Viscomi V. L., Rathmell J. P. and Pace N. L. *Anesth. Analg.* 1997, **84,** 1108–1112.
8 Park G. E. et al. *Anesth. Analg.* 1996, **83,** 299–303.
9 Saberski L. R., Kondamuri S. and Osinubi O. Y. O. *Regional Anesth.* 1997, **22,** 3–15.
10 Walker D. S. and Brock-Utne J. G. *Can. J. Anaesth.* 1997, **44,** 494–497.
11 Segal S., Eappen S. and Datta S. *J. Clin. Anesth.* 1997, **9,** 109–112.
12 Howie J. E. and Dutton D. A. In Reynolds F. (ed.) *Epidural and Spinal Analgesia in Obstetrics.* Bailliere Tindall, London, 1990, 162.
13 Marcus M. A. E. et al. *Anesth. Analg.* 1997, **84,** 1113–1116.
14 Carrie L. E. S. *Br. J. Anaesth.* 1990, **65,** 225.
15 Enever G. R. et al. *Anaesthesia* 1991, **46,** 169.
16 Baldwin A. M. et al. *Anaesth. Intensive Care* 1991, **19,** 246.
17 Lyons G., Columb M., Hawthorne L. and Dresner M. *Br. J. Anaesth.* 1997, **78,** 493–497.
18 James K. S., McGrady E. and Patrick A. *Br. J. Anaesth* 1997, **78,** 498–501.
19 Cox B. A. *Br. J. Anaesth.* 1997, **79,** 289–293.
20 Xuecheng J. et al. *Br. J. Anaesth.* 1997, **78,** 570–573.
21 McRae W. *Br. J .Anaesth.* 1997, **79,** 558–562.
22 Zaric D et al. *Regional Analg.* 1996, **21,** 14–25.
23 Fernando R. et al. *Anaesthesia* 1997, **52,** 517–534.
24 Campbell D. C. et al. *Anesthesiology* 1997, **86,** 525–531.

25 McSPI Europe Research Group *Anesthesiology*,1997, **86,** 346, 363.
26 Ala-Kokko T. I. et al. *Acta Anaesth. Scand.* 1997, **41,** 313–319.
27 Klant J. G. et al. *Anaesthesia* 1997, **52,** 547–551; Fernando R. et al. *Anaesthesia* 1997, **52,** 517–534.
28 Coda B., Bausch S., Haas M. and Chavkin C. *Regional Anesth.* 1997, **22,** 43–52.
29 Paw H. *Br. Med. J.* 1998, **316,** 160.
30 Russell R., Dundas R. and Reynolds F. *Br. Med. J.* 1996, **312,** 1384–1388; Reynolds F. and Russell R. *Br. Med. J.* 1998, **316,** 69–70.
31 Lanska D. J. and Kryscio R. J. *Obstet. Gynecol.* 1997, **89,** 413–418.
32 Morgan B. *Anaesthesia* 1990, **45,** 148.
33 Cesarini M et al. *Anaesthesia* 1990, **45,** 656.
34 Broadley S. A. and Fuller G. N. *Br. Med. J.* 1997, **315,** 1324–1325.
35 Ferouz F. et al. *Anesthesiology* 1997, **86,** 592–598.
36 Morgan M. *Anaesthesia* 1986, **41,** 689.
37 Report on Confidential Enquiry into Maternal Deaths in the United Kingdom 1994–1996 (1996). HMSO, London.
38 Lapinsky S. E., Kriczynsky K., Seaward D. R., Farine D. and Grossman R. F. *Can. J. Anaesth.* 1997, **44,** 325–329.
39 Mendelson C. L. *Am. J. Obstet. Gynecol.* 1946, **52,** 191 (reprinted in 'Classical File', *Surv. Anesthesiol.* 1966, **10,** 599).
40 Hahn R. G., Drobin D. and Stahle L. *Br. J. Anaesth.* 1997, **78,** 144–148.
41 Marcus M. A. E. et al. *Anesth. Analg.* 1997, **84,** 1113–1116.
42 Campbell D. C. et al. *Anesthesiology* 1997, **86,** 525–531.
43 Lyons G., Columb M., Hawthorne L. and Dresner M. *Br. J. Anaesth.* 1997, 78, 493–497.
44 Dahlgren G. et al. *Anesth. Analg.* 1997, **85,** 1288–1293.
45 Broadley S. A. and Fuller G. N. *Br. Med. J.* 1997, **315,** 1324–1325.
46 Thomas R. and Nanson J. *Anaesthesia* 1998, **53,** 613.
47 Chung C. J., Bae S. H., Chae K. Y. and Chin Y. J. *Br. J. Anaesth.* 1996, **77,** 145–149.
48 Lang D. J., Wafai Y. and Salem M. R. *Anesthesiology* 1996, **85,** 246–253.
49 Lockey D. J. *Anaesthesia* 1997, **52,** 242–243.
50 Baraka A. S., Sayyid S. S. and Assaf B. A. *Anesth. Analg.* 1997, **84,** 1104–1107.
51 Yentis S. M. and Dob D. P. *Anaesthesia* 1998, **53,** 606–607.
52 Brahms D. *Anaesthesia* 1990, **45,**161.
53 Alahuhta S., Kangas-Saarela T., Hollmin A.I. and Edstrom H. H. *Acta Anaesth. Scand.* 1990, **34,** 99.
54 Yentis S. M. and Dob D. P. *Anaesthesia* 1998, **53,** 606–607.
55 McCartney A. and Dirk R. *Anaesthesia* 1998, **53,** 308–309; McIndoe A., Hammond E., Babbington P. C. *Br. J. Anaesth.* 1995, **75,** 97–101.
56 Brighouse D. et al. *Anaesthesia* 1998, **53,** 107–112.
57 Jayaram A., Bowen M. P., Deshpande S. and Carp H. M. *Anesth Analg.* 1997, **84,** 522–526.
58 Hippocrates 4th Century BC.
59 Patterson K. W. and O'Toole D. P. *Br. J. Anaesth.* 1991, **66,** 513.
60 Schindler M. et al. *Anaesth. Intensive Care* 1990, **18,** 1691.

61 Loevingen E. H. et al. *Obstet. Gynecol.* 1985, **65,** 281.
62 Tillman H. A. *Can. Anaesth. Soc. J.* 1984, **31,** 210.
63 Curry S. C., Carlton M. W. and Raschke R. A. *Anesth. Analg.* 1997, **84,** 1121–1126.
64 Saunders N. and Hammesley B. *Lancet* 1995, **345,** 788–789.
65 Ramathan J. et al. *Am. J. Obstet. Gynecol.* 1988, **158,** 40.
66 Lapinsky S. E., Kriczynsky K., Seaward D. R., Farine D. and Grossman R. F. *Can. J. Anaesth.* 1997, **44,** 325–329.
67 Mather S. J. and Hughes D. G. *A Handbook of Paediatric Anaesthesia.* Oxford University Press, Oxford,1996.
68 Marshall Hall (1790–1857). *Lancet* 1856, **2,** 601 (reprinted in 'Classical File'. *Surv. Anesthesiol.* 1977, **21,** 398).
69 Curet L. B., Izquierdo L. A., Gilson G. J., Schneider J. M., Perelman R. and Converse J. *J. Perinatol.* 1997, **17,** 113–115.
70 Mercier F. J., Dounas M., Bouaziz H., Lhuissier C. and Benhamou D. *Anesth. Analg.* 1997, **84,** 1117–1120.
71 Head H. *J. Physiol. (Lond.)* 1889, **10,** 1 and 279.
72 McDowall E. *Elect. Rep. Analyt. Rev.* 1817, **7,** 242.
73 Sims J. M. (1813–1883) *Am. J. Med. Sci.* 1852, **23,** 59.
74 Tait L. *Med. Times Gaz.* 1881, **2,** 654.
76 Rosendaal F. R. *Semin. Haematol.* 1997, **34,** 171–187.
77 Jacobeus H. C. *Münch. Med. Wochenschr.* 1910, **57,** 2090.
78 Harris M. N. E. et al. *Br. J. Anaesth.* 1984, **56,** 1214.
79 Calverly R. K. and Jenkins L. C. *Can. Anaesth. Soc. J.* 1973, **20,** 679.
80 Haldane G., Stott S. and McMenemin I. *Anaesthesia* 1998, **53,** 598–603.

Chapter 4.4

Trauma and multiple injuries[1]

'SCOOP AND RUN' VERSUS 'STAY-AND-STABILIZE'

For individual patients, these two ends of the first-aid spectrum have now given way to more precise protocols dealing with specific situations. Immediate oxygenation with protection of the airway is the first priority, followed by circulatory support. Need for inotropes during transfer is a poor prognostic sign.

Head injured patients, especially children, have cervical support (collar, sandbags, Hines splint, etc.) until there is proof of cervical stability.[2]

FIELD EQUIPMENT

1 Box, bag or rucksac.
2 Intravenous fluids, of value even days after the event[3] (crystalloids, colloids and bags for group-compatible blood if ready-grouped donors are available, i.e. 'blood on the hoof'), cannulae, adhesive tape, bandages, support splints, etc. Crystalloids may be marginally better than colloids.[4]
3 Airways and tracheal tubes, larygoscopes, self-inflating ventilation bags.
4 Drugs: analgesics, opioids, especially nalbuphine 20–30 mg in spring-loaded self-administration syringes (and naloxone to differentiate opioid stupor from head-injury coma), ketamine with midazolam, entonox, sublingual buprenorphine, atropine, ephedrine, local analgesics; syringes, needles.
5 Triservice apparatus and foot-operated sucker for the field hospital; O_2, portable O_2 concentrator,[5] with thiopentone, etomidate, halothane, vecuronium, sterilizing system for tracheal tubes, etc.

A total intravenous anaesthesia (TIVA) technique has been described:[6] midazolam 5 mg, ketamine 200 mg, vecuronium 12 mg in 50 ml saline, infused at 0.5 ml/kg/h. The mixture is stable for at least 24 h and finds special application in a theatre sealed against chemical weapon attack.

ORGANIZATION IN THE ACCIDENT RECEPTION CENTRE[7]

The major accident plan is activated. The appointed 'controllers' (medical, theatres, nursing, administrative, and triage officer) are informed, and all resident staff alerted, plus medical records staff, porters, mortuary technician, chaplains. Each reports to the control room for identity and action cards. Non-resident staff are informed by private telephone (i.e. not via the hospital switchboard).

Each staff member has a designated and defined job.

Disaster equipment is packaged and labelled ready for use.

Ketamine has a place in anaesthetic management of painful treatments, at the site, or in the accident department, when more usual methods are overwhelmed by numbers or unavailable for other reasons. Clinical monitoring assumes greater importance, but genuinely portable instrumental monitoring is important.

Secondary triage is undertaken.

Takeover of other hospital areas and facilities is planned and agreed in advance (the emergency medicine 'buffer ward' is useful in accidents of small numbers).

Ventilation facilities in the intensive therapy unit (ITU) should be expandable (in equipment personnel and space).

EARLY MANAGEMENT OF THE SEVERELY INJURED PATIENT[8]

Head injury is common and should be considered in any trauma case. Treatment of head injury (an adequate supply of oxygenated blood flow), preventing secondary brain insult, takes priority over most other considerations. Maintaining cerebral perfusion pressure above 70 mmHg is the target.[9]

Basic trauma life support

A simple scheme remembering priorities in basic trauma life support (BTLS) is as follows:

1 *Airway* – is it clear? Extend head, open and clear mouth, lift jaw, insert airway or intubate etc. Endotracheal intubation in the field improves survival in patients with severe head injury.[10] Does the patient need intubating?

2 *Breathing* – is the patient doing it? If not, the operator institutes intermittent positive-pressure ventilation (IPPV). Is the patient being oxygenated? This is an absolute priority. Pulse oximetry is needed.
3 *Circulation* – pressure control of external haemorrhage, elevate legs (or MAST pants), cardiac massage if necessary.

Circulation is usually improved by setting up an infusion of warmed crystalloid or colloid immediately, and by stopping haemorrhage. Monitoring needed; capillary refill. Is a pulse palpable? What is the arterial pressure? Are the jugular veins full?

Advanced trauma life support

For advanced trauma life support (ATLS), check A, B, C, as above plus intravenous cannulation, central venous pressure (CVP); is the circulation to any part of the body compromised? The legs are elevated and intravenous infusions run at full speed if the patient is hypovolaemic. Prevention of hypotension (and hypertension) are important.

1 Disability assessment: includes Glasgow Coma Score; identify all the injuries.
2 Expose the whole body and perform a whole-body search for traumatic damage. This is never more difficult than in blunt chest trauma where diagnosis and treatment are testing even in specialist centres.[11]
3 Has haemostasis been achieved, e.g. by external pressure?
4 Is the patient being kept warm? Hypothermia is a potent cause of coagulopathy in trauma. Monitoring is needed.
5 Is urine still being produced?
6 Is there dyspnoea? Pneumothorax? Are chest drains needed?

Many patients are reasonably stable for the first hour after injury, with oxygenation and intravenous resuscitation ('*The golden hour*'). This is the time available for completing the optimization of the patient's physiology. After this time, decompensation and organ failure is progressively more common. Patients intoxicated with alcohol[12] are more likely to have full stomachs, brain injuries, inhaled vomit, and hypotension.

Haemmorrhage, overt or concealed, is another major feature of trauma. Acute hypovolaemia may cause cardiac ischaemia with segmental wall motion abnormalities.[13]

Analgesia is important. The pain management team has a role here. A label is attached to every patient who receives analgesics.

Maximization of O_2 delivery is a primary goal.[14]

Breaking bad news to relatives requires skill and sensitivity,[15] and the help of hospital chaplains. It is not unknown for anaesthetists to be left to do this task.

> **Key problems of blunt chest trauma**
>
> 1 Fractured ribs, haemothorax, pneumothorax, chylothorax, direct lung trauma.
>
> 2 Diaphragmatic rupture.
>
> 3 Myocardial injury causing failure (Holness R. and Waxman K. *Crit. Care Med.* 1990, **18**, 1)).
>
> 4 Immediate or delayed rupture of aorta.
>
> 5 Bronchial tears may give rise to large leaks requiring negative pressure to intercostal drains.
>
> 6 Mediastinal surgical emphysema or haematoma.

CHEST INJURIES

Hypoxia occurs with airway or pleural bleeding. Blood clot, saliva, stomach content and other debris may be inhaled to produce suffocation. The flail chest also causes hypoxia as paradoxical respiration occurs. Pain from fractured ribs also prevents proper respiration. Analgesia without respiratory depression is thus important (e.g. non-steroidal anti-inflammatory drugs (NSAIDs), low-dose ketamine, intercostal blocks,[16] thoracic epidural). Up to a quarter of these patients require IPPV, one-fifth are severely shocked and about one-third will have other (especially head) injuries. Pneumothorax must be kept in mind.

Pulmonary contusion is another potent cause of prolonged hypoxia.[17]

In major thoracic injury the first priority is to treat hypoxia and hypovolaemia. By the time a haemothorax is visible on chest X-ray, well over a litre of blood is present. An arterial cannula is inserted if possible.

Pneumothorax may not always be diagnosed by X-ray; a computed tomography (CT) scan may be needed.[18]

Monitoring

Pulse oximetry, direct arterial pressure, CVP for concealed haemorrhage and cardiac tamponade, chest X-rays, pulmonary artery catheter, Urine flow, Glasgow Coma Score.

Intensive therapy is likely to be required.

HEAD INJURIES (*see also* CHAPTER 4.1 'NEUROANAESTHESIA')

Responsible for two-thirds of trauma deaths in hospital, up to half ITU occupancy, and a third of scans.

Pathophysiology

Primary injury from impact. The brain may be damaged by contusion or haemorrhage.

Secondary injury from bleeding in the brain, and oedematous swelling of undamaged brain after impact. Local or global ischaemia, with diffuse axonal injury, may follow hypoxia, hypotension, low cerebral perfusion pressure and hyperthermia.

Tertiary injury from compression due to oedema around a haematoma or pressure from outside, e.g. subdural haematoma.

It is vital that proper oxygenation of the brain is maintained. Primary efforts should therefore be directed to maintenance of the airway and adequate pulmonary ventilation, arrest of any serious haemorrhage and maintenance of an adequate blood circulation. Uncomplicated head injury should not prevent the treatment of abdominal injuries, compound limb fractures or haemothorax, though faciomaxillary fractures can usually be left to a later date. Hyperglycaemia (and hypoglycaemia) increases the infarction associated with ischaemia, especially with brain lactate levels above 16 mmol/kg.

Intermittent positive-pressure ventilation is normally instituted in significant head injury to control the $PaCO_2$ at 3.5–4 kPa. Very low $PaCO_2$ is avoided (*see* Chapter 4.1 'Neuroanaesthesia').

The most important physical signs are:

1 progressive deterioration of consciousness;
2 progressive dilatation of a previously normal pupil;
3 progressive bradycardia, perhaps with a rising systolic blood pressure;
4 progressive weakness of the face, arm and even leg on the side opposite to the injury;
5 apnoea – this sign carries the gravest prognosis, even when instantly remedied by IPPV;
6 fits.

Management

To prevent or limit secondary brain damage: immediate restoration of cerebral perfusion pressure and oxygenation.

First aid

Airway management, oxygenation and avoiding delays in treatment. Lateral position in anticipation of vomiting, control of haemorrhage, speedy hospitalization, with in-line neck support (then intubation and IPPV).

Monitoring

1 Clinical signs and symptoms – Glasgow Coma Score.
2 Instrumental, arterial pressure, CVP, pulse oximetry, capnography.
3 Monitoring of cerebral function within the controlled neurosurgical environment, by intracranial pressure (ICP) recording (and ICP waveform analysis), electroencephalogram (EEG) and cerebral function monitoring, brainstem auditory evoked potentials (BSAEP), evoked potentials, cerebral blood flow, cerebral O_2 consumption ($CMRO_2$), normally 3–4 ml/100 g/min, cerebral arteriovenous O_2 difference (A-JDO_2), normally 6–7 vol%, phosphorus spectroscopy, positron emission tomography, etc. The cerebral function monitor should produce a waveform between 5 and 15 μV. A fall below 5 μV may indicate reduced cerebral perfusion; EEG, near infra-red spectroscopy and jugular venous oximetry.
4 Scans, e.g. CT and magnetic resonance imaging (MRI).

Prevention of secondary cerebral injury

By oxygenation, maintenance of cerebral perfusion pressure, IPPV, mild head-up tilt, and reduction of cerebral oedema.

Full diagnosis

Diagnose injuries (*see above*). Is the head injury localized or diffuse? Glasgow Coma Scale recording is established and an agreed flow chart commenced. Skull, cervical spine and chest X-rays, CT scan, MRI scan may be taken. Other injuries are treated, especially haemorrhage. Central venous pressure lines are inserted. (In many head injuries, the neck is also damaged, and not suitable for inserting CVP lines. The subclavian route may be needed.)

Note that relaxants and propofol infusion used in head injury make the clinical diagnosis of other injuries more difficult, and extra use may have to be made of scans.

Reduction of raised intracranial pressure

By intubation, IPPV, etc. Prevention of coughing and vomiting is an important component of this. Mannitol may be needed, for hyperosmotic effect and reduction of blood viscosity. The patient may be nursed 15 degrees head up.

Control of clinical or subclinical fits

As shown on the EEG, by propofol[19] in low-dose infusion, e.g. a bolus dose of 0.2 mg/kg i.v., with infusion at 1 mg/kg/h, with target blood level of 1.5 μg/ml. Barbiturates and benzodiazepines are also used. Sedation reduces the ICP, provided that pulmonary ventilation is maintained.

Cerebral protection

1 Moderate hypothermia (but care is needed to maintain insulin levels).
2 Thiopentone (once discredited[20] but now revived, provided that the blood pressure and cerebral blood flow can be maintained during its use, e.g. by adrenaline, dobutamine, etc.).
3 Nimodipine and N-type presynaptic calcium-channel blockers, 21-aminosteroid lipid peroxidase inhibitors, phenytoin, prostacyclin, naloxone, magnesium chloride.

Managing the reperfusion phenomenon

By antagonizing O_2 radicals and tissue damage mediators, e.g. with indomethacin 30 mg/kg/h.

General intensive care

Early enteral feeding, H2 blockers, and antacids prevent gastric ulceration.

Transfer to neurosurgical units

TRANSPORTATION OF NEUROSURGICAL PATIENTS[21]

Indications for neurosurgical referral

Immediate

Fractured skull plus Glasgow Coma Score <15. Focal neurological signs; fits; or symptoms.

or   Reducing consciousness or coma.

or   Focal neurological signs alone.

Urgent

Continuing confusion.

Compound depressed fracture.

Cerebrospinal fluid (CSF) leak.

Worsening headache and vomiting.

Uncontrollable convulsions.

1 Intubation and IPPV. Oxygen and ventilator should be alongside the patient.
2 One or two intravenous cannulae are in place before leaving. A pressure infusor will be required because of the limited head-room in helicopters for elevation of the fluid container.
3 Invasive arterial, CVP, electrocardiogram (ECG), SpO_2 and CO_2 monitoring.
4 Slight head-up tilt.
5 The doctor and nurse are advised to take travel sickness pills.
6 The following drugs should be carried: atropine, propofol, thiopentone, suxamethonium, ephedrine, dexamethasone and diuretics. Cardiopulmonary resuscitation (CPR) equipment must be to hand.
7 Full documentation.

Brainstem death

First described clinically in 1959.

Preconditions: no depressant drugs, no paralysis, no hypothermia, electrolyte abormalities or hypoglycaemia, no wax in the ears, normal $PaCO_2$ and PaO_2. Not within 24 h of cardiac arrest.

For this diagnosis all the following signs must be present, in addition to a clear diagnosis of the underlying condition, for at least 12 h. Pupils have no response to light. Oculovestibular reflex absent. The 'doll's-eye reflex' does not mean that there is brain death. Corneal reflex absent. Gag reflex absent. Carinal reflex absent. No response to pain inflicted on head. No spontaneous respiration for 4 min in the absence of hypothermia, and anoxia, with a normal ($ > 6.6$ kPa) $PaCO_2$. Positive end-expiratory pressure (PEEP) is useful here. Electroencephalogram confirmation is useful but opinions vary concerning its necessity.

Such a diagnosis is made by two doctors independently, one of 5 years' qualification, the other a consultant. It should be noted that spinal reflexes may persist after brain death.

SPINAL INJURIES

The utmost care is necessary during transport and movement.

Early management

Should tracheal intubation be necessary to procure a patent airway, the production of muscle relaxation with suxamethonium may remove the protective splinting provided by the support muscles allowing subluxation and spinal cord damage.[22] This is prevented by in-line cervical collars, some of which have opening front flaps for cricoid pressure. The most dangerous neck

---

Anaesthesia problems after cervical spine transection

1 Autonomic hyperreflexia, prevented by spinal analgesia; controlled by autonomic blocking drugs.

2 Suxamethonium hyperkalaemia 3 days to 3 months after injury.

3 Impaired autonomic control with hypotension and hypothermia.

4 Risk of pulmonary embolism.

5 Respiratory failure: poor coughing; respiratory depressants are avoided; nerve blocks if indeed analgesia is needed. Physiotherapy vital.

6 Chest and urinary infections are common.

---

movement is flexion. The Bullard laryngoscope has been designed for this situation. Emergency cricothyrotomy may be needed.

Spinal analgesia will control hyperreflexia in patients with chronic spinal cord injury.[23]

Fat embolism[24]

This was first described in humans by Friedrich Albert Zenker (1825–1898) in 1862,[25] with full clinical description by von Bergmann (1836–1907) in 1873,[26] and may be wrongly diagnosed as shock. Due to escape of droplets of fat into the circulation, and their deposition in the lungs, brain or skin. Often associated with fractures of lower-limb bones. Onset of symptoms may rapidly follow the injury or may be delayed for 2 or 3 days.

Pulmonary signs and symptoms include dyspnoea, pallor, cyanosis, pyrexia and frothy sputum. Bilateral shadowing is seen in chest X-rays. Fat globules may be seen in sputum and urine.

Cerebral changes (really signs of cerebral microhypoxia) usually seen in the first 24 h after operation or injury, with pyrexia, and there may be restlessness, leading to coma, convulsions and paralysis; deep coma carries a bad prognosis; fat emboli may sometimes be seen in the retinal vessels with an ophthalmoscope.

Skin signs are likely to be a purpuric eruption with petechiae over the upper front chest, neck and conjunctivae and are seen on the second or third day.

Metabolic signs: hypoxaemia, acidosis, hypocalcaemia, anaemia and thrombocytopenia.

Renal signs: acute renal failure may occur.

The lung manifestations are the most common and constitute the major threat to life. Hypoxia is due to ventilation/perfusion imbalance. If the patient's respiratory exchange can be maintained, the prognosis is good.

Treatment

All therapeutic measures depend upon proper respiratory management. Intermittent positive-pressure ventilation is often necessary, with PEEP, and continuous positive airway pressure (CPAP) in the weaning phase. Steroids are useful in the first 24 h but harmful thereafter.

Fulminant fat embolism syndrome: onset within a few hours of the injury or operation with rapid progress to a fatal conclusion.[27] It has been said that collapse in the second hour after injury is likely to be due to shock; in the second day, to fat embolism; in the second week, to pulmonary embolism.

ANAESTHESIA FOR THE ACUTELY INJURED PATIENT

Resuscitation and preparation

There is emphasis on prevention of shock by volume replacement, analgesia, and maximizing O_2 delivery[28] (e.g. > 600 ml/min/m^2). In practice this means energetic intravenous replacement of losses, O_2 and the use of inotropes such as dobutamine. Preoperative pulse rate is not usually helpful in assessing blood volume.

The military or other outdoor patient, e.g. mountaineer, is likely to be moderately to severely dehydrated, especially in hot climates. A large crystalloid infusion is appropriate here as preanaesthetic resuscitation, in addition to colloid or blood replacement of haemorrhage losses. Such patients may also be dehydrated from burns exudation. Maintenance of renal function is high priority, started as soon after trauma as possible.

Anaesthesia

Spinal block is not often appropriate because of unstable circulation. General anaesthetic: minimal doses of anaesthetic drugs, enabled by relaxants and IPPV.

Monitoring

Usually normal monitoring plus CVP. Arterial blood gases, coagulation and lactate levels are needed in the severe case. Any head injury, of course, will need monitoring.

Operations in chemical/biological warfare isolation theatres presents special problems of anaesthetic pollution, poor lighting (pulse oximetry is invaluable), lack of temperature control (for the staff as well as the patient!) and air conditioning, water supply, and facilities for clearing up of spilt blood and other waste (sand is useful for this). A total intravenous technique is useful, using the triservice equipment for added oxygenation and IPPV.

Diagnosis of CO poisoning

1 Cherry red skin.

2 Headache and nausea (HbCO of 15–20%).

3 Coma (at levels COHb > 40%).

4 HbCO estimation on CO-oximeter.

5 Electrocardiogram (ischaemia).

6 Full blood count, electrolytes, arterial blood gases.

It should be remembered that there is altered (usually reduced) drug clearance after trauma.[29]

BURNS

In the military situation, burns and limb injuries form the largest group of patients and in chemical warfare burns with mustard gas, may be a problem. Initial assessment of burns patients includes fluid needs, extent of burn (extent, and depth of skin burn, and respiratory injury); need for pain relief; incipient sepsis; chemical injury (e.g. CO, cyanide, chlorine, phosgene); other physical injury.

The rule of 9s and Lund and Browder charts are used to assess percentage burn. Blood is taken for cross-matching. Evidence of other medical conditions is actively sought, e.g. epilepsy, stroke, diabetes, overdose, child abuse.

Is there a respiratory burn? (Mortality 50%.) Is there upper airways obstruction? (Usually due to dry heat.) Coughing, soot in nostrils or sputum, pulmonary oedema, cyanosis, dyspnoea, tachypnoea, stridor, hoarseness, swelling of lips, tongue, pharynx or larynx. (Tracheal intubation should not be undertaken without very good indication, but when indicated should be done immediately under local analgesia.)

Is there lower airway injury due to chemical burn (HCN, Cl_2, phosgene) or later ARDS? Expiratory ronchi are heard. Even in the absence of respiratory burn, hypoxia may occur due to fluid shifts and ARDS.

Is there CO poisoning? (The 'cherry red' colour is unreliable for diagnosis.) Greater than 15% COHb is significant and requires ECG monitoring.

In circumferential thoracic burn, is escharotomy indicated?

Monitoring of respiratory injury

Immediate peak expiratory flow rate (PFR), blood gases, blood carboxyhaemoglobin expressed as % concentration (cyanide levels are also increased in those with raised carboxyhaemoglobin), packed cell volume (PCV), urea

---

Treatment of CO poisoning

1 One hundred per cent O_2 inhalation immediately.

2 Airway support; IPPV if in coma (ABC).

3 Monitoring ECG, blood pressure, $EtCO_2$ arterial blood gases, COHb.

4 Inotropic support of poisoned heart.

5 Correction of metabolic acidosis.

6 Hyperbaric O_2 if COHb $>$30–40% or if pregnant.

7 Mannitol or dexamethasone if cerebral oedema is diagnosed.

---

and electrolytes, ECG (high incidence of silent ischaemia in CO poisoning), chest X-ray.

Early management of the burns patient

1 Pain relief for partial-thickness burns by intravenous opioids or Entonox.
2 Oxygen inhalation, with high humidification; this reduces the half-life of HbCO to $<$1 h, and improves O_2 delivery to the tissues. The mitochondria are also poisoned. HbCO estimation repeated after 4 h.
3 Intravenous fluid replacement is of greatest importance in first 48 h. First 500 ml is normal saline, then colloid (e.g. 5% albumin in saline). Volume (ml) required in first 4 h:

$$\frac{\text{Wt in kg} \times \text{\% burn}}{2}$$

If only crystalloid is used, volume (ml) = wt in kg $\times$ % burn.

Central venous pressure monitoring indicated in the elderly and those arriving after long delays. After first 4 h, intravenous fluids judged by hourly microhaematocrit (target 35%) until stable.

In war or disaster situations, a mixture of Hartmann's solution and gelatin solution has been used.[30]
4 Catheterization of the bladder to assess urine flow and osmolality. (Target flow 0.5 ml/kg/h may take a day or so to achieve because of high anti-diuretic hormone (ADH) levels.) Initial urine osmolality may be high (900 mosmol), unless high-output renal failure occurs (300 mosmol). Samples are sent for protein and 'casts'. Black urine indicates myoglobinuria. Renal failure is common.
5 If intubation is needed for severe upper airway obstruction, it is done immediately under local analgesia with possible fibreoptic laryngoscope help. Cuff pressure is rechecked hourly and the patient kept sitting if possible to reduce pulmonary oedema. Apnoeic, acidotic patients are of

course intubated immediately, and may well have cyanide poisoning, requiring dicobalt edetate and sodium thiosulphate.

6 'Burns encephalopathy' is sought (hyperpyrexia, irritability, vomiting, twitching, coma, hyponatraemia).

Later management

1 Infections are treated as they arise. Aminoglycosides, ticarcillin, azlocillin are commonly used.
2 ARDS.
3 Deep venous thrombosis (DVT) (60% incidence) and pulmonary embolism (PE) (5% incidence) are treated.
4 Blood transfusion often needed.
5 Nutritional care needed if burn > 15% in adults or 10% in children, because of:
   (a) reduced intake;
   (b) increased calorie need and nitrogen loss;
   (c) diarrhoea and vomiting are common.
   Protein need = 1 g/kg + 2 g/% burn area.
   Calorie need = 20 kcal/kg + 50 kcal/% burn area.

Metabolic needs may be reduced by preventing hyperpyrexia and adequate analgesia. A weight loss of 10% is common, and is monitored.

The rise in metabolic rate following burns is greater than after other forms of trauma. There is loss of body heat, disturbance of the vasoconstrictor mechanism, and a reset of the hypothalamic thermostat, all exacerbated by pain and apprehension. There is a rise in plasma catecholamines, cortisol and glucagon. Hyperglycaemia is common and there is probably enhanced degradation of insulin. Energy requirement may be as high as 17 MJ/24 h (4000 kcal). Palatable food is best but will often need to be supplemented by enteral tube feeding and sometimes parenteral nutrition if alimentary function is disturbed. During anaesthesia, hypermetabolism is reflected in the need for increased alveolar ventilation.

Clinical pharmacology in burns

1 Aminoglycoside losses are increased, so increased doses required for adequate blood levels.
2 Cimetidine losses are increased, partly due to decreased protein binding from hypoproteinaemia.
3 Benzodiazepines (normally highly protein bound) have more free drug available and may be initially more potent. They are, however, distributed into a larger volume than usual.
4 Suxamethonium causes hyperkalaemia due to increased numbers of extra-junctional receptors.

5 Resistance to non-depolarizing relaxants, ED_{95} is doubled (peak effect 2 weeks after burn), possibly due to increased number of neuromuscular junction receptors.

DROWNING

About 700 fatalities from drowning occur in the UK every year, about a quarter in the sea. There are pathophysiological differences between fresh- and salt-water drowning, although these are largely of academic interest since survivors who reach hospital need similar therapeutic measures in both situations.

Fresh water

Due to the difference in osmotic pressure, water passes rapidly from the lungs to the general circulation. There may be a 50% increase in circulatory volume within 3 min. This results in haemolysis, and ventricular fibrillation, resistant to treatment, occurs at an early stage. The heart is submitted to hypoxia, over-filling, potassium excess and sodium deficit. The clinical features can be demonstrated readily in animals, but there is evidence that the haemodilution is much less in humans, and it is possible that some other factor may be operative. The prognosis is poor.

Salt water

The osmotic effect is exerted in the opposite direction. Fluid passes out from the circulation into the alveoli to produce pulmonary oedema. In practice, fresh and salt water drowning are clinically very similar.

Vagal inhibition

Death from vagal inhibition can occur without entrance of fluid into the lungs. A precordial thump may be successful in this case, and atropine is given as soon as possible.

Other effects

Drowning is likely to be complicated by:

1 hypothermia (*see also* Chapter 2.8);
2 acute pulmonary oedema;
3 respiratory distress syndrome;

4 pulmonary infection;
5 cerebral oedema (not a common complication).

Monitoring

Glasgow Coma Score, temperature, blood pressure, pulse oximetry, blood gases, chest auscultation, CVP, and possibly ICP and cerebral perfusion pressure.

Treatment

Speed is vital. Treatment should consist of:

1 very quick efforts to clear the mouth and pharynx of debris and efforts to drain the lungs in salt water drowning;
2 artificial ventilation, if possible while the subject is still in the water;
3 external cardiac massage;
4 administration of pure O_2 as soon as practicable and transfer to hospital;
5 treatment of hypothermia, if present, by rapid rewarming in water at 37°C and intravenous glucose and steroid administration;
6 tracheal intubation and IPPV when possible;
7 Chest X-ray, blood and urine analysis, blood gas estimation and intensive therapy as indicated;
8 One litre of human albumin solution infused rapidly intravenously.

RESUSCITATION

Cardiac arrest

See The 1997 ILCOR Advisory statements[31] and Resuscitation Guidelines, European Resuscitation Council 1998.[32]

Coronary artery disease is the commonest cause of arrest in adults (while trauma is the commonest cause of death in the first four decades of life).

Causes of cardiac arrest

1 *Cardiac disease:*
   (a) myocardial ischaemia;
   (b) secondary to hypoxia – prognosis is very poor;
   (c) pulmonary (and air) embolism – prognosis is very poor;
   (d) in fixed-output states (tight valvular stenosis, constrictive pericarditis, severe pulmonary hypertension, cardiac tamponade) prognosis is very poor;
   (e) cardiomyopathies – prognosis is very poor;
   (f) acute myocarditis – prognosis is very poor;

    (g) other rare conditions, e.g. atrial myxoma or ball-valve thrombus with change of posture; pneumopericardium[33]; massive G-forces, as in motor racing accidents.

2 *Haemorrhage.*
3 *Hypotension from any cause.*
4 *Hypoxia*, e.g. due to pneumothorax.
5 *Electrocution* (a danger to the rescuer!).
6 *Drowning.*
7 *Hyperkalaemia, hypokalaemia, hypercalcaemia.*
8 *Effect of drugs:*
    (a) direct myocardial depression (specific impairment of contraction of the muscle fibres);
    (b) vagotonic effect (e.g. additive bradycardic effect of opioids and beta-blockers);
    (c) sympathetic stimulation;
    (d) increased excitability of ventricular muscle (e.g. tricyclic drug overdose).
9 *Hypercapnia.* Results in:
    (a) increase of circulating catecholamines;
    (b) increase of serum potassium level;
    (c) prolongation of the period of asystole induced by vagal stimulation.
In a healthy patient, moderate hypercapnia is well tolerated in the absence of hypoxia. (*See* the 4 Hs and 4 Ts of electromechanical dissociation (EMD) below.)
10 *Sudden infant death syndrome* (SIDS).
11 *Hypothermia. See* Chapter 2.8.
12 *Cardiac catheterization.*
13 *Vagal reflexes.* Sources of stimuli which may provoke bradycardia or asystole include the rectum, uterus and cervix, glottis, bronchial tree, bladder and urethra, mesentery, the carotid sinus, heart, biliary tract, traction on extraocular muscles (especially the medial rectus) and testis. Atropine may prevent them.
14 *Circulating catecholamines.* A rise in the blood catecholamine level occurs with injection of adrenaline, anxiety, adrenal tumours and after haemorrhage. Fenfluramine and ecstasy act as catecholamines.

Signs of cardiac arrest

1 Immediate loss of pulse.
2 Unconsciousness in about 15 s.
3 Respiratory arrest, which may be preceded by the last gasps, 1–3 min after the cardiac arrest.
4 The pupils dilate (also caused by adrenaline and atropine).
5 Absence of heart sounds on auscultation.
6 General appearance of the patient. Cyanosis, pallor and loss of capillary refill.
7 On ophthalmoscopy the veins of the fundus show segmentation of the blood columns.

The ECG is important in diagnosis and in the differential diagnosis between ventricular fibrillation (VF) and non-VF (asystole and EMD). But even a normal ECG can exist in EMD.

The effects of cardiac arrest on the brain

1 Unconsciousness.
2 Electroencephalogram changes occur in 4 s and the tracing is flat within 20–30 s.
3 Histological changes: diffuse neuronal damage is not restricted to any particular vascular territory of the brain. Petechial haemorrhages also occur. Brain damage may be diffuse or focal. The mildest structural damage is selective neuronal necrosis, but with more severe hypoxia neuroglial cells are affected also and areas of infarction may arise. (*See* also McDowall D. G. *Br. J. Anaesth.* 1985, **57**, 1.)

Treatment of cardiac arrest

BASIC LIFE SUPPORT

D for danger, R for response, A for airway, B for breathing, C for circulation ('DRABC').

1 Ensure safety of rescuer and victim.
2 Check the victim and assess for a response.
3 (a) If he or she responds by answering or moving: leave the victim in the position in which you find him or her (provided there is no further danger). Check his or her condition and get help if needed. Reassess regularly. Keep him or her warm.
  (b) If the victim does not respond: shout (or call by mobile phone) for help, remove any obvious foreign bodies in the mouth, and open the *airway* by extending the neck (avoid this if neck injury is suspected in trauma cases) and lifting the jaw forward. Look, listen and feel for *breathing*. If the victim is breathing, turn him or her into the recovery position (not if a neck injury is suspected). If he or she is not breathing, send someone for help, and start 'rescue breathing', e.g. mouth to mouth, or mouth to mask. Give two effective breaths.

Preliminaries to advanced cardiac life support (ACLS)

1 Check the patient is not connected to a live electrical circuit.
2 Make the diagnosis (*see above*).
3 Ascertain how long it has existed.
4 Shout for help.
5 Initiate treatment; loosen tight clothing, proceed with ACLS:

Movements of the chest should be observed with each breath to check that adequate expansion of the lungs has occurred. Assess the victim for signs of a *circulation* by checking for signs of life (movement, swallowing, breathing), and check for the carotid pulse. If no pulse is felt, start external chest compressions over the lower third of the sternum, 100 per minute; 15 compressions and 2 breaths, if alone; 5 compressions to one breath with second rescuer; the chest is compressed 4–5 cm.

ADVANCED LIFE SUPPORT

While basic life support (BLS) continues, intravenous access is set up. The patient is intubated, ventilated with 100% O_2 and monitored with ECG; if VF, defibrillation is carried out to restore rhythm, 200 J; if this fails, 200; and then if that fails, 360 J. Care is needed to disconnect the O_2 during defibrillation. Give shocks in batches of three, not removing the paddles from the chest wall and monitoring through the paddles. If a perfusing rhythm is obtained, remove paddles and check carotid pulse.

Drugs are required – intravenous adrenaline 1 mg is given every 3 min during resuscitation.

In asystole, which carries a worse prognosis, adrenaline is given every 3 min and BLS continued.

Correction of any of the following items is made: (5 Hs and 5 Ts) Hypoxia, Hypovolaemia, Hypo/hyperkalaemia, Hypothermia; Tension pneumothorax; cardiac Tamponade; Toxic/therapeutic disturbances; Thromboemboli. Alkalizing and/or antiarrhythmic agents may be needed.

External chest compression should be abandoned when it becomes clear that a perfusing rhythm cannot be obtained, or when the general condition of the patient including existence of pre-existing pathology does not justify its continuance. External chest compression may rarely cause visceral injuries, especially if not performed properly.

After restoration of rhythm, adrenaline may be used as an inotrope. Coronary perfusion is improved. The positive inotropic effect of adrenaline or isoprenaline infusion is opposed by metabolic acidosis and enhanced by alkalosis.

If congestive cardiac failure is present, isoprenaline is preferred. Acting almost exclusively on the β_1 receptors it is a potent cardiac stimulant. Ephedrine, 10 mg i.v., or dopamine[34] infusion (1–10 mg/kg/min), are also highly effective. Low-dose dopamine also improves renal blood flow and diuresis. Facilities for external pacing should be available. Hydrocortisone, 1 g i.v., may also have a pressor effect especially in arrest due to Addison's disease.

Calcium chloride 1 g by slow i.v. injection is also useful, but perivenous injection is very caustic.

Repeated defibrillation shocks may cause myocardial (epicardial) damage.

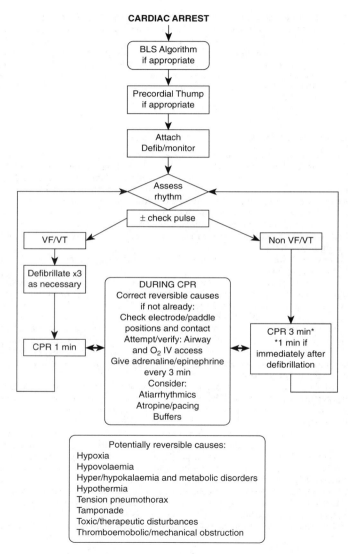

CARDIAC ARREST

BLS Algorithm
if appropriate

Precordial Thump
if appropriate

Attach
Defib/monitor

Assess
rhythm

± check pulse

VF/VT

Non VF/VT

Defibrillate x3
as necessary

DURING CPR
Correct reversible causes
if not already:
Check electrode/paddle
positions and contact
Attempt/verify: Airway
and O₂ IV access
Give adrenaline/epinephrine
every 3 min
Consider:
Atiarrhythmics
Atropine/pacing
Buffers

CPR 1 min

CPR 3 min*
*1 min if
immediately after
defibrillation

Potentially reversible causes:
Hypoxia
Hypovolaemia
Hyper/hypokalaemia and metabolic disorders
Hypothermia
Tension pneumothorax
Tamponade
Toxic/therapeutic disturbances
Thromboemobolic/mechanical obstruction

Figure 4.4.1 ALS algorithm (used by kind permission © ERC 1998)[32]

Prognosis after cardiac arrest

Factors improving outcome are as follows:

1 Witnessed arrest.

2 Ventricular fibrillation rhythm rather than asystole. (Physical cardiac damage and long-acting drug-induced arrest have worse prognosis.)

3 Early commencement of effective resuscitation (<2.5min).

4 Early defibrillation with good cardiac output.

5 Absence of need for inotropic drugs during transportation.

6 Spontaneous eye movements were present; pupil light reflex was present; corneal reflex was present.

7 Normothermia.

8 Immediate postresuscitation percutaneous coronary angioplasy following angiography (Spaulding E. M. et al. *N. Engl. J. Med.* 1997, **336**, 1629–1633).

9 Rapid return of end-tidal CO_2 (Levine R. L., Wayne M. A. and Miller C. C. *N. Engl. J. Med.* 1997, **337**, 301–306).

10 Normal or normalized blood glucose (Mullner M. et al. *J. Cereb. Blood Flow Metab.* 1997, **17**, 430–436).

11 Age of patient – the oldest and youngest have worse prognosis.

12 Absence of hypovolaemia.

Biochemical changes during cardiac arrest

These occur as a result of tissue hypoxia, hypercarbia and lactic acidosis. Even with external chest compression, the flow of blood (up to 1500 ml/min) is not sufficient to perfuse all the tissues normally. As a result of tissue hypoxia, there is anaerobic metabolism, hyperglycaemia (up to 20 mmol/l.), movement of water and sodium into the cells and of potassium ions out into extracellular fluid. This results in a rise in PCV and in plasma proteins, while plasma potassium concentration can reach levels as high as 7 mmol/l in a few minutes.

Even in the best situations, the successful resuscitation rate in only 40%.

After resuscitation, prevention of secondary cerebral injury requires full oxygenation with cerebral perfusion pressure > 70 mmHg. Hyperpyrexia must be controlled. The head is slightly elevated and IPPV used to maintain $PaCO_2$ at 3.5–4 kPa (25–28 mmHg).

MANAGEMENT OF CARDIAC ARREST IN INFANTS AND CHILDREN[35]

The immediate action is artificial ventilation and oxygenation, due to the following.

1 Hypoxia is the commonest cause of paediatric cardiac arrest.
2 Hypoxia develops faster because of high metabolic rate.
3 There is usually a longer period of hypoxia.
4 Hypoxic brain damage carries a worse prognosis.
5 Hypothermia carries a worse prognosis.
6 External chest compression is done by depression of sternum one-third to one-half of the resting chest diameter, with two to three fingers at 100/min. Five compressions to one breath.

As in adults, the response of the pupils is one guide to progress or lack of it, unless adrenaline has been given.

Uncontrollable rise of ICP after paediatric arrest has been treated by dihydroergotamine.[36]

Basic life support

1 Safe approach: Ensure safety of rescuer and victim (e.g. still attached to live electricity).
2 Stimulate the victim and see if he or she responds.
3 Shout for help.
4 (a) If the victim responds by answering or moving: leave the victim in the position in which you found him or her (provided he or she is not in further danger); check the victim's condition and get help if needed. Reassess regularly.
  (b) If the victim does not respond, remove any foreign bodies in the mouth, and open the airway by extending the neck (avoid this if neck injury is suspected) and holding the jaw forwards.
  Look, listen and feel for breathing. If the victim is breathing, turn him or her into the recovery position. If the victim is not breathing, send someone for help, turn him or her supine and start 'rescue breathing', mouth to mouth, five breaths.

Movements of the chest should be observed to check that adequate expansion of the lungs has occurred (as if the child were taking a deep breath).

Assess the victim for signs of a circulation by checking signs of life (movement, swallowing, breathing), and carotid pulse (brachial pulse in infant). If no pulse is felt, start chest compressions, 100/min (five compressions to one breath) lower third of sternum, compression one-third of resting diameter of chest.

Advanced life support

1 Intravenous access is gained.
2 Monitor cardiac rhythm (VF or non-VF).
3 Intubate and ventilate with 100% O_2. A laryngeal mask may be used if intubation fails.
4 Adrenaline 10 μg/kg is given.
5 For VF (rare in children) give precordial thump and defibrillate 2 J/kg two times; defibrillate 4 J/kg one time.
6 Adrenaline 10 μg/kg is given.
7 One more minute CPR; five compressions to one breath.
8 Defibrillate 4 J/kg three times (disconnecting staff and O_2 from the patient).
9 Correct hypothermia/hypovolaemia/electrolytes/acidosis.
10 Repeat adrenaline 100 μg/kg every 3 min.
11 Continue ventilation and cardiac massage.

After three loops without success, check intravenous access, intubation and paddle position. Consider correcting reversible causes: Hypoxia, Hypovolaemia, Hypokalaemia, hyperkalaemia, Hypothermia (5 Hs); Tension pneumothorax; Tamponade; Toxic/therapeutic disturbances; Thromboembolism (5 Ts). Alkalizing and/or antiarrhythmic agents may be needed.

For asystole

1 Adrenaline 10 μg/kg i.v. is given.
2 Three minutes CPR; five compressions to one breath.
3 Adrenaline 100 μg/kg may be given every 3 min.
4 Loop to CPR, checking the 5 Hs and 5 Ts as above.

Pulseless electrical activity (electromechanical dissociation)

Adrenaline 100 μg/kg may be given intravenously and possible causes are corrected as above.

When to stop resuscitation

It is very easy to start; not so easy knowing when to stop!

1 When it is discovered that the patient was about to die anyway, e.g. of terminal cancer, terminal senile dementia.
2 When the patient had requested not to be resuscitated ('Living will').
3 When a 'Do not attempt resuscitation' (DNAR) note has been written in the notes.
4 When chest compression does not produce any palpable pulse in spite of resuscitation.
5 After prolonged EMD, when the 5 Hs and 5 Ts have been checked.
6 Other completely hopeless situations, e.g. in obvious catastrophic head injury.

REFERENCES

1 Ramrakha P. S. and Moore K. P. *Oxford Handbook of Acute Medicine.* Oxford University Press, Oxford, 1998.
2 Crosby E. T. and Lui A. *Can. J. Anaesth.* 1990, **37,** 77.
3 Safar P. J. *Wld. Assoc. Emerg. Disaster Med.* 1986, **1–4,** 34–47.
4 Schierhout G. and Roberts I. *Br. Med. J.* 1998, **316,** 961–964.
5 Hall L. W., Kellagher R. E. B. and Fleet K. J. *Anaesthesia* 1986, **41,** 516–518.
6 Restall J. and Knight R. J. In Baskett P. J. F. and Weller R. M. *Medicine for Disasters.* Butterworth, Oxford, 1988.
7 Skinner D., Swain A., Perton D. and Robertson C. *Cambridge Textbook of Accident and Emergency Medicine.* Cambridge University Press, Cambridge, 1997; Illingworth K. and Simpson K. *Anaesthesia and Analgesia in Emergency Medicine,* Oxford University Press 1998, Oxford.
8 Colvin M. P., Healy M. T. and Samra G. S. *J. R. Soc. Med.* 1998, **91,** 26–29.
9 Chan K. H. et al. *Neurosurgery* 1993, **32,** 547–553.
10 Winchell R. J. and Hoyt D. B. *Arch. Surg.* 1997, **132,** 592–597.
11 Fabian T. C. and Richardson J. D. *J. Trauma, Injury, Infection and Critical Care* 1997, **42,** 374–380; Conn A.G. and Johnston A. J. *Anaesthesia* 1998, **53,** 612–613.
12 Yates D. W. et al, *J. R. Soc. Med.* 1987, **80,** 486–489.
13 Seeberger M. D. et al. *Anesth. Analg.* 1997, **85,** 1252–1257.
14 Shoemaker W. C. et al. *Chest* 1988, **94,** 1176–1186; Boyd O., Grounds R. M. and Bennett E. D. *J. Am. Med. Assoc.* 1993, **270,** 2699–2707.
15 McLaughlan C. A. J. *Br. Med. J.* 1990, **301,** 1145–1149.
16 Lee A. et al. *Anaesthesia* 1991, **45,** 1028–1031.
17 Cohn S. M. *J. Trauma* 1997, **42,** 973–979.
18 Conn A. G. and Johnston A. J. *Anaesthesia* 1998, **53,** 612–613.
19 Mackenzie S. J. et al. *Anaesthesia* 1991, **45,** 1043–1045.
20 Abramson M. S. et al. *N. Engl. J. Med.* 1986, **314,** 397–403.
21 *Guidelines For Transport Of The Critically Ill Patient,* Intensive Care Society, Tavistock Square, London, 1998.
22 Crosby E. T. and Lui A. *Can. J. Anaesth.* 1990, **37,** 77.
23 Barker I. et al. *Anaesthesia* 1985, **40,** 533.
24 Fabian T. C. et al. *Crit. Care Med.* 1990, **18,** 42.
25 Zenker F. A. *Beitrage zur Anatomie der Lungen.* G. Shonfeld's Buchhandlung, Dresden, 1862.
26 Von Bergmann E. *Berl. Med. Wochensch.* 1873, **10,** 385.
27 Hagley S. R. *Anaesth. Intensive Care* 1983, **11,** 162.
28 Boyd O., Grounds R. M. and Bennett E. D. *J. Am. Med. Assoc.* 1993, **270,** 2699–2707.
29 Shikuma L. R. et al. *Crit. Care Med.* 1990, **18,** 37.
30 Williams J. G. et al. *Br. Med. J.* 1983, **286,** 775.
31 The ILCOR Advisory Statements; Reports of Working Groups on Life Support, C. Robertson, P. Steen, J. Adgey, L. Bossaert, P. Carli,

A. Handley, D. Chamberlain, W. Dick, L. Ekstrom, S. Hapnes, S. Holmberg, R. Juchems, F. Kette, R. Koster, F. DeLatorre, K. Linder, N. Perales. The 1998 European Resuscitation Council Guidelines for adult advanced life support. *Resuscitation* 1997, **34**, 97–128.

32 The ILCOR Advisory Statements; Reports of Working Groups on Life Support, C. Robertson, P. Steen, J. Adgey, L. Bossaert, P. Carli, A. Handley, D. Chamberlain, W. Dick, L. Ekstrom, S. Hapnes, S. Holmberg, R. Juchems, F. Kette, R. Koster, F. DeLatorre, K. Linder, N. Perales. The 1998 European Resuscitation Council Guidelines for adult advanced life support. *Resuscitation* 1998, **37**, 81–90.

33 Djaiani G. and Major E. *Anaesthesia* 1998, **53**, 580–816; Rothwell P. M., Slattery J. and Warlow C. P. *Br. Med. J.* 1997, **315**, 1571–1577; *Eur. J. Anaesth.* 1998 **(Suppl.)** 51–52.

34 Thompson B. T. and Cockrill B. A. *Lancet* 1994, **344**, 7–8; Juste R. et al. *Intensive Care Med.* 1997, **23 (Suppl. 2),** S80.

35 *The 1997 Resuscitation Guidelines*, Resuscitation Council (UK), 1997.

36 Orliaguet G. A. et al. *Anesth. Analg.* 1997, **85**, 1218–1220.

Anaesthesia in abnormal environments

ABNORMAL AMBIENT PRESSURE

Low pressures – high altitude

Still measured in feet by pilots, but in metres by mountaineers. Barometric pressure (pb) decreases exponentially with altitude, halving every 18 000 ft (5.5 km). Temperature decreases linearly at 2°C per 1000 ft up to 40 000 ft, where it is minus 60°C. In a pressurized jet plane flying at 40 000 ft (12.2 km), or in Concorde up to 60 000 ft (18.3 km), passengers are in effect at about 5000–8000 ft (1.5–2.4 km). Unpressurized aircraft do not fly above 12 000 ft (3.7 km). *See* Table 4.5.1.

Problems of anaesthesia at high altitude

Well over 10 million people live at altitudes over 3000 m, and some hospitals in the Andes are above 5000 m. It is necessary to remember that partial pressure of anaesthetic gases and vapours, rather than concentration, determines their potency.

1 *Hypoxia*. Inspired and arterial PO_2 are low. High concentrations of O_2 (at least 40%) should be given both during and after anaesthesia. *Venturi oxygen masks* deliver the correct concentration at altitude, as the increased flow through the O_2 flowmeter (*see* 4 below) offsets the error that would otherwise occur. The PO_2 will of course be less.

2 *Nitrous oxide* is therefore limited to 60%, and the partial pressure of even this concentration decreases as pb decreases. Since its minimal alveolar concentration (MAC) is over 100% at sea level it is of little use as an anaesthetic at 1500 m and of no value whatsoever at 3000 m.

3 *Cylinder pressure gauges* are reliable as the pressures involved are so high compared with ambient.

4 *Flowmeters* read low at altitude because of the low gas density, especially at higher flows, when flow is turbulent around the bobbin. The error is about

20% at 3000 m. It should affect all gases to the same extent, but this may not be true at lower flows, where the laminar flow around the bobbin depends on the viscosity. Analysis of FIO_2 is essential.

5 *Vaporizers.* Since SVP of a vapour does not change with pb (but only with temperature), the amount (and hence partial pressure) of anaesthetic delivered at a given dial setting is the same whatever the altitude. However, its concentration will increase as pb decreases. Any changes in the splitting ratio are slight. So the clinical effect that can be expected from a given dial setting is the same at all ambient pressures.

6 *Gas and vapour analysers.* These all measure partial pressure, but often present the result as per cent concentration, by assuming pb is that of sea level. Thus, the true concentration will be underestimated at altitude.

7 *Low temperatures* are associated with altitude.

8 *Pathophysiology* of both the unacclimatized and acclimatized resident at high altitude. Changes include hyperventilation, respiratory alkalosis which gradually becomes compensated, polycythaemia, pulmonary hypertension, fluid retention, pulmonary or cerebral oedema. Acute pulmonary oedema requires descent to lower levels and intermittent positive-pressure ventilation (IPPV) if possible. Acetazolamide is often taken as prophylaxis against mountain sickness.

9 *Anaesthesia.* The hypoxic respiratory drive is important. Sensitivity to opiates may occur. There is a higher incidence of spinal headache. Other regional techniques are satisfactory.

High pressures – diving

Pressure increases linearly with depth, 1 atmosphere for each 10 m of sea water. Divers may fall ill or be injured when saturation diving, i.e. working for several days under pressures as high as 20–30 atmospheres absolute (ATA), which are those on the continental shelf 200–300 m deep. Doctors require training to work under these conditions. Surgery would take place in a large compression chamber back at base, with the medical team also at high pressure.

Problems of anaesthesia at depth (e.g. in a naval decompression chamber)

Many factors should be considered, including the following.

1 *Air-breathing over 50 m deep may cause nitrogen narcosis:* 15% loss of cognitive skills and 5% loss of manual dexterity at 6 ATA. Overcome by the use of oxygen–helium mixtures.

2 *Oxygen toxicity:* acute cerebral toxicity may cause convulsions if PIO_2 exceeds 2 ATA; chronic pulmonary O_2 toxicity may occur in saturation diving when the PIO_2 should not exceed $\frac{1}{2}$ ATA. This limits the FIO_2 to less than 2% at 25 ATA.

Table 4.5.1 Barometric pressure pb and moist inspired oxygen pressure P_IO_2 (mmHg), and the inspired O_2 concentration needed to make P_IO_2 its sea-level value of 150 mmHg (20 kPa), for various altitudes and depths. Note that alveolar water vapour tension is always 47 mmHg. In practice, pb on Everest's summit is slightly higher, and has been measured at 253 mmHg.[1] HPNS = high-pressure nervous syndrome.

Altitude		PB	P_IO_2	F_IO_2 needed for P_IO_2 to be 150 mmHg	
feet	km	mmHg	mmHg		
63 000	19.2	47	0	–	Blood boils
40 000	12.2	141	20	–	
29 028	8.848	236	40	79%	Everest summit
20 000	6.1	349	63	50%	May lose consciousness without O_2
18 000	5.5	380	70	45%	Barometric pressure halved
10 000	3.0	523	100	32%	
6 000	1.8	609	118	27%	
0	0	760	150	21%	
Depth (metres)					
10		1520	309	10%	
50		4 560	945	3.3%	Lower limit of air diving
200		15 960	–	0.9%	
500		38 760	–	0.4%	HPNS precludes diving lower than this

3 *High-pressure nervous syndrome:* tremor, loss of fine movement control, disorientation. Occurs at about 500 m, but may be less especially if compression is rapid (over 1 m/min). Caused by direct effects on enzymes.
4 *Rapid gas compression:* raises its temperature, and helium's high thermal capacity has a big effect on body heat balance.
5 *Blood samples:* decompressed before analysis outside the chamber.
6 *Pressure reversal:* affects all general anaesthetics, with around 30% loss of potency at 31 ATA.
7 *Cuffs:* on tracheal tubes and Foley catheters should be filled with water, not air.
8 *Voice communication:* with helium-containing mixtures is difficult.
9 *Glass containers:* e.g. of drugs may implode on compression; opening them beforehand may render them unsterile.
10 *Bubbles* of gas appearing in any local analgesic solution injected into the body.

11 *Colonization of the skin of divers:* Gram-negative organisms, such as Proteus and Pseudomonas.

Possible techniques:

1 ketamine, the anaesthetic agent least affected by pressure reversal, or propofol infusion;
2 intravenous regional analgesia for limb injuries;
3 for major procedures, morphine 2–3 mg/kg with muscle relaxants and IPPV with air.

Inhalational agents are precluded because the chamber atmosphere is recycled. A small ventilator powered by gas, e.g. Penlon, is suitable.

Hyperbaric chambers have a place in the treatment of conditions unrelated to diving, especially CO poisoning, osteomyelitis, other refractory tissue infections, especially with anaerobes, and compartment syndrome.[2] Facilities are naturally limited, and patients who might benefit from hyperbaric O_2 should be discussed with the nearest unit.

ABNORMAL AMBIENT TEMPERATURE

Low temperatures

These may be encountered at altitude, at sea or in polar regions, particularly under field conditions. Mean skin temperature below 33°C causes discomfort and shivering. The patient must be kept warm, and techniques of local analgesia are often unsatisfactory. Some liquid N_2O may form in Entonox cylinders below minus 7°C (*see* Chapter 2.3).

Tropical conditions

Many drugs deteriorate if stored at too high temperatures, e.g. atracurium, suxamethonium. The filling ratio (weight of gas in a 'full' cylinder as a ratio of the weight of water that the cylinder is capable of holding) of N_2O and CO_2 cylinders is 0.75 in temperate climates, but 0.67 in the tropics, to prevent excessive pressure if ambient temperature rises. Tropical conditions do not prevent the use of open ether. Rubber articles are liable to perish. Dehydration is common, and requires generous intravenous replacement.

SITUATIONS OF UNUSUAL DIFFICULTY

Anaesthesia may have to be administered without the facilities of the modern general hospital:

1 following major disasters (earthquake, nuclear explosions, mining and other industrial accidents, transport accidents);
2 on board ships at sea;
3 during exploration of remote regions;
4 in underdeveloped countries;
5 in military surgery.

Major accident procedures

Hospitals should have major accident procedures and rehearse them regularly. Emergency boxes contain resuscitation equipment, lights, distinctive protective clothing, etc. Anaesthetic equipment may include a self-inflating bag (e.g. Ambu), face masks, tracheal tubes, laryngoscopes, drugs, etc. Infusion fluids in plastic containers, cannulae, giving sets and a manual pressure pump are also included. Boxes should be lightweight, able to be carried by one person and have clear labelling and an inventory.

Apparatus for field use

Apparatus for intravenous anaesthesia is easily carried. Medical gases are likely to be in short supply. Volatile agents may be vaporized in air, or perhaps O_2-enriched air. Draw-over apparatus is useful, and should be light and portable. Ether remains a valuable agent in such circumstances. Tracheal tubes may make anaesthesia safer. Where laryngoscopes are not available, simple equipment can be improvised[3] or various blind techniques used. A Venturi system for O_2 enrichment is economical. A portable container of 1.2 litres of liquid O_2 (equivalent to 1000 litres of gas, and weighing just 4.3 kg when full) can deliver up to 15 l/min or power gas-driven ventilators.[4]

Inhalation apparatus

1 *Open masks.* In the first 80 years of general anaesthesia, many millions of patients were managed satisfactorily this way, which cannot be discarded even today. Halothane can be used for induction with ether for maintenance. Atropine should be given beforehand.
2 *Epstein–Macintosh Oxford vaporizer (EMO).*[5] A draw-over ether vaporizer, and can be used with Oxford bellows for IPPV. Has a water jacket heat sink and is temperature and level-compensated. Holds 450 ml of ether.
3 *Oxford Miniature vaporizer.*[6] Delivers up to 3.5% halothane and was designed to smooth induction with ether. Has a sealed water jacket but is not temperature compensated. Holds 20 ml.
4 *Flagg can.*[7] Devised during World War I. The patient breathes to and fro through a can containing ether. Such a simple device may be improvised from available material, e.g. coffee jar, food tins, and control over vapour strength achieved by admitting air as a diluent.[8]

5 *Triservice anaesthetic apparatus (Penlon)*. Consists of a Laerdal self-inflating bag, valve and mask resuscitator connected to two Oxford Miniature vaporizers (originally for trichloroethylene and halothane, but may be used with enflurane or isoflurane) and an O_2 supplementation attachment. The vaporizers are modified by the addition of feet and their capacity increased to 50 ml. In its box the apparatus weighs 25 kg and is rugged enough to be dropped by parachute. Has been much used by the services and for disasters. Low concentrations of isoflurane may be supplemented with intravenous ketamine, midazolam and alfentanil.[9] Arrangements for preoxygenation have been described.[10]

Techniques in the field

Intravenous apparatus, induction agents, muscle relaxants and self-inflating bags are easily carried and may be used in conjunction with tracheal tubes and portable apparatus as described above. Field hospitals are established.[11] Techniques include the following:

1 Thiopentone, muscle relaxant, either ether from an EMO vaporizer or halothane from an Oxford Miniature vaporizer, intubation and IPPV with air (possibly with added O_2) using the Oxford inflating bellows.[12]
2 Ketamine, i.v. or i.m., may be useful in the rare accident case where access to the airway is difficult, and when the patient may be shocked. A suitable agent where evacuation to hospital is not available.
3 Entonox is valuable for treatment of trapped casualties. Properly administered it produces good analgesia without reduction of blood pressure or loss of consciousness.

Anaesthesia in developing countries

The greatest challenge to practitioners of Western anaesthesia is to see that the most relevant information is brought to all those who need it. Gifts of books and journals may be more welcome than outdated complex equipment. Great skills of improvisation are seen in the developing countries. The anaesthesia will depend largely on the facilities available. Regional techniques are widely used, with or without other anaesthesia.

Anaesthesia in the dark

Diminution of room lighting, or near-total darkness, may be requested during microsurgery, endoscopy and radiological procedures. The patient is then exposed to the hazards of unrecognized cyanosis, respiratory obstruction, exhaustion of gas cylinders, etc. Monitoring is at its most valuable. When lights have to be reduced, the anaesthetist should pay particular attention to the following points:

1 spot lighting must be on continuously for inspection of the patient;
2 that gas cylinders, particularly O_2, contain adequate reserves;
3 tracheal intubation may reduce the danger of airway obstruction;
4 full monitoring;
5 in some anaesthetic machines, vital parts may be fluorescent.

REFERENCES

1 West J. B. et al. *J. Appl. Physiol.* 1983, **54,** 1188.
2 *Anaesthesia* 1998, **53(S)**: Wattel F. et al. p. 63; Bakker D. G. p. 65; Andel H. et al. p. 68.
3 O'Donohoe B. P. et al. *Anaesthesia* 1988, **43,** 970.
4 Ramage C. M. H. et al. *Anaesthesia* 1991, **46,** 395.
5 Epstein H. B. and Macintosh R. R. *Anaesthesia* 1956, **11,** 83.
6 Parkhouse J. *Anaesthesia* 1966, **21,** 498.
7 Flagg P. J. *The Art of Anaesthesia*, 7th edn. Lippincott, Philadelphia, 1954.
8 Boulton T. B. *Anaesthesia* 1966, **21,** 513.
9 Restall J. et al. *Anaesthesia* 1990, **45,** 965.
10 Lowe D. M. and McFadzean W. *Br. J. Anaesth.* 1991, **66,** 196.
11 Adley R. et al. *Anaesthesia* 1992, **47,** 996.
12 Boulton T. B. *Anaesthesia* 1978, **33,** 769.

Section 5
REGIONAL TECHNIQUES

Local anaesthetic agents

GENERAL CONSIDERATIONS

Local anaesthetics cause reversible blockade of peripheral nerve conduction or inhibition of excitation at nerve endings with resultant loss of sensation in the appropriate area of the body.

Local analgesic drugs are water-soluble salts of lipid-soluble alkaloids. Each molecule is composed of an aromatic portion, intermediate chain and an amide portion. Procaine, chloroprocaine and amethocaine have ester linking the aromatic end of the molecule and the intermediate chain; lignocaine, prilocaine, mepivacaine, bupivacaine, ropivacaine and etidocaine have an amide group between the aromatic part of the molecule and the intermediate chain. Ester-linked drugs are degraded by hydrolysis and amides by oxidative dealkylation in the liver. Overall clearance rate is fastest with prilocaine, then lignocaine, mepivacaine and finally bupivacaine and ropivacaine. Anaphylactoid reactions are well documented in the case of ester-linked agents, but extremely rare when amide-linked drugs are administered.

With the exception of cocaine (a vasoconstrictor) and lignocaine (no effect on vessels), local analgesic drugs are vasodilators. Vasoconstricting agents such as adrenaline (epinephrine) may be added to local analgesics to delay absorption and also to prevent haematoma formation if a small local vein is damaged by the needle. Adrenaline and noradrenaline do not prolong the action of local analgesic solution applied topically. Most of the local analgesic drugs are available as hydrochlorides in modified Ringer's solution. Those containing adrenaline are often acid with a pH of 4 or 5, and contain a reducing agent sodium metabisulphite to prevent oxidation of the adrenaline. In addition, a small amount of preservative and fungicide may be added.

Theories of impulse conduction along nerve fibres

The nerve membrane consists of a bimolecular framework of phospholipid molecules associated with a globular protein mosaic. Non-specific channels, one permeant to sodium and the other to potassium, are thought to be controlled by gates which are voltage-dependent. Myelinated nerves are protected by the myelin sheath which acts as an insulator. The impulse propagation has been studied in the squid axon because of its great size compared with the mammalian fibre. There is a resting potential of -70 mV on the outside of the membrane, which rises to about -55 mV, the firing threshold, before it jumps up to $+40$ mV to form an action potential which constitutes a change of over 100 mV.

This is associated with movement of sodium ions inwards and potassium ions outwards, through their respective channels. The membrane becomes depolarized. During recovery, the ions reverse the direction of their movement across the cell membrane. Local analgesic agents may prevent depolarization and so may prevent conduction of impulses.

Impulse blockade

The local analgesic solution prevents depolarization of the nerve membrane. As the concentration increases, the height of the action potential is reduced, the firing threshold is elevated, the spread of impulse conduction is slowed and the refractory period lengthened. Finally, nerve conduction is completely blocked.

It is thought that local analgesic drugs exert their effect by bonding to the internal mouth of the sodium channel. It is likely that specific receptors exist to which molecules of local analgesic drug become attached. Expansion of the membrane also occurs during impulse blockade; this may be the cause of conduction block or may just be an associated phenomenon.

The weak nerve block of perineural opioids is of a conduction type (although opioid receptors have been demostrated in peripheral nerves), is short-lived, and is not reversed by naloxone. (*See* Arendt-Nielsen L. et al. *Acta Anaesth. Scand.* 1991, **35,** 24; Gissen A. J. et al. *Anesth. Analg.* 1987, **66,** 1272.)

Site of action

The site of action of local analgesic drugs is at the surface membrane of cells of excitable tissues. In a myelinated nerve the site of action is the node of Ranvier. Two or three adjacent nodes must be affected to prevent conduction; at least 6 mm and perhaps 10 mm of nerve fibre must be exposed to the local analgesic agent or else a blocked segment may be jumped.

Differential block

The minimum concentration of local drug necessary to cause block of a nerve fibre of given diameter is known as the Cm. The thicker the diameter of a nerve fibre the greater the Cm required. The $A\delta$ fibres have a Cm about half that of $A\alpha$ fibres; it is therefore possible to block pain sensation while leaving sensation to pressure or position intact. The Cm of preganglionic autonomic B fibres is similar to that of small A so that sympathetic blockade is equivalent to analgesia in spinal analgesia. In practice, the sequence of block is autonomic, sensory, and finally motor block according to fibre diameter. Local analgesics affect not only nerve fibres but all types of excitable tissue, including smooth and striated muscle, e.g. in the myocardium vessels etc., probably by interfering with the cation fluxes across the muscle-cell membranes (as in nerve tissue). In moderate doses there is inhibition of activity of ventricular ectopic foci in the heart. The membrane-stabilizing effect is shared by other drugs such as phenothiazines, antihistamines, many beta-blockers, barbiturates, some antihypertensive agents, e.g. guanethidine.

Uptake

Local analgesic drugs are lipid-soluble bases, which act by penetrating lipo-protein cell membranes in the non-ionized state. In order to make a suitable solution for injection, the non-ionized base has to be converted to the ionized state.

The blocking quality of a local analgesic drug depends on its:

1 potency;
2 latency (time between its injection and maximum effect) – this in turn depends on nerve diameter, local pH, diffusion rate and concentration of the local drug;
3 duration of action;
4 regression time (time between commencement and completion of pain appreciation).

Dissociation constants

The dissociation constant (pKa) is the pH at which a local analgesic drug is 50% ionized and 50% non-ionized (base). So local analgesic drugs with pKa values close to physiological pH tend to have a rapid time of onset. The degree of ionization of a molecule is important and the pKa is a measure of this. It may be calculated from the Henderson–Hasselbalch equation, $pH = pKa + log\ base/cation$. Most local analgesic agents are weak bases with pKa between 7 and 9, and are relatively insoluble in water. Examples of pKa are: lignocaine, 7.87; amethocaine, 8.50; bupivacaine, 7.74; procaine, 8.92. They are usually prepared for clinical use as the acid salt. The un-ionized form is lipid soluble and can spread through tissues and penetrate membranes; the cation is the active agent to produce the pharmacological effect. pH of local analgesic solution may be lowered by addition of adrenaline (epinephrine), sodium metabisulphite (antioxidant) and glucose. When the buffering effect of the tissue is low, local analgesic drugs may be less effective. This occurs in inflamed tissues. Mucous membranes also have minimal buffer reserve and this is one reason why higher concentrations of drugs are needed for topical analgesia.

Carbonated local analgesic solutions

Available in Canada and Germany. Carbonated lignocaine and prilocaine produce a shorter latent period and more intense blockade than the hydrochloride salts,[1] but trials of carbonated bupivacaine proved disappointing.[2]

For further information about impulse conduction and impulse blockade by local analgesic drugs, *see* Covino B. G. In Wildsmith J. A. W. and McClure J. H. (eds) *Conduction Blockade for Postoperative Analgesia.* Edward Arnold, London, 1991; also Lee J. A. et al. (eds) *Lumbar Puncture and Spinal Analgesia; Intradural and Extradural,* 5th edn. Churchill Livingstone, Edinburgh, 1985.

Biotransformation

Ester-linked drugs are hydrolysed in the plasma by plasma cholinesterase, the rate depending on substitution in the aromatic ring of the molecule. Half-life in plasma varies from less than 1 min (chloroprocaine) to 8 min (amethocaine) and is prolonged in the presence of atypical cholinesterase. Amide-linked drugs undergo biotransformation in the liver, the rate of clearance being dependent on hepatic blood flow and drug extraction by the liver. Hepatic blood flow may be altered in general anaesthesia and as a result of administering vasoactive drugs. Extraction by the liver may be diminished in conditions such as cirrhosis, congestive cardiac failure, hypothermia and the administration of cimetidine. Half-life is likely to vary between 1.5 and 3 h.

Toxicity

Toxic signs are not always related to dosage. A study of plasma concentration of local analgesic drugs suggests that higher levels are reached after lignocaine than after prilocaine in equal dosage. Addition of adrenaline (epinephrine) to the local infiltration reduces the plasma concentration of lignocaine but not of

---

The following factors influence local analgesic toxicity

Quantity of solution.

Concentration of drug.

Presence or absence of adrenaline.

Vascularity of site of injection.

Rate of absorption of drug .

Rate of destruction of drug.

Hypersensitivity of patient.

Age, physical status and weight of patient.

prilocaine. Higher plasma levels are found after intercostal block than after extradural injection. Plasma concentrations of local analgesic drugs correspond very poorly with the patient's body weight. The site of injection is far more important. There is no maximum safe dose for all procedures. Skeletal injuries, including dislocation of the shoulder joint have been caused by convulsions due to the toxicity of local analgesic agents.[3]

Central nervous system

Central stimulation followed by depression, restlessness, hysterical behaviour, vertigo, tremor, convulsions and respiratory failure. *Treatment* consists of artificial ventilation with O_2 or air and intravenous injection of suxamethonium or just sufficient thiopentone to control convulsions (10–150 mg). Diazepam may be useful. A rise in $PaCO_2$ increases tendency to convulsions, so treatment should include hyperventilation with O_2.

Cardiovascular system

Hypotension. Acute collapse – primary cardiac failure, feeble pulse and cardiovascular collapse, bradycardia, pallor, sweating and hypotension. This has followed moderate amounts given intravenously of etidocaine and bupivacaine.[4] This type of intoxication may be due to a rapid absorption of the drug.

Treatment: elevate legs; give O_2 by intermittent positive-pressure ventilation (IPPV); rapid intravenous infusion; raise blood pressure; cardiac massage if necessary. Resuscitation after the longer-acting drugs, bupivacaine and etidocaine, may be difficult and lengthy.[5] High-energy shock electrical defibrillation may be required.[6]

Respiratory depression

This may progress to apnoea from medullary depression or respiratory muscle paralysis. It may have delayed onset.

Allergic phenomena

Allergy reactions are rare; may take form of bronchospasm, urticaria or angioneurotic oedema. Well documented in association with the use of ester-linked agents, including contact dermatitis in personnel handling procaine. Cross-sensitivity can occur. Allergy to amide-linked agents is extremely rare but has been reported.[7] Injections of adrenaline, hydrocortisone and oxygen therapy by IPPV and intravenous colloid solutions may be necessary.

Reactions to vasoconstrictor drugs include pallor, anxiety, palpitations, tachycardia, hypertension and tachypnoea and may respond to alpha-blocker. Care should be taken in patients receiving monoamine oxidase inhibitors or tricyclic antidepressants.

Toxicity may occur as a result of simple overdosage, by inadvertent intravenous injection, or because of susceptibility of the patient to normal dosage. Injection with a moving needle, together with frequent aspiration testing, minimizes risk of intravenous injection. No preservatives such as phenol, chlorocresol or sodium sulphite should be used when any large volume of local analgesic solution is to be injected. Allergic reactions may be due to methylparaben, sometimes used in commercial preparations of local analgesic solutions as a stabilizing agent.[8]

Toxic signs are often due to intravenous injection.

There is evidence that local analgesic drugs may have cytotoxic effects, although harmful clinical consequences are difficult to find.[9]

Improving duration and quality of local analgesia

Addition of adrenaline, e.g. 1 : 200 000 to 1 : 500 000 solution. Free base is liberated quickly due to rapid buffering and liberation of CO_2 which diffuses across cell membranes. Thus, the analgesic base is brought closer to nerve tissue more rapidly and in higher concentration, resulting in a more widespread and more intensive block (*see* Table 5.1.1). The amount of free base available determines the rate of diffusion of the local analgesic solution. Adjusting the pH to about 7 (alkalinization) reduces the time of onset and the duration of analgesia. Substitution of the carbonated salts of local analgesic drugs for the hydrochloride, the pH of carbonated salts (6.5) is relatively higher than other acid salts so that speedy buffering occurs with liberation of free base and CO_2 which diffuses to lower the pH inside the nerve sheath (diffusion trapping).[10]

Premedication

Adequate premedication is essential for successful local analgesia in major surgery. The subject is set out in Chapter 5.3.

Methods of local analgesia

1 Simple topical application of local analgesic to the operative site, e.g. on to the ovaries at ovarian cystectomy or into the knee at meniscectomy under general anaesthetic, for effective postoperative analgesia. Intrapleural analgesia is a modification of this.
2 Infiltration analgesia[11] to abolish the pain due to surgical intervention and to ease pain associated with trauma and the injection of irritant drugs. The direct injection of drugs into the area to be incised and between bone ends in fractures.
3 Field block. The injection of a local analgesic so as to create a zone of analgesia around the operative field.

Table 5.1.1 Some dosages of local analgesics

Drug	Minimum effective concentration	Maximum dose for 70 kg adult when used 'plain'	Maximum dose for 70 kg adult when used with adrenaline 1 : 200 000
Bupivacaine	0.125%	150 mg (30 ml of 0.5%)	150 mg (30 ml of 0.5%)
Lignocaine	0.25%	200 mg (40 ml of 0.5%)	500 mg (100 ml of 0.5%)
Prilocaine	0.5%	400 mg (80 ml of 0.5%)	600 mg (120 ml of 0.5%)
Ropivacaine	0.25%	250 mg (50 ml of 0.5%)	not yet defined

In children, the above adult doses do not apply, but the dose can be calculated on a 'dose for weight' basis, e.g. the maximum dose for a 7-kg child would be one-tenth of the adult dose.

4 Nerve block (conduction anaesthesia). The injection of a solution of local analgesic drug near the nerve or nerves supplying the area to be operated on. The use of a peripheral nerve stimulator increases the accuracy of needle placement and the success of the block.
5 Refrigeration analgesia.
6 Intravenous local analgesia (Chapter 5.2).
7 Topical or surface analgesia.
8 Central neural blockade (Chapter 5.3).

PHARMACODYNAMICS AND PHARMACOKINETICS OF DRUGS USED IN LOCAL ANALGESIA

A molecule of local analgesic drug possesses an aromatic or lipophilic group and a hydrophilic group with a linking chain between them which may be an ester (COO–) or an amide (NH.CO–).

Ester-linked drugs

Cocaine (Benzoyl methylecgonine hydrochloride)[12]

A naturally occurring plant extract. A derivative of the nitrogenous base ecgonine and an ester of benzoic acid. Alkaloid isolated in 1855 and synthesized in 1924. First use in surgery (of the cornea) in 1884.

Easily decomposed by heat sterilization. Cocaine is soluble in water and alcohol. It is an excellent surface analgesic and vasoconstrictor, 4% being a suitable strength. It is often toxic when injected.[13] A dangerous drug of addiction. Duration of effect, 20–30 min. Solutions should be protected from the light. pKa 8.7.

PHARMACODYNAMICS

Central nervous system
Stimulated from above downwards. In the cortex, excitement and restlessness are caused and mental powers increased. There is euphoria, agitation, decreased sleep, anxiety, hyperexcitability, psychosis, paranoia, suicidal tendency, violence and confusion. In higher dosage, convulsions (prevented by diazepam and reduced by D1 antagonists)[14] are followed by apnoea and death associated with hyperthermia. Calcium-channel blockers increase toxicity.[15]

The sympathetic nervous system is stimulated. As cocaine is a powerful vasoconstrictor, adrenaline added to it is not only unnecessary but also increases the risks of cardiac dysrhythmia and ventricular fibrillation. The two drugs should not be used together.[16]

It inhibits monoamine oxidase. It is not destroyed by cholinesterase.

Cardiovascular system
Small doses increase the pulse rate, raise the blood pressure and potentiate the effects of adrenaline on capillaries (dilatation or constriction). Dysrhythmias may occur, but can be reversed by beta-blockade. Cutaneous vasoconstriction prevents heat loss. Hypertension and vasospasm may lead to vascular accidents.

Eye
Mydriasis, perhaps due to sympathetic stimulation; there is blanching of the conjunctiva from vasoconstriction, clouding of the corneal epithelium and, rarely, ulceration, together with excellent analgesia. Used as 1% solution for analgesia. Eserine counteracts the mydriatic effect of cocaine and atropine increases it. Now rarely used in ophthalmology.

TREATMENT OF OVERDOSE[17]

Diazepam 5–10 mg slowly, repeated to control fits and agitation (other antiepileptic drugs have been used successfully), and oxygenation. Active cooling and rehydration may also be needed.

PHARMACOKINETICS

Absorption from all mucous membranes, including the urethra and bladder. There is some evidence that stronger solutions are absorbed less readily than weaker solutions, owing to the increased vasoconstriction they produce.

In nose and throat surgery used in 1–20% solution. Can be employed usefully as a spray to produce ischaemia of the nose, e.g. before nasal intubation.

*Excretion:*cocaine is detoxicated in the liver, one metabolite being ecognine, a cental nervous system (CNS) stimulant. About 10% is excreted by the kidneys, unchanged.

A safe dose of cocaine for surface analgesia is 2 ml of 4% solution. It was for years used to overcome drowsiness due to chronic morphine addiction in the treatment of severe pain in terminal disease (e.g. in the Brompton cocktail).

Procaine hydrochloride

Para-amino-benzoyl-diethyl amino-ethanol hydrochloride. pKa 8.9. The standard local analgesic agent until the advent of lignocaine. First synthesized in 1899. Like amethocaine, it inhibits the bacteriostatic action of *p*-aminosalicylic acid and the sulphonamides. Should be stored in a cool place to retard hydrolysis.

For infiltration the strength used is 0.25–1%; for nerve block, 1–2%. Procaine 5.05% in water is iso-osmotic, with pH of 6.4. Hydrolysed by serum cholinesterase, diethyl amino-ethanol and *p*-aminobenzoic acid being formed. Biotransformation requires absorption into the bloodstream as neural tissue and cerebrospinal fluid lack esterases.

Analgesia lasts from 45 to 90 min when adrenaline (epinephrine) is added. Relatively non-toxic.

Procaine has been recommended as the agent of choice for patients with a history of malignant hyperpyrexia.[18] A concentration of 5% may be necessary for successful extradural block.

Procaine intravenously has been recommended for the treatment of malignant hyperpyrexia, in almost toxic doses.

Chloroprocaine hydrochloride

An ester of *p*-aminobenzoic acid. Was in use in the US since 1952. Quick onset of effect, but analgesia may disappear suddenly. Rapid hydrolysis makes it relatively non-toxic and it is not easily transferred across the placenta. Effect lasts about 45 min. Used as a 2 or 3% solution, pKa 8.7. Initial dose for obstetrical extradural block 8–10 ml, which can be followed by bupivacaine or ropivacaine. The most acid of local analgesic agents commonly used (3% solution has pH of 3.3). Paraplegia has been reported following its use, particularly after intradural injection for which it is not recommended. This may be due to sodium metabisulphite in the commercial solution.

Amethocaine hydrochloride

First synthesized in 1928. pKa 8.2. Solutions prepared under sterile conditions remain sterile and bactericidal. Like cocaine, it may cause cardiac asystole or ventricular fibrillation. Used for topical and corneal analgesia in 0.5% solution. The solution can be boiled once or twice without deterioration, but is rendered inactive by alkalis. It should be protected from light. For infiltration the usual strength is 1 : 2000 to 1 : 4000, preferably with adrenaline (epinephrine). Up to 200 ml of 1 : 2000 solution with adrenaline (epinephrine) can safely be used for infiltration analgesia. It is hydrolysed completely by serum cholinesterase but four times more slowly than is procaine. None is found in bile or urine. Used for intradural block.

The maximum dose is 100 mg or 1.5 mg/kg of body weight. Large doses are unwise and maximum for surface analgesia should be 8 ml of 0.5% solution in two or three divided doses with an interval of 5 min between each dose. A lozenge containing 60 mg amethocaine is available. Absorption from the bronchial tree, when analgesia for bronchoscopy is being induced, is almost as rapid as that following intravenous injection. A 4% gel (Ametop) is available for topical analgesia in children. Onset of cutaneous analgesia is rapid ($\sim$ 30 mins).

Amethocaine's effect lasts longer than that of procaine and lignocaine, roughly 1.5–3 h. Onset of analgesia slow. For intradural block, 0.5–1% solution may be used; for extradural block 0.25–0.5% with adrenaline (epinephrine). The addition of adrenaline greatly reduces its toxicity, toxic signs being similar in appearance and treatment to those of cocaine.

Oxybuprocaine

Available in Europe and Japan. Bradycardia may be a problem,[19] but unlikely when used for surface analgesia for tonometry (0.4% solution less irritant to the conjunctiva than amethocaine; duration 5 min).

Amide-linked drugs

Lignocaine hydrochloride

The most commonly used local analgesic agent in the UK today. A tertiary amide, synthesized in 1943 in Sweden.[20] First used by Gordh in 1948.[21] Very stable, not decomposed by boiling, acids or alkalis. The pKa is 7.86. Solutions of 0.25–0.5% for infiltration, with adrenaline (epinephrine) 1 : 250 000; 4% for topical analgesia, in surgery of throat, larynx, pharynx, etc. For nerve block 1.5–2% with adrenaline (epinephrine), and for extradural block 1.2–2% with adrenaline (epinephrine). For corneal analgesia 4%; this causes no mydriasis, vasoconstriction or cycloplegia. For urethral analgesia 1–2% in jelly and for tracheal tubes 5% as an ointment. Toxicity not great, but cardiovascular and central nervous symptoms of poisoning may occur. Can be toxic when ingested orally.

The clearance of lignocaine is reduced in the presence of propranolol, with increased risk of toxicity. As in the case of prilocaine, the metabolism of lignocaine can give rise to the formation of methaemoglobin. It is not a vasodilator nor does it interfere with the vasoconstrictive action of adrenaline (epinephrine). It has a cerebral effect, causing drowsiness and amnesia. It is metabolized by oxidases and amidases from microsomes in the liver, but this is retarded in chronic liver disease.[22] It is excreted renally, hastened when the urine is acid.

Duration of effect of 1% solution, 1 h; with adrenaline (epinephrine), 1.5–2 h. Has rapid onset. Has been given intravenously in 40-mg doses at 5-min intervals, to potentiate the analgesia of thiopentone–gas–O_2–relaxant combination, and also intramuscularly in 250-mg doses in 2% solution. Has been used in the treatment of status epilepticus, and due to its cell membrane-stabilizing effect on cardiac tissue for ventricular dysrhythmias, by intravenous injection. As lignocaine may facilitate the release of calcium from sarcoplasmic reticulum, it should not be used in patients susceptible to malignant hyperpyrexia. Its use in the treatment of cardiac infarction is not proven. While it controls the non-dangerous unifocal ectopics, it is far less successful in cases of multifocal ectopics. Suggested maximum safe dose of lignocaine for a 70-kg man; with adrenaline (epinephrine) – 500 mg, i.e. 7 mg/kg; without adrenaline (epinephrine) – 200 mg, i.e. 3 mg/kg body weight (*see* Table 5.1.1).

The carbonate of lignocaine (and prilocaine) has been investigated[23] and found to give greater speed of onset and intensity of both sensory and motor block, in comparison with the hydrochloride salt, especially in the L5 and S1 segments. On injection the CO_2 diffuses out of the drug, so lowering the tissue pH and increasing the concentration of the non-ionized base.[24]

Alkalinized lignocaine may have an even faster onset. Bicarbonate buffering of the solution to pH 7.4 reduces stinging on injection, especially important around the eyes.

Toxic effects of lignocaine are twitching, convulsions, apnoea and acute cardiac failure.

Mepivacaine

A tertiary amine; synthesized and first used in 1956. It is clinically comparable with lignocaine. It is resistant to acid and alkaline hydrolysis. The pKa is 7.8. Seventy per cent of the drug becomes protein bound (greater than in the case of lignocaine but less than with bupivacaine). Most of the drug is metabolized in the liver and some has been recovered from the urine (increased by acidification). Unlike lignocaine, it is not metabolized by neonates; eliminated via the kidneys. It is claimed to be a little less toxic than lignocaine while its local analgesic effects last rather longer. The subconvulsive dose in humans is 5 mg/kg. When injected into the extradural space of patients in labour it passes rather rapidly into the fetal circulation where it may cause harm. It would appear to have few advantages over lignocaine. A dose of 400 mg should not be exceeded (about 5 mg/kg body weight). For extradural analgesia 15 ml of 2% or 20 ml of 1.5% solution; for intradural block 1–2 ml of 'heavy' 4% solution. Has antidysrhythmic properties. Onset may be speeded by alkalinization. (*See* Tetzlaff J. E. et al. *Reg. Anaesth.* 1990, **15**, 242.)

Bupivacaine

This amide-type local analgesic drug was synthesized 1957,[25] and used clinically in 1963.[26] The base is not very soluble but the hydrochloride readily dissolves in water. The pKa is 8.2. It is very stable both to repeated auto-claving and to acids and alkalis, but solutions containing adrenaline (epi-nephrine) should not be autoclaved more than twice. It is reputed to be four times as potent as both mepivacaine and lignocaine, so that a 0.5% solu-tion is roughly equivalent to 2% lignocaine. More cardiotoxic than lignocaine and this is made worse by hypoxia, hypercapnia and by pregnancy.[27] It causes more sensory than motor block. It is not recommended for intravenous regio-nal analgesia as leakage past the tourniquet into the bloodstream may cause toxic or even fatal complications. Duration of effect is between 5 and 16 h, one of the longest acting local analgesics known. This may be more related to binding to nerve tissue than to its overall retention in the body. Duration of action of a local analgesic drug correlates with binding to plasma lipopro-teins. There are two major binding proteins in serum; albumin and $\alpha - 1$ acid glycoprotein the latter of which is absent in the fetus. The duration may be prolonged by mixing the drug with dextran.

A small percentage of a given dose of bupivacaine is excreted unchanged in the urine. The remainder is metabolized in the liver. The N-dealkylated meta-bolite, pipecolyloxylidine, is found in the urine.[28] Maximal dose is 2 mg/kg body weight (25–30 ml of 0.5% solution) and the strength used is 0.125–0.75% with or without adrenaline (epinephrine) 1 : 200 000 or 1 : 400 000; adrenaline (epinephrine) does not greatly prolong its effect but reduces its toxicity (*see* Table 5.1.1). The carbonated form probably has few advantages over the hydrochloride salt. A plain solution of 0.5% has been much used for intradural block, either alone or made hyperbaric with dextrose, and for extradural analgesia. The pH of the 0.5% solution with adrenaline (epi-nephrine) is 3.5 and its density 0.997 g/ml at 37°C.

Etidocaine hydrochloride

A long-acting local analgesic drug related chemically to lignocaine; described in 1972. It is a stable compound and can be autoclaved up to five times with-out deterioration. The onset of action is rapid and the duration of action is long (comparable to bupivacaine or ropivacaine). It is very lipid soluble and almost completely protein bound; metabolic pathways not yet deter-mined. Probably retained in the body longer than other local analgesic drugs. Less toxic than bupivacaine but more toxic than lignocaine. Gives good motor block. pKa 7.7.

The drug has been used in extradural block but in obstetric analgesia has the disadvantage that motor block is readily produced. It has been used in 0.25 and 0.5% concentration. The former may give inadequate analgesia, the latter inappropriate motor block. Concentrations of up to 15% have been used with success in extradural block for surgical operations. Maximal dose: 4 mg/kg.

It is a useful topical analgesic, similar to bupivacaine or ropivacaine and stronger than lignocaine.

Prilocaine hydrochloride

A close relation of lignocaine to which it is clinically comparable. A secondary amide. First used clinically in 1959. A very stable compound, pharmacologically resembling lignocaine but less toxic. pKa 7.9. Whereas lignocaine is metabolized in the liver, prilocaine is metabolized also in the kidneys and lungs and more rapidly, partly by amidase. Little drug reaches the urine. This rapid metabolism may account for the methaemoglobinaemia sometimes seen after its use, if more than 600 mg are injected.[29] A maximal safe dose without adrenaline (epinephrine) is 400 mg; with adrenaline 600 mg.

Methaemoglobin is continuously formed during red-cell metabolism but normally does not exceed 1% of the haemoglobin at any one time. The cause of this oxidation of haemoglobin to methaemoglobin is not prilocaine itself but one of its degradation products. The degree of cyanosis due to methaemoglobin following prilocaine varies with erythrocyte methaemoglobin reductase[30] and usually disappears spontaneously in 24 h. It is of little clinical importance unless there is severe anaemia or circulatory impairment. The presence of cyanosis indicates that 1.5 g/dl or more of the haemoglobin is circulating as methaemoglobin. There is an associated shift of the O_2 dissociation curve of the remaining haemoglobin which hinders O_2 liberation at tissue level. Methaemoglobin crosses the placenta. A dose of 6 mg/kg or more is necessary to cause symptoms of hypoxia and is only likely to be seen after extradural block with repeated injections through a catheter. Congenital or acquired methaemoglobinaemia are probably contraindications to the use of the agent.

Treatment is by intravenous injection of 1% methylene blue, 1–2 mg/kg.

In extradural block the drug has been shown to give a slower onset and spread with a longer duration of effect and greater intensity than lignocaine, with less toxicity. The addition of adrenaline (epinephrine) prolongs the duration of effect less with prilocaine than with lignocaine (*see* Table 5.1.1).

It is most useful when high dosage and strong concentration are required of a local analgesic drug as when injection is into vascular areas, e.g. pudendal block and blocks about the face and neck, and for Bier's intravenous local analgesia in 0.5% solution, for which it is most suitable,[31] and for which it can be alkalinized.[32] For topical analgesia 10 ml of 4% solution is reasonable. A rough guide to dosage is to regard 4 mg/kg as reasonably safe.

Cinchocaine hydrochloride

Synthesized in 1925. Used for many years for spinal analgesia (intradural), and also for infiltration and surface analgesia. No longer commercially available in the UK.

Ropivacaine

An amide local anaesthetic; introduced as a safer alternative to bupivacaine. Chemically similar to bupivacaine with butyl group being replaced by propyl group. A single *s*-enantiomer drug rather than a racemic mixture (as is bupivacaine). Has differential effect on motor and sensory nerves at low concentrations. Most[33,34] but not all studies[35,36] have found that onset and duration of sensory block in epidural analgesia is similar to bupivacaine whilst motor block is slower in onset, shorter in duration and less intense with ropivacaine. Indeed, in one study 1.0% ropivacaine produced more reliable motor block than 0.5% bupivacaine.[36] In animal studies ropivacaine is less cardiodepressant, less arrhythmogenic and less toxic to the CNS than bupivacaine. These findings have been confirmed in a human volunteer study.[37]

PHARMACOKINETICS

The greater lipid solubility of bupivacaine compared with ropivacaine may explain the greater peak plasma concentration and the shorter half-life of ropivacaine.[34] Plasma clearance is similar for both drugs.[34] Peak blood levels of about 1 mg/l are found after injection of nearly 200 mg ropivacaine, unaffected by addition of adrenaline (epinephrine).[38] (See also Katz J. A. et al. *Anesth. Analg.* 1990, **70**, 16.)

Has been used in many techniques (labour, hip replacement and varicose vein surgery) with good results.[33-36]

A dose of 250 mg should not be exceeded (about 3.5 mg/kg body weight); up to 20 ml of 1.0 % solution for extradural analgesia and up to 10 ml/h of 0.2% solution as a continuous infusion (*see* Table 5.1.1).

Novel local anaesthetic drugs

Lecithin-coated microdroplets of methoxyflurane produce long-lasting local analgesia which is stable and localized.[39]

Autoclaving of local analgesic drugs

The commonly used agents are very stable chemical compounds. Ampoules of the hydrochloride salts of lignocaine, prilocaine, mepivacaine, bupivacaine or ropivacaine, etidocaine and procaine can all be autoclaved and thereafter show no chemical change on chromatographic analysis. They are not inactivated by γ radiation (25 Mrad).

DRUGS USED FOR VASOCONSTRICTION

Vasoconstrictor drugs have been used in local analgesia since Braun introduced adrenaline in 1902.[40] The adrenaline-induced contraction of the smooth muscle of vessel walls is modified to different degrees by the same molar concentrations of different local analgesic agents and by different concentrations of the same agent. The vascularity of the tissues receiving the injection is also a factor to be considered in estimating the optimal concentration in a given case. Vasoconstrictors are employed:

1 to retard absorption and reduce toxicity;
2 to prolong analgesic activity;
3 to produce ischaemia.

Adrenaline (epinephrine)

The tartrate, which is synthetic, is used for injection and contains a stabilizer, potassium metabitartrite, 0.1%, which increases the acidity of the solution. Many workers add their own adrenaline (epinephrine) to local analgesic solutions, preferring this to the commercially available mixtures, in extradural block. It is used less frequently in intradural block. The hydrochloride, which is of animal origin, is for topical application. For infiltration it is probably unnecessary to use a strength greater than 1 : 200 000, although dentists employ 1 : 80 000. Discoloration indicates decomposition; it can be autoclaved once but not repeatedly. For infiltration to produce ischaemia before incision the usual amount added is 1 mg to 250–500 ml of saline, giving a 1 : 250 000 to 1 : 500 000 solution. It is probably unwise to inject more than 0.5 mg at one time. The addition of adrenaline (epinephrine) reduces the uptake of lignocaine by the circulation more than that of the other amide-linked agents.

It is an α- and β-adrenergic stimulant and may produce pallor, tachycardia and syncope. It should be used with the greatest care if halothane is to be given, lest the combination should cause ventricular fibrillation. It has been suggested that, providing there is no hypercapnia or hypoxia, 10 ml of 1 : 100 000 adrenaline solution can be injected with safety in any 10-min period and not more than 30 ml/h. Vasoconstrictors help to produce a dry operative field. Adverse reactions to adrenaline (epinephrine) and noradrenaline are most likely to occur following intravascular injection, especially in patients with diabetes, heart disease, thyrotoxicosis, epilepsy and those receiving some halogenated anaesthetics or drug therapy involving tricyclic antidepressants or adrenergic neuron-blocking drugs.

Phenylephrine

Used for vasoconstriction during local analgesia, 0.25–0.5 ml of 1% solution added to each 100 ml of local analgesic solution. Causes no cerebral stimulation or tachycardia.

Noradrenaline (norepinephrine)

This can be used to produce local vasoconstriction but is less effective than adrenaline as it is a weaker α-receptor stimulant. Does not stimulate the α-receptors in muscle so causes no ischaemia there. It is oxidized in the body more rapidly by amine oxidase than is adrenaline. Tricyclic antidepressants increase its pressor effects.

Felypressin

This is 2-phenylalanine-8-lysine vasopressin and is a good local vasoconstrictor for use along with halothane, cyclopropane, trichloroethylene. It is a synthetic derivative of the octapeptide hormone, vasopressin, from the posterior pituitary. It causes constriction of all smooth muscle but has little oxytocic or antidiuretic effect. May result in coronary arterial constriction, but has little influence on cardiac rhythm. Unlike adrenaline (epinephrine) it does not alter cardiac rate or rhythm in dental surgery. Available with 3% prilocaine for dental use.

REFERENCES

1 Bromage P. R. et al. *Br. J. Anaesth.* 1967, **39,** 197.
2 Appleyard J. N. et al. *Br. J. Anaesth.* 1974, **46,** 530.
3 Pagden D. et al. *Anesth. Analg. (Cleve.)* 1986, **65,** 1063.
4 Editorial, *Anesthesiology* 1979, **51,** 285.
5 Albright G. A. *Anesthesiology* 1979, **51,** 285.
6 Scott D. B. *Br. J. Anaesth.* 1984, **56,** 437.
7 Brown D. T. et al. *Br. J. Anaesth.* 1981, **53,** 435; Fisher M. McD. and Pennington J. C. *Br. J. Anaesth.* 1982, **54,** 893; Reynolds F. *Br. J. Anaesth.* 1982, **54,** 901.
8 Nagel J. F. and Fuscaldo J. T. *J. Am. Med. Assoc.* 1977, **237,** 1594.
9 Sturrock J. E. and Nunn J. F. *Br. J. Anaesth.* 1979, **51,** 273.
10 Bromage P. R. et al. *Br. J. Anaesth.* 1967, **39,** 197; Catchlove R. F. H. *Br. J. Anaesth.* 1973, **45,** 471; Soderman M. and Duke P. C. *Can. Anaesth. Soc. J.* 1983, **30,** S71; Bokesch P. M. et al. *Anesth. Analg. (Cleve.)* 1987, **66,** 9.
11 Cook J. H. *Ann. R. Coll. Surg. Engl.* 1987, **69,** 3; Owen H. et al. *Ann. R. Coll. Surg. Engl.* 1985, **67,** 114; Pybus P. K. *Ann. R. Coll. Surg. Engl.* 1988, **70,** 260; Foate J. A. et al. *Ann. R. Coll. Surg. Engl.* 1989, **71,** 72.
12 Pearman T. *J. Laryngol. Otol.* 1979, **93,** 1191.
13 Van Essen E. J. and Ploeger E. J. *Anaesthesia* 1981, **36,** 713.
14 Withkin J. M. et al. *Life Sci.* 1989, **44,** 1289.
15 Derlet R. W. and Albertson T. E. *Am. J. Emerg. Med.* 1989, **7,** 464.
16 Delikan A. E. et al. *Anaesth. Intensive Care* 1978, **6,** 328.
17 Choy-Kwong M. and Lipton R. B. *Neurology* 1989, **39,** 425.
18 Cousins M. J. and Mather L. E. *Anaesth. Intensive Care* 1980, **6,** 270.
19 Christensen C. *Acta Anaesth. Scand.* 1990, **34,** 165.
20 Lofgren N. *Xylocaine.* Haeggstroms, Stockholm, 1948; *Archiv. Kemi Mineral Geol.* 1946, **18,** 22A.

Relative contraindications to regional analgesia, when used alone

1 In young children (aged < 10 years).
2 In uncooperative or restless patients.
3 In some psychiatric patients
4 In long operations when the patient may become uncomfortable and restless.

In addition there are some rare patients in whom local anaesthetics appear not to produce analgesia.

Practical considerations when using regional analgesia

Regional analgesia is used less frequently than it might be because of:

1 time taken to establish block (0.5 h with bupivacaine or ropivacaine, but faster with lignocaine);
2 the fear of failure;
3 the fear of neurological complications;
4 the unpopularity of the awake patient at operation.

'One-shot' blocks provide postoperative analgesia which wears off in a few hours. This can be overcome, almost anywhere in the body, by inserting an ordinary epidural catheter at the block site which can be 'topped up' with local anaesthetic as often as needed.

Regional analgesia is supremely useful and effective in postoperative pain relief. Sensory block, without motor block, is indicated, and the smaller the area of the body blocked, the better, since some patients do not like having large numb or paralysed areas. Either longer-acting analgesics, or regular top-ups using a catheter placed at the block site, or both, are most effective.

Before any local anaesthetic is given

An indwelling intravenous cannula.

A tilting table or trolley.

Facilities for intermittent positive-pressure ventilation (IPPV) with O_2.

Suction equipment and catheters.

Syringes, needles and ampoules of thiopentone, suxamethonium, diazepam and pressor drugs.

Fluid for infusion.

Resuscitation equipment.

Standard minimal monitoring.

Trained help.

Sedation and supplementation of regional analgesia

Dangers of intravenous sedation in regional blockade include undetected (even fatal) respiratory insufficiency. It should only be used in those cases which are impossible without it; with minimal doses, extreme care, and full monitoring. This situation is an example of the differences between the ideal world (no sedation needed) and the real world (some patients are terrified and the procedure cannot be done without it).

Purposes

1 To allay anxiety and control restlessness – opioids (e.g. remifentanil infusion) and benzodiazepines (e.g. midazolam 1 mg i.v.), or propofol infusion (target level 1 μg/ml).
2 Extra analgesia for less-than-perfect blocks, e.g. short-acting opioids, nonsteroidal anti-inflammatory drugs (NSAIDs) or N_2O (sedoanalgesia or relative analgesia).[1] Also for where pain is already severe, e.g. fractures. Low-dose intravenous ketamine is an excellent extra analgesic for these situations. Note that opioids may produce problems as well as prevent them, e.g. nausea, vomiting, bradycardia, hypotension, respiratory depression, bronchospasm.
3 To prevent vasovagal faints during the procedure.[2]

These sedatives may be given as premedication, as boluses or infusions. Propofol and remifentanil have the advantage of rapid recovery.

Sedation is chosen with care or omitted in obstetric regional blocks. Children may require more sedation, including light anaesthesia.

Relaxing music may be played through headphones, or the anaesthetist may give reassuring conversation.

Uses of vasoconstrictors in patients on other drugs

The commonest concentration of adrenaline in premixed local anaesthetic–adrenaline solutions is 1 : 200 000. Dental cartridges contain adrenaline 1 : 80 000 solution (but felypressin may be substituted).

If volatile anaesthetic agents are being given at the same time, suitable beta-blocking agents should be available. Hypoxia and hypercapnia should, as always, be avoided.

With tricyclic antidepressants and monoamine oxidase inhibitors (MAOIs), the cardiovascular effects of catecholamines may be increased. They should not be used together.

Identification of nerves

Use of a nerve stimulator will facilitate localization of the nerve in many nerve blocks. An electric current (1–5 mA, 1–2 Hz) is administered via a short-bevel needle, insulated apart from its tip. Muscular contraction shows proximity to nerve.[3] Nerves can be located using voltages high enough to stimulate motor fibres without causing sensory discomfort as sensory stimulation requires a higher voltage than motor stimulation.[4]

Topical analgesia[5]

From the Greek topos, 'a place'. Can be applied:

1 on gauze swabs;
2 as a liquid in a spray;
3 as a cream, gel, or ointment, e.g. EMLA, amethocaine and lignocaine gels;
4 as an aerosol;
5 by direct instillation, e.g. conjunctival sac, nose and trachea.

Sites

1 The conjunctival sac; stinging pain on instillation can be eased if the drug is dissolved in methyl cellulose.
2 The external ear, mouth, nose, throat, trachea, genitalia and urethra.
3 Before open wound closure.[6]

Infiltration analgesia

A weal is raised in the skin with a fine needle and through this weal a larger needle is used to inject the main bulk of solution. Prilocaine or lignocaine 0.5–1% solution, each with adrenaline, is ideal for this procedure. *For painless skin incisions, infiltration should be intradermal as well as subcutaneous.* For maximal intradermal analgesia the adrenaline should be omitted.[7] A slow, gentle technique is important, and the solution should be injected while the needle is moving to reduce the chances of intravenous injection.

As with all forms of local analgesia, the effect is not instantaneous and a proper interval must elapse between injection and incision.

Patients taking some adrenergic neurone-blocking drugs for hypertension may develop total ischaemia in areas infiltrated with local anaesthetic–adrenaline solutions.[8]

Transverse injection anaesthesia

A name given by Russian surgeons to a method (Vishnevsky technique) in which a transverse disk of tissue of a limb is infiltrated from skin to bone with a large volume of a dilute solution of an analgesic drug such as 0.5% procaine. In the vernacular 'the squirt-and-cut' technique.

HEAD AND NECK

Field block of scalp and cranium

Anatomy

The trigeminal nerve supplies the anterior two-thirds, the posterior divisions of cervical nerves the posterior third (Fig. 5.2.1).

There are five sensory nerves in front of the ear and four behind it. These nerves all converge towards the vertex of the scalp, so that a band of infiltration passing just above the ear through the glabella and the occiput will block them all.

Technique

Injections of 0.5% lignocaine with adrenaline solution must be made in three layers:

1 the skin, intradermal;
2 the subcutaneous tissues superficial to the epicranial aponeurosis in which the nerves and vessels lie, and also below the aponeurosis;
3 the periosteum.

In addition, solution should be injected into the substance of the temporalis muscle. The dura is insensitive except at the base of the skull.

For removal of sebaceous cysts or suturing of small wounds, a zone of infiltration surrounds the area. Periosteal injection is only necessary if bone is to be removed.

Useful in some cases of acute head injury and also to reduce haemorrhage in intracranial operations under general anaesthesia.

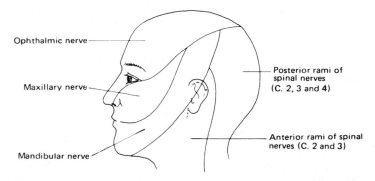

Figure 5.2.1 Showing the cutaneous nerve areas of the face and scalp. (From *Gray's Anatomy*, by kind permission of the Editor).

Nerve block for eye operations

Retrobulbar, and periocular (peribulbar)[9] blocks are used (*see* Chapter 4.1, 'Anaesthesia for ophthalmic surgery').

Nerve block for ear operations

Greater auricular nerve block

This nerve is blocked by infiltration of local anaesthetic solution over the mastoid process in the skin fold behind the back of the ear.

Auriculotemporal nerve block

This nerve is blocked by infiltration of local anaesthetic solution into the skin over the auditory canal in front of the ear.

Blockade of the auriculotemporal and greater auricular nerves together is used for pinnaplasty.

Paracentesis of the eardrum

Two or three metered (10-mg) doses of lignocaine aerosol spray are applied to the superior wall of the external auditory canal and allowed to trickle down onto the eardrum. This is repeated after 2 min and the incision can be made 3 min later.

Nerve block for nose operations

Anatomy

The nerve supply is from the first (ophthalmic) division and from the second (maxillary) division of the trigeminal (V cranial) nerve.

The skin of the nose is supplied by the supratrochlear branch of frontal nerve of the ophthalmic; the anterior ethmoidal branch of the nasociliary (ophthalmic) and the infraorbital branch of the maxillary. The maxillary nerve via the sphenopalatine ganglion supplies the lining of the maxillary antrum. The frontal nerve, a branch of the ophthalmic, supplies the frontal sinus. The anterior and posterior ethmoidal branches of the nasociliary supply the ethmoid region.

The anterior ethmoidal branch of the nasociliary nerve (division 1) supplies sensation to the anterior one-third of the nasal septum and lateral wall of the nasal cavity. The long sphenopalatine nerves from the sphenopalatine ganglion (division 2) supply sensation to posterior two-thirds of the nasal septum and lateral walls of the nasal cavity.

Injections into the nose or orbit have, exceptionally rarely, resulted in total spinal block (cf. rhinorrhoea after fractured base of skull).

Techniques

MAXILLARY NERVE AND SPHENOPALATINE GANGLION BLOCK

Useful for operations on antrum (e.g. Caldwell–Luc) and on upper lip, palate and upper teeth as far as the bicuspids.

Technique: A weal is raised 0.5 cm below the mid-point of the zygoma, which is over the anterior border of the coronoid process. Through it a needle is introduced at right angles to the median plane of the head until it strikes the lateral plate of the pterygoid process at a depth of about 4 cm. Set marker 1 cm from skin surface and reinsert needle slightly anteriorly (pointing towards opposite eyeball) so that its point glances past the anterior margin of the external pterygoid plate and advances as far as the marker. The needle point should be in the pterygomaxillary fissure where the spheno-palatine ganglion joins the nerve. The needle has been known to enter the pharynx or the orbit. If aspiration test is negative, 3–4 ml of 1.5% solution of lignocaine is injected and a similar amount as the needle is slowly with-drawn (Fig. 5.2.2).

Transient paralysis of the sixth cranial nerve may result.

ANTERIOR ETHMOIDAL (MEDIAN ORBITAL) NERVE BLOCK

This is a branch of the nasociliary nerve and is blocked in the medial wall of the orbit as the nerve passes through the anterior ethmoidal foramen. A weal

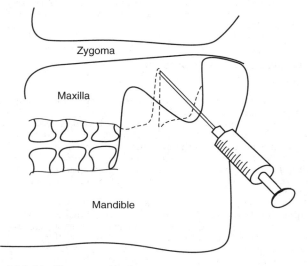

Figure 5.2.2 Maxillary nerve block

is raised 1 cm above the caruncle at the inner canthus of the eye. A small needle is introduced along the upper medial angle of the orbit for 3.5 cm keeping near the bone. Two millilitres of analgesic is usually sufficient.

FRONTAL NERVE BLOCK

From the same weal as in anterior ethmoid block, the needle is introduced more laterally towards the central part of the roof of the orbit where the frontal nerve lies between the periosteum and the levator palpebrae superioris. analgesic solution is injected close to the bone.

INFRAORBITAL NERVE BLOCK

The infraorbital nerve, the terminal portion of the maxillary nerve, supplies the side of the nose, the lower eyelid, the upper lip and its mucosa. The infraorbital foramen is in line with the supraorbital notch and canine fossa both of which are palpable or the second upper and lower premolar teeth and the mental foramen; it is 1 cm below the margin of the orbit, below the pupil when the eyes look forwards.

A needle is inserted through a weal 1 cm below the middle of the lower orbital margin, a finger-breadth lateral to the ala of the nose. Lignocaine, 2 ml of 2% solution, is deposited near the nerve as it issues from the foramen (not while it is in the foramen).

For radical operation on the antrum, a maxillary block is indicated, together with local infiltration inside the upper lip, over the canine fossa.

For radical operation on the frontal sinus, anterior ethmoidal and frontal blocks are necessary.

For operations for dacryocystitis, anterior ethmoidal and infraorbital blocks are required.

Topical analgesia of the nasal cavities

Useful in cooperative patients with reasonably patent nares.

Packing: the nasal cavities are first sprayed with 4–10% lignocaine, any excess solution being rejected and not swallowed. The cavity is then packed with gauze soaked in 4–5% lignocaine. In places where cocaine is used, adrenaline is not necessary as it is a powerful vasoconstrictor. Trauma must be avoided. After 10 min the packing is removed and the mucosa will be found to be avascular.

Use of cocaine paste:[10] cocaine is toxic; care must be taken to limit the amount of paste used to 2 mg/kg.

Moffett's method:[11] the solution is a mixture of 2 ml of 8% cocaine hydrochloride, 2 ml of 1% sodium bicarbonate, 1 ml of 1 : 1000 adrenaline solution. It can also be used as 4% cocaine, omitting bicarbonate and adrenaline. A 2-ml syringe with bent or curved cannula is required (Fig. 5.2.3).

Position 1: patient lies with the head tilted right back at angle of 45 degrees with horizontal. Analgesic solution is squirted into each naris along the floor of the nose via a cannula. If the septum is to be operated on, 2 ml of 1%

lignocaine–adrenaline should be injected into the columella and base of septum in addition, as this area is covered by squamous epithelium which will not absorb the topical agent.

The method gives good analgesia, free from the unpleasantness of gauze packing and its resulting mild trauma.

Nerve block for maxillofacial operations

The oral mucosa may be sprayed with topical lignocaine before needle insertion, for greater comfort.

Local infiltration for dental extraction

This can be done for all teeth with the possible exception of the lower molars. Lignocaine 2% with 1 : 80 000 adrenaline solution is commonly used, alternatively 3% prilocaine with felypressin. A 26-G needle is inserted at the junction of the adherent mucoperiosteum of the gum with the free mucous membrane of the cheek and directed parallel to the long axis of the tooth; 0.5–1 ml of solution is injected superficial to the periosteum on the buccal and either the lingual or palatal side. Analgesia is tested for after 5 min by pushing the needle down the periodontal membrane on each side of the tooth to be

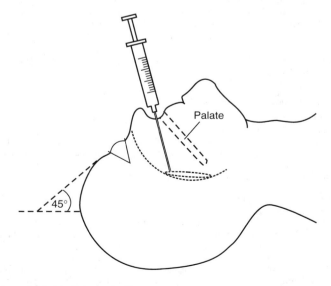

Figure 5.2.3 Moffet's method

extracted. If required more solution can be injected. Where there is infection involving teeth in the lower jaw, a 5% solution may give better analgesia than the usual 2%. It has a shorter latency but a similar duration of activity.

Mandibular (inferior dental) block

A single well-placed injection renders one-half of the lower jaw and tongue analgesic, except for the central incisor which receives some nerve supply from the other side and the lateral buccal fold and molar buccal alveolar margin and gum supplied from the buccinator nerve. Both of these areas can be infiltrated with a small volume of solution to make them painless.

With the mouth open palpate the anterior border of the ramus of the mandible, the retromolar fossa and the internal oblique ridge. The needle is inserted just medial to this ridge lateral to the pterygomandibular ligament for a distance of 1.5 cm, keeping the syringe parallel to the occlusal plane of the lower teeth with its barrel over the premolar teeth of the opposite side; 2 or 3 ml of solution is now injected.

In patients whose orbital blood supply is derived from the middle meningeal artery (a rare anomaly), mandibular nerve block may result in transient amaurosis. This may be due to intra-arterial injection of the local anaesthetic–adrenaline solution.

Unusual reactions to lignocaine in dental surgery (fixed drug eruption) may occur.[12]

Lingual nerve block

The lingual nerve is the only sensory nerve supplying the floor of the mouth between the alveolar margin and the midline.

A finger in the retromolar fossa of the mandible will palpate the internal oblique line. The lingual nerve can be injected, just medial to this line, with 2 ml of analgesic. A useful method of analgesia for removing calculi from the submaxillary duct.

Intraoral nerve block for extraoral lesions[13]

Useful for repair of lacerations of face and removal of skin lesions. There is no tissue distortion and injections are less painful than through the skin.

INFRAORBITAL NERVE

Injection in mucobuccal fold, just medial to canine tooth; 1–2 ml of local anaesthetic solution is injected, advancing needle 1 cm. The entire upper lip is anaesthetized. Can be bilateral.

MENTAL NERVE

Injection between apices of premolar teeth of lower jaw of 1–2 ml of local anaesthetic solution will anaesthetize the lower lip.

LONG BUCCAL NERVE

Can be blocked as it crosses the anterior border of mandible. Injection immediately in front of the ramus, in the mucobuccal fold opposite the first molar tooth. Needle is inserted just anterior to the margin of the mandible and 2–3 ml of solution injected while needle is withdrawn. Useful for blocking 'cross-over' fibres.

Facial nerve block

For hemifacial spasm.[14] The nerve is blocked as it crosses the neck of the mandible.

Nerve block for throat operations

Glossopharyngeal nerve block[15]

1 Head fully rotated to opposite side with patient lying supine. At mid-point of a line joining the tip of the mastoid process to the angle of the jaw a needle inserted vertical to the skin makes contact with the styloid process 2–4 cm deep. Needle partially withdrawn and reinserted 0.5 cm deep to and posterior to styloid process. Injection of 6 ml of solution at this point will produce analgesia of posterior one-third of tongue.
2 An alternative technique is to deposit solution near the jugular foramen. A 5-cm needle is introduced through a weal just below the external auditory meatus, anterior to the mastoid process. It is advanced perpendicularly to the skin until it meets the styloid process 1.5–2 cm deep and passes it posteriorly for a further 2 cm. Analgesia involves the IXth to XIIth nerves inclusive and has been maintained with a long-acting drug in cases of malignant disease in the posterior third of the tongue, and in severe cases of neuralgia. Successful block results in analgesia of the posterior one-third of the tongue, uvula, soft palate and pharynx. There is no motor block. The gag reflex is suppressed. Also used in differential diagnosis between glossopharyngeal and atypical trigeminal neuralgias.
3 Injection in the base of the posterior pillar of the fauces.[16]

Superior laryngeal nerve block

The internal laryngeal nerve passes forwards and downwards and pierces the thyrohyoid membrane to reach the space between the epiglottis and the pharyngeal mucosa posteriorly and the membrane in front. Its terminal twigs convey sensation from the larynx above the cords, the epiglottis, vallecula and the base of the tongue. This nerve is blocked at its point of division into the internal and external laryngeal nerve, slightly below and anterior to the greater cornu of the hyoid bone. Block of the internal branch causes analgesia of the lower pharynx, the laryngeal aspect of the epiglottis, the vallecula, the vestibule of the larynx, the aryepiglottic fold and the posterior part of the rima glottidis. There is no motor block.

A weal is raised between the superior cornu of the thyroid and the greater cornu of the hyoid. Through the weal, a needle is introduced laterally and solution is injected. A further few millilitres of solution are injected as the needle is withdrawn. A similar procedure is carried out on the other side.[17]

This block causes analgesia of the posterior surface of the epiglottis and of the larynx above the cords, so that food and drink must be prohibited for an adequate period depending on the drug and strength used.

It is useful, in conjunction with topical analgesia of the nose and pharynx, to enable awake fibreoptic intubation.

Topical analgesia, coupled with superior laryngeal and glossopharyngeal nerve block, gives good results for awake intubation, tonsillectomy and bronchoscopy.[18] *See below.*

Transtracheal block

See Benumof J. L. *Anesthesiology* 1991, **75,** 1087, and 'Anaesthesia for fibreoptic intubation and bronchoscopy', below.

Vagus nerve block

This was described as a method of analgesia for broncho-oesophagoscopy and in the diagnosis of pain arising in the thorax. Now seldom used.[19]

Field block for tonsillectomy

ANATOMY

The lesser palatine (from maxillary), the lingual (from mandibular) nerves, and the glossopharyngeal nerve, via the pharyngeal plexus, which gives off filaments that form a plexus called the circulus tonsillaris, supply the tonsil and its immediate surroundings.

TECHNIQUE

Half an hour before the analgesia is commenced, a local anaesthetic lozenge is given, after which the mouth and pharynx should be sprayed with 4–10% lignocaine solution; some operators object to this preferring to the keep the cough reflex active throughout. Injections of 3–5 ml of 1.5% lignocaine and adrenaline are now made:

1 into the upper part of the posterior pillar;
2 into the upper part of the anterior pillar – both pillars must be made oedematous throughout their whole extent;
3 into the triangular fold, near the lower pole;
4 into the supratonsillar fossa, after drawing the tonsil towards the middle line.

The patient is sitting, well supported, in a chair. Adequate time must be given for the analgesic to act. Fainting is sometimes seen, while the depression of the tongue by the spatula may cause discomfort.

Accessory nerve block

The nerve has both cranial and spinal roots. It leaves the skull through the jugular foramen, enters the deep surface of the sternomastoid, pierces it and emerges just above the mid-point of its posterior margin. It crosses the posterior triangle of the neck and enters the anterior border of the trapezius, giving motor fibres to it and to the sternomastoid.

TECHNIQUE

Needle inserted 2 cm below the tip of the mastoid and 5–10 ml of solution injected into muscle.

INDICATIONS

To relax sternomastoid and trapezius muscles during physiotherapy for pain in the shoulder and neck, e.g. torticollis.

Cervical plexus block (C1–4)

This is paravertebral cervical analgesia. It is convenient for the removal of superficial tumours and cysts from the neck.

ANATOMY

Formed by the anterior primary divisions of the upper four cervical nerves, each of which comes to lie in the sulcus between the anterior and posterior tubercles of the transverse process of the appropriate cervical vertebra. The posterior primary divisions of the cervical nerves supply skin and muscles of the middle of the back of the neck. Their cutaneous distribution spreads like a cape over the upper thorax and shoulders, and this area is made insensitive in cervical plexus block.

Superficial branches emerge posterior to the lateral border of the sternomastoid, near its midpoint. They are as follows.

1 Ascending branches. Lesser occipital (C2) and great auricular (C2 and C3). They supply skin of the occipitomastoid region, auricle, and parotid.
2 Transverse branch. The anterior cutaneous nerve of the neck (C2 and C3) supplying skin of anterior part of neck between the lower jaw and the sternum.
3 Descending branches. The supraclavicular nerves (C3 and C4) supplying skin of shoulder, upper pectoral region and breast.

Deep branches of the plexus are the phrenic nerve – C3, C4 and C5; muscular branches to sternomastoid, levator scapulae, trapezius and scalenus medius.
Communicating branches are:

1 sympathetic – from the superior cervical ganglion;
2 to vagus;
3 branch to hypoglossal nerve from C1 and C2, the descendens hypoglossi which joins the descendens cervicalis (C2–C3) to form the ansa hypoglossi.

Nerve supply of thyroid is from middle and inferior cervical sympathetic ganglion; of the oesophagus, the vagus (and sympathetic); of the trachea, recurrent laryngeal (and sympathetic); of the sternomastoid, the XIth cranial, and second and third cervical nerves.

TECHNIQUE

Cervical block requires the deposition of analgesic solution just lateral to the transverse processes of the second, third and fourth cervical vertebrae (the sixth, seventh and eighth nerves having no sensory branches in the neck, and the first is purely motor). These are easily felt in the middle of the side of the neck. A needle is inserted to a depth of 1.5–2 cm pointing slightly caudally (to avoid the vertebral artery and spinal canal) so that the transverse processes are contacted (Fig. 5.2.4).

In addition, 20 ml of local anaesthetic solution is injected between skin and muscle along the posterior border of the sternomastoid near its mid-point,

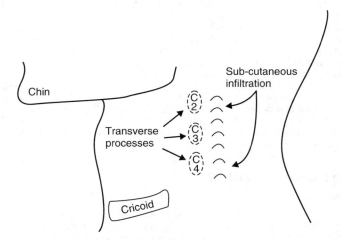

Figure 5.2.4 Cervical plexus block

usually just below the position where it is crossed by the external jugular vein, so as to cut off impulses from the ascending, transverse and descending superficial branches of the plexus.

Cervical plexus block gives analgesia of the front and back of the neck, the occipital region, and a cape-like area over the shoulders to below the clavicle, the skin above the third rib anteriorly and above the upper border of the scapula posteriorly.

Complications include:

1 phrenic block;
2 intrathecal or intravascular injection;
3 vagus and/or recurrent laryngeal nerve block, causing aphonia;
4 cervical sympathetic block and Horner's syndrome.

SHOULDER AND UPPER EXTREMITY

Suprascapular nerve block (C5–6)[20]

The nerve is the pathway of somatic pain from the shoulder and acromioclavicular joints and structures surrounding them. The block does not result in any skin analgesia, but when successful, relieves pain in the shoulder joint.

Technique

The patient should be sitting with arms to the sides and head and shoulders slightly flexed. With a skin pencil the spine of the scapula is lined in: the inferior scapular angle is located and bisected by a line which crosses the first line. A weal is raised one finger-breadth from the crossing, in the upper outer angle, and a needle inserted downwards and medially to make contact with the bone of the supraspinatus fossa, just lateral to the notch. Needle then withdrawn and reintroduced more medially until its point lies in the notch. Stimulation paraesthesiae takes the form of pain at the tip of the shoulder, and after aspiration 10 ml of analgesic solution are injected. The block must be at the suprascapular notch as there the nerve is accessible to a needle and no afferent branches leave it before it passes through the notch. Types of shoulder pain relieved by this block include subacromial bursitis, painful abduction of the arm; calcified deposits about the capsule of the shoulder joint. Used for pain relief, not surgery.

Brachial plexus block (C5–T1)[21,22]

Anatomy

The brachial plexus is formed from the anterior primary divisions of C5, C6, C7, C8 and T1. It forms the entire motor and almost the entire sensory nerve supply of the arm. It receives communicating branches from C4 and T2. These roots unite to form three trunks, which pass between the scalenus anterior and the scalenus medius, joined by the subclavian artery, invaginate the scalene fascia to form a neurovascular space. This fascia then becomes the brachial plexus sheath or axillary sheath which may be entered at any level; a single injection into it will produce analgesia, the extent of which will depend on the volume of solution injected and the level of injection. Each trunk divides, behind the clavicle, into anterior and posterior divisions, which unite in the axilla to form cords which then divide into nerves.

The anterior relations of the plexus are the skin, superficial fascia, platysma and supraclavicular branches of the cervical plexus, the deep fascia and external jugular vein; the clavicle is in front of its lower part, the scalenus anterior is in front of its upper part. Its posterior relations are the scalenus medius and the long thoracic nerve. Its inferior relations are the first rib, where the plexus lies between the subclavian artery anteriorly and the scalenus medius behind.

The roots each receive grey rami from the sympathetic ganglia.

Branches from roots: the nerve (of Bell) to the serratus anterior from C5, C6 and C7. Dorsalis scapulae nerve from C5. Muscular branches to the longus cervicis (C5–C8) and the three scaleni (C5–C8), the rhomboids (C5) and a branch to the phrenic (C5).

Branches from trunks: suprascapular nerve (C5 and C6). Nerve to subclavius (C5 and C6).

Branches from cords: From lateral cord (three) – lateral pectoral (C5–C7); lateral head of the median (C5–C7); musculocutaneous (C5, C6, C7). From the posterior cord (five) – radial (C5, C6, C7 C8 and T1); axillary (C5 and C6); thoracodorsal nerve to the latissimus dorsi (C6, C7, C8); upper and lower subscapular nerves (C5 and C6). From the medial cord (five) – medial head of the median; medial pectoral; ulnar; medial cutaneous of the forearm (all from C8 and T1); medial cutaneous of the arm (T1).

Connective tissue septa between the components of the plexus make the sheath multicompartmental and the compartments do not always intercommunicate. (Thus, using any technique of block, certain nerves may remain unblocked.[23]) (Fig. 5.2.5.)

Technique

SUPRACLAVICULAR APPROACH

The patient should be sitting or lying supine. The head is rotated to the other side and the arm and shoulder depressed. A weal is raised 1 cm above the midpoint of the clavicle, a position:

1 midway between the sternoclavicular and acromioclavicular joints;
2 crossed by a line produced downwards from the external jugular vein, made prominent by blowing out the cheeks;
3 just lateral to the pulsating subclavian artery, often palpable;
4 lateral to the outer border of the scalenus anterior, sometimes palpable under cover of the sternomastoid.

In thin subjects, the cords of the plexus can be easily rolled on the first rib by the finger, giving clear location of the plexus.

A nerve stimulator set at 1–5 mA is attached to the insulated needle and inserted through the weal *downwards, inwards and backwards*, so that it is pointing to the spine of the second to fourth thoracic vertebra, a finger meanwhile guarding the subclavian artery and drawing it slightly medially. A cough from the patient is a warning that the pleura is being irritated by the needle. If stimulation or motor jerk is felt, the needle is steadied and after a negative aspiration test, 30 ml of the solution are injected. The following nerves are blocked: the median, the musculocutaneous, the radial, the axillary, the ulnar, the media cutaneous nerve of the arm and the medial cutaneous nerve of the forearm.

If stimuli or jerks are not felt in the arm and hand after one or two needle thrusts, the upper surface of the first rib is contacted and the needle inserted on to it so that the pulsations of the subclavian artery are transmitted to the needle. This is at a depth of 1.2–2.5 cm. If stimulation is felt in the second, third or fourth fingers, a successful block results in over 90% of cases. It may be incomplete if only the first and fifth fingers react to stimulation.[24] A feeling of warmth and 'pins and needles' often precedes analgesia, while motor paralysis, when it occurs, follows analgesia.

An area of skin over the point of the shoulder and another on the inner aspect of the upper arm from the axilla to its mid-point (intercostohumeral T2) is not made insensitive. A subcutaneous band of injection downwards from the acromioclavicular joint and surrounding the shoulder will render these areas analgesic. Occasionally, median nerve block at the wrist is necessary, as the palm of the hand, supplied by the middle trunk (C7) of the plexus via the median nerve, is the most resistant area to successful block.

Toxic and ill or feeble patients should have the strength of solution and not the volume reduced.

Continuous brachial plexus block[25] is convenient using an epidural catheter. Complications include the following:

1 Paralysis of phrenic nerve.[26] Such a block is usually harmless but if the patient has a respiratory problem, the possibility of diaphragmatic paralysis must be borne in mind. There is a high hemidiaphragm on X-ray examination.
2 Puncture of vessels, including subclavian artery. A haematoma may form. Intravascular injection must be avoided.
3 Pneumothorax. Due to piercing Sibsons fascia. A chest drain is likely to be needed. The axillary approach avoids this complication. Silent pneumothorax is unlikely as a needle in the pleura is usually accompanied by pain. Surgical emphysema may be seen, probably due to wounding of the lung by the needle. Pain in the chest during needling may also be due to irritation of the nerve to the serratus anterior.
4 Toxic effect of drug injected. Slow injection lessens chance of this.
5 Postoperative disability following brachial plexus block is rare, although the paralysing effects of bupivacaine or ropivacaine may last many hours.[27]
6 *Horner's syndrome* may or may not follow injection. It is due to paralysis of the cervical sympathetic chain. For details, *see above*.

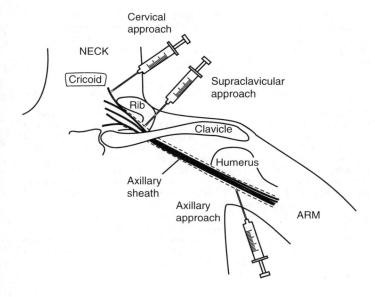

Figure 5.2.5 Brachial plexus bock

INTERSCALENE (CERVICAL APPROACH)[28]

Described by Labat in 1927[29] and Alon Winnie.[30] The sheath of the plexus can be entered via the interscalene space between the anterior and middle scalene muscles at the level of C6 (cricoid). At the edge of the sternomastoid muscle the palpating finger lies on the scalenus anterior muscle and more laterally the groove between the anterior and middle scalene muscles can be felt. A stimulating needle is inserted perpendicular to the skin, pointing slightly caudally, bypassing the external jugular vein, and advanced to touch the transverse process. After careful aspiration tests the desired volume of analgesic solution is injected (e.g. 25–40 ml). For complete analgesia of the inner aspect of the upper arm, block of the intercostohumeral nerve (T12) may be required. Permanent neurological damage has been reported.[31]

Although the dangers of pneumothorax are avoided, there is risk of injection into the extradural space, into cerebrospinal fluid (CSF) or the vertebral artery and bilateral block of the cervical and brachial plexuses.[32] The needle should not be inserted more than 3 cm[33] and pointed slightly caudally. Successful injection blocks both the cervical and brachial plexuses. Suitable

620 Lee's Synopsis of Anaesthesia

for operations on the shoulder joint and for the reduction of fractures. The complications are the same as may arise from cervical plexus block. Thirty millilitres of analgesic may be used. Complete onset of block may take 30 min. An acute exacerbation of asthma has been reported in an asthmatic patient.[34]

THE SUBCLAVIAN (SUPRACLAVICULAR) PERIVASCULAR TECHNIQUE

The tip of the anaesthetist's index finger is placed posterior to the lateral border of the relaxed sternomastoid at the level of C6 (cricoid cartilage). The tip of the finger moves medially behind the belly of the sternomastoid, enters the interscalene groove and is edged inferiorly. The interscalene groove is palpated, and followed down until the subclavian artery is felt pulsating, and in the thin subject the cords of the plexus rolled beneath the finger on the hard rib. At this point, a stimulating needle is inserted through the clavicular head of sternomastoid, and pushed downwards (caudally) until it enters the perivascular space, shown by stimulation or jerks in the arm (not the shoulder as this may be due to irritation of the suprascapular nerve) or by a click as the needle pierces the fascia. After aspiration, 20–40 ml of solution is injected slowly. The intercostobrachial and the medial brachial cutaneous nerve (C8–T1) must in addition be blocked by a few millilitres of solution injected subcutaneously over the axillary artery if a tourniquet is to be applied.

AXILLARY APPROACH TO BRACHIAL PLEXUS[35]

In the axilla, the brachial plexus and artery are still enclosed in a fascial sheath. The median and musculocutaneous nerves together with their sensory branches are anterior or anterolateral, i.e. above and beyond the artery; the ulnar nerve is inferior; the radial nerve is posterolateral or below and behind the vessel. The musculocutaneous and axillary nerves are given off high in the axilla.

Technique: The patient lies supine with the arm abducted to a right angle, the humerus externally rotated and the elbow flexed. The skin of the axilla is not shaved but is well cleaned and a weal is raised where arterial pulsation is felt. A stimulating needle[36] is inserted until a click shows that the neurovascular sheath has been entered; a stimulus or jerk shows that the point has entered the sheath. It is easy to push the needle too deeply and to thus miss the sheath. Twenty millilitres of local analgesic solution is placed in each quadrant surrounding the vessel. The addition of potassium chloride to 0.25% solution of bupivacaine (but not to prilocaine) causes a more rapid onset of sensory block.[37] To prevent dissipation of the solution downwards in the neurovascular space firm finger pressure may be applied below the needle during and after the injection. Occasionally the musculocutaneous nerve (C6), which is a continuation of the lateral cord of the plexus, is given off higher than usual and consequently escapes the effects of local analgesic solution deposited in the neurovascular space. In such cases it can be dealt with by the injection of 10–15 ml of solution from a point 2.5 cm distal to the crease of the elbow joint in the cleft between the tendon of the biceps and the brachioradialis where it becomes the lateral antebrachial cutaneous nerve, or 5 ml of solution injected into the substance of the coracobrachialis muscle. Similarly, a few drops of solution may be deposited medial to the neuro-vascular bundle, to block the intercostobrachial nerve which supplies the inner and outer aspects of the upper arm. An area of skin over the point of the shoulder supplied by the intercostohumeral nerve (T1 and T2) is not blocked by this approach.

An alternative approach is to enter the neurovascular sheath at the lowest point of the axilla just posterior to the head of biceps, where pulsation is felt. The plexus is quite superficial at this point.

Extent of block by axillary approach: complete analgesia below the elbow joint. Good sympathetic block of arm. Shoulder joint, supplied by the supra-scapular nerve (C5 and C6), not made insensitive.

Advantages: only one landmark, the axillary artery. No pneumothorax, stel-late ganglion block, recurrent laryngeal nerve block or phrenic nerve block. Difficult in obesity or when the arm cannot be abducted. Continuous block, using a catheter, eases pain following trauma to the arm.[38]

Brachial plexus block is a most satisfactory method of analgesia though less popular since the reintroduction of intravenous regional analgesia. For dis-locations of the shoulder joint or elbow joint, for tendon suture, for manipu-lation of fractures under the X-ray screen, for suturing of lacerations, etc., the method is excellent.

Injury to the brachial plexus following brachial plexus block may be due to lack of support for the anaesthetized limb after operation.[39]

Intravenous regional analgesia

This was first described by Bier in 1908.[40] Intravenous injection of local analgesic agents has been used for:

1 general anaesthesia;
2 in the treatment of cardiac dysrhythmias;
3 to produce local analgesia.

Local analgesia involves the injection of a local analgesic solution into a vein of a limb which has been made ischaemic by a tourniquet. Most useful for operations on arms but can also be used in the leg.

Technique

A cannula is inserted into a vein on the dorsum of the hand (preferably not in the forearm) and very firmly secured; another should be in a vein in the other limb in case of toxic signs. The limb is drained of blood by elevation for 5 min, with or without compression of the brachial artery. An Esmarch bandage, the Rhys–Davies exsanguinator (an inflatable pneumatic cylinder which is easier to apply and less uncomfortable)[41] or an orthopaedic pneumatic splint[42] can all be used for this purpose. Two narrow sphygmomanometer cuffs are securely placed on the upper arm, one proximal to the other, and the upper one inflated to 50 mmHg above the systolic blood pressure, before removal of the compression or pneumatic bandage (if used). Forty millilitres of the local analgesic solution is now injected, and after 5–10 min, the lower cuff is inflated and the upper one released, to minimize discomfort. A tourniquet that does not occlude the brachial artery throughout the operation may result in congestion of the limb, absorption of the drug and imperfect analgesia. Close attention to detail and to the efficiency of the apparatus is most important. The patient is ready for operation after an interval of 10 min. Analgesia continues while the tourniquet remains inflated. The block has been used successfully in children, and also on the lower extremity, in which case the cuff should be placed on the mid-calf.[43] The tourniquet is released for 1 min, reinflated for 5 min, and then released again.

Note that tourniquet release can cause changes in the blood concentrations of drugs other than the local analgesic.[44] The information derived from angiography of the upper limb may be increased if guanethidine is used to produce sympathetic block, using the Bier technique.[45]

Local analgesic solutions

Preservative-free 0.5% lignocaine and prilocaine are effective and relatively safe;[46] the usual volume required is 3–4 mg/kg. In contrast, 0.2% bupivacaine is efficient but potentially toxic and should not be used.

The site of action of the drug is on the peripheral nerve endings, and also on nerve trunks if stronger solutions are used.

Cuff deflation is done in stages,[47] with reinflation if toxic signs occur over the next 10 mins: (drowsiness, convulsions, hypotension, asystole).

Contraindications

These may include Raynaud's disease, sickle-cell anaemia and scleroderma. Reactionary oedema may follow release of the cuff, so that, in fractures, a plaster-of-Paris back splint should be applied and the cast completed later. Intravenous regional analgesia of one finger has been reported.[48]

Intra-arterial local analgesia

A pneumatic cuff is applied to the upper arm, and a fine, short-bevel needle, attached to a 20-ml syringe containing 0.5% lignocaine solution, is introduced into the brachial artery near the elbow. The cuff is then inflated until arterial pulsations are occluded and the solution injected intra-arterially 5 ml at a time until the desired analgesic effect is obtained. The average dose in adults is 14–15 ml, considerably less than would be required in intravenous regional analgesia. Unsuccessful attempts at intra-arterial injection may cause temporary vascular spasm, but no other complications were seen in a series of 300 cases.[49]

Distal nerve blocks

Elbow block

Intradermal and subcutaneous circles of infiltration are made just proximal to the internal epicondyle.

MEDIAN BLOCK

Obtained by injecting through a weal placed midway between the outer side of the tendon of the biceps and the medial epicondyle or from a weal 1 cm medial to the brachial artery at the bend of the elbow. The needle should be inserted in an upward direction. If stimuli or jerks are felt, success is likely: 5 ml of solution is used. The median nerve supplies the lateral part of the palm and fingers.

ULNAR BLOCK

Performed 2 or 3 cm proximal to the point where the nerve can be palpated behind the medial epicondyle using 2–4 ml of solution. The ulnar nerve supplies skin on the medial side of the palmar and dorsal aspects of the hand and fifth and medial part of fourth fingers.

RADIAL BLOCK

Block of the radial and lateral cutaneous nerve of the forearm (the sensory continuation of the musculocutaneous nerve), is performed through a weal 1 cm lateral to the tendon of the biceps at the line of the bend of the elbow. The needle is directed upwards to reach the front of the outer surface of the lateral epicondyle and solution deposited between the bone and the skin. Alternatively, a weal is raised four finger-breadths proximal to the lateral epicondyle of the humerus which overlies the point at which the nerve pierces the intermuscular septum and is close to the bone. The needle is advanced perpendicularly to the skin towards the bone and 20 ml of analgesic solution are deposited above and below this point.

Wrist block

Circular lines of intradermal and subcutaneous infiltration are carried out just above the wrist joint.

Median nerve (C5–T1): the median nerve at the wrist lies deeply between the flexor carpi radialis laterally and the palmaris longus and flexor digitorum sublimis medially. It is injected with 5 ml of analgesic immediately lateral to the tendon of the palmaris longus with the hand dorsiflexed. Attempts to elicit stimuli are made, but if unsuccessful the solution is injected nevertheless.

The median nerve supplies the skin of the thenar eminence and of the anterior aspects of the lateral three and a half fingers together with the skin over the dorsal aspects of their terminal phalanges. Median nerve block at the wrist or elbow may be followed by neuritis.

Ulnar nerve (C7–T1) divides (5 cm) above the wrist joint into superficial terminal or palmar (mixed), and dorsal (sensory) branches.

The superficial terminal branch lies between the flexor carpi ulnaris tendon and the ulnar artery. It supplies the medial part of the palm of the hand and the palmar aspect of the fifth and medial side of the ring finger. The pisiform bone is immediately medial to it. Its sensory branch is blocked from a weal immediately lateral to the flexor carpi ulnaris.

The dorsal branch is anaesthetized by intradermal and subcutaneous injection along a line at the level of the ulnar styloid from the medial side of the tendon of the flexor carpi ulnaris to the middle of the back of the wrist. It supplies the ulnar border of the dorsum of the hand.

Radial or musculospiral nerve (C5–T1) is the sensory nerve of the lateral part of the back of the hand. After accompanying the radial artery along the medial border of the brachioradialis, it passes 6–7 cm above the wrist joint beneath the tendon of that muscle and comes to lie beneath the skin on the extensor aspect of the lower forearm and wrist. It can be blocked by infiltrating between the skin and the bone on the posterolateral aspect of the radius near the base of the thumb lateral to the radial artery, 2–3 cm proximal to the radial styloid.

Wrist block, with a finger tourniquet, is useful for surgery of the hand, especially if motor function is required during the operation. It does not remove the discomfort of an Esmarch bandage on the forearm.

Elbow and wrist block are often unwise in the presence of neuritis or carpal tunnel syndrome, unlike intravenous regional analgesia and local infiltration, which are not contraindicated.

The palm can be blocked at the wrist and the sole at the ankle.

Digital block (fingers or toes)

Two palmar and two dorsal nerves supply each digit. With a fine (25-G) needle an intradermal weal is raised on the dorsum of the finger near its base. Two millilitres of 1 or 2% lignocaine (or one of its congeners) solution are injected into the substance of the finger through this weal between the bone and the skin and repeated on the other side of the digit. The weals should be connected by 1 ml of solution between skin and bone on the dorsal aspect. Analgesia may take 15 min to become established. The palmar/plantar skin is not pierced. *Adrenaline should not be used* (Fig. 5.2.6).

Metacarpal/metatarsal block

Another method of blocking the finger is to deposit 5–7 ml of 1% lignocaine solution in the interosseous spaces at each side of the metacarpal bone, entering from the dorsal aspect and carrying the needle almost to the palmar/

plantar skin. Spread of infection due to this technique is very rare, providing that solution is not injected into infected tissue.

If a tourniquet is used, no more than 3 ml of solution should be injected; a tourniquet must not remain on the finger for more than 15 min and not used at all in patients with Raynaud's disease.

A similar technique using less solution can be employed on the toe. Intravenous regional analgesia of one finger has been reported.[49]

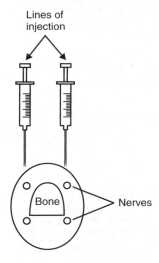

Figure 5.2.6 Cross-section of digit for digital block

THORAX

Breast surgery

Major operations on the breast are not satisfactory under regional analgesia, but biopsies can be obtained without pain using lignocaine and adrenaline.[50]

Paravertebral nerve blockade

Involves injecting a local analgesic close to the vertebral column where the nerve trunks emerge from the intervertebral foramina.

The paravertebral space is a wedge-shaped compartment, bounded above and below by the heads and necks of adjoining ribs; posteriorly by the superior costotransverse ligament; medially it communicates with the extra-dural space through the intervertebral foramen; laterally its apex leads into the intercostal space. The posterolateral aspect of the body of the vertebra and the intervertebral foramen and its contents forms the base.[51]

There is no direct communication between one paravertebral space and another, but an indirect communication exists medially through the inter-vertebral foramen with the extradural space. Spread from one paravertebral space to another, across the extradural space, is frequent and may involve nerves on the same or on the opposite side of the body.

When the first thoracic to second lumbar nerve roots are blocked, their rami communicantes are blocked too.

Paravertebral cervical block

Described under cervical plexus block.

Paravertebral thoracic block

Indicated for operations on the chest or abdominal wall, for relief of post-operative pain, post-herpetic pain and the pain of fractured ribs.

TECHNIQUE

Skin weals are raised 4 cm from the midline, opposite the lower borders of the vertebral spines. Through each weal, a needle is inserted perpendicularly to strike bone near the lateral extremity of the transverse process. It is then redirected to pass upwards and slightly medially over the upper border of the transverse process and at this point local analgesic solution is injected. Aspiration tests should be made to ensure that the needle point has not entered a vessel or the dura. Puncture of the pleura is also possible.

Intercostal nerve block

The cutaneous nerves of the trunk (Figs 5.2.7–5.2.10)

ANTERIORLY

1 The lateral, intermediate and medial supraclavicular branches of the super-ficial division of the cervical plexus (C3–C4) to the second interspace.
2 The anterior rami of the thoracic nerves, excluding T1 to the thorax and abdomen.
3 The iliohypogastric and ilio-inguinal nerves (L1) to the groin.

POSTERIORLY

The posterior rami of C2–C5; T1–T12; L1–L3; the five sacral and the coccy-geal nerves to the midline of the back.

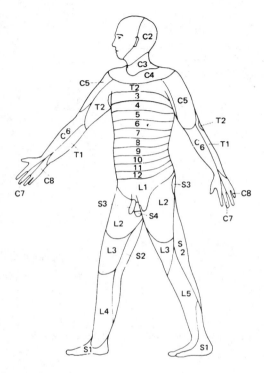

Figure 5.2.7

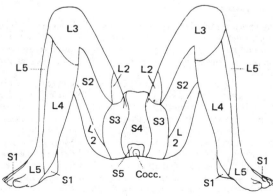

Figure 5.2.8

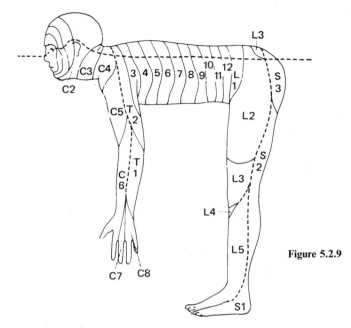

Figures 5.2.7–5.2.9 Distribution of cutaneous nerves. (After Foerster O. *Brain* 1933, **56**, 1.)

Anatomy of spinal nerves

Typical intercostal nerves are the third to sixth inclusive. Each nerve is formed by the union of the anterior (motor) and the posterior (sensory) root: the latter has a ganglion on it. The mixed spinal nerve soon divides into anterior and posterior primary divisions (rami). The thoracic or dorsal nerves then are distributed as follows:

The posterior rami are smaller than the anterior. They turn backwards and divide into medial and lateral branches (except C1, S4 and S5, coccygeal) and supply the muscles and skin of the midline of the back.

The anterior rami in the thoracic region of the second to sixth nerves are each connected to the lateral sympathetic chain by a grey and a white ramus communicans. Each crosses the paravertebral space between the necks of contiguous ribs and then enters the subcostal groove where it lies below the vein and artery in a triangular space, bounded above by the rib, the posterior intercostal membrane and the internal intercostal muscle (intercostal intima)[52] until it reaches the anterior axillary line, at which point the nerves come into direct relationship with the pleura, as the innermost intercostal muscle terminates. There is a communication between each space and those contiguous to it, and analgesic solution may spread medially from here to surround the sympathetic chain in the paravertebral space.[52] Each intercostal nerve supplies muscular branches to the intercostal muscles and lateral and anterior cutaneous branches to supply the skin of the chest and abdomen. The seventh to eleventh nerves pass below and behind the costal cartilages, between the slips of the diaphragm running between the internal oblique and transversus muscles (again between the second and third layers) to enter the posterior layer of the rectus sheath. They run deep into the rectus, pierce and supply it, and end as anterior cutaneous nerves supplying the middle of the front of the chest.

The lateral cutaneous branches emerge in the mid-axillary line, and divide into anterior and posterior branches which supply the skin on the lateral wall of the chest as far forward as the nipple line (Fig. 5.2.10).

Exceptions: the first intercostal nerve parts with most of its fibres to the brachial plexus. The lateral cutaneous branch of the second intercostal nerve crosses the axilla and becomes the intercostobrachial nerve supplying the skin on the medial aspect of the arm. The lateral cutaneous branch of the 12th thoracic nerve, which does not divide into anterior and posterior branches, crosses the iliac crest to supply the skin of the upper part of the buttock as far as the greater trochanter.

The 10th nerve, lateral and anterior cutaneous branches, supplies the area of the umbilicus.

The ninth, eighth and seventh nerves supply the skin between the umbilicus and the xiphisternum.

The 11th, 12th and first lumbar nerves supply the skin between the umbilicus and the pubis.

Technique

At the angle of the ribs: at this point the nerve becomes relatively superficial, lateral to the erector spinae muscle. In this technique the local analgesic solution tracking may block the rami communicantes conveying afferent impulses medially but splanchnic analgesia will be necessary in addition for intra-abdominal surgery. The patient is arranged in the lateral spinal position with the back well arched over the edge of the table. After swabbing with antiseptic and fixing sterile towels, two lines are drawn, one on each side four finger-breadths from the middle line, the lines should extend from the spines of the scapulae to the iliac crests. At a point where the lower border of the 11th rib on the patient's upper side crosses the line, a stimulating needle is introduced (through an intradermal weal if necessary) until it makes contact with the rib. It is then partially withdrawn and advanced until it slips past the lower border of the rib for 3 mm; 2–3 ml of local analgesic solution with adrenaline are then injected, while the needle point is slightly advanced and withdrawn so as to surround the nerve with analgesic solution. The needle should be attached to a syringe (so that should the pleura be punctured no air will enter the pleural cavity).

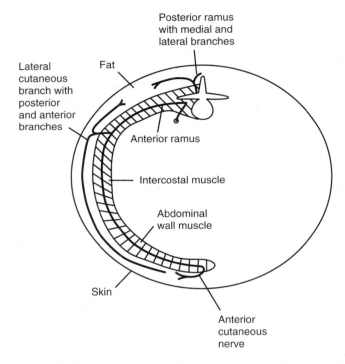

Figure 5.2.10 Oblique cross-section of body wall showing 10th intercostal nerve

The 10th to the 6th nerves are now injected on the upper side, followed, after turning, by the same nerves on the other side. The 12th nerves are deeper and require special care. Before the sixth and seventh nerves can be injected the patient's scapulae must be drawn laterally by crossing the arms over the chest. The needle pierces the trapezius, the latissimus dorsi and the two intercostal muscles. Bupivacaine or ropivacaine should produce good analgesia for up to 12 h.[53] For paramedian or midline incisions, bilateral block is necessary.[52] A possible complication is pneumothorax.

Posterior splanchnic block can be performed with the patient in the same position if the abdomen is to be opened without general anaesthesia.

A block in the mid-axillary line misses the lateral cutaneous nerve. Local analgesic solution injected via an extradural catheter can spread several spaces above and below the point of injection, external to the pleura.[54] Massive haematoma formation has been reported.[52]

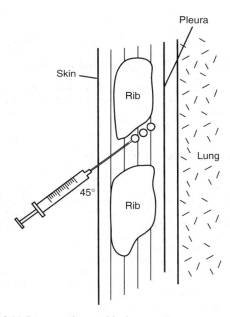

Figure 5.2.11 Intercostal nerve block

Indications

Blocking of the lower seven intercostal nerves on each side results in analgesia of the anterior abdominal wall from just below the nipple line to a level just above the pubic bone. In addition, it produces analgesia of the parietal peritoneum and relaxation of the muscles of the anterior abdominal wall.

Although intercostal block is useful in enabling deep breathing and coughing to take place in patients with postoperative abdominal pain or with fractured ribs it does not always produce good results.[55]

Blood levels of local analgesic solutions injected near the intercostal nerves rise rapidly.

Freezing an intercostal nerve within the thorax using a cryoprobe is now rarely used to reduce post-thoracotomy pain.

It has been proposed that more complications follow intercostal nerve block performed from inside the thorax than percutaneously.[56]

Intercostal block for rib resection and insertion of a drain

The surgeon is asked to mark out the position of the incision, and it is infil-trated intradermally and subcutaneously with 0.5–1% lignocaine solution.

An intradermal and subcutaneous line of infiltration is carried out one rib above and one below the length of rib to be removed. Their lines extend 2.5 cm in front and 2.5 cm behind the proposed incision, and the extremities are joined by intradermal and subcutaneous infiltrations, so that a rectangle is marked out. The intercostal nerves within this rectangle are blocked at their posterior extremities (Fig. 5.2.11).

Local block is usually the preferred method of anaesthesia in these operations. Patients who are well enough should sit sideways across the table, to prevent them drowning in their own pus if the abscess ruptures into a bronchus.

Interpleural block for intercostal nerves[57-60]

The analgesic solution is given as a single injection, or as an infusion through a cannula inserted between the ribs into the pleural space. Identifying the pleural space without causing a pneumothorax requires care. A skin weal is raised just above a rib (at the angle of the rib, or in the axillary line). A semi-blunt needle, e.g. Tuohy, attached to a saline- or local analgesic-filled syringe is inserted and loss of resistance used to identify the interpleural space. Spontaneous respiration makes puncture of the lung less likely at this point. The needle hub is occluded beween detaching the syringe and inserting the catheter, to prevent air rushing in. Various systems are available for this. Twenty millilitres of 0.5% bupivacaine or ropivacaine will produce a block lasting up to 4 h. Continuous infusion is less effective than intermittent injection, possibly due to regional interpleural pressure profiles (Fig. 5.2.12).

The technique is frequently used to control postcholecystectomy pain,[61] and after other abdominal operations. It has been used in chronic pain.[62]

Toxic effects are rare after boluses of 20 ml of 0.5% bupivacaine or ropivacaine.

Complications

Pneumothorax, damage to intercostal vessels during insertion, toxic signs of abnormally rapid absorption of drug from pleural space.[63,64]

ABDOMEN AND PERINEUM

Abdominal field block

Sensory nerve supply of abdominal wall: see spinal nerves, above.

Vessels of the abdominal wall: the only vessels likely to be injured by the anaesthetist are the superior and inferior epigastric arteries and veins. The superior artery is the termination of the internal mammary and enters the rectus sheath posterior to the seventh costal cartilage. The inferior epigastric artery arises from the external iliac artery and enters the rectus sheath behind the arcuate line of Douglas.

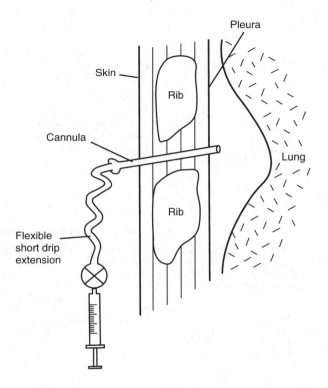

Figure 5.2.12 Interpleural block

Surface markings: the xiphoid is on a level with the body of T9. The subcostal plane is at L3. The highest part of the iliac crest is on a level with L4 or the L4–L5. interspace.

Technique

In all operations performed under field block analgesia it is necessary to infiltrate the line of incision both subcutaneously and intradermally. The injections should be commenced 15–20 min before the incision is to be made.

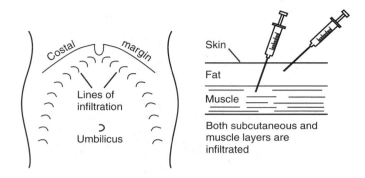

Figure 5.2.13 Subcostal abdominal field block

SUBCOSTAL BLOCK OF ABDOMINAL WALL FOR LAPAROTOMY (COSTO-ILIAC BLOCK)

This is an extremely easy, quick and useful block for all types of laparotomy, to enhance relaxation and give postoperative pain relief.

Weals are raised on each side along the costal margin and vertically downward to the iliac crest. Solution is deposited, from needles passed through these weals, into the subcutaneous and muscular layers of the abdominal wall, remembering that laterally the intercostal nerves lie between the transversalis and internal oblique. The weals are joined together by subcutaneous and intramuscular infiltration, using a long needle (50–100 mm). In addition, solution can be injected into the rectus sheath. The volume of solution required is 20–40 ml (Fig. 5.2.13).

NERVE BLOCK FOR UMBILICAL HERNIORRAPHY

A more localized version of the subcostal block may be used. An inverted V-shaped infiltration of analgesic is made above and at the sides of the hernia in both the subcutaneous and muscular layers of the abdominal wall (from one entry point, if a 9 cm needle is used). More local analgesic may need to be injected into the peritoneal sac by the surgeon. Excellent for postoperative analgesia.

RECTUS-SHEATH BLOCK

An excellent method of producing muscular relaxation when combined with a light general anaesthetic, and if the incision is to be midline or paramedian it is usual to do both sides. Perforation of the peritoneum should be avoided, but in the absence of peritonitis or adhesions no serious harm is likely to result. The anterior layer of the rectus sheath is often leathery and easily detected by the needle throughout its whole extent, but the posterior layer only for about 7.5 cm above and below the umbilicus. Solution is placed between rectus muscle and the posterior rectus sheath. If the abdomen shows the scar of a previous operation, abdominal field block may be difficult as the sole anaesthetic, and intercostal block or paravertebral block may be indicated if the operation is to be performed under local analgesia.

Intermittent injection or infusion through a small plastic catheter in each sheath can be used to produce good postoperative analgesia for midline incisions.

Abdominal field block renders the abdominal wall and its underlying parietal peritoneum insensitive. To block pain impulses from the viscera, and posterolateral parietal peritoneum, either light general anaesthesia or a splanchnic block and posterior intercostal and vagal block, is required.

Regional analgesia for intra-abdominal surgery is popular as an adjunct to general anaesthesia, giving greatly enhanced abdominal relaxation, and excellent postoperative analgesia. In remote and difficult situations, it enables much reduced concentrations of ether, with few side-effects.

Ilioinguinal block for repair of inguinal hernia

Anatomy

The nerve supply of the inguinal region is from the last two thoracic and the first two lumbar nerves via the iliohypogastric, the ilio-inguinal and the genitofemoral.

The last two thoracic nerves run downwards and inwards, just above the anterior superior iliac spine, between the internal oblique and transversus muscles. They end by piercing the rectus sheath.

The iliohypogastric and ilio-inguinal nerves come from the first lumbar root. They are inferior to the last two thoracic nerves and curve round the body just above the iliac crest, gradually piercing the muscles and ending superficially; the ilio-inguinal nerve traverses the inguinal canal, lying anterior to the spermatic cord, and becomes superficial through the external ring and supplies the skin of the scrotum. The iliohypogastric nerve, after running between the internal oblique and the transversus abdominis, pierces the internal oblique just above the anterior superior iliac spine and supplies the skin over the pubis.

The genitofemoral nerve comes from the first and second lumbar nerves and divides into a genital and a femoral branch. The former enters the inguinal canal from behind through the internal ring.

Indications

1 To avoid the risks of general anaesthesia or the possible risks of hypotension associated with intra- or extradural analgesia in slim, elderly, poor-risk patients.
2 To reduce the risks of aspiration of intestinal contents in cases of strangulation, by having a fully awake patient (however, bowel resection usually requires general anaesthesia).

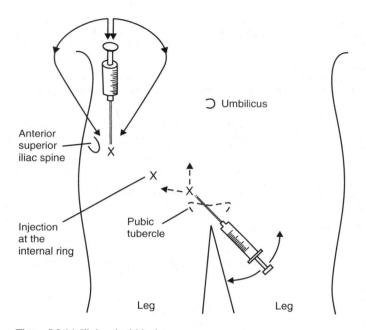

Figure 5.2.14 Ilioinguinal block

3 For day-stay surgery.[65]
4 For postoperative pain relief.
5 Used routinely by some surgeons.[66]

Contraindications to using the technique on its own

Obesity (successful block is very difficult in fat patients), coagulopathy, lack of cooperation by the surgeon, and nervousness of the patient.

Technique

Three weals are made as follows:

1 A finger-breadth internal to the anterior superior iliac spine.
2 Over the spine of the pubis.
3 One and a half centimetres above the mid-point of the inguinal ligament.

Through weal 1 a larger needle is introduced vertically backwards until it is felt to pierce the aponeurosis of the external oblique with a slight click.

After aspiration, 20–30 ml of solution are injected so that both the ilio-inguinal and iliohypogastric nerves are surrounded. At this point a needle introduced perpendicularly to the skin will not pierce the peritoneum. Solution is deposited in all layers including that small area of tissue between the weal and the anterior superior spine.

Through weal 2 a larger needle deposits solution in the intradermal and subcutaneous layers in the direction of the umbilicus. This blocks nerve twigs overlapping from the opposite side.

Through weal 3 a needle is inserted perpendicularly to the skin until it pierces the aponeurosis of the external oblique. At this level 20 ml of solution is injected so that the genital branch of the genitofemoral nerve is blocked. Note: this is immediately in front of the femoral artery!

Intradermal and subcutaneous infiltration along the line of the incision may be necessary to get perfect analgesia; in addition, infiltration of the periosteum near the pubic tubercle and Astley Cooper's ligament, the conjoint tendon and the lateral border of the rectus abdominis muscle should be performed in cases of direct inguinal hernia (Fig. 5.2.14).

The use of 0.5% solution of prilocaine with adrenaline allows a generous volume of relatively non-toxic local analgesic solution to be employed. Otherwise 0.25% bupivacaine or 0.5% lignocaine, both with adrenaline, are suitable. Dose of bupivacaine should not exceed 2 mg/kg. Mixing the analgesic with dextran 70 or 150 has been used to prolong local analgesic effect.[67]

If the hernia is strangulated or irreducible, the surgeon, under vision, should inject deeper layers, as he or she goes along.

The patient may complain of temporary discomfort when the neck of the sac is being dissected; this can often be relieved by infiltration of local analgesic solution around the neck. Infiltration analgesia is a perfectly acceptable method of pain relief in elective inguinal and femoral hernias and patients require less postoperative analgesia and vomit less than after general anaesthesia.[65,66]

A protocol, based on extensive surgical experience, for performing this operation under local analgesia has been described.[68] Preoperative weight reduction is advisable. Procaine 2% solution (for those over 70 years, 1–1.5%) without adrenaline; total volume 150 ml (i.e. a big dose); 80–100 ml subcutaneously with a further 10–20 ml beneath the external oblique aponeurosis, with a similar volume round the internal ring, avoiding the inferior epigastric vessels.

Advantages of regional analgesia: avoids the risks of general anaesthesia; makes the surgeon gentle; patient can cough during the operation if required; surgeon uses less tension in his sutures; patient can walk off the table and be treated as a day-stay case; and a quicker turn-round of cases.

Systemic absorption of local analgesic is measurable.[69]

Ilioinguinal block is helpful for postoperative analgesia.[70]

Complications

1 Haematoma.

2 Femoral nerve block, from tracking of solution back to the lumbar plexus, or forwards to the femoral nerve in the groin. (Weaker solutions, giving only sensory block, are used, so that if this complication occurs, the leg will not be paralysed for the duration of the analgesic.)

Field block for repair of femoral hernia

The technique is similar to that for repair of inguinal hernia, with the addition that the lump in the thigh is surrounded by subcutaneous and intradermal weals.

Paravertebral block from T10 to L3 may also be carried out; it is a suitable procedure for operation on strangulated inguinal and femoral herniae.

Iliac crest block

A weal is raised 4 cm from the anterior superior iliac spine on a line joining this spine to the xiphisternum. A needle is inserted laterally, first just beneath the skin and then deeper until the ilium is touched. Solution is injected so that it anaesthetizes the 12th thoracic, iliohypogastric and ilio-inguinal nerves as they lie between the internal oblique and the transversus abdominis muscles.

Field block for appendicectomy

This can be useful in interval cases, but is seldom successful in operation for acute appendicitis.

Two weals are raised, one just above and behind the anterior superior iliac spine, the second below the costal margin at the tip of the 10th rib on the right side. The tissues between the skin and peritoneum in this line are infiltrated, and subcutaneous infiltration is made between the two weals and downwards between the lower weal and the iliac bone. Thus, the 10th, 11th and 12th thoracic nerves are blocked, together with the ilio-inguinal and iliohypogastric.

Splanchnic block or topical lignocaine in the peritoneal cavity are usually necessary, except in the very simplest operations on thin subjects.

Field block for operations on the anal canal

A weal is made on each side of the anus and 2.5 cm away from it. From these weals a subcutaneous rhomboidal zone of infiltration is made, using 20 ml of 0.5% bupivacaine and adrenaline. Deep injections are now made from the infiltrated zone into each quadrant, 5 ml into each with a finger in the rectum preventing perforation of the mucous membrane. The nerve to the external anal sphincter is the perineal branch of the fourth sacral nerve. The operation can be done satisfactorily with the patient in the prone position with the pelvis raised. Premedication should be employed.

Penile block; field block for circumcision

Anatomy

The sensory nerves of the penis are derived from the terminal branches of the internal pudendal nerves. The dorsal nerves of the penis travel beneath the pubic bone, one on each side of the midline, lying against the dorsal surface of the corpus cavernosum. The skin at the base of the organ is supplied by the ilio-inguinal and perhaps the genitofemoral nerves. In addition, the posterior scrotal branches of the perineal nerves run para-urethrally to the ventral surface and fraenum, so four nerves have to be blocked.

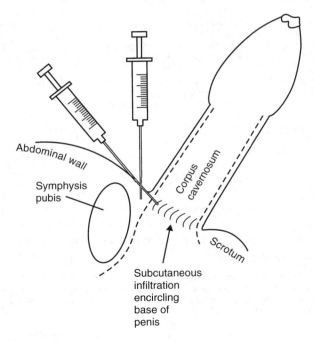

Figure 5.2.15 Penile block

This is a satisfactory alternative to extradural sacral block, with fewer complications.[71]

Technique

An intradermal and subcutaneous ring weal is raised around the base of the penis; the subcutaneous infiltration should precede the intradermal. The dorsal nerve is next blocked on each side by injecting 5 ml of solution into the dorsum of the organ just below but not deep to the symphysis so that the needle point lies against the corpus cavernosum. If the needle pierces the corpus cavernosum, pain is experienced and blood can be aspirated. For the ventral injection of the para-urethral branches, the penis should be pulled upwards and 2 ml of solution injected near the base of the organ into the groove formed by the corpora cavernosa and the corpus spongiosum. Infiltration of 5 ml of 1% plain lignocaine or 0.5% plain bupivacaine into each dorsal nerve provides good postoperative analgesia[72] (Fig. 5.2.15). In infants, smaller volumes are used. Postoperative pain can be relieved by repeated penile block in awake patients, even in children, without undue discomfort.[73,74]

Adrenaline must not be used lest necrosis of tissue results, as the arteries of the penis are end-arteries.

The smallest possible needle is used to prevent haematoma formation. If one begins, pressure is applied for 5 min to stop it. Subpubic injection must be avoided.[75]

Lignocaine spray, EMLA or amethocaine gel, applied topically gives useful relief for pain following circumcision.

Pudendal block

Injection is made through the lateral walls of the vagina above and below the ischial spines.

HIP AND LOWER EXTREMITY

Nerve block at the upper part of the thigh

Anatomy of lumbar plexus

The ventral rami of the lumbar nerves form the lumbar plexus lying in the psoas major, anterior to the transverse process of the lumbar vertebrae. A branch from the fourth unites with the fifth nerve to form the lumbosacral trunk which joins the sacral plexus.

The branches of the lumbar plexus are as follows.

The femoral nerve from L2, L3 and L4 (posterior divisions): passes between psoas and the iliacus, enters the thigh behind the inguinal ligament and just lateral to the femoral artery, from which it is here separated by a slip of the psoas major. It has anterior and posterior divisions, the latter giving rise to the saphenous nerve and the medial and intermediate cutaneous nerves of the thigh. The femoral nerve supplies the quadriceps, the femur, hip joint and knee joint, the skin of the anterior part of the thigh and the anteromedial part of the leg.

The obturator nerve from L2, L3 and L4 (anterior divisions): runs down the medial border of the psoas, pierces the obturator canal, and divides into anterior and posterior branches; the former supplies the adductor longus and brevis and the gracilis, with a twig going to the hip joint; the posterior branch supplies the adductor magnus and the hip joint. It supplies an area of skin on the medial aspect of the thigh and sends a small branch to the knee joint. An accessory obturator nerve is present in about 25% of people and runs a variable course across the superior pubic ramus and not via the obturator foramen; it comes from L3 and L4 (anterior divisions).

The iliohypogastric nerve from L1 leaves the psoas major, crosses the quadratus lumborum, perforates the transversus abdominis and then divides into lateral and anterior cutaneous branches. Its lateral cutaneous branch supplies the skin on the anterior part of the gluteal region after piercing the internal and external oblique muscles 5 cm behind the anterior superior iliac spine and just above the iliac crest, while the terminal part of the nerve supplies the skin over the pubic bone after piercing the aponeurosis of the external oblique, 2 cm medial to the anterior superior iliac spine.

The ilio-inguinal nerve from L1 accompanies the iliohypogastric nerve, in its early course, lying just inferior to it in close relationship to the iliac crest. It then passes with the spermatic cord through the inguinal canal and supplies the skin of the upper and medial part of the thigh and the adjacent skin covering the genitalia.

The genitofemoral nerve from L1 and L2: Travels with psoas to the groin. The genital branch supplies the skin of the scrotum or labium majus, and the cremaster muscle. The femoral branch supplies an area of skin on the middle of the anterior surface of the upper part of the thigh.

The lateral cutaneous nerve of the thigh from L2 and L3 (posterior divisions): supplies the skin of the anterolateral aspect of the thigh as far as the knee anteriorly, but laterally not quite so low after passing behind the inguinal ligament, just medial to the anterior superior iliac spine (Figs 5.2.16–17).

Femoral nerve block

A weal is raised a finger-breadth to the outer side of the femoral artery, just below the inguinal ligament. A needle is inserted for 3–4 cm so that the pulsations of the artery are transferred to the needle and 20 ml of analgesic are injected. The nerve lies beneath the deep fascia. Femoral nerve block, following injection of solution lateral and deep to the femoral artery, greatly reduces pain, following fractured neck of the femur during movement in adults and children.[76]

Sciatic and femoral nerve blocks in combination are useful in operations on the leg and foot from a point 5 cm below the patella. Operations on or above

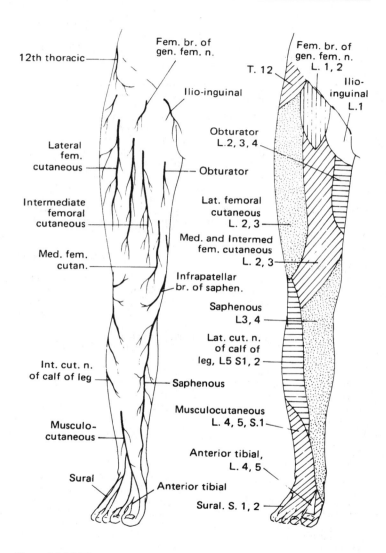

Figure 5.2.16 The cutaneous nerves and segmental distribution of the right lower extremity. Anterior aspect

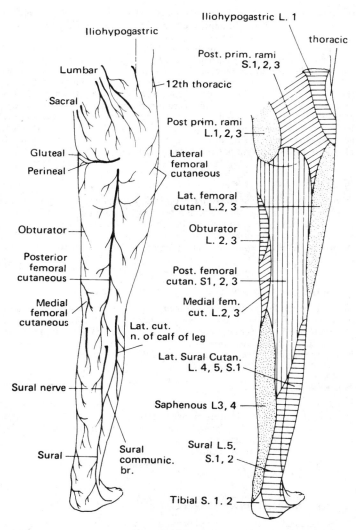

Figure 5.2.17 The segmental distribution of the cutaneous nerves of the right lower extremity. Posterior aspect (After *Gray's Anatomy* by kind permission.)

the knee require, in addition, lateral femoral cutaneous and obturator block, the latter being difficult. Manipulations of the lower half of the femur can, however, be carried out under sciatic and femoral block.

Nerve to quadratus femoris: this branch of the femoral nerve supplies the hip joint. To block it the patient is placed in the prone position with leg externally rotated. A line is drawn with a skin pencil joining the posterior superior iliac spine and the sacrococcygeal joint. The junction of the middle and lower thirds is marked. A weal is raised 5 cm posterior to the greater trochanter on a level with the lower end of the sacrum and a 14-cm 16-G needle inserted at 45 degrees to the horizontal towards the point previously marked until it hits bone. The needle point is worked medially 1–2 cm while 20 ml of solution are deposited along the flat surface of the body of the ischium. Useful for relief of pain in the hip joint in patients with osteoarthritis.

'Regional hip blockade'

Regional hip blockade involves injection into the region of the nerve to the quadratus femoris and the obturator nerve, with the aim of ameliorating severe pain due to osteoarthritis of the hip joint. Some workers have found the block of doubtful utility.[77]

(Some pain relief also follows the injection into the hip joint of 10 ml of 0.5% bupivacaine.)[78]

The 'three-in-one block' (inguinal perivascular block)[79]

Injection of 25–40 ml of solution into the region of the femoral nerve and psoas muscle, from just below the inguinal ligament, will block the femoral, obturator and lateral femoral cutaneous nerves. The analgesic travels up to the lumbar plexus in the substance of psoas. Useful together with sciatic block for analgesia of the leg (Fig. 5.2.18).

Saphenous nerve block

This is the terminal branch of the femoral nerve and becomes subcutaneous immediately below the sartorius muscle at the medial side of the knee joint; it accompanies the long saphenous vein to the medial malleolus. It can be blocked by a subcutaneous injection of 10–15 ml of local analgesic solution in the close vicinity of the vein just below the knee joint, taking care to avoid intravenous injection. Useful for long saphenous vein stripping under regional analgesia.

Lateral cutaneous nerve of thigh block[80]

A weal is raised one finger-breadth below and medial to the anterior superior spine of the ilium. A needle is inserted perpendicularly to the skin and local analgesic is deposited between the skin and the iliac bone and along the pelvic brim for two finger-breadths internally to the anterior superior spine;

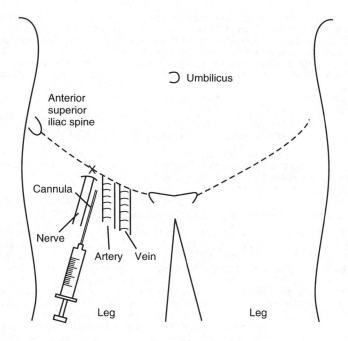

Figure 5.2.18 Three-in-one block

10–15 ml of solution are used. The nerve lies deep to the fascia lata of the thigh.

When associated with femoral block, adequate analgesia is produced for taking skin grafts from the front of the thigh. Alternatively, infiltration analgesia of the skin of the front of the thigh can be performed, using intra-dermal and subcutaneous injections to cover the desired area.

Obturator nerve block

Block is required for operations involving the knee joint, the medial aspect of the thigh, and may be necessary to make application of an arterial tourniquet above the knee tolerable.

With a nerve stimulator, the nerve is located as it lies in the obturator canal below the superior ramus of the pubis, between the pectineus and the obturator externus.

A weal is raised 1 cm below and lateral to the pubic tubercle and through it a 8–10-cm needle is inserted to meet the body of the pubic bone. The point is now moved gently laterally until it enters the obturator foramen. Stimuli or jerks indicate proximity to the nerve. Ten millilitres of solution are injected. An additional similar volume is finally injected as the needle is withdrawn. Successful block is shown by weakness when the patient attempts to adduct the leg.

It can also be used for the treatment of pain in the region of the hip joint or of adductor spasm.

LOCAL INFILTRATION FOR NAILING ETC. A FRACTURED NECK OF FEMUR

The line of incision is infiltrated down to the bone with 0.5% lignocaine or 1:2000 amethocaine. Solution is injected between the ends of the fractured neck from above the great trochanter and from a point just external to the pulsating femoral artery.

Psoas compartment block (lumbar plexus block)[81]

A single injection of solution or serial injections through a catheter introduced via an insulated stimulating needle from a weal 5 cm lateral to the upper border of the fourth lumbar vertebra (in the middle of a triangle made by the spines, the 12th rib, and the iliac crest). The 10-cm needle is inserted perpendicularly to the skin until contact with the transverse process is made. It is then partially withdrawn and glided over the transverse process. When the nerve stimulator produces stimuli or jerks, 40 ml of 0.25% bupivacaine solution are placed within the Psoas compartment (Figs 5.2.19–20). This is said to be safe and is recommended for surgery of the hip and knee, including arthroplasty together with light general anaesthesia.[82] It is excellent for postoperative analgesia. This is a useful block in the management of fractured femur before, during and after operation and during transport. The three-in-one block achieves the same result.

ANATOMY OF SACRAL PLEXUS

The sacral plexus is composed of the lumbosacral trunk (L4 and L5) and the ventral rami of the upper four sacral nerves. They lie on the posterior wall of the pelvic cavity between the piriformis and the pelvic fascia and have in front the ureter, internal iliac vessels, and the sigmoid colon on the left.

The following branches are given off.

The sciatic nerve (L4 and L5; S1–S3) supplies the skin at the back of the leg and sole of the foot. It leaves the pelvis through the greater sciatic foramen, and occupies the space between the ischial tuberosity and the greater trochanter. It supplies the back of the thigh. At or near the popliteal fossa it splits into:

1 the tibial nerve, which gives origin to the sural, supplies the back of the calf and divides near the ankle into the medial and lateral plantar branches, supplying the sole of the foot;

2 the common peroneal nerve, which crosses the neck of the fibula, supplying the peroneal compartment. From it originate the deep (anterior tibial) and superficial peroneal (musculocutaneous) nerves, supplying the front of the foot.

The pudendal nerve leaves the pelvis through the greater sciatic foramen, crosses the ischial spine medial to the pudendal vessels and goes through the lesser sciatic foramen. With the pudendal vessels it passes upwards and forwards along the lateral wall of the ischiorectal fossa, in Alcock's canal, a sheath of the obturator fascia. It supplies:

1 the external anal sphincter and the skin around the anus;
2 the scrotum or labium majus;
3 the penis, clitoris, vagina;
4 visceral branches supplying the rectum and bladder, from the second, third and fourth sacral nerves;
5 the pelvic splanchnic nerves supplying bladder, prostate, rectum and anus. The fourth sacral nerve supplies the levator ani and the coccygeus, and also the external anal sphincter.

The posterior femoral cutaneous nerve (S1–S3) supplies the skin of the lower part of the gluteal region, the perineum and the back of the thigh and leg.
The perforating cutaneous nerve (S2 and S3) supplies the skin over the medial and lower parts of the gluteus maximus.

Sciatic nerve block[83]

POSTERIOR APPROACHES

The patient lies on sound side with hip slightly flexed. *A nerve stimulator is attached to a 100-mm insulated needle.*
Technique:

1 A line connecting the sacral hiatus with the most prominent part of the greater trochanter is drawn and a weal raised at its mid-point. The needle is inserted at right angles to the skin and down to touch the bone at the back of the acetabulum. Through it 10–15 ml of plain local analgesic is injected.
2 A line is traced between the upper extremity of the great trochanter and the posterior superior iliac spine. From mid-point of this line a perpendicular is dropped 3–5 cm long, and at its end a weal is raised and a needle introduced at right angles to the skin plane until it reaches the ischial spine, 5–7.5 cm from the skin surface. The nerve lies on this area of bone so that stimuli or jerks must be elicited before the needle strikes bone; 10–15 ml of plain analgesic is then injected. Intraneural injection is painful and undesirable.
3 A surface marking is the junction of the medial third with the lateral two-thirds of a line joining the ischial tuberosity to the greater femoral trochanter – the needle being inserted at right angles to the skin surface until stimuli or jerks are felt (Fig. 5.2.21).

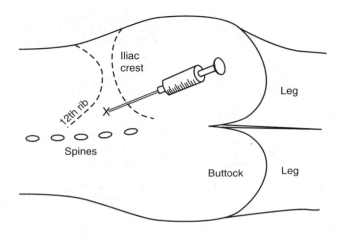

Figure 5.2.19 Landmarks for Psoas compartment block

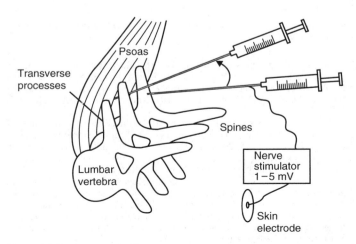

Figure 5.2.20 Approach to Psoas compartment

The block is useful for reduction of fractures around the ankle, combined if necessary with a saphenous nerve block just below the knee joint as it accompanies the long saphenous vein. It can be used together with femoral block for ligation of varicose veins on the front of the leg.

An alternative for operations below the knee is injection into the region of the tibial and common peroneal nerves in the popliteal fossa, and the saphenous nerve adjacent to the knee.

A peripheral nerve stimulator is essential for accuracy here.

The block also causes vasoconstrictor paralysis of the foot. A rise in skin temperature starts in 10 min and is maximal in 20–30 min. Sciatic nerve block gives analgesia of the whole foot with the exception of an area of skin over the medial malleolus supplied by the saphenous branch of the femoral nerve. The pain caused by gangrene of the foot has been relieved by continuous sciatic nerve block in which a catheter was inserted into the neurovascular sheath by the posterior approach.[84]

ANTERIOR APPROACH[85]

This may be useful when the patient cannot be easily moved from the supine position and when intervention on the foot or lower leg is required. Other nerve blocks in the leg may be combined with it. The stimulating insulated needle passes between the sartorius laterally and the rectus femoris medially and reaches the sciatic nerve close to the posteromedial edge of the femur, below the lesser trochanter.

For technique of lateral approach with the patient supine *see* Dalens B. et al. *Anesth. Analg.* 1990, **70,** 131.

Regional analgesia for the knee

This is not easy and often not satisfactory unless a spinal block is performed. 'L3 supplies the knee.'

Methods:

1 lumbar plexus and sciatic block;
2 Biers block (large doses needed);
3 intra- and extradural analgesia;[86]
4 for arthroscopy of the knee – femoral and lateral femoral cutaneous nerve block has been recommended;[87]
5 Doppler localization of the popliteal artery combined with nerve localization with a peripheral nerve stimulator facilitates block of the sciatic, tibial, peroneal and geniculate nerves in the politeal fossa.[88]

Ankle block

A subcutaneous and intradermal weal is raised circumferentially around the ankle just above the medial malleolus. *Five nerves must be blocked.*

The deep peroneal (anterior tibial; S1 and S2): blocked by inserting a needle midway between the most prominent points of the medial and lateral malleoli, on the circular line of infiltration in front of the ankle joint. It is directed medially towards the anterior border of the medial malleolus and solution is injected between the bone and the skin; nerve stimulation should be used if possible. Instead of blocking this nerve at the ankle, its parent trunk, the common peroneal nerve, can be blocked at the neck of the fibula where it can be rolled under the finger: the only palpable nerve in the leg. It supplies the skin on adjacent sides of the first and second toes, dorsal aspect. The amount of solution used should be 10–15 ml.

The superficial peroneal (musculocutaneous, S1 and S2): a branch from the common peroneal nerve, can be blocked immediately above the ankle joint by a subcutaneous weal extending from the front of the tibia to the lateral malleolus. It supplies the dorsum of the foot (with the exception of the small area innervated by the tibial nerve).

The sural nerve (L5; S1 and S2): formed with branches from the tibial and common peroneal nerves and descends with the short saphenous vein below and posterior to the lateral malleolus to supply the outer part of the foot and heel. It is blocked by subcutaneous infiltration between the tendo Achillis and the prominence of the lateral malleolus, using 5–10 ml of solution.

The saphenous nerve (L3 and L4): this is the terminal branch of the femoral nerve and accompanies the long saphenous vein anterior to the medial malleolus where it can be blocked by the injection of 10 ml of local analgesic solution. It supplies an area of skin just below and above the media malleolus.

The tibial nerve (S1 and S2) passes behind the medial malleolus to divide into medial and lateral plantar nerves after giving off the medial calcaneal

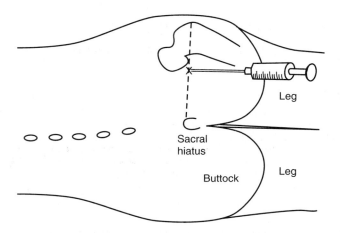

Figure 5.2.21 Bryce-Smith approach to sciatic nerve block

branch. With the patient in the prone position it is blocked by 10 ml of solution introduced through a point on the circular weal just internal to the tendo Achillis, deep to the flexor retinaculum near the palpable posterior tibial artery. It is easiest with the patient lying prone. The needle is inserted forwards and slightly outwards towards the posterior aspect of the tibia, near which the solution is deposited.

Tibial block alone is useful for testing for potential vasodilatation of the foot.

Block for hallux valgus

A weal is raised near the proximal end of the first intermetatarsal space, superior surface, and, from this, solution is deposited between the two layers of skin, dorsal and plantar, as far forwards as the web between the toes. More solution is injected between the dorsal skin and the first metatarsal bone. A second weal medial to the first one, on the internal aspect of the metatarsal, is raised, and injection made between it and the bone between the plantar skin and the bone. A 10–15-min pause is made before the operation is commenced. From 15 to 20 ml of solution are used (e.g. 1–1.5% lignocaine).

Local analgesia of the foot[89]

Sole of the foot

Supplied by the medial (L4 and L5) and lateral (S1 and S2) plantar branches of the tibial nerve, supplying the media and lateral anterior part of the sole; the sural nerve supplying the posterior and lateral part of the sole and heel; and the tibial nerve (S1 and S2) supplying the medial part of the heel. Calcaneal branches of the tibial nerve supply the plantar surface of the heel, but not by the sural nerve.

Dorsum of the foot

Supplied by medial terminal branch of deep peroneal nerve (the adjacent sides of the first and second toes). The sural innervates the lateral side of the fifth toe, the superficial peroneal supplies the remainder. Mid-tarsal block for surgery of the forefoot (*see* Sharrock N. E. et al. *Br. J. Anaesth.* 1986, **58,** 37).

Medial side of the foot: supplied by saphenous nerve from the femoral nerve. Also from the medial plantar branch of the tibial nerve.

Lateral side of the foot: supplied by sural nerve from the tibial and common peroneal, which goes to fifth toe and lateral side of foot.

Ring block of the toe

Lignocaine plain, 1.5 ml of 2% solution, to be injected into each side of the proximal phalanx near its base. Injection from dorsal aspect with small amount of solution across from side to side. After an interval of 7–10 min the operation can commence.

Local analgesia for reduction of closed fractures

After localizing the exact site of fracture by means of X-rays, a weal is raised near the fracture and a needle introduced into the haematoma between the broken bone ends. *Full aseptic technique must be perfect.* Aspiration of old blood confirms the position and must be obtained: injection is then made of 1.5 or 2% lignocaine without adrenaline. Colles' fracture the amount required is 15–20 ml; injection should be made from the extensor aspect of the wrist and, in addition, a few millilitres should infiltrate the ulnar styloid. The method is easier, quicker and does not carry the possible risks of intravenous local analgesia; although pain relief is superior with the latter. For Pott's fracture, 10–20 ml of solution with hyaluronidase can be used; for fractured femur, 20–30 ml. These are high doses so the possibility of toxic signs must be borne in mind. Cases of recent fracture are the most suitable for this method of reduction, especially fractures of the metatarsal or metacarpal bones. Good results are claimed for the addition of 1000 units of hyaluronidase to each 20 ml of solution. With lignocaine, analgesia comes on after 10 min. and lasts 2–3 h. This technique does not produce complete pain relief but may be employed when dealing with mass casualities or when anaesthetists are not available.

BLOCKS OF THE SYMPATHETIC NERVOUS SYSTEM

Sympathetic block is most commonly carried out:

1 in the neck (stellate ganglion block);
2 in the upper and lower limbs (intravenous sympathetic block);
3 in the lumbar region (L1–L4);
4 in the abdomen (splanchnic or coeliac plexus block).

Stellate ganglion block[90]

The stellate ganglion is formed by the fusion of the lowest of the three cervical ganglia with the first thoracic ganglion. It is irregular in size and position, being usually 13 cm long, and differs in the same individual on the two sides.

Stellate ganglion block is also referred to as cervicothoracic sympathetic block, because when 10–15 ml of analgesic solution is injected into the correct plane at the base of the neck, the middle cervical, stellate and the second, third and usually the fourth thoracic ganglia and their rami are blocked. This results in interruption of all sympathetic fibres to most of the thorax, head, neck and arm (except possibly the nerve of Kuntz). Certain visceral afferent fibres are also blocked, e.g. the cervical cardiac nerves.

The stellate ganglion may be blocked by spill-over from supraclavicular brachial plexus block.

Anatomy

The cervical sympathetic chain and its three ganglia lie in front of the head of the first rib and the seventh cervical and first thoracic transverse process, just behind the subclavian artery and origin of the vertebral artery. It lies posterior to the carotid sheath on the longus colli and longus cervicis muscles. It is anterior to the eighth cervical and first thoracic nerves, so paraesthesia involving these nerves shows, if stellate ganglion block is done from the front, that the needle is too deeply placed. On the right side, the apex of the lung and the dome of the pleura are anterior relations; on the left side these structures are 2.5 cm lower and so are not in such close relationship to the ganglion. Vasoconstrictor fibres pass from the stellate and the other cervical sympathetic ganglia to a plexus around the carotid arteries. Branches from the second and sometimes also from the third thoracic sympathetic ganglion often go directly to the upper extremity via the first thoracic nerve, thus bypassing the stellate ganglion (the nerve of Kuntz). But this nerve is usually blocked by spread of the analgesic solution down to the region of the fourth thoracic ganglion.

It sends grey rami to the seventh and eighth cervical nerves, gives origin to the inferior cervical cardiac nerve, and supplies branches to the vessels in its vicinity. It may communicate with the vagus.

Its most frequent indication is to release vascular tone, and it may need to be repeated several times.

Postganglionic sympathetic fibres are also distributed to the arm with the somatic nerves of the brachial plexus and are distributed from them to the vessels, supplying vasoconstrictor impulses to the whole limb.

Indications

1 Sympathetic block of head, neck and upper limb (e.g. after intra-arterial thiopentone).
2 It has been used to treat acute deafness[91] and quinine blindness.[92,93]
3 Has been used for relief of the acute pain due to herpes zoster ophthalmicus.[94]
4 Chronic pain, e.g. complex regional pain syndrome.[95]

Technique

Block of right and left ganglia should not be carried out at the same time.

1 *Paratracheal approach:*[96] the patient lies supine, chin forwards, neck extended without a pillow. A weal is raised two finger-breadths lateral to the suprasternal notch and a similar distance above the clavicle, which is on the medial border of the sternomastoid overlying the transverse process of the seventh cervical vertebra. The position can be checked by palpating

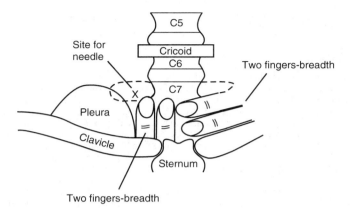

Figure 5.2.22 Stellate ganglion block; paratracheal approach

the tubercle of Chassaignac (difficult) or the cricoid cartilage, both of which
are at the level of the sixth cervical transverse process, i.e. a little higher
than the weal. A fine 5–8-cm needle is inserted directly backwards through
the weal, while downward and backward pressure is exerted on the sternomastoid to draw the muscle and the carotid sheath laterally. When contact
is made with bone (C7) the needle is withdrawn 0.5–1 cm so that its point
lies in front of the longus colli muscle and, after careful aspiration for blood
(the vertebral artery is very near) and for cerebrospinal fluid, 15–20 ml of
0.5% lignocaine or similar solution are injected. This will, if correctly
placed, diffuse up and down in the fascial plane and will block the ganglia
and rami from C2 to T4 inclusive. Thirty minutes may elapse before
Horner's syndrome and vasodilatation of the arm appear (Fig. 5.2.22).

2 *Anterior approach* (Apgar).[97]
3 *Lateral approach* (Goinard).[98]
4 *Posterior approach.*
5 *Tissue displacement method.*[99]

Signs of successful block

1 Horner's syndrome: miosis, enophthalmos and ptosis. This does not
   guarantee sympathetic paralysis of the vessels of the arm.
2 Flushing of the cheek, face and neck and arm. Engorged veins of arm.
   Increase in skin temperature.
3 Flushing of the conjunctiva and sclera.
4 Anhidrosis of the face and neck.
5 Lacrimation.
6 Stuffiness of the nostril (Guttmann's sign).
7 Mueller's syndrome: injection of tympanic membrane and warmth of face.

Sympathetic block can be assessed by the cobalt blue and ninhydrin sweat tests which are more informative than the sympatho-galvanic response.[100]

Complications and dangers of the block

1 Stellate ganglion block performed on a patient with a coagulopathy may result in a large haematoma in the deep planes of the neck.
2 Perforation of the oesophagus, with infection.
3 Intrathecal injection causing a total spinal block.
4 Intravascular injection, e.g. sending volume of solution via the vertebral artery straight up to the medulla.
5 Pneumothorax.
6 Cardiac arrest – very rare, although it has resulted from surgical cervicothoracic sympathectomy (a permanent stellate block).[101]
7 Alteration of voice from recurrent laryngeal nerve block.
8 Phrenic nerve block.
9 Brachial plexus block.
10 Extradural or intradural block.
11 Mediastinitis.
12 Intercostal neuralgia.[102]

Intravenous sympathetic block

Guanethidine 10–20 mg with 500 units of heparin in 25 ml of saline is injected intravenously in the exsanguinated limb with tourniquet and left in place for 20–30 min. Arterial pressure readings are made at minute intervals when the tourniquet is released. If hypotension occurs during the next 20–30 min, an intravenous infusion and vasoconstrictor may be injected via the indwelling needle in the other arm.

Used to reduce chronic pain *see* Chapter 6.1; a form of regional blockade.[103]

Lumbar sympathetic block

Surgical lumbar sympathectomy was first described in 1934. A technique using phenol dissolved in a radio-opaque medium and an image intensifier has been used.[104]

Anatomy

The sympathetic trunk in the lumbar region consists of four ganglia and their interconnecting fibres. It lies on the anterolateral aspect of the bodies of the lumbar vertebrae, immediately medial to the psoas muscle, which fills the triangular space between the vertebral bodies and the transverse processes. A tendinous arch, which gives part origin to the psoas muscle, connects the upper and lower borders of each lumbar vertebra and forms a tunnel around the side of the bone in which the lumbar vessels and the grey ramus communicans run. The lumbar arteries are posterior but the veins may be anterior. The fatty tissue occupying this tunnel is an extension of that in the extradural space and it passes through the intervertebral foramina as far forward as the sympathetic chain. The chain lies in a fascial plane bounded by the vertebral column, the psoas sheath and the parietal peritoneum. L1 is on a level with the intersection of the last rib and the outer border of the erector spinae. The L4/L5 interspace corresponds to the highest point of the iliac crests in many patients.

In the sacral region, each chain consists of four ganglia with intervening fibres lying medial to the anterior sacral foramina. Preganglionic fibres (white rami) are derived from the anterior primary rami from T4 to T12 and each ganglion gives off a grey ramus to the corresponding sacral nerve, to supply sympathetic innervation to the lower limbs. On the coccyx, the two chains unite to form the ganglion impar.

Disturbances of function of the sympathetic nervous system can produce vasospasm, pain and visceral dysfunction. Sympathetic block can remedy all of these, either temporarily, for diagnosis, or permanently, by interrupting a vicious circle.

Indications

See Chapter 6.1.

Technique

Use of X-ray control with an image intensifier greatly adds to the accuracy of needle placement.

Posterior approach:[105] the patient is placed in the prone position, with two pillows flexing the lumbar spine, or in lateral spinal position with the affected side uppermost and the spine flexed. He or she should be premedicated with a sedative. The procedure can be carried out in the patient's bed if necessary.

Skin weals are raised at points 5 cm lateral to the upper borders of the spinous processes of the second, third and fourth lumbar vertebrae. Successful injection at these points blocks all the vasoconstrictor impulses to the lower limb. These points lie immediately above the transverse processes of the corresponding vertebrae. A 12–16-cm needle is introduced through each weal at right angles to the skin for 4–5 cm and should encounter the transverse process; it is slightly withdrawn and directed upwards so that it passes between the transverse processes; it is also directed slightly inwards. After travelling 3–4 cm from the transverse process, the needle should make contact with the anterolateral aspect of the body of the vertebra. After careful aspiration to exclude both blood and cerebrospinal fluid, 10 ml of 1% lignocaine are injected at each site. (If force is required, needle tip is in anterior vertebral ligament or the psoas muscle and should be slightly withdrawn.) It spreads out in the retroperitoneal tissue. The spinal lumbar nerves run midway between the spinous processes, so if the needle point is kept in relation to the upper border of the transverse process, pain from hitting a nerve should be avoided. The lumbar arteries, branches of the aorta, with their veins must also be avoided. After 5–20 min the leg becomes less painful, its temperature increases and it becomes dry, its superficial veins dilate, and there is hyposensitivity to pin-prick.

Results of chemical lumbar sympathectomy can be assessed by taking infra-red thermograms before and after the injections.[106]

Complications

1 Intradural injection and spinal analgesia.
2 Intravascular injection.
3 Hypotension.
4 Haemorrhage into the sheath of the psoas muscle with pain referred to the groin and upper and inner part of the thigh.
5 Neuritis of the genitofemoral nerve.
6 Caudal block gives the same results but is not unilateral: it produces, in addition to sympathetic paralysis, motor paresis and analgesia which may be useful objective signs of successful sympathetic block.

Coeliac plexus block; splanchnic analgesia

Anatomy[107]

Semilunar or coeliac plexus: two in number, one on each side of the midline, lying on the aorta and the crura of the diaphragm just above the pancreas, at the level of the first lumbar vertebra between the adrenal glands and behind the stomach and lesser sac. The renal vessels are inferior to the plexus while the vessels to the adrenals often pass through it. They are connected with each other and with their associated ganglia (superior mesenteric and inferior mesenteric, etc.) by a network of nerve fibres around the coeliac artery. These fibres are postganglionic fibres of the greater and lesser splanchnic nerves. From this mass of retroperitoneal nerve tissue fibres pass with the arteries to the abdominal viscera. These plexuses also receive twigs from the right vagus and the phrenic nerves. The semilunar or coeliac ganglia with the aorticorenal and superior mesenteric ganglia together make up the solar or epigastric plexus.

Afferent fibres from the abdominal viscera, both sympathetic and parasympathetic (vagus), pass through the coeliac ganglia. Afferent fibres from the pelvic viscera, travelling through the nervi erigentes (S2–S4) do not.

Greater splanchnic nerve (the superior thoracic splanchnic nerve): like the lesser and the lowest splanchnic, is composed of pre-ganglionic fibres which are, in effect, elongated white rami. The majority of its fibres are myelinated. It rises from the union of four or five roots coming from the thoracic sympathetic ganglia which receive white rami from the fifth to the 10th thoracic nerves, sometimes higher. The nerve enters the abdomen through the crus of the diaphragm on each side, with the lesser and lowest splanchnic nerves, and enters the corresponding semilunar ganglion. It mainly contains visceral afferent fibres. Within the abdomen the nerve lies between the diaphragm and the adrenal gland on each side.

Lesser splanchnic nerve (the middle thoracic splanchnic nerve): this arises from the lower thoracic ganglia of the sympathetic cord, connected with the 10th and 11th thoracic nerves. It enters the corresponding aorticorenal ganglion.

Lowest splanchnic nerve (the inferior thoracic splanchnic nerve): this arises from the last thoracic ganglion and enters the renal plexus and the posterior renal ganglion.

The lumbar splanchnic nerves are presumably blocked when the coeliac plexus is blocked, by spreading of solution. The first lumbar splanchnic nerve arises from the first lumbar ganglion; the second from the second and third ganglia (they join the coeliac plexus): the third from the second, third and fourth ganglia; the fourth from the fourth and fifth ganglia. The last two join the superior hypogastric plexus.

The hypogastric nerve (presacral nerves) extends from the third lumbar vertebra to the first sacral where it ends by dividing into the right and left hypogastric nerves or plexuses. It lies in front of the lower part of the abdominal aorta, behind the peritoneum.

THE SUPERIOR HYPOGASTRIC PLEXUS

Formerly known as the presacral nerve. It is retroperitoneal, lying on the body of the fifth lumbar vertebra. It receives fibres from the sympathetic trunk via lumbar ganglia 3 and 4; fibres known as the intermesenteric plexus coming from the coeliac, mesenteric and pararenal plexuses; and parasympathetic fibres. From it are derived fibres supplying, via the inferior mesenteric artery the transverse, descending and sigmoid colon; the inferior hypogastric nerves to the rectum and ureters which contain both sympathetic and parasympathetic elements.

THE INFERIOR HYPOGASTRIC PLEXUS

A collection of ganglia and nerve fibres where preganglionic sympathetic fibres synapse. It receives fibres from the inferior hypogastric nerves, together with parasympathetic fibres and supplies the viscera of the female pelvis (except the ovaries). Its sympathetic element provides sensory and motor fibres to the urinary and anal sphincters; the parasympathetic fibres are motor to the bladder and rectum. These fibres travel with blood vessels.

Many of these structures are damaged in pelvic operations. Division of the superior hypogastric plexus (presacral neurectomy) is used in the treatment of dysmenorrhoea.

AFFERENT PATHWAYS FROM UPPER ABDOMINAL VISCERA

These visceral afferents travel from sensory nerve endings in the walls of the viscera, mesentery, etc. via the splanchnic nerves and enter the cord with the white rami of the lower seven thoracic nerves (and sometimes higher), having their cell stations in the posterior root ganglia of these nerves. Afferent impulses also travel up in the vagi and the phrenic nerves (e.g. from the gall bladder).

Visceral afferent fibres, travelling with the sympathetic, enter the cord at the following levels: stomach, T6–10; small gut, T9–10; large gut to middle of transverse colon T11–L1; distal colon, L1–2; liver and biliary tract T7–9; pancreas T6–10; kidney and ureter T10–L1–2; bladder and prostate T11–12; testis and ovary T10–11; uterus T10–11.

NERVE SUPPLY TO ADRENAL GLANDS

Preganglionic fibres do not synapse in coeliac or other pre-aortic plexuses, but pass directly to end around chromaffin cells of the medulla. In addition to the lesser splanchnic, fibres go to the adrenals from the 10th thoracic to second lumbar nerves.

Technique

Splanchnic block can be performed during laparotomy.[108] The liver is gently retracted upwards and the stomach is drawn to the left. The anterior aspect of the body of the first lumbar vertebra is located medial to the lesser curvature of the stomach; the aorta is retracted laterally and the long Braun needle is inserted down to the bone and 50 ml of solution injected (e.g. 0.5%ligno-caine).

Percutaneous method:[109] the patient is in the spinal position, sitting or lying prone. The fourth interspace is located, lying on or before the intercristal line; by counting upward, the spine of the first lumbar vertebra is identified. Weals are raised four finger-breadths from this spine, one in each side of the midline. The weals must be below the 12th rib.

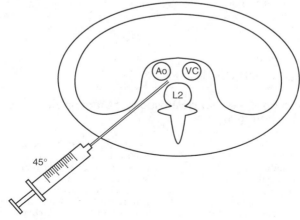

Figure 5.2.23 Coeliac plexus block

A 150-mm needle is inserted at an angle of 45 degrees to the median plane through this weal with its bevel facing inwards. It is directed slightly upwards and inserted under image intensifier control until it makes contact with the body of the first lumbar vertebra. It is then partly withdrawn and its point directed more laterally until its bevel is felt to glance past the lateral aspect of the body of the vertebra. The needle is then advanced a further 1 cm and, after a most careful aspiration test, 20–40 ml of solution are injected. The average distance between the skin and the plexus is 7–10 cm. If blood is aspirated into the syringe, the needle point may be in the vena cava or the aorta and must be moved until it is free of these vessels. Bilateral block is probably unnecessary. Computed tomography guided coeliac plexus block has been described.[110] Insertion of the needle at the level of L2 has been advocated (Fig. 5.2.23).

The usual strengths of solution employed are prilocaine, 0.5%; lignocaine, 0.5%; amethocaine, 1 : 2000 to 1 : 4000. Adrenaline should be added.

Splanchnic block causes a profound fall in blood pressure which can be partially controlled by an intravenous infusion of fluid or by ephedrine or one of its congeners, should it be considered necessary. It produces analgesia of the abdominal viscera, with the exception of the pelvic viscera, i.e. the sigmoid colon, rectum, bladder and reproductive organs. The bowel becomes contracted and ribbon-like. The patient must be particularly well premedicated, intravenous narcotic analgesic being given until his or her mental state is calm. The surgeon must be light-handed, especially when the peritoneal cavity is being explored, as its lateral walls are not rendered insensitive either by the splanchnic block or the abdominal field block (but by posterior intercostal block).

Therapeutically, splanchnic block is useful in the treatment of carcinoma of the pancreas.[111] The block may be repeated if desirable. It has also been used in the terminal stages of upper abdominal cancer to relieve pain. Alcohol in saline, 50%, preceded by local analgesic solution, has been employed. Paraplegia has followed this block.[112]

TOPICAL ANALGESIA

Topical analgesia for gastroscopy, fibreoptic endoscopy and oesophagoscopy

The patient is given a tablet of amethocaine (60 mg) or lignocaine to suck. Intravenous diazepam or midazolam may be necessary, 1 mg i.v. each minute until ptosis or dysarthria occurs. In cirrhotic patients, diazepam may result in hepatic coma. Chlormethiazole (Heminevrin) may be used instead in hypotensive patients. The gums, tongue, palate and pharynx are now sprayed with 4% lignocaine, 4% cocaine, 1% amethocaine or some other suitable analgesic solution. Patients can be given amethocaine hydrochloride 2% to gargle, or Xylocaine Viscous to swallow, a 2% solution in a mucilage base, very pleasantly flavoured. In active bleeding, topical analgesia increases the risk of aspiration.[113]

Gargling with 4% lignocaine makes the passage of the small fibreoptic endoscope tolerable in over 90% of patients, without premedication or intravenous sedatives.

Many operators have now discarded the use of local analgesia prior to fibreoptic gastroscopy, relying on the use of intravenous sedative and/or analgesic drugs alone.

Topical analgesia for fibreoptic intubation and bronchoscopy[114]

1 Uppermost zone (mouth or nose, pharynx): the gums, tongue, palate and pharynx are sprayed with lignocaine (e.g. 4%) on two occasions, a few minutes apart; or the glossopharyngeal nerve is blocked in the posterior pillar of the fauces.
2 Upper part of larynx:
   (a) spraying lignocaine at the epiglottis and the cords, blind or under direct vision using a laryngoscope;
   (b) after a short interval, the piriform fossae and the terminal twigs of the internal laryngeal nerve beneath its mucosa are made analgesic by application of swabs soaked in lignocaine, applied on Krause's laryngeal forceps;
   (c) the superior laryngeal nerve may be blocked percutaneously between the upper cornu of the laryngeal cartilage and the greater cornu of the hyoid.
3 Lower part of larynx and trachea:
   (a) spraying lignocaine through the glottis;
   (b) a needle or fine intravenous cannula is inserted through the cricothyroid membrane into the trachea. Aspiration of air confirms its position in the trachea. An injection of 2–3 ml of 4% lignocaine is now made after a deep expiration.
4 Extra O_2 is administered (via this cannula if necessary).
5 The patient is advised not to eat or drink for at least 3 h.

Topical analgesia of the peritoneal cavity

Lignocaine, 0.15%, or prilocaine, 0.25%, is used. Volume 200 ml. This is poured into the peritoneal cavity and the peritoneal edges are drawn together. After 5–8 min the solution is sucked out. Results: slackening of the peritoneum, contraction of the bowel, absence of reflex response from visceral trauma. Toxic reactions are said to be rare. Good results are not seen in cases of peritonitis or where the bowel is grossly distended.

REFERENCES

1 Edmunds D. H. and Rosen M. *Anaesthesia*, 1984, **39**, 138–142, 279. Austin T. R. *Anaesthesia* 1980, **35**, 391.
2 McClure J. H. et al. *Br. J. Anaesth.* 1983, **55**, 1089.
3 Montgomery M. B. et al. *Anesth. Analg.* 1973, **52**, 827; Raj P. P. et al. *Anesth. Analg.* 1973, **52**, 897; Zeh D. W. et al. *Anesth. Analg.* 1978, **57**, 13; Ford D. J. et al. *Anesth. Analg. (Cleve.)* 1984, **63**, 925.
4 Smith D. C. and Miah H. *Anesthesiology* 1985, **60**, 569.
5 Boulton T. B. *Anaesthesia* 1967, **22**, 101.
6 Cook J. H. *Ann. R. Coll. Surg.* 1987, **69**, 4.
7 Morris R. W. and Whish D. K. M. *Anaesth. Intensive Care* 1984, **12**, 113.
8 French A. J. and Patel Y. U. *Lancet* 1980, **2**, 482.
9 Fry R. A. and Henderson J. *Anaesthesia* 1990, **45**, 14.
10 Barton R. P. E. and Gray R. F. E. *J. Laryngol. Otol.* 1979, **93**, 1201.
11 Moffett A. J. *Anaesthesia* 1947, **2**, 31.
12 Curley R. K. et al. *Br. Dent. J.* 1987, **162**, 113.
13 Macht S. D. et al. *Surg. Gynecol. Obstet.* 1978, **146**, 87.
14 Takahashi T. and Dohi S. *Br. J. Anaesth.* 1983, **55**, 333.
15 Rovenstine E. A. and Papper E. M. *Am. J. Surg.* 1948, **75**, 713; Montgomery W. and Cousins M. J. *Br. J. Anaesth.* 1972, **44**, 383.
16 Barton S. and Williams J. D. *Arch. Otolaryngol.* 1971, **93**, 186.
17 Gaskill J. R. and Gillies D. R. *Arch. Otolaryngol.* 1966, **84**, 654; Gaskill J. R. *Arch. Otolaryngol.* 1967, **86**, 697; Coghlan C. J. *Anesth. Analg. Curr. Res.* 1966, **45**, 290; Young T. M. *Anaesthesia* 1976, **31**, 570.
18 Cooper M. and Watson R. L. *Anesthesiology* 1975, **43**, 377. Isaac P. A. et al. *Anaesthesia* 1990, **45**, 46.
19 Mushin W. W. and Macintosh R. R. *Proc. R. Soc. Med.* 1945, **38**, 308.
20 Wertheim H. M. and Rovenstine E. A. *Anesthesiology* 1941, **2**, 541; Milougky J. and Rovenstine E. A. *Anesthesiology* 1948, **9**, 76.
21 Macintosh R. R. and Mushin W. W. *Local Anaesthesia: Brachial Plexus*, 4th edn. Blackwell Scientific Publications, Oxford, 1967. (1st edn. 1943.)
22 Winnie A. P. *Plexus Anesthesia, Vol. 1.* Churchill Livingstone, Edinburgh, 1983.
23 Thompson G. E. and Rorie D. K. *Anesthesiology* 1983, **59**, 117.
24 Yasuda I. et al. *Br. J. Anaesth.* 1980, **52**, 409.
25 Randalls B. *Anaesthesia* 1990, **45**, 143.
26 Knoblanche G. E. *Anaesth. Intensive Care* 1979, **7**, 346.
27 Moraitis K. *Anaesthesia* 1977, **32**, 161.
28 Mulley K. *Beitr. z. Clin. Chirurg.* 1919, **114**, 666; Etienne J. (1925), *see* Vidal-Lopez F. *Anesth. Analg. (Cleve.)* 1977, **56**, 486; Winnie A. P. *Anesth. Analg. (Cleve.)* 1970, **49**, 455; Ward M. E *Anaesthesia* 1974, **29**, 147; Winnie A. P. *Surg. Clin. North Am.* 1975, **55**, 874; Vester-Andersen T. et al. *Acta Anaesth. Scand.* 1981, **35**, 81.
29 Labat G. *Br. J. Anaesth.* 1927, **4**, 174.
30 Winnie A. P. *Anesth. Analg. (Cleve.)* 1970, **49**, 455; Mathews P. J. and Hughes T. J. *Anaesthesia* 1983, **38**, 813.

31 Barutell C. et al. *Anaesthesia* 1980, **35,** 365.
32 Huang K. C. et al. *Anaesth. Intensive Care* 1986, **14,** 87.
33 Edde R. R. et al. *Anesth. Analg. (Cleve.)* 1977, **54,** 446.
34 Lim E. K. *Anaesthesia* 1979, **34,** 370.
35 Brockway M. S. and Wildsmith J. A. W. *Br. J. Anaesth.* 1990, **64,** 224.
36 Toumineu M. K. et al. *Anaesthesia* 1987, **42,** 20.
37 Parris M. R. and Chambers W. A. *Br. J. Anaesth.* 1986, **58,** 297.
38 Rosenblatt R. et al. *Anesthesiology* 1979, **51,** 565; Winnie A. P. *Surg. Clin. North Am.* 1975, **55,** 861.
39 Boures J. B. *Anaesthesia* 1984, **39,** 1250.
40 Bier A. *Arch. Klin. Chir.* 1908, **86,** 1007 (translated and reprinted in 'Classical File', *Surv. Anesthesiol.* 1967, **11,** 294).
41 Rhys-Davies N. and Stotter A. T. *Ann. R. Coll. Surg. Engl.* 1985, **67,** 193.
42 Finlay H. *Anaesthesia* 1977, **32,** 357.
43 Wallace W. A. et al. *Hosp. Update* 1978, **17,** 999; Davis J. A. H. and Walford A. J. *Acta Anaesth. Scand.* 1986, **30,** 145; Valli H. and Rosenberg P. H. *Anaesthesia* 1986, **41,** 1196; Nusbaum L. M. and Hamelberg W. *Anesthesiology* 1986, **64,** 91; Turner P. L. et al. *Aust. NZ. J. Surg.* 1986, **56,** 153.
44 Schmitt H., Batz G., Knoll R., Danner U. and Brandl M. *Acta Anaesth. Scand.* 1990, **34,** 104.
45 Vaughan R. S. et al. *Ann. R. Coll. Surg. Engl.* 1985, **67,** 309.
46 Armstrong P., Brockway M. and Wildsmith J. A. W. *Anaesthesia* 1990, **45,** 11.
47 Tucker G. T. and Boas R. A. *Anesthesiology* 1971, **34,** 538.
48 Ryding F. N. *Anaesthesia* 1981, **36,** 969.
49 Van Niekerk J. P. de V. and Coetzee T. *Lancet*, 1965, **1,** 1353.
50 Dixon J. M. and Crofts T. J. *J. R. Coll. Surg. Edinb.* 1983, **28,** 292.
51 Macintosh R. R. and Bryce-Smith R. *Local Analgesia: Abdominal Surgery*, 2nd edn. Churchill Livingstone, Edinburgh, 1962.
52 Nunn J. F. and Slavin G. *Br. J. Anaesth.* 1980, **52,** 253; Cronin K. D. and Davies M. J. *Anaesth. Intensive Care* 1976, **4,** 259.
53 Cronin K. D. et al. *Anaesth. Intensive Care* 1976, **4,** 259.
54 Sellheim H. *Verh. Dtsch. Ges. Gyn. Anaesth.* 1987, **59,** 149.
55 Ross W. N. et al. *Br. J. Surg.* 1987, **74,** 63; Baxter A. D. et al. *Br. J. Anaesth.* 1987, **59,** 162.
56 Shretting P. *Br. J. Anaesth.* 1981, **53,** 527; Moore D. C. *Br. J. Anaesth.* 1981, **53,** 1235.
57 Reiestad F, Stromskag J. E. *Regional Anesthesia* 1986, **11,** 89.
58 Vadeboncoeur T. R. et al, *Anesthesiology* 1989, **71,** 339; Blake D. W. et al. *Anaesth. Intensive Care* 1989, **17,** 269; Lee A. et al, *Anaesthesia* 1990, **46,** 1028.
59 Lee A. et al. *Anaesthesia* 1991, **45,** 1028–1031; Frenette L. et al, *Can. J. Anaesth.* 1991, **38,** 71; Scott P. V. *Br. J. Anaesth.* 1991, **66,** 131.
60 Scheinin B. et al. *Acta Anaesth. Scand.* 1989, **33,** 156.
61 McIlvaine W. B. et al. *Anesthesiology* 1988, **69,** 261.
62 Ahlburg P. et al. *Acta Anaesth. Scand.* 1990, **34,** 156.
63 Miserocchi G. et al. *J. Appl. Physiol.* 1984, **56,** 526.

64 Kambam J. R. et al. *Can. J. Anaesth.* 1989, **36,** 106.
65 Glassow F. *Ann. R. Coll. Surg. Engl.* 1976, **58,** 133; Flanagan L. and Bascom J. V. *Surg. Gynecol. Obstet.* 1981, **153,** 557.
66 Alexander-Williams J. and Keithley M. R. B. *Ann. R. Coll. Surg. Engl.* 1979, **61,** 251.
67 Armstrong D. N. and Kingsnorth A. N. *Ann. R. Coll. Surg.* 1986, **68,** 207.
68 Glassow F. *Ann. Surg.* 1976, **58,** 134; Glassow F. *Ann. R. Coll. Surg. Engl.* 1984, **66,** 382.
69 Hayse-Gregson P. B., Achola K. J. and Smith G. *Anaesthesia* 1990, **45,** 7.
70 Tverskoy M. et al. *Anesth. Analg.* 1990, **70,** 29.
71 Yeoman P. M. et al. *Anaesthesia* 1983, **38,** 862.
72 Bacon A. L. C. *Anaesth. Intensive Care* 1977, **5,** 63; White J. et al. *Br. Med. J.* 1983, **266,** 1934; Yeoman P. M. et al. *Anaesthesia* 1983, **38,** 862.
73 Muir J. G. *Anaesthesia* 1985, **40,** 1021.
74 Soliman M. G. and Trembley N. A. *Anesth. Analg. (Cleve.)* 1978, **57,** 495; Goldberg P. J. *J. Urol.* 1981, **126,** 337.
75 Sara C. A. and Lowry C. J. *Anaesth. Intensive Care* 1985, **13,** 79.
76 Berry F. R. *Anaesthesia* 1977, **32,** 576; Khoo S. T. and Brown T. C. K. *Anaesth. Intensive Care* 1984, **11,** 40; Grossbard G. D. and Love B. R. T. *Aust. NZ. J. Surg.* 1979, **49,** 592.
77 Coates D. P. et al. *Anaesthesia* 1983, **38,** 588.
78 Casale F. F. and Thomas T. L. *Anaesthesia* 1983, **38,** 1090.
79 Winnie A. P. et al. *Anesth. Analg.* 1973, **52,** 989; Winnie A. P. *Surg. Clin. North Am.* 1975, **55,** 881.
80 Brown T. C. K. and Dickens D. R. V. *Anaesth. Intensive Care* 1986, **14,** 126.
81 Chayen D. et al. *Anesthesiology* 1976, **45,** 95; Brands E. et al. *Anaesth. Intensive Care* 1978, **6,** 256.
82 Odoom J. A. et al. *Anaesthesia* 1986, **41,** 155.
83 Dalens B., Tanguy A. and Vanneuville G. *Anesth. Analg.* 1990, **70,** 131.
84 Smith B. E. et al. *Anaesthesia* 1984, **39,** 155.
85 Beck G. P. *Anesthesiology* 1963, **24,** 222; Winnie A. P. *Surg. Clin. North Am.* 1975, **45,** 887.
86 Atkinson R. S. and Lee J. A. *Anaesthesia* 1985, **40,** 1059.
87 Patel N. *Regional Anesth.* 1985, **10,** 40.
88 Wedel D. J. et al. *Regional Anesth.* 1985, **10,** 48.
89 Schurman D. J. *Anesthesiology* 1976, **44,** 348.
90 *See* Moore D. C. *Stellate Ganglion Block.* Thomas, Springfield, 1954.
91 Cook T. G. et al. *Anesthesiology* 1981, **54,** 421.
92 Valman H. B. et al. *Br. Med. J.* 1977, **1,** 1065; Boscoe M. J. et al. *Anaesthesia* 1983, **38,** 669; Bateman D. N. et al. *Anaesthesia* 1984, **39,** 71; Robertson D. B. *Anaesthesia* 1984, **39,** 603.
93 Dyson F. H. et al. *Br. Med. J.* 1985, **291,** 31.
94 Harding S. F. et al. *Br. Med. J.* 1986, **292,** 1428.
95 Glynn C. *Pain Reviews* 1995, **2,** 292–297.
96 Moore D. C. *Stellate Ganglion Block.* Thomas, Springfield, 1954, 83.

97 Apgar V. *Anesth. Analg. Curr. Res.* 1948, **27,** 49.

98 Goinard P. *Acad. di. Chir.* 1936, 258.

99 Smith D. W. *Am. J. Surg.* 1951, **82,** 344.

100 Benzon H. T. et al. *Anesth. Analg. (Cleve.)* 1985, **64,** 415.

101 Zee R. F. Y. *Anaesth. Intensive Care* 1977, **5,** 76.

102 McCallum M. I. and Glynn C. G. *Anaesthesia* 1986, **41,** 850.

103 Hannington-Kiff J. G. *Lancet* 1984, **1,** 2019. *See also* Kepes E. R. et al. *Regional Anaesth.* 1982, **7,** 92.

104 Sanderson C. J. *Ann. R. Coll. Surg. Engl.* 1981, **63,** 420; Correspondence, *Ann. R. Coll. Surg. Engl.* 1982, **64,** 135.

105 Mandl F. *Paravertebral Block*. Heinemann (Medical Books) Ltd, London, 1928 (translated into English, 1947); Parke F. W. and Chalmers J. A. *J. Obstet. Gynaecol. Br. Commonw.* 1957, **64,** 420.

106 McCollum P. T. and Spence V. A. *Br. J. Anaesth.* 1985, **57,** 1146.

107 Nauss L. A. et al. *Anesthesiology* 1979, **51,** Suppl. 237; Ward E. M. et al. *Anesth. Analg. (Cleve.)* 1979, **58,** 465.

108 Braun H. *Beitr. Klin. Chir.* 1919, **115,** 161; Braun H. *Die Lokal Anaesthesie.* Leipzig, 1905, p. 311; Kappis, K. M. *Bruns. Beitr. Klin. Chirg.* 1919, **115,** 161.

109 Kappis M. *Zentbl. Chir.* 1920, **47,** 98; *Dtsch. Med. Wochenschr.* 1920, **40,** 535; *Klin. Wochenschr.* 1923, **2,** 1441.

110 Filshie J. et al. *Anaesthesia* 1983, **38,** 498.

111 Gardner A. M. H. and Soloman G. *Ann. R. Coll. Surg. Engl.* 1984, **66,** 498.

112 Cherry D. A. and Lamberty J. *Anaesth. Intensive Care* 1984, **12,** 59.

113 Hoare A. M. *Br. J. Hosp. Med.* 1980, **23,** 347.

114 Ikeda S. et al. *Keio J. Med.* 1968, **17,** 1.

Spinal analgesia: intradural and extradural

May be used for:

1 the relief of pain during and/or following surgical operations;
2 the relief of pain during labour;
3 supplementing light general anaesthesia, e.g. propofol infusion;[1]
4 suppressing the transmission of afferent impulses and resulting hormonal and autonomic responses to surgery;
5 it can provide relaxation of the abdomen without the use of relaxants.

ANATOMY

Some useful surface markings

The vertebra prominens (spine of C7) is easily palpable. The tip of the spine of T3 is opposite the roots of the spines of the scapula, with the arms at the sides of the body.

The tip of the spine of T7 is opposite the inferior angle of the scapula, with the arms to the sides.

The highest points of the iliac crests are usually on a line crossing the spine of L4 or the L4/5 interspace.

The dimples overlying the posterior superior iliac spines are on a line crossing the second, posterior sacral foramina and at this level the dural sac in the adult usually ends. The lower end of the spinal cord terminates at the level of the upper border of the body of L2.

The vertebral canal

Bounded in front by bodies of the vertebrae and intervertebral disks with the posterior longitudinal ligament; posteriorly by the laminae, ligamenta flava and the arch which bears spinous processes and by ligaments between them called the interspinous; laterally by pedicles and laminae. Size and shape vary, but is larger in cervical and lumbar regions.

Between the spinal dura and the vertebral canal is the extradural (epidural, peridural) space. Its average depth is 0.5 cm and it is widest in the midline posteriorly in the lumbar region.

Contents of epidural space

The contents include the dural sac and the spinal nerve roots, the extradural plexus of veins and the spinal arteries, lymphatics and fat. The valveless veins become distended when the patient strains or coughs. They connect the pelvic veins below with the intracranial veins above, so that air or local analgesic solution injected into one of them may ascend straight to the cranium. They drain into the inferior vena cava via the azygos vein, so that when there is obstruction to vena caval flow, as with large abdominal tumours, advanced pregnancy, etc., they form an alternative venous pathway and become distended. The shape of the space is triangular with the apex dorsomedial. A dorsomedial fold of dura mater occasionally divides the space into a ventral and two dorsomedial compartments which do not always communicate freely with each other causing patchy analgesia or inadvertent dural puncture when the midline approach is used.

The dura mater is attached to the margins of the foramen magnum, but this does not prevent the passage of analgesic drug into the cranial cavity. It is also attached to the second and third cervical vertebrae and to the posterior longitudinal ligament. In adults it ends at the upper border of the second sacral vertebra, and becomes the filum terminale. Prolongations of the dura surround the spinal nerve roots and fuse with the epineurium of the complete spinal nerves, as they traverse the intervertebral foramina. Extradural block includes blocking of the sympathetic fibres travelling with the anterior or ventral roots, which soon become the white rami. The distance between skin and lumbar extradural space is 4–5 cm.

Contents of intradural space

1 Roots of spinal nerves.
2 Spinal membranes with their enclosed cord and cerebrospinal fluid (CSF).

The narrowest part is between T4 and T9.

Spinal stenosis (e.g. in patients with 'back trouble') may make spinal blocks more difficult and cause cord compression after central neural blockade.[2] This may be intensified should there be extradural haemorrhage.[3]

The subdural space

This is a potential space between the dura and the pia-arachnoid into which a catheter, contrast medium or local analgesic solution may track.[4] Injection into it of local analgesic solution may cause inadequate block, abnormally high block or even total central neural blockade.[5] It does not communicate with the subarachnoid space but is in free communication with the lymph spaces of the nerves.

The vertebral ligaments bounding the canal

1 *Supraspinous ligament*, passes longitudinally over tips of spinous processes from C7 to the sacrum.
2 *Interspinous ligaments*, joining spinous processes together. Cyst formation in the interspinous ligament may result in a false-positive sign of entry into the intradural space.
3 *Ligamenta flava*, running from lamina to lamina, composed of yellow elastic fibres. Half of the substance of the posterior wall of the vertebral canal is composed of the bony laminae, half by the ligamenta flava. They become progressively thicker from above downwards.
4 *Posterior longitudinal ligament*, within the vertebral canal on posterior surfaces of bodies of vertebrae, from which it is separated by the basivertebral veins.
5 *Anterior longitudinal ligament*, runs along the front of the vertebral bodies and disks to which it is adherent.

The spinal cord

The cord is nominally divided into segments by the pairs of spinal nerves which arise from it. These pairs are 31 in number and are as follows: (i) 8 cervical; (ii) 12 thoracic; (iii) 5 lumbar; (iv) 5 sacral; (v) 1 coccygeal.

Spinal nerves

Anterior root is efferent and motor and include sympathetic preganglionic axons from cells in the intermediolateral horn of the spinal cord from T1 to L2 inclusive. Blockade of these fibres influences the response of the adrenal glands to surgical stress.

The posterior root is largely sensory. Each posterior root has a ganglion and conveys fibres of:

1 pain;
2 tactile;
3 thermal sensation;
4 deep or muscle sensation from bones, joints, tendons, etc.;
5 afferents from the viscera (accompanying sympathetic);
6 vasodilator fibres.

Pain and temperature fibres enter the posterior horn where they synapse around cells in laminae I–VII; fibres then cross to the contralateral side within three segments and ascend in the lateral spinothalamic tract to the thalamus.

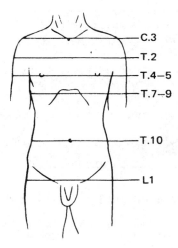

Figure 5.3.1 Segmental levels

Tactile impulses ascend in the ventral spinothalamic tract to the thalamus. Deep or muscle sensory impulses ascend in the posterior columns and spinocerebellar tracts. Vibration impulses ascend in the posterior columns.

The anterior and posterior roots each with its covering of pia-arachnoid and dura cross the extradural space and unite in the intervertebral foramina to form the main spinal nerve trunks, which soon divide into anterior and posterior primary divisions – mixed nerves. Analgesic drugs affect autonomic, sensory and motor fibres in that order, while fibres which block easily hold the drug longest; thus sensory block lasts longer than motor and usually ascends two segments higher up the cord than motor block.

Segmental levels (Fig. 5.3.1)

Perineum, S1–S4; inguinal region, L1; umbilicus, T10; subcostal arch, T6–T8; nipple line, T4 and T5; second intercostal space, T2; clavicle, C3–C4.

Segmental levels of spinal reflexes: epigastric, T7 and T8; abdominal, T9 and T12; cremasteric, L1 and L2; plantar, S1 and S2; knee jerk, L2–L4; ankle jerk, S1 and S2; anal sphincter and wink reflexes, S4–S5.

Movement of joints: hip flexion, L1–L3; extension, L5, S1; knee flexion, L5, S1; extension, L2–L3; ankle flexion, L4–L5; extension, S1–S2.

Factors affecting analgesic toxicity

1 Nature of local anaesthetic, e.g. bupivacaine more toxic than prilocaine; esters have greater allergy potential.

2 Route of administration; especially intravenous; vascular sites and nose, leading to absorption from gastrointestinal tract.

3 The dose given.

4 Patient factors: age, size, cardiovascular disease, epilepsy, history of allergies.

5 Addition of vasoconstrictors usually reduces absorption and systemic toxicity.

Blood supply to spinal cord

The posterior spinal arteries, two on each side, branch from the posterior inferior cerebellar arteries at the level of the foramen magnum. They supply the posterior columns of the cord.

The anterior spinal artery, a single vessel lying in the substance of the pia mater overlying the anterior median fissure, arises at the level of the foramen magnum from the junction of a small branch from each vertebral artery. It receives communications from the intercostal, lumbar and other small arteries. It supplies the lateral and the anterior columns, three-quarters of the substance of the cord. Thrombosis of this artery causes the anterior spinal artery syndrome in which there is paralysis sparing the posterior columns (joint, position, touch, vibration sense). Communicating branches at the level of T1 and T11 are larger than the others and help to supply the enlargements of the cord (the arteries of Adamkiewicz).[6] The artery at T11 supplies the cord both upwards and downwards; that at T1 only downwards from this level. There are thus three vascular areas in the cord with no anastomosis between them.[7] Normal intraspinal capillary pressure is 30–35 mmHg. Deprivation of blood supply for 2–3 min may result in infarction of the cord.[8]

DRUGS USED TO PRODUCE SPINAL ANALGESIA

Note that dosage of drugs for spinal analgesia varies from place to place. The reasons for this are unclear. When an anaesthetist moves to a new location, it is wise to take local advice on the appropriate dosage.

Bupivacaine (Marcain) is a long-acting drug which has been used in 0.05–0.5% concentration, without adrenaline, giving analgesia for up to 8 h. Epidural volumes, e.g. 20 ml need to be given in increments. Motor block is not quite so intense as that produced by 1.5% lignocaine. In obstetrics, 0.0625–0.375% solutions (often with fentanyl 2–3 µg/kg) are popular, giving analgesia without paralysis, allowing ambulatory labour. For surgical operations, 0.75% has been used, but neurotoxic sequelae have been reported.[9]

Intradural dose up to 4 ml of 0.5% solution; this should be reduced in the elderly. (*See also*, Tuominen M. *Acta Anaesth. Scand.* 1991, **35**, 1.)

Levobupivacaine may be used.

Lignocaine has a rapid onset in about 10 min and gives good relaxation. Duration of effect 1–1.5 h, depending on strength of solution employed: 0.5% solution gives good sensory without motor block (differential block); 1.5% solution gives good motor block. In very muscular patients, 2% solution may produce more intense muscular relaxation. Widely used in US. With epidural infusions, the shorter action makes no difference to duration, and adds a safety factor in the event of an intradural misplacement. A common practice is to give the initial dose of lignocaine as 5 ml of 0.5% solution. (If the epidural catheter is in fact subarachnoid, an effective but safe spinal block will develop very rapidly.) If the epidural catheter tip is in the epidural space, a second, third and even fourth 5 ml are given at intervals to complete the epidural block.

Lignocaine and bupivacaine can be given in a mixture[10] as a bolus, to gain motor block for operating time of 1–2 h, followed by sensory block for 6–12 h. This may then be extended by further injections via an epidural catheter. Such an approach has been superseded by the common use of epidural infusions (where a shorter duration of action is a safety factor), e.g. 10 ml/h in adults.

Ropivacaine hydrochloride is similar to bupivacaine in terms of speed of onset and duration, but ropivacaine is slightly less potent, has a slightly shorter duration of action (plasma half-life 1.8 h) and better differential block.[11] It has been used in concentrations between 0.5 and 0.1% solution (entirely sensory); 0.3% solution (sensory with moderate motor block); 1% solution (sensory with profound motor block).[12]

Prilocaine: rapid onset of action. Strengths of 0.5–4%, have been used. Less toxic than lignocaine, but doses in excess of 10 mg/kg may cause mild methaemoglobinaemia.

Etidocaine 1 or 1.5% solution. Results in greater motor block than bupivacaine.

Chloroprocaine hydrochloride: used mainly in the US as 2–3% solution. Short latency and duration of activity (about 45 min), its effects ceasing suddenly. It antagonizes fentanyl (binds to µ and κ receptors).[13]

Other agents: midazolam spinal anaesthesia is effective with midazolam 0.1%. (in the rat).[14] Magnesium sulphate has shown no intrathecal neurotoxicity in 6.3% and 12.6% MgSO$_4$ in rat model and is fully reversible.[15] Neostigmine has been used to control postoperative pain.[16]

A host of other compounds are being tried in an attempt to find the ideal agent which safely and reliably produces pure analgesia, including extenders – liposomes, microcrystals and microsomes.

Vasoconstrictors are seldom used in the intradural space for fear of compromising the blood supply of the cord, or in the extradural space, except in test doses.

PREPARATION FOR SPINAL BLOCK

1 Assessment, clinical history, explanation, consent and examination of patient.
2 Is the patient on anticoagulants or aspirin? Cases of epidural haematomas continue to occur in spite of reassurances about the average responses of patients to these drugs. However, in practice, the anaesthetist cares not only for patients with a median response to drugs, but also for those whose response is two or more standard deviations from the mean. Aspirin medication in particular shows a very diverse response.

   Prophylactic *heparin* for deep venous thrombosis (DVT): an APTT ratio up to 2 is safe ground for an epidural.

   Prophylactic *coumarin (e.g. warfarin)* for DVT: an INR up to 2 is safe ground for an epidural.

   Aspirin: the vital questions in the history are: (i) do you take aspirin? and (ii) how much and how often do you take it? Regular or large-dose aspirin may call for the bleeding time test to be performed. While this test is not accurate enough for research purposes, a bleeding time greater than 10 min is so abnormal that spinal block is questionable. A delay of 10 days or a platelet transfusion should restore normal platelet function. (*See* Wildsmith J. A. W. and Checketts M. R. *Brit. J. Anaesth.* 1992, **82,** 164–167.
3 Safety factors:
   (a) an intravenous drip is set up and a preload of crystalloid or colloid given, up to 1 litre in fit patients;
   (b) resuscitation equipment, including defibrillator is made available;
   (c) full 'minimal monitoring' is applied to awaken the patient.
4 Possible anxiolysis with low-dose benzodiazepine (*see below*).
5 Choice of equipment:
   (a) disposable sets;
   (b) sterilization of reusable packs (in many parts of the world);
   (c) choice of needle, e.g. Whitacre, Sprotte, Quinke, (26 or 29 G[17] passed through an introducer which is prepositioned in the interspinous ligament. In young patients there is a greater chance of postspinal headache. The Tuohy needle is chosen when a catheter is to be inserted. The greater the gauge of the needle the easier it is to appreciate loss of resistance, but the greater the hole if an inadvertent dural puncture occurs. The Tuohy needle is less likely to puncture the dura than a sharper pointed needle, because of the rounded Huber point. The needle should be suitably marked to enable the depth of the point to be instantly recognized[18] (Fig. 5.3.2).

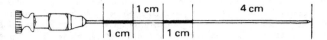

Figure 5.3.2 The Lee marked needle (*Medical & Industrial Equipment*).

CONCERN FOR THE COMFORT OF THE PATIENT

Cardiac arrest during spinal anaesthesia is often related to sedation techniques. However, patients who come to the theatre in an anxious state of mind can be helped by very small intravenous doses of a suitable benzodiazepine – not sufficient to cause sedation. The smoothness of an otherwise correct technical procedure may be undermined if the patient moves or coughs a lot. Careful maintenance of airway and full monitoring of respiratory rate, oxygenation and CO_2 are mandatory.

Ketamine 0.2–0.5 mg/kg i.v. is excellent when positioning causes pain, as in fractured hip, and is also useful in the 'failed block drill'. Memantine and dextromethorphan have a similar use.

TECHNIQUE

The lumbar puncture must be done in a good light on a bed or table which can be tilted. Pain can be minimized by the infiltration of local analgesic solution into the subcutaneous and deeper tissues, especially, during the paramedian approach, near the lamina.

Lumbar puncture is contraindicated in patients with:

1 raised intracranial pressure (papilloedema, cerebral oedema, tumours in the posterior fossa, suspected subarachnoid haemorrhage, unless disproved by a computed tomography (CT) scan;[19]
2 coagulopathy, blood dyscrasias and those patients on full anticoagulant therapy;
3 skin sepsis and marked spinal deformity.

Lumbar puncture

Midline approach

Puncture in the sitting position: the patient sits on the table or bed with feet resting comfortably on a stool; spine should be flexed with chin pressed on to sternum. A pillow on the knees gives helpful support to the arms. Flexion of the spine rather than flexion of the hips is the aim.

Puncture in the *left lateral* position: the awake patient should be supported by a nurse and positioned with back at edge of table and parallel to it, knees flexed on to abdomen, head brought down to knees, and hips and shoulders vertical to the table to avoid rotation of the vertebral column. In the obese the median crease sags downwards sometimes as much as 2.5 cm, so the point of the needle should be inserted above the crease in these cases.

The line joining the highest points of the iliac crests crosses either the spine of the fourth lumbar vertebra or the interspace between L4 and L5. Precise identification of the lumbar spines may be impossible, but this does not matter so long as the first lumbar interspace (and those above this level) are avoided, unless a thoracic block is intended. When the chosen (often the widest interspinal distance) interspace is located the intradermal needle is inserted after careful palpation, midway between the two spines, and a small weal of analgesic solution is raised. A small incision is made in the skin with a larger needle to prevent a tough skin from grasping the spinal needle tightly and to prevent a core of skin being carried into the intra- or extradural space with the lumbar puncture needle.[20] The needle is then slowly advanced at right angles to the back, with its bevel in the plane to separate and not to divide the longitudinal fibres of the dura.

If bone is met or nerve pain is felt, it is necessary to withdraw and slightly alter direction either upwards or downwards (or laterally in cases of scoliosis). Paraesthesia is a signal to withdraw and redirect the needle immediately to avoid damage to the cauda equina.

Paramedian approach

A needle is inserted 1.5 cm from the midline directly opposite the centre of the interspace, and at an angle of 25 degrees to the midline. With this approach, flexion of the back is not so important. It is said to cause minimal pain as tough ligaments are avoided and the sense of touch and needle control are more accurate. Sometimes it is successful when attempts using midline approach have failed.

Some advantages of the paramedian approach:

1 the inter- and supraspinous ligaments, sometimes bony hard, are not penetrated, so possibly less backache;
2 the lamina, if touched by the needle, indicates the depth of the extradural space if a marked needle is used;
3 flexion of the back is not as important as with the median approach: this may be beneficial in late pregnancy.

Skin puncture in the lumbar region requires no after-treatment other than a spray or adhesive dressing. Infection seldom occurs in the skin and subcutaneous tissues.

In *intradural block*, after injection of the drug, the patient is turned into the supine position; the injected analgesic drug is now at the apex of the lumbar curve and the direction of movement of 'heavy' solutions then depends on which way the patient is tilted.

It is advisable to place the patient in the required position without delay so that fixation of the drug occurs after the desired spread has taken place. For almost any work inside the abdominal cavity analgesia should reach to the subcostal arch (T6–T8). Upper abdominal procedures require block to T4–T5. Any sensory test is useful in estimating height of block.

In *epidural block*, the following points suggest that a needle tip is in the extradural space.

1 Identification of epidural space by sudden ease of injection of saline through the advancing needle (the complications of air injection include pneumocephalus, headache nausea, hemiparesis, delayed awakening after N_2O, nerve root compression, subcutaneous emphysema, retroperitoneal air after extracorporeal shock wave lithotripsy (ECSWL), venous air embolism, all rare.[21]

2 A false-positive test may result if the needle point enters a small cyst in the yellow ligament.

3 X-ray and ultrasonic localization – mainly in pain clinic work.

All of the solution injected, even by experienced anaesthetists, after a positive loss of resistance test, does not always enter the extradural space.[22]

Injection must only commence when position of needle point is certain.

Epidural test dose

An initial injection is made (following aspiration test) of either 1 ml of lignocaine with adrenaline or 2 ml of 0.5% bupivacaine with adrenaline, or with isoproterenol 5 mg (which, in obstetrics, increases maternal heart rate and uterine blood flow, no effect of fetal heart rate or umbilical blood flow, while adrenaline lowers uterine bloodflow[23]). If in 5 min there is no evidence of intradural block, e.g. inability to move the feet, or tachycardia from possible intravenous injection of adrenaline, the main injection can be made.

Procedure if dura is pierced by an 'epidural' needle

Although dural puncture is usually due to lack of delicacy in technique, it may result from previous manipulations at the same site or spinal stenosis (which can also cause intermittent claudication of the cauda equina.) The choice is as follows:

1 Leave needle in theca so that it occludes the dural puncture and attempt to locate the extradural space from a higher or lower level. Withdraw first needle after injection of local analgesic solution through the second needle into the extradural space.

2 Convert the block into an intradural (subarachnoid) one.

3 Abandon the method and use general anaesthesia.

Post-dural puncture headache (PDPH) is a risk, depending on the size and point of the needle.[24] Blood patch will be needed in about half of these cases. It works by tamponade, shown by magnetic resonance imaging (MRI) to spread four to five spaces.[25]

Cerebrospinal fluid dripping from the needle can be differentiated from local analgesic solution by:

1 difference in temperature;
2 testing for glucose and protein on urine-testing paper strips;
3 allowing a few drops to fall onto thiopentone solution, when local analgesic solution causes turbidity (pH of thiopentone is 10; of analgesic solution, about 5).[26]

A filter may be used to prevent injection of foreign material into the extradural space. The presence of a filter does, however, make aspiration tests difficult.

Management of the very difficult case

More difficulty is encountered in the very elderly, those with ankylosing spondylitis, previous lumbar spinal surgery, obesity and scoliosis.

Failure at one interspace can often be made successful at an adjacent interspace. The interspace with the largest gap between spines is often the easiest one to attempt regardless of the desired level of block. If finding the interlaminar space with a fine needle is difficult, it may be easier to 'walk' the point of a thicker needle (e.g. 20–22 G) along the laminae and so find the space. If the midline approach proves impossible, the paramedian approach may be tried. In scoliosis an oblique approach to the twisted spine may be required. Even after detailed consultation of the X-ray of the spine, this needs skilled spatial orientation!

If there is repeated failure to access the epidural space, the operator should ask 'Is this spinal block essential, or merely desirable?' If merely desirable, spinal block may be abandoned and general anaesthesia or other technique begun.

If the block is essential and the whole lumbar spine is impossible for access, the sacral hiatus is a possible entry point, although larger (extradural) volumes will be needed to reach up to the upper lumbar or lower thoracic segments. It is unlikely (but not impossible) that the thoracic spine will be easier than the lumbar spine.

Difficulty due to morbid obesity requires longer needles, e.g. 150 mm. Finding the midline is made easier by sitting the patient up and even measuring the mid-point between the iliac crests with a ruler. In the obese, the vertebra prominens is often palpable and a line can be drawn between this and the sacral hiatus to locate the midline. Ask the patient to point to the midline.

Thoracic extradural block

The ideal puncture site for thoracic operations is T2–T6; for upper abdominal operations, T8, and the paramedian approach is recommended. A skin weal is placed just lateral to the spinous process at the inferior aspect of the interspace and the needle directed 10 degrees medially and 45 degrees cephalad. After identification of the space and the usual aspiration test, a test dose may be injected, followed by the insertion of an extradural catheter. Puncture of the theca is less likely than in the lumbar region because of the angulation of the needle and the tendency of the Huber point to 'toboggan' over the dura mater. The dose of solution may vary from 3 to 5 ml of 1.5% lignocaine or 0.5% bupivacaine for a block of two to four segments, or up to 10–15 ml when a greater zone of analgesia is required as in abdominal surgery. An infusion of 0.125% bupivacaine at 10–15 ml/h is commonly used.

Cervical extradural block

Used for the management of intractable pain and by some enthusiasts, for thyroidectomy and for carotid endarterectomy. Differential block is used, i.e. the concentration of solution should be such as to provide sensory block without motor block of the phrenic nerves, e.g. lignocaine 0.5% or bupivacaine 0.125%. For the injection the patient sits with the head and neck flexed forward. The C7/T1 interspace (vertebra prominens) is identified and a skin weal made over it in the midline. The needle is advanced slowly, inclined at an angle of 30 degrees cephalad. Usual dose is 6–8 ml of analgesic solution for neck analgesia. Technically, this block is easy, although potentially very harmful, should the cord be pithed. Nonetheless, experienced workers advocate it. The extradural space is relatively superficial and the ligamentum flavum thin.

Conduct of spinal analgesia with safety steps (Mulroy M., Norris M. C. and Liu S. S. *Anesth. Analg.* 1997, **85**, 1346–1356)

1 A quiet operating room, the use of ear muffs and comfort on the table for the patient.

2 There must always be an intravenous infusion.

3 Full frequent monitoring of circulation and respiration.

4 Oxygen inhalation.

5 Intravenous light sedation for anxious patients, e.g. midazolam 1 mg i.v., or propofol infusion, at 1 mg/kg/h, with target blood level of 1 μm/ml.

6 Nausea and vomiting are controlled by antiemetics but can necessitate general anaesthesia and rapid-sequence intubation.

7 Correction of acute hypotension.

8 If analgesia ascends high up the body, consciousness may be lost, as afferent impulses reaching the cortex become fewer and fewer.

9 Pressor drugs are always at hand (very clearly labelled).

Differential blockade

Weaker solutions produce only sensory and autonomic block. If it is desirable to avoid motor block, then the solution strengths should be less than 0.25% bupivacaine; 1% lignocaine; 0.125% ropivacaine,[27] or 1% prilocaine.

Specimen dosage for adults

Doses quoted in the following section are for guidance only. All experienced workers in this field have found the spread of solutions within the intradural space capricious, so that exact levels of analgesia following injection of a given dose cannot always be forecast. Correct dosages also vary from place to place, and local advice should be sought when moving location.

Perineal operations: intradural, 1–2 ml of a heavy solution sitting up; extradural, 5–15 ml of solution via sacral route.

Prostate bladder and thigh operations: intradural, 2–3 ml and head-down tilt; block to T10 (to remove unpleasant sensation of bladder fullness); extradural, 20 ml of solution via mid to upper lumbar route.

Knee operations require block of L3 (intradural, 2–3 ml), but total knee replacement requires block up to T10 (intradural, 2–3 ml and head-down tilt) to (rather hopefully) block the pain of high tourniquet.

Inguinal hernia operations require block to T10 (intradural, 2–3 ml and head-down tilt); extradural, 20 ml of solution via mid to upper lumbar route.

Umbilical operations require block to T7 (intradural, 3 ml and head-down tilt).

Lower abdominal operations, incision below umbilicus (e.g. hysterectomy), require block to T7 (intradural, 3 ml and head-down tilt).

Upper abdominal surgery (gastrectomy, transverse colectomy) analgesia must reach T4 (note risk of bradycardia) (intradural, 4 ml and head-down tilt); raising the head and shoulders to limit cephalad spread.

For operations on the gut, afferent stimuli may still pass up vagal fibres, requiring the surgeon to perform para-oesophageal block of the vagus, or light general anaesthesia with tracheal intubation. Central neural bockade gives an ischaemic field, gut retraction, good relaxation, reduction of stress and (with a catheter) excellent postoperative analgesia.

Epidural catheters

These are very frequently used (with bacterial filters), as they allow accurate incremental dosing or infusion, with prolonged analgesia, e.g. in postoperative and obstetrics. Multiport catheters have less unilateral analgesia and unblocked segments than single port catheters.[28]

Intradural catheters

A 32-G catheter is inserted (via a 26-G spinal needle) with about 3 cm in the intradural space. Infusion of 1–2 ml plain bupivacaine per hour has been used.[29] There may be problems threading such a fine catheter until the skill has been acquired.[30]

Microcatheters also have a place in the administration of narcotic drugs for pain control.

Difficulties (and their prevention) during operation

The following troublesome symptoms and signs may occur:

1 nausea (antiemetics);
2 vomiting (requires emergency intubation);
3 headache (simple analgesics);
4 precordial discomfort (remove the surgeon's elbow!);
5 paraesthesiae in the limbs (reassurance);
6 difficulty in phonation (reassurance);
7 hypotension (intravenous fluids and vasocostrictors);
8 restlessness (reassurance, benzodiazepines, or even general anaesthesia);
9 inability to cough effectively (reassurance);
10 repeated coughing by the patient with COPD (codeine 30–60 mg i.m., adult);
11 hiccups (metoclopramide 20 mg i.v., adult; or even general anaesthesia).

PHYSIOLOGY OF CENTRAL NEURAL BLOCKADE

Order of blocking nerve fibres:

1 autonomic preganglionic B fibres;
2 temperature fibres – cold before warm;
3 pin-prick fibres;
4 pain fibres;
5 touch fibres;
6 deep pressure fibres;
7 somatic motor fibres;
8 fibres conveying vibratory sense and proprioceptive impulses.

Recovery is in roughly the reverse order.

In spinal analgesia, entirely adequate for surgery of a lower limb, a patient may complain of pain due to the tourniquet. A concentration of a solution of local analgesic drug may give excellent analgesia for ordinary sensation, conveyed by small nerve fibres, but may not be adequate to block transmission in larger fibres transmitting pressure–pain sensation. An increased concentration will avoid this. Another explanation of bizarre pains occurring during otherwise adequate low spinal analgesia may be that some pain fibres pass with sympathetic nerves to reach the cord at a higher level.

Local analgesic drugs act mainly on the nerve roots leaving the cord, though opioids reach its substance. Opioid movement depends on:

1 diffusion across the dura and pia;
2 lipid solubility (fentanyl is lipophilic and tends to remain localized, morphine is hydrophilic and tends to move freely in the CSF).

Local analgesics act on neuronal voltage-sensitive Ca^{2+} channel-binding sites[31] in correlation with anaesthetic potency and lipid solubility.

The drugs are removed from the extradural space via the extradural veins.

Effect of spinal block on the cardiovascular system

The side-effects of spinal block are mainly on the cardiovascular system:

1 vasodilatation of arteriolar resistance vessels (reducing afterload) and venous capacitance vessels (lowering venous return); the resulting coupling of blood volume to cardiac output is a fundamental destabilizer of the circulation;
2 block of cardiac efferent sympathetic fibres (T1–T4) resulting in loss of chronotropic and inotropic drive, bradycardia and fall in cardiac output;
3 the atrial or Bainbridge reflex causing bradycardia;
4 the operation of Marey's law causing tachycardia;
5 systemic absorption of the local analgesic drug causing vasodilatation and myocardial depression (in some circumstances moderate levels of plasma lignocaine may be associated with increased cardiac output, arterial pressure and heart rate, but this is probably a central mechanism dependent upon an intact autonomic system);[32]
6 block of sympathetic supply to adrenals (splanchnic nerves), with consequent catecholamine depletion;
7 adrenaline effect (if used) following absorption, resulting in beta-stimulation and associated rise in cardiac output and reduction in peripheral resistance. The overall effect is a rise in mean arterial pressure (MAP). The tachycardia produced by added adrenaline is a useful sign (but not in obstetrics) when a 'test dose' is intravascular.[33]

Spinal block may not cause hypotension in fit young adults, though the elderly risk significant hypotension. Hypotension is also likely in the debilitated or hypovolaemic subject, and this may lead to cardiac arrest. When there is cardiac decompensation, removal of sympathetic tone may be dangerous causing cerebral ischaemia and hypoxia.

Mild hypotension is seldom a cause for anxiety in young, fit patients, where the usual limits of minimum MAP of 70 mmHg apply. In the elderly, normotension is the target using vasoconstrictors, intravenous 'loading' infusion and leg elevation to maintain arterial pressure. However, inotropic and chronotropic drugs may increase subendocardial O_2 demand as well as O_2 supply, and are used with caution.

8 Compression of the great vessels within the abdomen by the pregnant uterus, large abdominal tumours or abdominal packs may cause severe hypotension in the presence of central neural blockade.

Management of hypotension during spinal analgesia

Rapid intravenous fluid infusion up to 2 litres crystalloid or colloid;[34] 100% O_2 inhalation; injection of pressor drug (e.g. ephedrine 10–25 mg; meta-raminol, or noradrenaline); with elevation of the legs. When there is brady-cardia, correction by atropine 0.2–0.5 mg will often also elevate blood pressure. Vasopressors may be used prophylactically in high blocks and high-risk cases.

Intra-arterial and central venous pressure are monitored.

The vasoconstrictor reflex in haemorrhage is abolished by spinal block, in proportion to the height of the block, so that the patient is unable to protect against this stress. This contraindicates spinal analgesia in hypovolaemic shock and the acute abdomen. Early and rapid volume replacement is necessary if haemorrhage occurs during surgery under spinal analgesia.

Respiratory system

Remarkably little disturbance, making regional block ideal for patients with respiratory problems.

There is no change in FRC, $\dot{V}/\dot{Q}$ ratio, or pulmonary gas exchange. Vital capacity and forced expiratory volume may be reduced, especially in smokers. Intercostal paralysis is compensated for by increased descent of the dia-phragm which is made easier by the lax abdominal wall. This is not accompa-nied by hypoxia or hypercapnia though the effectiveness of cough is impaired. (Coughing is a nuisance during laparotomies under spinal analgesia.) Oxygen therapy is routine in spinal block. In obstructive airways disease there is some reflex (baroreceptor) bronchodilatation. There is decreased pulmonary blood volume and pulmonary arterial blood pressure.

Postoperatively, respiratory function is better if the pain of the operation is relieved by extradural block, rather than by parenteral opioids. There is less reduction of FRC and consequent physiological shunting which may arise from airways closure.

Management of apnoea during spinal analgesia

1 Immediate diagnosis by careful monitoring throughout the procedure.
2 The cause must be elucidated. This may be:
   (a) total spinal analgesia, blocking C3, 4, 5 roots if strong solutions of local analgesics are used;

    (b)   massive epidural spread, e.g. in spinal stenosis;
    (c)   accidental subdural injection – a small volume of solution may travel to an unexpectedly high level in this potential space;
    (d)   toxic effects of the local analgesic drug;
    (e)   injection of narcotic analgesic drug (*see below*);
    (f)   inadequate medullary blood flow due to inadequate cardiac output – a serious situation demanding immediate cardiorespiratory support.
3 Ventilation of lungs by 100% O_2/intubation.
4 Monitoring of other vital signs, e.g. arterial pressure, pulse oximetry, capnography, level of consciousness, level of block, pupil size, skin rashes auscultation of the chest.

Gastrointestinal system

Nausea and vomiting due to hypotension may occur and usually come on in waves lasting a minute or so and then passing away spontaneously. Upper abdominal sensation may ascend along the unblocked vagi and phrenic nerves, and cause aching discomfort. Para-oesophageal infiltration of local analgesic solution may prevent this by blocking vagal afferents. Colonic blood supply and oxygenation are increased in animals following spinal analgesia,[35] perhaps an important factor in the prevention of endotoxinaemia.

Endocrine system

Spinal block prevents adrenal response to trauma (catecholamine and glucocorticoid secretion) and antidiuretic hormone release during surgery is suppressed. Postoperative lymphocytosis and granulocytosis are suppressed.[36]

    Because spinal block suppresses the hyperglycaemic response to surgery and trauma it is useful in diabetic patients.[37] Insulin resistance is prevented. Infused glucose is well utilized.

Stress responses

The most effective method of avoiding stress responses to surgery is probably continuous extradural block, although even this is not very effective following upper abdominal operations, because some afferent pathways (e.g. vagus) remain unblocked.

Genito-urinary system

The sympathetic supply to kidneys is from T11 to L1, via the lowest splanchnic nerves.

    Sphincters of bladder not relaxed, so soiling of table by urine is not seen, and tone of ureters not greatly altered. The penis is often engorged and flaccid due to paralysis of the nervi erigentes (S2 and S3); this is a useful positive sign

---

Failed spinal drill

Partial failure may be due to the following.

1 Failure to fully access the subarachnoid or epidural space.

2 Insufficient dosage (or patient not tilted enough when heavy solutions are used in the intradural space).

3 Webs and septa, preventing spread. Unilateral block can occur; its cause is obscure. Occasionally, one or more nerve roots remain unblocked.

4 Resistance to local analgesics.

5 The surgeon has gone beyond his or her stated zone of operation.

Action

1 The surgeon is asked to pause for a few minutes.

2 Intravenous analgesia may be sufficient, e.g. short-acting opioids; low-dose intravenous ketamine (with a little benzodiazepine) is rapid and very effective.

3 Proceed to general anaesthesia if relaxation is required.

   Note that the patient may be complaining of pain in a different part of the body to the site of operation, e.g. shoulders or neck.

---

of successful block. Postspinal retention of urine may be moderately prolonged as L2 and L3 contain small autonomic fibres and their paralysis lasts longer than that of the larger sensory and motor fibres. During continuous lumbosacral blockade, the bladder must be routinely palpated with catheterization when necessary. Spermatorrhoea is sometimes seen.

   Uterine tone is unchanged after spinal analgesia in pregnancy.

Body temperature

Vasodilatation after spinal block causes hypothermia, requiring preventive measures.[38] However, absence of sweating favours hyperpyrexia in hot environments.

Factors influencing height of analgesia in intradural block

1 *Dose of drug injected.* The greater the dosage and concentration, the higher and longer the block. When opioids are used, lipid solubility of the drug

influences spread, e.g. lipid-soluble fentanyl[39] tends to remain localized whereas water-soluble morphine tends to spread by diffusing in the CSF.

2 *Volume of fluid injected.*

3 *Specific gravity of solution.* Addition of glucose 5–8% makes the intradural solution hyperbaric ('heavy'). Head-down tilt results in the block extending a few segments higher. This may make all the difference between success and failure in spinal analgesia for abdominal surgery, where the analgesic should reach the middle of the thoracic curve (T5). Posture has little effect when plain solutions are used.

4 Choice of interspace.

5 Patient factors. These include age (higher segmental block likely for a given dose),[40] height, pregnancy (the effect is marginal), spinal stenosis (wider spread).

IMMEDIATE COMPLICATIONS OF SPINAL BLOCK (AND MANAGEMENT THEREOF)

1 *Hypotension* due to sympathetic block: this means that the blood volume and cardiac output are tightly coupled – a fundamentally unsafe situation unless there is a good intravenous infusion in place to manipulate the circulating volume. (Head-down tilt, fast intravenous infusion, vaso-constrictors.) *See also above.*

2 *Hypotension* due to bradycardia, due to block of T4. (intravenous atropine).

3 *Hypotension* due to inadequate coronary perfusion due to low diastolic pressure (the electrocardiogram (ECG) may or may not be abnormal):
   (a) lungs are ventilated with 100% O_2;
   (b) legs are raised to promote venous return;
   (c) vasoconstrictors are injected cautiously, e.g. aramine;
   (d) colloids are infused fast until the central venous pressure (CVP) is restored to normal.

4 Following epidural – *total spinal analgesia*: the possibility of this must always be present in the mind of the anaesthetist performing an extradural block. While it usually comes on soon after the injection, it may be delayed for 30–45 min.[41] If this has occurred the patient is likely to show, within 3 min of injection of the analgesic drug:
   (a) marked hypotension;
   (b) apnoea;
   (c) dilated pupils;
   (d) loss of consciousness.

There is grave danger of death from asphyxia. Management: intubate and ventilate the lungs with 100% O_2, elevate legs, inject a pressor drug intra-venously, give 2–3 litres of intravenous colloid. These will in most cases rescue the patient. The operation can then proceed and spontaneous

---

Key features of a true PDPH

A headache after a spinal block may be a 'postspinal headache' if:

1 it is different from any headache previously experienced by the patient;

2 it is initiated or made worse by adoption of the sitting or erect posture;

3 it has occipital and nuchal components;

4 it is relieved by abdominal compression, which raises the venous pressure.

---

respiration will probably recommence within the hour. Unpleasant sequelae are unlikely.

5 *Toxicity* due to intravascular injection or by absorption of the local analgesic. The signs are excitement, disorientation, going on to twitching, convulsions and perhaps apnoea, with severe cardiac depression. Bupivacaine tends to produce more cardiac depression and arrythmias. These usually come on soon after injection but may be delayed. Management consists of injecting a small dose of barbiturate (e.g. thiopentone, 50 mg) or diazepam into the drip; the administration of O_2 by intermittent positive-pressure ventilation (IPPV); protection of the patient's teeth and tongue from the trauma of the fits, which are usually self-limiting, but of longer duration with bupivacaine.

6 *Hypoventilation* due to brainstem hypoxia. (Lungs are ventilated with 100% O_2 and arterial pressure is immediately raised to normal as above[42].)

7 *Hypoventilation* due to block of phrenic nerve roots (one sign of a 'total spinal' with severe hypotension). (Lungs are ventilated with 100% O_2.)

8 *Allergic response to injected drug* (O_2, intravenous adrenaline 0.1 mg and fast intravenous colloid infusion).

9 *Hypothermia.*[43]

10 *Epidurocutaneous fistula* (successfully treated by a blood patch).[44]

11 *Prolonged analgesia may occur.*

LATER COMPLICATIONS

Headache[45]

This may occur after deliberate or accidental dural puncture, or even after uncomplicated epidural block. More common in young adults.

It occurs much less when fine pencil-point needles are employed. Onset within 3 days. Usually worse when the patient sits or stands. Often occipital and associated with pain and stiffness in neck; may be vertical or frontal, can cause pain in the orbit.[46] Headaches also occur after simple lumbar puncture (the incidence of post-lumbar puncture headache in medical wards was estimated at 30%.[47] The average causative leakage of CSF into epidural space is about 10 ml/h and healing may take 3 weeks. Air travel, soon after dural puncture, may cause a recurrence of headache.[48] Headache may last days, weeks or months, but usually 1–2 weeks. Loss of up to 10 ml of fluid during lumbar puncture probably has no effect on subsequent headaches. Dural tap has also brought to light unsuspected arteriovenous malformations, with delayed neurological signs.[49]

It may be caused by low CSF pressure. The commonest cause of this is loss of CSF through a dural hole. The rate of leakage of CSF exceeds its rate of formation, and this results in changes in the hydrodynamics of the fluid, with loss of cushioning of the brain and pressure or traction on vessels and sensitive brain structures, basal dura, tentorium, etc. In cases of traumatic leakage of CSF, the choroid plexus can form 500 ml/day.

Differential diagnosis

Migraine, meningitis, tumour, dehydration, hyponatraemia. It is important to consider these every time a PDPH occurs.

Treatment

This is both prophylactic and therapeutic.

PROPHYLACTIC

1 Avoidance of spinal block in unsuitable patients, including those with a history of frequent severe headaches.
2 Use of fine needles. The smaller the needle gauge the lower the incidence of headache, but the greater the difficulty in its insertion.
3 Choice of needle point. The Whitacre needle has a pencil point and separates rather than tears the fibres. The orifice is not at the tip. Its use reduces the incidence of headache.[50] The Sprotte needle[51] differs from the Whitacre in the shape and size of the orifice, which is also not at the needle tip, but is also effective in reducing the incidence of headache;[52] the orientation of pencil-point needle aperture is not important for the spread of the spinal.[53]
4 Prevention of dehydration, straining and coughing in the perioperative period.

THERAPY FOR ESTABLISHED HEADACHE

1 Full hydration of the patient (in the very resistant case, DDAVP 4 mg/day has been used).
2 Simple analgesics.

3 Maintain the supine position.
4 A continuous drip of Hartmann's solution, via a catheter in the lumbar extradural space, for 24 h;[54]
5 'Blood patch', injection of 10–20 ml (adult) of autologous blood into the extradural space, to form a blood patch for sealing the dural puncture has over 90% success rate and spreads four to five segments.[55] An extradural needle is sited at the same level as the original spinal puncture, while a colleague takes 30 ml of venous blood under aseptic conditions, using 20 ml for injection into the spinal canal (and 10 ml for blood culture). This is occasionally followed by minor neurological changes.[56] Failure of a blood patch to ease headache may be due to
   (a) headache caused by something else;
   (b) incorrect position of the injection; or
   (c) too small a volume of injected blood.

Central nervous system complications of spinal anaesthetics

These are related to trauma, ischaemia, infection or neurotoxicity. Pre-existing neurological disease has been found to occur in 10% of patients receiving spinal anaesthesia. Needle placement associated paraesthesiae occurred in 6.3% with 1 in 50 of these feeling pain or hyperaesthesiae later. Needle placement associated paraesthesiae was a risk factor for PDPH, as was younger age, urological and obstetric operations.[57]

Backache

Probably not much more common after spinal than after general anaesthesia (or delivery, in obstetrics).[58] A small pillow under the lumbar region reduces incidence of postoperative backache irrespective of method of anaesthesia.

Retention of urine

Resolves when the block wears off (may also be due to postoperative opioids). Rarely prolonged retention due to spasm of vesical sphincter consequent on spinal analgesia is seen, which may respond to simple catheterization.

Meningitis/arachnoiditis

This may occur even with a seemingly flawless technique.[59] Aseptic meningitis has been reported.[60]

Contamination with chemical antiseptics, starch powder from gloves, detergents, higher concentrations of the drug and variations in pH have all been blamed. The need remains for careful adherence to aseptic technique when blocks are carried out.

Paralysis of the sixth cranial nerve

Palsy of external rectus causes diplopia. First reported in 1907.[61] Onset commonly between fifth and 11th postoperative days and associated with headache. May be delayed for 3 weeks. Even simple lumbar puncture without injection of analgesic solution can cause it. Has been said to occur in about 1 in 300 cases of spinal analgesia. Paralysis is never complete and is a different entity from the total paralysis associated with such conditions as skull fracture.

It may be caused by mechanical, inflammatory, or toxic effects of drug acting on an unstable binocular vision mechanism, phylogenetically a recently acquired one; a similar condition is seen in acute alcoholic intoxication.

While the condition persists, dark glasses may be worn. About 50% of cases recover within a month. If after 2 years spontaneous recovery of function has not occurred, operative cure may be considered. About 25% of the cases show bilateral nerve involvement.

Paralysis of every cranial nerve except the first, ninth and 10th has been reported after spinal analgesia, and transient deafness or tinnitus is not uncommon. Diplopia occurs following general anaesthesia and after the use of relaxants and may also persist for some time.

Other neurological lesions

Pruritus following intradural block, in patients with peripheral neuropathy has been seen.[62] The addition of sodium metabisulphite as an antioxidant, to solutions for intradural injection (e.g. chloroprocaine) may cause neurological damage,[63] and should be avoided.

Unexplained pain during injection.[64] This should raise suspicion of potential direct nerve trauma, and the injection is stopped immediately.

Trigeminal nerve palsy has followed lumbar extradural analgesia.[65]

Transient lesions of cauda equina cause abnormalities of leg reflexes, incontinence of faeces, retention of urine, loss of sexual function, sensory loss in lumbosacral distribution and temporary paralysis of peroneal nerve. Most of these clear up spontaneously. Radiculitis, ascending myelitis, transient transverse myelitis, adhesive arachnoiditis, paraplegia, meningoencephalitis and bulbar involvement have all been reported. Their cause is not fully understood nor is it always due to the method of pain relief. Localized haematoma formation may be a cause of symptoms due to pressure on the cord.[66] Severe back pain with paraplegia requires emergency neurological referral, CT scan and, if necessary, surgical exploration. Ischaemia of the cord may be caused by severe hypotension, or the use of high concentrations of local vasoconstrictors. Electromyographic studies enable lesions of the lower motor neuron type due to spinal analgesia to be differentiated from other neurological and myopathic conditions. An extradural abscess following several spinal blocks, without causing either sensory or motor impairment, only localized pain, in a diabetic patient with an infected leg, has been reported.[67]

Extradural abscess,[68] which may take up to 16 days to develop, may be metastatic. Extradural haematoma has been reported in a patient, 3 days after delivery who received neither extradural block nor anticoagulants.[69] Extradural abscess must be drained immediately after diagnosis, otherwise paraplegia may result.

Existing spinal stenosis may also be responsible for neurological sequelae.[70]

Anterior spinal artery syndrome produces a lower motor neuron paralysis (paraplegia) without involvement of the posterior columns of the spinal cord, subserving joint position sense, touch and vibration sensibility and has followed spinal analgesia.[71]

Horner's syndrome has been reported following extradural sacral block.[72] Intracerebral haematoma formation causing hemiparesis, coincident with a lumbar puncture with a 19-G needle, in a previously fit patient, has been reported.[73]

Other conditions which may cause signs and symptoms referable to the central nervous system in any postoperative patient may include: vascular, neoplastic, infective or viral disease, myopathies, neuropathies, operative trauma, e.g. due to the position of the patient on the table, retractors, etc. Careful clinical and electromyographic investigation is always necessary. Subdural haematoma with delayed neurological signs, ending in death, has also occurred.[74] Spinal infarction may occur independently of central neural blockade. An infarcted cord does not recover.[75]

Epidermoid spinal tumours have been reported.[76]

Intraocular haemorrhage has been reported after the rapid injection of 30 ml.[77] This may raise the CSF pressure with resulting subhyaloid bleeding.

In the past, up to 20 ml of thiopentone[78] and 160 ml of parenteral nutritional solution[79] have been accidentally injected into the extradural space, both without harm. Accidental injection of 5 ml ether led to pain followed by temporary paraplegia with full recovery in 4 h.[80]

Neurological complications following operations under spinal analgesia are not necessarily due to the method, while similar complications following surgical operations may be seen in patients who have had general anaesthesia.

BROKEN NEEDLES AND CATHETERS

If a needle breaks, the proximal part and the stylet should, if possible, be left in place to serve as a guide to the distal part. If the proximal part has already been removed, another needle is thrust along the track of the first one for purposes of localization. Removal should be attempted at once under image intensifier. Should a catheter break, it should be noted and the neurosurgeon informed. It is seldom justified to carry out exploration.

THE CHOICE BETWEEN SPINAL (INTRA- AND EXTRADURAL) ANALGESIA AND GENERAL ANAESTHESIA

Advantages of spinal analgesia

1 Obviates the need for general anaesthesia, which may be problematic in some patients.
2 Profound muscle relaxation.
3 Spontaneous respiration, with good abdominal relaxation (useful in patients with respiratory disease).
4 Cheap.
5 Avoids need for intubation where this is likely to be difficult.
6 Reduction of surgical haemorrhage, e.g. at prostatectomy.
7 In hip surgery, epidural block is associated with a smaller incidence of DVT than general anaesthesia,[81] and normal fibrinolysis during and after surgery.[82]
8 Excellent postoperative analgesia.
9 Good cardiovascular stability in peripheral vascular surgery,[83] with reduced stress response,[84] and myocardial protection.[85]

Intradural block can be said to have the following advantages over extradural

1 It is easier.
2 It is quicker.
3 It provides slightly better relaxation of the abdomen.
4 The danger of toxic signs due to the drug are negligible.

Disadvantages of spinal analgesia

1 It may destabilize the circulation in patients with cardiac disease.
2 It may destabilize the circulation in shock.
3 Postoperative headache may occur.
4 Some patients prefer to be asleep during surgery.

Indications for 'spinal' analgesia (intradural and extradural)

1 Operations in lower half of body.
2 Operations in patients with significant pulmonary disease.
3 Avoidance of use of muscle relaxants.
4 Avoidance of use of general anaesthesia when intubation is known to be very difficult.
5 Postoperative and obstetric analgesia.
6 Reduction of surgical stress[86] (for the patient!).

Skilled workers may meet fewer difficulties with central neural blockade than with general anaesthesia in the morbidly obese patient, using a thoracic blockade. Extra-long needles may be required.

Contraindications to spinal blockade

These may be absolute or relative and are listed below.

Absolute

1 Patient refusal – to proceed is trespass.
2 Local infection – may introduce bacteria to the epidural space.
3 Shock – large doses of local anaesthetic should not be used until corrected, as sympathetic blockade may cause cardiovascular collapse; hypovolaemia; dehydration; hypotension below 80–90 mmHg systolic; gross hypertension.[87]
4 Uncorrected coagulopathy or anticoagulation – may promote the occurrence of epidural haematoma.
5 Fixed cardiac output states, e.g. severe aortic stenosis, heart block, medication with beta-blocking drugs, etc., and therefore unable to respond to vasodilatation, sudden blood loss, etc.
6 Inexperienced/unsupervised practitioner.
7 Inadequate facilities/resuscitation equipment.
8 Raised intracranial pressure – dural puncture carries the risk of tentorial/medullary herniation.

Relative

1 Systemic infection (by haematogenous spread) with potential abscess formation.
2 Cardiac disease – myocardial degeneration, toxaemia; severe ischaemic heart disease, especially with history of cardiac infarction.
3 Neurological disease, e.g. cerebral ischaemic attacks. In general there is little evidence that epidurals may cause any exacerbation but any deterioration may be attributed to the epidural. Patients who are chronic sufferers from headaches will in all probability get a headache of moderate severity after operation following intradural block.
4 Major spinal abnormalities or previous surgery – may make the procedure difficult.
5 Mechanical. Patients with a splinted diaphragm which interferes with breathing, due to hydramnios, large ovarian tumours, gross ascites, gross omental obesity. Dangers to be considered include hypoxia due to respiratory inadequacy and aortocaval compression by the tumour mass. Lateral tilt, O_2 and IPPV should be used when indicated. Dosage should be reduced in such patients. This is a relative contraindication related to the size of the abdominal tumour.

6 The acute abdomen. The patient is often shocked with cardiovascular instability, and would be unable to cope with a regurgitation during operation, even if fully conscious.

7 Genito-urinary. In renal artery stenosis, hypotension is to be avoided, either by avoiding spinal analgesia or by actively preventing hypotension during it.

8 Patients with deformed backs. Because of difficulty in the performance of lumbar puncture.

9 Operations for lesions of the spinal cord or cauda equina (on medicolegal grounds).

10 Bleeding disorders.

   (a) Full anticoagulation with heparin: within 6 h of full anticoagulation, spinal block is not performed, nor are epidural catheters removed. An epidural catheter may be sited an hour or more before full anticoagulation, e.g. in vascular surgery.

   (b) Thrombosis prophylaxis with coumarins: not contraindicated if INR is less than 1.5.

   (c) Thrombosis prophylaxis with low-dose heparin: the last dose before the spinal is omitted.

   (d) Thrombosis prophylaxis with low-dose, low-molecular-weight heparin, e.g. clexane: 12 h elapses between the last dose and the spinal (or removal of a spinal catheter);[88] the APTT ratio should be less than 2.

   (e) Low-dose aspirin therapy: acceptable unless bleeding time is abnormal (this is not a very accurate test, but it does show up those seriously prolonged times which present a risk in spinal analgesia).

   It should be remembered that extradural haematoma can occur spontaneously.[89] Vigilance is needed for postoperative epidural haematoma (good prognosis if treated early).

11 In cases of dehydration. These are bad risks and must be fully rehydrated before instituting a spinal block.

SPINAL ANALGESIA IN CHILDREN

Risk of circulatory depression is low because of excellent compensation of their cardiovascular systems. Puncture should be in the L4/L5 interspace because cord extends lower in children than in adults.

THERAPEUTIC USE OF EXTRADURAL INJECTIONS

1 Prolonged postoperative pain relief, e.g. 48–96 h, and for prevention of postoperative chest complications in patients with respiratory failure.

2 In the management of fractured ribs, allowing spontaneous respiration.

3 In eclampsia, to control arterial pressure, increase placental blood flow, and prevent pain-induced hypertension.
4 To control chronic pain.
5 In acute occlusive vascular conditions to promote vasodilatation in the lower half of the body.
6 In obstetrics for pain relief.
7 In the treatment of postspinal headache (blood patch).

EXTRADURAL SACRAL BLOCK (CAUDAL BLOCK)

This method of analgesia was introduced by Cathelin[90] and Sicard[91] (1872–1929) of Paris in 1901. It has been used in animals, especially in cattle, since 1925. Very suitable for block of the sacral and lumbar nerves. For higher block the lumbar approach to the extradural space is preferable as less solution will thereby be used.

Anatomy of the sacrum

The sacrum is a large triangular bone formed by the fusion of the five sacral vertebrae, articulating above with the fifth lumbar vertebra and below with the coccyx.

The posterior surface is convex and down its middle line runs the median sacral crest with its three or four rudimentary spinous processes. The laminae of the fifth and sometimes of the fourth sacral vertebrae fail to fuse in the midline; the deficiency thus formed is known as the sacral hiatus. The tubercles representing the inferior articular processes of the fifth sacral vertebra are prolonged downwards as the sacral cornua. These cornua, with the rudimentary spine of the fouth vertebra above, bound the sacral hiatus. Four posterior sacral foramina correspond with the anterior foramina. Each transmits a sacral nerve posterior ramus and communicates with the sacral canal.

The apex is directed downwards and articulates with the coccyx.

The coccyx represents four rudimentary vertebrae (sometimes three or five).

The sacral canal is a prismatic cavity running through the length of the bone and following its curves from the lumbar canal to the sacral hiatus (closed by the posterior sacrococcygeal membrane). Fibrous strands sometimes occur in the canal and divide the extradural space into compartments. These may account for some cases of failure to produce uniform analgesia. Its anterior wall is the sacral vertebrae; its posterior wall, the laminae. Laterally four foraminae are present. The anterior wall is sometimes very thin, easily pierced by a needle, which then enters a marrow cavity. Aspiration reveals blood and injected drug rapidly enters the venous system.

The contents of the sacral canal are as follows:

1 The dural sac which ends at the upper border of the second sacral vertebra, on a line joining the posterior superior iliac spines. The pia mater is continued as the filum terminale.
2 The sacral nerves and the coccygeal nerve, with their dorsal root ganglia.
3 A venous plexus formed by the lower end of the internal vertebral plexus. These vessels are more numerous anteriorly than posteriorly and so the needle point should be kept as far posteriorly as possible.
4 Areolar and fatty tissue – more dense in males than in females.

The sacral hiatus is a triangular opening, caused by failure of the fifth (and sometimes of the fourth) laminar arch to fuse, with rounded apex formed by the fourth sacral spine, and a sacral cornu on each side below and laterally. It is covered over by the sacrococcygeal membrane which is pierced by the coccygeal and fifth sacral nerves. It is superior to the sacrococcygeal junction, usually about 3.8–5 cm from the tip of the coccyx and directly beneath the upper limit of the intergluteal cleft.

Anatomical abnormalities of the sacrum are not uncommon. They include:

1 upward or downward displacement of the hiatus;
2 pronounced narrowing or partial obliteration of the sacral canal, making needle insertion difficult;
3 ossification of the sacrococcygeal membrane;
4 absence of the bony posterior wall of the sacral canal, due to failure of laminae to fuse,
5 dural extension to the level of S3–S4 in 2% of patients, quoted by Louis,[92] or even to the sacrococcygeal membrane itself;[93]
6 the hiatus may be of many different shapes, ranging from long and narrow to broad and shallow. The epidural space deep to it may range from being deep to excessively shallow. It may have a variable relationship to the tubercles.

The average capacity of the sacral canal is 34 ml in males and 32 ml in females. Its average length is 10–15 cm.

Technique

A needle is inserted through the sacrococcygeal membrane at about 90 degrees to the skin surface in females and 45 degrees in males. Only after penetrating the membrane is the needle hub depressed towards the intergluteal cleft and the needle is advanced into the sacral canal. Moving the needle in this way *before* piercing the membrane will lead the needle point into the subcutaneous tissues rather than the sacral canal. The point must not ascend higher than the line joining the posterior superior iliac spines lest the dura, which ends at this level, be pierced. Occasionally (e.g. in children) the dural sac extends lower than S2. The mean distance between the apex of the hiatus and the dural sac is 4.5 cm.

After aspiration tests for blood and CSF have been proved negative, a test dose can be injected if thought necessary. Should blood flow back through the needle, its tip is probably in the marrow cavity of the body of the vertebra, and must be re-sited correctly in the sacral canal. Should CSF appear, a decision must be made either to proceed to intradural injection, the proper amount of drug being introduced into the theca through the sacral needle, or to abandon the technique.

As a further test of entry to the sacral canal, 1 ml of air may be injected via the needle while an assistant listens over the lumbar spine with a stethoscope. A whoosh of air is clearly heard via the stethoscope.

Five minutes after the test injection of 3 ml of 1% lignocaine with adrenaline 1 : 200 000, movement of the toes is called for; if this is present, an intradural block has not resulted and the needle point is not in the theca; further injection is then made. When the needle is correctly placed, injection is easy, no great force being required to depress the plunger of the syringe (except in patients with spinal stenosis). If the needle is subcutaneous, injection of a few millilitres of air will produce surgical emphysema with its crepitus, or a tumour is raised over the sacrum as the injection proceeds (only seen in thin patients). If the needle point comes to lie between periosteum and bone the force needed for injection will be great – a sure sign of an incorrect position.

Indications

1 Haemorrhoidectomy and other perianal operations.
2 Forceps delivery in obstetrics.
3 Operations on the lower limbs and transurethral operations, e.g. lignocaine 6 mg/kg of 2% solution or bupivacaine 2.2 mg/kg of 0.5% solution.
4 Analgesia for circumcision and herniorraphy.

The extradural injection of large volumes of bupivacaine, e.g. 30 ml of 0.5% solution or other agents, is extensively used for the relief of skeletal pain.

Sacral extradural block in infants and children

Advantages: excellent postoperative analgesia is obtained. Bolus dose of bupivacaine 0.25%, 0.5 ml/kg. Popular for postoperative analgesia in children, e.g. after circumcision and orchidopexy.

Disadvantages include:

1 risk of inadvertent subarachnoid injection, if dura extends downwards;
2 hypotension and possible signs of drug toxicity with large doses;
3 it produces complete flaccidity of the anal sphincters, a condition unpopular with some surgeons doing operations for fissure and fistula-in-ano.

EXTRADURAL AND INTRADURAL OPIOID ANALGESICS

There is no doubt that intrathecal opioids are associated with a much higher incidence of severe respiratory depression than when the drugs are given extradurally, and apnoea has been described many hours later.[94] Close respiratory monitoring of patients is therefore required and naloxone should be available for immediate use in case of respiratory depression. The danger is less if hyperbaric solutions are used and head-up tilt maintained.

Pharmacokinetics and pharmacodynamics

Analgesic drug injected into the extradural space has to pass through the dura into the intradural space to reach the opioid receptors in the cord.

Factors affecting molecular movement include molecular weight, molecular shape, solubility in fat and the concentration of the drug. Fentanyl and diamorphine are relatively highly lipophilic. Morphine is much more water soluble and dissolves more easily in CSF. The drugs act on the spinal cord.

In animals, following extradural injection of morphine, the concentration in lumbar CSF can peak at high levels after 2 h. There is a considerable concentration gradient in the CSF with very low concentrations near the fourth ventricle. Activities such as coughing can, however, disturb the equilibrium, allowing much higher concentrations to reach the brain.[95] The volume in which the drug is dissolved is also probably important.[96]

The danger of respiratory depression is greater when a patient has recently received an intramuscular injection of a narcotic analgesic drug.

Clinical use

Extradural catheter allows the use of repeated doses and infusions. The correct positioning may be validated by injection of local analgesic solution. The segmental level of injection should be as near to the cord segment where analgesia is desired as possible. This is higher than would be required when local analgesic drugs are used. Narcotic analgesic drug without preservative is used.

Fentanyl is often given by infusion; 2–3 μg/ml, infused at 0.1–0.2 ml/kg/h. Ketamine 4 mg in 10 ml of 5% dextrose in water injected into the extradural space also provides potent analgesia postoperatively, without side-effects.[97] Extradural opiates do not directly influence the metabolic response to surgery, but decrease the cortisol response postoperatively, secondary to improved analgesia.[98]

Advantages

1 Reduced dosage compared to intramuscular injection (about 10% of the intramuscular dose).

2 Good and prolonged analgesia without depression of consciousness, skin numbness or motor block.
3 Cardiovascular stability due to lack of sympathetic block.
4 Absence of constipation.

Complications

1 Severe respiratory depression, sometimes delayed up to 10 h, can occur.[99]
2 Itching, particularly in the area supplied by the fifth cranial nerve; sub-hypnotic propofol relieves spinal morphine pruritis,[100] e.g. at 1 mg/kg/h, with target blood level of 1 μg/ml.
3 Some nausea and dizziness has been reported.
4 Urinary retention may occur[101] but is difficult to assess. Urinary retention after extradural morphine may be relieved or prevented by four oral doses of phenoxybenzamine 10 mg given before and after surgery.[102]
5 May cause temporary inability to ejaculate in males.[103]

Choice of drug

Some drug doses which have been recommended for extradural injection for pain relief include: morphine, 2–4 mg; diamorphine, 0.1 mg/kg; methadone, 5–6 mg (top-up dose 4 mg); fentanyl, 0.2 μg/kg (bolus), infusion, 0.2 μg/kg/h); optimal fentanyl concentration is 3 μg/ml to reduce need for local analgesic by 50%;[104] buprenorphine, 0.3 mg; pethidine 10 mg; sufentanil 10 μg.[105] It is common to use an infusion via an epidural catheter.

Other agents have been used, e.g. midazolam.[106]

If opioids are given intradurally extreme caution must be exercised to actively monitor respiration for at least 12 h.

REFERENCES

1 Irwin M. G., Thompson M. and Kenny G. N. C. *Anaesthesia* 1997, **52,** 525–530.
2 Critchley E. M. R. *Br. Med. J.* 1982, **284,** 1588.
3 Newman B. *Anaesthesia* 1983, **38,** 350.
4 Norman P. F. *Br. J. Anaesth.* 1975, **47,** 1111.
5 Reynolds F. and Speedy H. M. *Anaesthesia* 1990, **45,** 120.
6 Adamkiewicz A. *Sber. Akad. Wiss. Wien. Abt. II* 1882, **85,** 101.
7 Djindjian R. *Proc. R. Soc. Med.* 1970, **63,** 181.
8 Dommisse G. F. *Ann. R. Coll. Surg.* 1980, **62,** 369; Dommisse G. F. *Arteries and Veins of the Human Spinal Cord from Birth.* Churchill Livingstone, Edinburgh, 1976.
9 Dunne N. M. and Kox W. J. *Br. J. Anaesth.* 1991, **66,** 617.
10 Magee D. A. et al. *Can. Anaesth. Soc. J.* 1983, **30,** 174.

11 Brockway M. S. et al. *Br. J. Anaesth.* 1991, **66,** 31.

12 Zaric D. et al. *Regional Analg.* 1996, **21,** 14–25.

13 Coda B., Bausch S., Haas M. and Chavkin C. *Regional Anesth.* 1997, **22,** 43–52.

14 Bahar M., Cohen M. L., Grinshpon Y. and Chanimov M. *Can. J. Anaesth.* 1997, **44,** 208–215.

15 Chanimov M. et al. *Anaesthesia* 1997, **52,** 223–228.

16 Klant J. G. et al. *Anaesthesia* 1997, **52,** 547–551.

17 Dahl J. B. et al. *Br. J. Anaesth.* 1990, **64,** 178; Flatter A. et. al. *Br. J. Anaesth.* 1990, **65,** 294.

18 Lee J. A. *Anaesthesia* 1960, **l5,** 186.

19 Dufy G. P. *Br. Med. J.* 1982, **285,** 1163.

20 Charlebois P. A. *Can. Anaesth. Soc. J.* 1966, **13,** 585.

21 Saberski L. R., Kondamuri S. and Osinubi O. Y. O. *Regional Anesth.* 1997, **22,** 3–15.

22 Mehta M. and Salmon N. *Anaesthesia* 1985, **40,** 1009.

23 Marcus M. A. E. et al. *Anesth Analg.* 1997, **84,** 1113–1116.

24 Lambert D. H., Hurley R. J., Hertwig L. and Datta S. *Regional Anesth.* 1997, **22,** 66–72.

25 Vakharia S. B., Thomas P. S., Rosenbaum A. E., Wasenko J. J., Fellows D. G. *Anesth. Analg.* 1997, **84,** 585–590.

26 Walker D. S. and Brock-Utne J. G. *Can. J. Anaesth.* 1997, **44,** 494–497.

27 Zaric D. et al. *Regional Anaesth.* 1996, **21,** 14–25.

28 Segal S., Eappen S. and Datta S. *J. Clin. Anesth.* 1997, **9,** 109–112.

29 Kestin I. G. *Br. J. Anaesth.* 1990, **65,** 280.

30 Kestin I. G. et al. *Br. J. Anaesth.* 1991, **66,** 232; Kestin I. G. and Goodman N. W. *Anaesthesia* 1991, **46,** 93.

31 Hirota K., Browne T., Appadu B. L. and Lambert D. G. *Br. J. Anaesth.* 1997, **78,** 185–188.

32 McWhirter W. R. et al. *Anesthesiology* 1973, **39,** 398.

33 Marcus M. A. E. et al. *Anesth. Analg.* 1997, **84,** 1113–1116.

34 Schierhout G. and Roberts I. *Br. Med. J.* 1998, **316,** 961–964.

35 Aitkenhead A. R. et al. *Br. J. Anaesth.* 1980, **52,** 1071.

36 Rem J. et al. *Lancet* 1980, **1,** 283.

37 Moller I. W. et al. *Acta Anaesth. Scand.* 1982, **58,** Traynor C. et al. *Br. J. Anaesth.* 1982, **54,** 319; Buckley F. P. et al. *Br. J. Anaesth.* 1982, **54,** 325.

38 Ben-David B. and Solomon E. *Anesth. Analg.* 1997, **85,** 1357–1358.

39 Fernando R. et al. *Anaesthesia* 1997, **52,** 517–534.

40 Igarashi T. et al. *Br. J. Anaesth.*, 1997, **78,** 149–152.

41 Woerth S. D. et al. *Anesthesiology* 1977, **47,** 380.

42 Cornish P. B. *Anesth. Analg.* 1997, **84,** 1387–1388; Liu S. S. et al. *Anesth. Analg.* 1997, **85,** 1416.

43 Ben-David B. and Solomon E. *Anesth. Analg.* 1997, **85,** 1357–1358.

44 Longmire S. and Joyce T. H. *Anesthesiology* 1984, **39,** 1115.

45 Fink B. R. *Anesth. Analg.* 1990, **71,** 208.

46 Kumar C. M. and Dennison B. *Anaesthesia* 1986, **41,** 556.

47 Gibb W. R. G. and Wen P. *Br. Med. J.* 1984, **289,** 530; Broadley S. A. and Fuller G. N. *Br. Med. J.* 1997, **315,** 1324–1325.

48 Vacanti J. J. *Anesthesiology* 1972, **37**, 358; Mulroy M. F. *Anesthesiology* 1979, **51**, 479.
49 Wark R. J. *Anaesthesia* 1977, **32**, 336.
50 Thomas T. A. and Noble H. A. *Anaesthesia* 1990, **45**, 459.
51 Sprotte G. *Regional Anaesth.* 1987, **10**, 104.
52 Broadley S. A. and Fuller G. N. *Br. Med. J.* 1997, **315**, 1324–1325.
53 Ferouz F. et al. *Anesthesiology* 1997, **86**, 592–598.
54 Crawford J. S. *Br. J. Anaesth.* 1972, **44**, 598.
55 Vakharia S. B., Thomas P. S., Rosenbaum A. E., Wasenko J. J. and Fellows D.G. *Anesth. Analg.* 1997, **84**, 585–590.
56 Rainbird A. and Pfitzner J. *Anaesthesia* 1983, **38**, 481.
57 Horlocker T. T. et al. *Anesth. Analg.* 1997, **84**, 578–584.
58 Russell R., Dundas R. and Reynolds F. *Br. Med. J.* 1996, **312**, 1384–1388; Reynolds F. and Russell R. *Br. Med. J.* 1998, **316**, 69–70.
59 Roberts S. P. and Petts H. V. *Anaesthesia* 1990, **45**, 377; Lee J J and Parry H. *Br. J. Anaesth.* 1991, **66**, 383.
60 Seigne T. D. *Anaesthesia* 1970, **25**, 402; Phillips O. C. *Anesth. Analg.* 1970, **25**, 402.
61 Venua E. *Wien. Klin. Wochenschr.* 1907, **20**, 566.
62 Cashman J. N. *Anaesthesia* 1984, **39**, 248.
63 Wang. B. C. et al. *Regional Anesth.* 1982, **7**, 85.
64 Edwards G. M. and Sprigge J. *Anaesthesia* 1984, **38**, 194.
65 Shigematsu L. et al. *Anesth. Analg. (Cleve.)* 1985, **64**, 653.
66 Scott D. B. *Br. Med. J.* 1982, **285**, 1048.
67 Beaudoin M. G. and Klein L. *Anaesth. Intensive Care* 1984, **12**, 163.
68 Chaudhari L. S. et al. *Anaesthesia* 1978, **33**, 722; Loarie D. J. and Fairley H. B. *Anesth. Analg. Curr. Res.* 1978, **57**, 351.
69 Crawford J. S. *Br. J. Anaesth.* 1975, **47**, 412.
70 Yates D. A. H. *J. R. Soc. Med.* 1981, **74**, 334; Hawkes C. H. and Roberts G. M. *Br. J. Hosp. Med.* 1980, **23**, 498.
71 Bhuiyan M. S., Mallick A. and Parsloe M. *Anaesthesia* 1998, **53**, 583–586.
72 Paw H. *Br. Med. J.* 1998, **316**, 160.
73 Wedel D. J. and Mulroy M. F. *Anesthesiology* 1983, **59**, 475.
74 Edelman J. D. and Wingard D. W. *Anesthesiology* 1980, **52**, 166.
75 Silver J. R. and Buxton J. H. *Brain* 1974, **97 (III)**, 539; Annotation *Lancet* 1974, **2**, 1299.
76 Rifaat M. *J. Neurosurg.* 1973, **38**, 366; Shaywitz B. A. *J. Pediatr.* 1972, **80**, 638; Batnitzky S. et al. *Lancet* 1977, **1**, 635.
77 Clark C. J. and Whitwell J. *Br. Med. J.* 1961, **2**, 1612.
78 Cay D. L. *Anaesth. Intensive Care* 1984, **12**, 61.
79 Patel P. C. et al. *Anaesthesia* 1984, **39**, 383.
80 Mappes A. and Schaer H. M. *Anaesthesia* 1991, **46**, 435.
81 Thorburn J. et al. *Br. J. Anaesth.* 1980, **52**, 1117.
82 Rosenfield B. A. et al. *Anesthesiology* 1993, **79**, 435–443.
83 Christopherson R. et al., *J. Clin. Anaesth.* 1996, **8**, 578–584.
84 Parker S. D. et al. *Crit. Care Med.* 1994, **23** 1954–1961.
85 Meibner A., Rolf N. and Van Aken H. *Anesth. Analg.* 1997, **85**, 517–528.

86 Parker S. D. et al. *Crit. Care Med.* 1994, **23,** 1954–1961.

87 Dagnino J. and Prys-Roberts C. *Br. J. Anaesth.* 1984, **56,** 1065.

88 Horlocker T. T. and Heit J. A. *Anesth. Analg.* 1997, **85,** 874–885.

89 *See also* Macdonald R. *Br. J. Anaesth.* 1991, **66,** 1; Wildsmith J. A. W. and McClure J. H. *Anaesthesia* 1991, **46,** 613.

90 Cathelin F. C. *R. Soc. Biol. (Paris)* 1901, **53,** 452.

91 Sicard J. A. C. *R. Soc. Biol. (Paris)* 1901, **53,** 396 (both Cathelin's and Sicard's papers are translated and reprinted in 'Classical File'. *Surv. Anesthesiol.* 1979, **23,** 271).

92 Nolte H. and Farrar M. D. *Anaesthesia* 1984, **39,** 1142.

93 Meyer R. J. *Anaesthesia* 1984, **39,** 610.

94 Daines G. K. et al. *Anesthesiology* 1980, **52,** 280; Davies G. K. *Anaesthesia* 1980, **35,** 1080.

95 Kafer E. R. et al. *Anesthesiology* 1983, **58,** 418.

96 Chrabasik J. et al. *Lancet* 1984, **1,** 793.

97 Islas J. A. et al. *Anesth. Analg. (Cleve.)* 1985, **64,** 1161.

98 Normandale J. P. et al. *Anaesthesia* 1985, **40,** 748.

99 Sidi A. et al. *Anaesthesia* 1981, **36,** 1044.

100 Warwick J. P., Kearns C. F. and Scott W. E. *Anaesthesia* 1997, **52,** 265–275.

101 Torda T. A. et al. *Br. J. Anaesth.* 1980, **52,** 939.

102 Evron S. et al. *Br. Med. J.* 1984, **288,** 190.

103 Torda T. A. et al. *Br. J. Anaesth.* 1980, **52,** 939.

104 Lyons G., Columb M., Hawthorne L. and Dresner M. *Br. J. Anaesth.* 1997, **78,** 493–497.

105 Campbell D. C. et al. *Anesthesiology* 1997,**86,** 525–531.

106 Niv D. et al. *Br. J. Anaesth.* 1983, **55,** 541.

Section 6
CHRONIC PAIN

Chronic pain

S.J. Dolin, Pain Clinic, St Richard's Hospital, Chichester

Pain is defined as 'an unpleasant sensory and emotional experience associated with actual or potential tissue damage, or described in terms of such' (International Association for the Study of Pain (IASP) definition). Chronic pain is pain that persists beyond a reasonable time that one would expect the pain from an acute injury to settle. The origin of the pain can be from ongoing tissue damage, such as arthritis or cancer (nociceptive), as a result of nerve injury (neuropathic) or the pain can be of unknown origin. For all pain types, both the pre-existing psychological make-up of the patient and the psychological response to ongoing pain can make an important contribution to the clinical picture.

The pain clinic

Pain clinics are usually headed by anaesthetists in conjunction with other specialties, including rheumatology, neurology, neurosurgery, psychiatry and other disciplines including nursing, physiotherapy, occupational therapy and clinical psychology. They are generally run as a multidisciplinary team.

The role of the pain clinic in patient care can be summed up as:

1 decrease subjective pain experience;
2 increase general level of activity;
3 decrease drug consumption;
4 return to employment or full quality of life;
5 decrease further use of health care resources.

Facilities required for a successful pain clinic should include a dedicated space for the multidisciplinary team to work together. This should include dedicated office space, consulting rooms, space for group-based pain management, and one-to-one treatments such as transcutaneous electrical nerve stimulation (TENS) and physiotherapy. Access to a X-ray imaging in a suitable room with monitoring and resuscitation is also required: many pain clinics make use of the day-surgery unit which is ideally suited for nerve blocks. Essential pain clinic equipment will include suitable imaging, suitable monitoring for sedation, radio-frequency lesion generator, cryoprobe machine and peripheral nerve stimulator. Access to in-patient beds is an excellent option for those requiring complex medication changes, or therapies requiring prolonged drug administration via complex routes, e.g. epidural or intrathecal.

Pain clinics have been shown to be effective, both for nerve block treatments[1] and for psychologically based therapies.[2]

The pain patient

Chronic pain is common, affecting an estimated 20–30% of the population. As the pain clinic approach is that of symptom control, referrals should ideally come from other specialties, where previous diagnostic work-up has been completed and after appropriate surgical and medical therapy. Most common referral is for back pain, mostly via rheumatology and orthopaedic clinics. Other routes of referral are from general medical and surgical firms, as well as neurology and the palliative care service. Some general practice referrals can be accepted, as long as complex diagnostic work-up is not required.

The patient will have already tried a variety of analgesic drugs, usually with only modest success. Others may be using benzodiazepines and antidepressants. Most will have tried physiotherapy and other alternative therapies often with limited success. Anxiety and depression are commonly found in chronic pain patients, and it is often unclear whether these are primary or secondary to persistent pain. Other emotions include anger and blame. Post-traumatic stress disorder commonly follows chronic pain due to trauma.[3] Litigation for personal injury or medical negligence is increasingly common. The patient may be in receipt of benefits for unemployment and disability.

Assessment of pain

Important aspects of pain assessment are as follows.

1 Site of pain. Body maps indicate extent of pain, and often request patient to identify the primary pain site. Total body pain is a surprisingly common presentation.
2 Severity of pain using visual analogue pain scales (VAS 100 mm continuous line) or numerical rating scale (scale of 0–10) or categorical rating (mild/moderate/severe).
3 Duration of pain.
4 Cause of pain, and diagnosis if known. Pain of unknown aetiology is common. Precipitating episode (surgery, trauma) or spontaneous onset.
5 Past history of pain: previous investigations, surgery, injections and other pain clinic treatments.
6 Pattern of pain: continuous, intermittent or flare-up pattern.
7 What makes the pain worse?
8 What makes the pain better?

9 Medications, TENS and other therapies. How effective are they ?
10 What words do they use to describe the pain?
11 Ask about depression and anxiety: sleep pattern, mood, fatigue, tearfulness, guilt feelings, future outlook, and any past history of depression, how treated and if successful.
12 Current levels of activity and employment. What does the pain stop the patient doing? How far can he or she walk, drive ? Is the patient independent for dressing, bathing ?
13 Home situation. Who is at home? Are they all well? Is the patient a carer or does he or she have a carer?
14 Is litigation active?

Commonly used pain questionnaires are the Brief Pain Inventory, and the McGill Pain Questionnaire. Many other questionnaires have been devised for research purposes but are occasionally useful for clinical practice (Beck Depression Inventory, MMPI). Patient pain diaries are commonly used by pain clinics.

Pain clinics are not intended for diagnostic assessment. If the pain clinician is at all unclear of the explanation for symptoms re-referral to appropriate specialist is in order. Many complex pain problems, however, elude a diagnosis, in spite of extensive investigations. Many pain clinics run joint clinics with other specialties, especially rheumatology, orthopaedics, maxillofacial surgery and psychiatry.

GENERALIZED PAIN PATTERNS

Neuropathic pain

Neuropathic pain is initiated or caused by primary lesion in the peripheral nervous system. It includes neuralgia and painful peripheral neuropathy. Neuralgia is pain in the distribution of a nerve or nerves, including trigeminal and post-herpetic neuralgia, scar pain. Painful polyneuropathies are usually symmetric and distal, affecting the feet and sometimes the hands, including diabetic and ischaemic neuropathy. These conditions may present with or without paraesthesiae, hypoaesthesia, hyperalgesia (excessive pain with noxious stimulus) and allodynia (touch is perceived as pain).

The mechanism of neuropathic pain is different to nociceptive pain. Peripheral mechanisms involve abnormal C-fibre function which can become sensitized to sympathetic stimulation. Axon sprouts develop where primary afferent neurons have been damaged. These may show abnormal sensitivity to mechanical, noradrenergic and thermal stimulation, and may also fire independent of any sensory input. Adjacent neurons may develop abnormal connections which may be recruited into the exaggerated response to stimuli. Central mechanisms involve changes in the long-term excitability of dorsal horn cells. These are mediated through the NMDA subtype of glutamate receptor, known as 'wind-up'. Damage to peripheral or central neurons can lead to loss of coordination of neuronal inhibitory processes.

Treatment of neuropathic pain is as follows:[4]

1 Tricyclic antidepressants are drugs of first choice with most neuropathic pains. Commonly used examples are dothiepin, amitriptyline, doxepin, nortripyline, imipramine (at daily doses of 25–75 mg) orally. Sedation is a problem, but lower doses generally well tolerated.
2 Anticonvulsants, including carbamazepine, phenytoin and clonazepam are often effective second-line drugs. Sedation and ataxia may limit their use.
3 Sodium-channel blockers lignocaine (intravenous and topical) and mexilitene (orally) can be effective.
4 Opioids (oral, intrathecal) can be effective in some but not all cases of neuropathic pain.
5 Capsaicin cream has been used on affected areas of skin, but its effectiveness is still uncertain.
6 Non-steroidals (oral and topical) have been effective in some studies, but not others.
7 Ketamine (intravenous and epidural) is effective but route of administration limits its use.
8 Clonidine (topical, oral, epidural) is also useful, but side-effects include sedation and hypotension.
9 Lumbar sympathectomy (chemical or radiofrequency) are often used to treat ischaemic leg pain, but it is unclear if they work by improving blood flow or reducing neuropathic pain.
10 Electrical stimulation (spinal cord stimulation) has been used successfully for some forms of neuropathic pain.[5]

Post-herpetic neuralgia is one of the more common forms of neuropathic pain seen in pain clinics. the herpes zoster virus causes an acute painful attack with skin lesions which gradually resolve over several weeks. In a small percentage of cases chronic pain and associated numbness occurs in the area of the scar. Clinical symptoms are pain, dysaesthesia, paraesthesia, allodynia and paroxysms of lancinating pain. The most common sites are the cranial nerves and the thoracic dermatomes. Early recognition and prompt treatment with an antiviral agent can be effective in preventing the development of post-herpetic neuralgia. Treatment is as for other neuropathic pain. Response to treatment is unpredictable and a few patients will be left with severe intractable pain, especially in the elderly.

Phantom pain occurs following amputation of limbs, but has also been described following mastectomy and anterior–posterior bowel resection. The aetiology is unclear. Most patients experience transient phantom sensations following amputation but only some patients experience phantoms as painful. Prophylactic treatment appears to be effective. Establishing epidural analgesia prior to amputation appears to diminish the incidence of phantom limb pain.[6] Other problems such as painful neuroma and muscle spasms can complicate the management of amputation pain. Treatment is as for other neuropathic pains.

Central (post-stroke) pain, also known as thalamic pain, occurs occasionally after a cerebrovascular accident, usually of the cerebral cortex. There may be associated sensory deficit. There is usually a background steady pain and occasionally an intermittent or lancinating pain.[7]

Scar pain can occur after any operation, but is most common after thoracotomy, inguinal hernia repair and mastectomy. It is due to neuroma formation where nerves have regenerated in an abnormal manner. Treatment is by local infiltration of the neuroma or the nerve supplying the area. If unsuccessful in the long term, cryoanalgesia can be helpful.

Complex regional pain syndromes (reflex sympathetic dystrophy)

The terms complex regional pain syndromes (CRPS) Type I and Type II are used to describe a syndrome of pain and sudomotor or vasomotor instability.

CRPS Type I (reflex sympathetic dystrophy) is defined as a syndrome that usually starts after a noxious event, is not limited to the distribution of a single peripheral nerve, and is disproportionate to the inciting event. The diagnosis requires:

1 pain, allodynia, or hyperalgesia disproportionate to the injury;
2 evidence at some time of oedema, changes in skin blood flow, or abnormal sudomotor activity in the region of the pain;
3 no other condition that would otherwise account for the degree of pain and dysfunction.

CRPS Type II (causalgia) is defined as a syndrome that starts after a nerve injury, and is not necessarily limited to the distribution of the injured nerve. The diagnostic criteria are the same as CRPS I. The difference between CRPS II and neuropathic pain is that CRPS II diagnosis requires evidence of oedema, cutaneous blood flow changes, or abnormal sudomotor activity.

Treatment of CRPS is as follows.

1 Medical therapies as for neuropathic pain (above).
2 Intravenous regional sympathetic blockade using guanethidine (10–20 mg) in prilocaine on three or more occasions. While still commonly used, doubt has recently been cast on the effectiveness of this therapy.
3 Intravenous regional techniques using ketanserin or bretylium have been shown to be effective, but are probably not widely used.
4 Oral corticosteroids have been shown to be effective, but again are probably not widely used.
5 Transcutaneous electrical nerve stimulation may be helpful.
6 Physiotherapy should be combined with pain-relieving treatments in an attempt to restore function. Specialist hand physiotherapists are worth seeking out here as the residual dysfunction can be significant. Hand rehabilitation may need to be prolonged.

Sympathetic blocks (lumbar chemical or radio-frequency sympathectomy or cervical/thoracic sympathectomy done by percutaneous radio-frequency or diathermy using a transthoracic approach) have been used but effectiveness is as yet unproven.

Muscle/soft-tissue pain

Fibromyalgia is a chronic pain disorder characterized by diffuse musculo-skeletal pain, stiffness, tenderness, fatigue and sleep disturbance. It occurs most commonly in women in the 20–40-year age group. Patients may describe their symptoms as total body pain, and the most striking feature on clinical examination is widespread muscle tenderness on palpation. Fibromyalgia is similar in presentation to chronic fatigue syndrome (ME), but in the latter, fatigue rather than pain is the predominant presenting symptom. Treatment of fibromyalgia is as for many pain syndromes. Regular analgesia can be help-ful. Low-dose tricyclic antidepressants can help restore sleep patterns and in addition have analgesic properties. Pain management programmes may be helpful. Physiotherapy based on pacing physical activity is more likely to be successful than fitness programmes. Prognosis is generally guarded, although the natural history of this condition is not well described.[8]

Myofascial pain syndrome is a regional pain disorder characterized by a local area of deep muscle tenderness called a trigger point, and a reference zone of pain, which is worsened by palpation of the trigger point. Each muscle group has characteristic trigger points and pain pattern. The most common muscles groups seen in the pain clinic with identifiable myofascial pain patterns are quadratus lumborum, gluteals, quadriceps femoris, levator scapulae and trapezius. Treatment is by avoidance of perpetuating factors such as repetitive muscle use, trigger point injection and a technique called a 'spray and stretch', which involves stretching the affected muscle group. Prognosis is generally good.[9]

Pain of advanced cancer

Pain occurs in 70% of patients with advanced cancer. Problems related to advanced cancer are dealt with mostly by palliative care services but there is often a large overlap with pain clinics. Clinical features of cancer pain syndromes are as follows.

1 Bone metastases from lung, breast or prostate produce multiple pain sites, worse on movement.
2 Invasion of hollow viscus (stomach, colon) by tumour produces colicky abdominal pain, worse with eating, improved by vomiting.
3 Liver metastases from bowel, lung or breast produce upper quadrant abdominal pain and hepatomegaly.
4 Bladder spasm from bladder or prostate cancer produces colicky supra-pubic pain. Infection or blood clots may need specific treatment.
5 Ureteric colic can occur with carcinoma of ureter or bladder, and will produce loin pain radiating to the groin.
6 Chest-wall or rib pain occurs with carcinoma of the lung and meso-thelioma.
7 Abdominal metastases occur with carcinoma of ovary and colon, and result in diffuse abdominal pain and tenderness.

8 Neuropathic pain occurs when nerves are damaged by tumour, as occurs in Pancoast's syndrome or invasion of the sacral plexus.
9 Headache occurs when tumours result in raised intracranial pressure, and when cranial nerves are involved, such as trigeminal neuralgia associated with meningioma and acoustic neuroma.
10 Spinal cord involvement can result from spinal metastases and can result in radicular pain as well as progressive sensory and motor deficit and sphincter dysfunction.
11 Painful muscle spasm can result from bony metastases and following hemiplegia.
12 Infection of fungating tumours produces severe pain.

Treatment of pain of advanced cancer includes active treatments such as radiotherapy which is especially effective for bony metastases, chemotherapy, hormone manipulation, orthopaedic correction of pathological fractures, surgical correction of bowel obstruction and neurosurgical decompression of cranium or spinal cord. Dexamethasone is commonly used to reduce painful tissue oedema.

Analgesic therapies are based on the WHO analgesic ladder, which involves a progression from a non-opioid analgesic such as paracetamol, to a weak opioid such as Co-proxamol (paracetamol plus dextropropoxyphene) to a strong opioid, such as morphine.

When pain of advanced cancer is not adequately treated by active treatments (above) or weak opioids the following options can be used.

1 Morphine, given orally as an elixir (Oramorph), which is quick acting but relatively short duration, tablets (Sevredol) which are also quick acting, slow-release tablets given either twice a day (MST) or once a day (MXL). Most patients manage on doses up to 200 mg/day, although some patients may require much higher doses. Oral diamorphine can be used as an alternative, but is not generally available outside the UK.
2 Methadone orally given 8–12-hourly can be a useful alternative when morphine becomes less effective (known as opioid rotation).
3 Fentanyl patches (Durogesic) with 72-h duration have become a popular alternative especially when vomiting precludes the oral route.
4 Diamorphine given subcutaneously by syringe driver is a commonly used technique for patients with vomiting, dysphagia and coma. Antiemetics such as cyclizine are often added when vomiting is a problem, and midazolam can also be added to treat terminal anxiety and distress.
5 Co-analgesics are often added to augment opioids and examples include non-steroidal anti-inflammatory drugs (NSAIDs), tricyclic antidepressants and other drugs used to treat neuropathic pain (*see above*).
6 Epidural catheter analgesia using bupivacaine plus diamorphine by continuous infusion can be used when oral opioid analgesia is unsuccessful. It can be used in the hospice as well as at home, but will require a large-volume (250-ml) portable pump and good coordination of staff.
7 Intrathecal catheter analgesia using diamorphine, clonidine and bupivacaine gives more widespread and better quality analgesia than the epidural

route. These can be tunnelled and externalized and connected to a portable pump, or fully implantable systems are available.

8 Other catheter techniques such as interpleural, brachial and lumbar plexus infusions using bupivacaine have been used.

A number of neurolytic techniques are in common practice for pain of advanced cancer.

1 Coeliac plexus block using alcohol or phenol is widely used for carcinoma of pancreas, but is also useful for pain emanating from stomach, liver and small intestine. The coeliac plexus transmits the majority of pain fibres from the upper abdomen via the splanchnic nerves and sympathetic trunks to T5–T12. The plexus lies anterior to the aorta at T12/L1 level. It can be approached either posteriorly through the crura of the diaphragm or directly through the aorta, or anteriorly through the liver or stomach. The technique is usually done under X-ray fluoroscopy but can be ultrasound or computed tomography (CT) guided. Side-effects include transient pain on injection, hypotension and diarrhoea.[10]

2 Splanchnic nerve blocks using phenol or alcohol are performed above the diaphragm at T11/T12, and used for similar indication as coeliac plexus blocks.

3 Chemical sympathectomy, either lumbar of presacral, can be used for refractory lower limb or pelvic pain.

4 Cordotomy done via radio-frequency of the spinothalamic tract at C2 is used mostly for mesothelioma which can be resistant to many other therapies.[11]

5 Intrathecal neurolysis using phenol or alcohol is an occasionally used technique for trunk pain. It carries the complication of sphincter and motor paralysis. Epidural neurolysis has also been described but results are variable.

CHRONIC PAIN BY ANATOMICAL LOCATION

Headache

Migraine is periodic unilateral headache. Pain is described as throbbing. Associated symptoms include nausea, vomiting and diarrhoea. Photophobia is common as is a visual aura that may precede the pain. Duration is usually about 4 h but can last longer. Occasionally focal neurological deficits occur. Treatment is to abort the current attack and to prevent the occurrence of migraine in the future.

Abortive therapies include:

1 sumatriptan is a 5-hydroxytryptamine (5-HT) analogue, given parenterally;
2 NSAIDs and antiemetics can also be effective;
3 ergotamine was the drug of first choice in the past but is contraindicated in coronary and cerebrovascular disease;

4 nerve blocks including sphenopalatine ganglion block have been used to terminate an attack.

Prophylactic treatment includes:

1 pizotifen, a 5-HT and histamine antagonist;
2 beta-adrenergic antagonists, propranalol and metoprolol;
3 calcium-channel antagonist verapamil;
4 serial sphenopalatine ganglion blocks have been described.

Cervicogenic headache is predominantly unilateral often with neck and arm pain. There are signs of cervical spondylosis with pain on movement and limited range of movement. Pain typically starts at the back of the head but may also involve the face, whereas migraine mostly starts at the front of the head, often centred behind the eye. There is a close anatomical relationship between upper cervical neurones and the trigeminal spinal nucleus. When the C2 nerve root is involved the headache is over the occiput and can be relieved by greater occipital nerve block. Injection of cervical facet joints can relieve pain in some circumstances and are diagnostic for radio-frequency cervical facet denervation. *Myofascial pain syndromes* involving posterior cervical muscles groups and sternomastoid can present as headache and can respond to injection and stretching (*see* 'Mysofascial pain syndrome' above).

Face pain

Temporomandibular joint dysfunction is a common chronic pain syndrome, more often seen in maxillofacial units. It is characterized by pain arising from the joints with joint noises and trismus. The pain radiates widely to the temporal, mastoid and occipital areas as well as the neck. The pain arises from arthritic changes in the joint and muscle spasm. There will be palpable and audible clicking and limited jaw opening. Auriculotemporal nerve block may be diagnostic. Treatment options are:

1 reassurance and simple analgesia including NSAIDs;
2 low-dose tricyclic antidepressants;
3 local anaesthetic injections into the joint and associated muscle groups (masseter, temporalis and lateral pterygoid) can be used to relieve muscle spasm.
4 psychological therapies including biofeedback have been used to teach muscle relaxation;
5 botulinum toxin has been injected in small doses into the affected muscle groups, but this work remains unproved;
6 occasionally arthroscopy and surgery is performed but this is reserved for the more severe, refractory cases.

Facial neuralgias involve the trigeminal, glossopharyngeal and superior laryngeal nerves. The following are examples:

1 Mental nerve compression in the bony canal of the mandible can occur in Paget's disease, and may require surgical decompression. In elderly

edentulous patients the nerve can become exposed as the mandible resorbs and may need to be repositioned.

2 Following tooth extraction, particularly third molar extraction, the mandibular nerve can be traumatized resulting in peripheral neuropathic pain (*see above*). Mandibular nerve blocks may be helpful temporarily and may lead onto cryotherapy of the affected nerve.

3 Post-herpetic neuralgia can occur in the various divisions of the trigeminal nerve and can represent a great therapeutic challenge (*see below*).

4 Intracranial neuralgias can result from lesions such as meningioma and acoustic neuroma which can involve the cranial nerves as they exit the skull.

Atypical face pain is a common presentation to pain clinics. It is important that a thorough diagnostic work-up is performed to exclude oral and maxillo-facial pathology. Investigations may include an odontopantogram and facial and maxillary CT imaging. Atypical face pain is continuous chronic face pain that occurs in the absence of demonstrable pathology. The aetiology is unknown. Treatment options are:

1 low-dose tricyclic antidepressants, dothiepin 25–75 mg orally nocte;
2 low-dose phenothiazines, trifluoperazine, can be added to the tricyclics;
3 TENS can be useful;
4 acupuncture is widely used for this condition;
5 the value of psychological therapies is unknown.

Temporal arteritis is an important condition to recognize. It can present as acute temporal pain, often with a tender inflamed temporal artery. Diagnosis is usually made by a high erythrocyte sedimentation rate (ESR). It is important to recognize and treat this condition promptly with high-dose steroids (prednisolone up to 60 mg/day), as delay can result in involvement of the ophthalmic artery and blindness.

Trigeminal neuralgia is not a specific disease but a symptom often caused by pathology involving the fifth cranial nerve. A loop of artery has been observed to impinge upon the nerve and surgical reposition of the artery can alleviate symptoms. The causative link, however, remains speculative. Trigeminal neuralgia can also occur in multiple sclerosis, aneurysm and in cerebello-pontine angle tumours (acoustic neuroma, meningioma). Most cases remain idiopathic.

Clinical features of trigeminal neuralgia are as follows:

1 Episodic recurrent unilateral face pain described as a sudden high intensity jab or electric shock.
2 Duration is just a few seconds with repetitive bursts over minutes. Frequent episodes may occur over several weeks, followed by prolonged pain-free intervals.
3 Occurs in the mandibular and maxillary divisions of the trigeminal nerve, while ophthalmic pain is less common.
4 Pain is triggered by stimulation of face, lips or mouth, and patients will avoid stimulation.

5 Cranial nerve examination is usually normal. If a trigeminal neurological deficit is found, magnetic resonance imaging (MRI) is indicated to exclude underlying pathology.

Treatment options for trigeminal neuralgia are as follows:

1 Carbamazepine up to 1000 mg/day. Most cases will respond to this therapy alone. Side-effects are sedation and ataxia which may limit their value in the elderly. Bone marrow suppression, liver and renal impairment occur with prolonged therapy and will require monitoring.
2 Second-line drug therapy includes phenytoin, baclofen and clonazepam.
3 Radio-frequency trigeminal ganglion thermocoagulation is performed in many pain clinics. It involves placing an insulated needle through the foramen ovale under fluoroscopy. Placement is assessed by stimulation down the needle, using both motor (muscles of mastication) and sensory testing. When the correct dermatome is located a radio-frequency heat lesion (75°C for 60 s) is perfomed in the trigeminal ganglion. Some numbness will occur in the face but this is usually self-limiting. This is probably the technique of choice when medical therapy fails.[12]
4 Injection of glycerol into the trigeminal ganglion is also used but less commonly than thermocoagulation.
5 Cryotherpy of the peripheral branches of the trigeminal nerve, especially mental and infraorbital nerve is commonly done in maxillofacial units. This is a useful short-term procedure but repeated freezing becomes difficult due to scarring.
6 Microvascular decompression is a neurosurgical technique which is recommended in younger patients. It does have a mortality and morbidity rate which are generally not seen with the percutaneous techniques, but long-term results may be better.

Neck pain

Whiplash injury is common and occurs after deceleration injury to the cervical spine. Most whiplash injuries settle spontaneously within 3 months regardless of treatment. Those that persist beyond 3 months become chronic. Pre-existing neck problems including spondylosis and speed of impact contribute to chronicity. Structures involved in whiplash injuries are the cervical facet (zygopophyseal joints) and the intervertebral discs. The pain is predominantly unilateral as rotation of the spine often occurs during the injury. There may also be marked muscle spasm secondary to the facet joint injury. Patients may also complain of headaches, arm pain and numbness, especially in the medial fingers reflecting trauma to the nerves that contribute to the ulnar nerve where they cross the first rib. The following are treatment options.

1 Regular analgesia and TENS.
2 Radio-frequency cervical facet denervation of the affected facet joints. This is done percutaneously under fluoroscopy and involves thermocoagulation

of the posterior ramus of the cervical nerves, usually C3–C5. The levels may need to be determined by selective diagnostic facet joint blocks.

3 Physiotherapy and muscle stretching may be needed following cervical facet denervation.[13]

Cervical radiculopathy can occur with cervical disc prolapse or due to cervical spondylosis, often precipitated by minor trauma, if the intervertebral foramen is already narrowed by osteophytes. The pain is typically dermatomal and neuropathic, often described as burning or lancinating. Treatment options are as follows:

1 Cervical epidural or nerve root injections via the intervertebral foramen.
2 Radio-frequency partial dorsal root ganglion rhizolysis via the foramen. This will require repeated diagnostic nerve blocks to determine the correct level.
3 Surgical decompression is occasionally required but this is done infrequently compared with the lumbar spine.[14]

Thoracic pain

Costochondritis presents as pain in the anterior chest wall. Involved sites are tender to palpation without inflammation. It is a benign, usually self-limiting disorder that may respond to simple analgesia, but may require infiltration of tender points with local anaesthetic and steroid or repeated cryoanalgesia.

Osteoporotic crush fractures present commonly to pain clinics. Osteoporosis alone tends not to be painful but spontaneous crush fractures of the thoracic vertebrae occurs with advanced osteoporosis. It usually occurs in elderly women or in those on prolonged steroid therapy. There is sudden onset of thoracic back pain, often with unilateral thoracic root pain. The diagnosis is confirmed by plain radiograph. It is important to exclude malignancy (myeloma) as a possible cause. Prophylactic treatment is aimed at preventing the progression of the disease but will not affect pain associated with the crush fracture. The pain tends to diminish spontaneously over several months but can be severe. Treatment consists or oral analgesia, TENS, thoracic epidural injection at the level of the fracture, nerve root injection and possibly dorsal root ganglion rhizotomy for root pain.

Postmastectomy and post-thoracotomy pain are common after surgery, although the frequency is often under-appreciated by surgeons. These are neuropathic pains and treatment is described above.

Abdominal pain

Abdominal wall pain is characterized by local tender points in the abdominal wall, particularly in the rectus abdominis muscle. Carnett's sign is elicited by asking the patient to tense the abdominal wall by lifting the legs off the couch or to attempt to sit from the supine position. Aggravation of pain confirms the muscle as the site of pain. Exclusion of other cause of abdominal pain is of course essential, the diagnosis being one of exclusion. Treatment is by repeated injection of tender points with local anaesthetic and steroid or cryo-analgesia. A common variation of this is pain after inguinal hernia repair, which usually responds to a series of injections around the ilio-inguinal and iliohypogastric nerves. Cryoanalgesia may also be useful here.

Pelvic pain can be caused by a variety of gynaecological, urological and gastroenterological diseases, but referral to pain clinics will be for pelvic pain of unknown aetiology, following extensive investigation, medical treatment and previous surgery. Initial treatment should be simple regular analgesia, tricyclic antidepressants at low dose, psychological therapies (*see below*). Some nerve blocks may be useful including sacral nerve blocks and presacral sympathectomy.[15]

Back pain and sciatica

Mechanical back pain is endemic in our society, and is perhaps best viewed as a design fault rather than a disease. Peak incidence is 45–55 years and the most common abnormality is degenerative osteoarthritis, although this is found universally in this age group. The pain is typically worse on movement and better with rest and may interfere with employment at a time when return to work may become difficult. There is a substantial disability due to back pain which has grown rapidly in recent years, partly related to changes in benefits and propensity for litigation. Initial assessment is based on history and examination. Routine radiographs of the spine provide relatively little useful information, and CT and MRI scans are probably best reserved for those being considered for spinal surgery. Back pain emanates from four possible sites in the spine.

1 Lumbar facet joints are thought to account for about 30% of back pain. These joints may be injured by violent rotation of the spine such as a sporting injury or trauma. The pain is often one-sided and aggravated by extension and rotation of the spine. Diagnostic facet joint injections with local anaesthetic can provide useful information.
2 Muscle pain is a common cause of back pain. Muscle groups may be painful to palpation and muscle spasm may be visible on examination. The most commonly affected muscles are quadratus lumborum and the gluteals.
3 Lumbar discs can be painful. Disc degeneration is commonly seen in radiographs and MRI scans of patients with back pain. Provocative discography involves injecting saline into individual discs in an attempt to reproduce pain, but the validity of this has been questioned.
4 Spinal nerve roots can produce leg pain when trapped by a prolapsed intervertebral disc. If the L5 or S1 nerve roots are affected the patient experiences posterior leg pain to the foot, known as sciatica. The ankle jerk may be diminished in S1 entrapment. L3 and L4 entrapment result in anterior thigh pain. A diminished knee jerk is indicative of an L4 lesion. Spinal stenosis occurs as part of the ageing process and combined with disc degeneration can produce critical narrowing of the spinal canal. In

the elderly this will present as unilateral leg pain with claudication. There is usually an absence of neurological signs in the leg.

Treatment options include the following:

1 Simple regular analgesia.
2 Physiotherapy including hydrotherapy and exercise regimes can be helpful. Increasingly physiotherapy departments are creating structured out-patient programmes based on exercise, fitness and education. They may have input from occupational therapy and psychology to create a multidisciplinary team.
3 Transcutaneous electrical nerve stimulation.
4 Facet joint treatment includes lumbar facet joint injections with local anaesthetic, and depot steroids (Depo-medrone, triamcinalone) are widely used but are unproven as long-term therapy.[16] Radio-frequency lumbar facet denervation involves thermocoagulation of the medial branch of the posterior ramus of L3–S1. Long-term outcomes appear to be reasonable.[17]
5 Muscle pain can be treated as per myofascial pain syndromes (*see above*). Hydrotherapy can also be useful. Rehabilitation of the spine with an indwelling epidural catheter can also enable refractory muscle pain to settle.[18]
6 Lumbar disc pain is more difficult to treat successfully. Local anaesthetic injection into the disc can be helpful in the short term. Radio-frequency lesion of the disc has been reported but experience is limited.[19] In theory, interruption of the sympathetic outflow at L2 should interfere with the pain pathways from the lumbar disc.[20] This can be achieved by dorsal root ganglion rhizotomy, but experience is limited. Spinal surgeons will consider spinal fusion of isolated disc degeneration, using either a bone graft or instrumented fusion. Long-term results are variable.
7 Nerve root compression by prolapsed intervertebral disc is best treated initially by lumbar epidural. This treatment is generally considered effective, although agreement is not universal.[21] Epidural injections are usually done with local anaesthetic and depot steroid (Depo-medrone, triamcinalone). The caudal approach is commonly performed by orthopaedic surgeons and rheumatologists, although the technical failure rate is probably high. Loss of resistance techniques enable closer access to the site of the lesions and perhaps allow lower volumes to be injected. Previous surgery will necessitate a transforaminal approach under fluoroscopy. Microdiscectomy is commonly performed for prolapsed intervertebral disc but usually after failure of epidural techniques. Surgical decompression of spinal stenosis is sometimes performed for intractable spinal claudication.

Coccydinia describes pain in the region of the coccyx, usually worse on sitting. It may follow a fall which results in a fracture of the coccyx, but there may also not be a history of trauma. Treatment options available include the following:

1 Regular simple oral analgesia.
2 Rubber cushions may help distribute weight from the coccyx.

3 Infiltration of the sacral nerve roots via the sacral hiatus with local anaesthetic and steroid. This may need to be done on several occasions, and is generally successful.

4 Sacral cryoanalgesia around the coccyx and sacral nerve routes can be a useful long-term therapy in refractory cases.

5 Occasionally coccygectomy is attempted, but success is not guaranteed.

Postspinal surgery pain (failed back syndrome) represents a great challenge for pain clinicians. The incidence of persistent pain following spinal surgery is probably in the region of 30–40%. The cause is unclear. There is not always a good link between observed spinal pathology and patient's symptoms. Advances in MRI scanning have led to an 'explosion of the false positive' as up to 70% of the normal population have lumbar disc bulges without symptoms. Patients present as having either persistent back pain or leg pain as the predominant complaint, although the two often coexist. Scarring has been demonstrated around nerve roots following spinal surgery. The nerve root can become tethered and any spinal movement can result in traction on the nerve. It is thought that complicated changes (known as 'wind-up') occur within the central nervous system as a consequence of nerve injury which results in chronic pain (*see under* 'Neuropathic pain'). There may be some residual compression of the nerve roots not adequately relieved by surgery. Facet joint disruption can occur and may lead to persistent back pain, with secondary arthritic change. Paraspinal muscle atrophy can occur if the posterior ramus has been injured as part of the disease process or as a consequence of surgery. This leads to loss of functional support of the spine and mechanical stresses on other structures.

Treatment options for failed back syndrome are as follows:

1 Simple regular analgesia.

2 If leg pain is predominant it is worth treating as neuropathic pain, especially if a neurological deficit is present (*see above*).

3 Nerve root blocks of the affected level can be achieved by directing a needle through the intervertebral foramen. Injection of local anaesthetic and steroid around the nerve root can provide useful symptomatic relief.

4 Lumbar facet denervation has been used successfully for persistent low back pain.[17]

5 Physical reactivation through graded exercise regime can be used alone or to follow on from injection therapy. This is best done within a multidisciplinary setting with input from physiotherapy, occupational therapy and clinical psychology. An epidural catheter may allow physical rehabilitation to occur when pain is limiting.[22]

6 Pain management programmes based on cognitive–behavioural therapy can be useful ways of patients learning to better manage their symptoms and disability (*see below*).

7 Implanted pain-relieving devices, such as spinal cord stimulation and implanted intrathecal pumps can be considered in patients whose pain and disability is not relieved by non-invasive techniques.

PSYCHOLOGICAL THERAPIES AND PAIN MANAGEMENT PROGRAMMES

Following diagnosis (where possible) and subsequent treatment involving drug therapy, injection therapy, physiotherapy and possibly surgery, some patients will be left with pain that cannot be cured. In these patients it is worth considering psychological therapies, either on an individual basis or part of a group programme. A number of conditions may be worth treating with psychological therapies from the start: examples include fibromyalgia and irritable bowel syndrome.

Psychological therapies include the following:

1 Operant conditioning works by removing secondary gain that may be obtained by maintaining pain behaviour. Gain can be positive such as getting attention or permission to rest or negative when pain allows avoidance of unpleasant situations. The technique works by eliminating reward for pain behaviour and reinforcing well behaviour.
2 Behavioural therapy involves manipulating the environment by taking analgesia on a time-determined basis, physical pacing, social feedback based on achievement not pain, education about the nature of pain and relaxation training.
3 Cognitive therapy involves changing negative thoughts to more positive ones, coping skills training by stress management, relaxation and imagery, and improving problem-solving skills.
4 Biofeedback is the use of increased awareness of physiological changes (heart rate, muscle tension) to enhance the learning of relaxation techniques. This may be particularly helpful for patients with increased muscle tension.
5 Hypnosis can be particularly helpful for pain. It involves relaxation, substitution of another sensory modality which is more acceptable (warmth), displacement of perceived site pain to a more peripheral body part and dissociation to a more pleasant location (e.g. a sunny day at the beach).

Pain management programmes have become increasingly well established in pain clinics. They are run by multidisciplinary teams involving clinical psychologists, physiotherapists and occupational therapists. General principles involves physical reactivation, based on physical pacing, rationalization of drug consumption, teaching goal setting, improving coping strategies, education, reducing illness behaviour. Programmes are either in-patient or outpatient and are run on a group basis over several weeks. They are not designed to treat pain directly but help patients to better manage their symptoms. Many patients come to terms with their chronic pain and decide to stop being patients by no longer seeking medical assistance.[23]

RECOMMENDED FURTHER READING

Wall P. D. and Melzack R. (eds) *Textbook of Pain*, 3rd edn. Churchill Living-stone, Edinburgh, 1994.

McQuay H. and Moore A. *An Evidence Based Resource for Pain Relief*. Oxford University Press, Oxford, 1998.

Dolin S., Padfield N. and Pateman J. *Pain Clinic Manual*. Butterworth Heine-mann, Oxford, 1996.

World Health Organization. *Cancer Pain Relief and Palliative Care: Report of a WHO Expert Committee*. WHO, Geneva, 1990.

REFERENCES

1 Davies H. et al. *Pain* 1997, **70,** 203–208
2 Flor H. et al. *Pain* 1992, **49,** 221–230
3 Dolin S. *Anaesthesia* 1998, **53,** 212–213.
4 Kingery W. *Pain* 1997, **73,** 123–139; McQuay H. and Moore A. *see* recom-mended reading; North R. et al. *Pain* 1991, **44,** 119–130.
5 North R. *Pain* 1991, **44,** 119–130
6 Bach S. *Pain* 1988, **33,** 297–301; Shug S. *Regional Anaesth.* 1995, **20,** 256.
7 Anderson G. *Pain* 1995, **61,** 187–193.
8 Wolfe F. *Rheum. Dis. Clin. North Am.* 1989, **15,** 1–29.
9 Travell J. and Simons D. *Myofascial Pain and Dysfunction: the Trigger Point Manual*. Williams & Wilkins, Baltimore, 1983.
10 Eisenberg E. *Anesth. Analg.* 1995, **80,** 290–295.
11 Nagaro T. *Pain* 1994, **58,** 325–330.
12 Sweet W. *J. Neurosurgery* 1981, **36,** 1129–1131.
13 Barnsley L. *Pain* 1994, **58,** 283–307; Wallis B. *Pain* 1997, **73,** 15–22; Lord S. *N. Engl. J. Med.* 1996, **335,** 1721–1726.
14 Castagnera L. *Pain* 1994, **58,** 239–243; Vervest A. *Pain Clin.* 1991, **4,** 103–112.
15 Wesselmann U. *Pain* 1997, **73,** 269–294.
16 Lippett A. *Spine* 1984, **7,** 746–750; Carette S. *N. Engl. J. Med.* 1991, **325,** 1002–1007.
17 North R. *Pain* 1994, **57,** 77–83; Gallagher *J. Pain Clin.* 1994, **7,** 193–198.
18 Dolin S. *Disab. Rehab.* 1998, **20,** 151–157
19 Van Cleef M. *Pain Clin.* 1996, **9,** 259–268.
20 Nakamura S. J. *Bone Joint Surg.* 1996, **78B,** 606–611.
21 Koes B. *Pain* 1995, **63,** 279–288.
22 Dolin S. *Disab. Rehab.* 1998, **20,** 151–157
23 Williams A. *Pain* 1996, **66,** 13–22.

Appendix

SI UNITS (LE SYSTÈME INTERNATIONAL D'UNITÉS)

Physical quantity	*SI unit*	*Symbol*
Length	metre	m
Mass	kilogram	kg
Volume	cubic metre	m^3
	The litre (l or L) is also acceptable.	
	It is 0.001 m^3 or 1 dm^3	
Time	second	s
Electric current	ampere	A
Thermodynamic temperature	kelvin	K
Luminous intensity	candela	cd
Amount of substance	mole	mol
Energy, work, quantity of heat	joule	J
Force	newton	N
Power	watt	W
Pressure	pascal	Pa
Electrical charge	coulomb	C
Electrical potential difference	volt	V
Electrical resistance	ohm	Ω
Electrical conductance	siemens	S
Electrical capacitance	farad	F
Inductance	henry	H
Magnetic flux	weber	Wb
Magnetic flux density	tesla	T
Luminous flux	lumen	lm
Illuminance	lux	lx
Frequency	hertz	Hz

Ampère, André Marie (1775–1836), French mathematician
Coulomb, Charles Augustin de (1736–1806), French physicist
Faraday, Michael (1791–1867), English experimental physicist
Henry, William (1797–1884), English chemist and mathematician
Hertz, Heinrich (1857–1894), Bavarian physicist
Joule, James Prescott (1818–1889), English physicist
Kelvin, William, First Lord Kelvin of Largs (1824–1907), Ulster-Scottish physicist
Newton, Sir Isaac (1642–1727), English mathematician
Ohm, Georg Simon (1787–1854), Bavarian physicist and mathematician
Pascal, Blaise (1623–1662), French philosopher and mathematician
Siemens, Sir William (1823–1883), German born, naturalized British, inventor and engineer
Tesla, Nikola (1856–1943), Croatian–American electrical engineer
Volta, Alessandro (1745–1827), Italian mathematician and physicist
Watt, James (1736–1819), Scottish mathematical instrument maker and inventor
Weber, Wilhelm Eduard (1804–1891), German physicist

Pressure is force per unit area. 1 pascal = 1 newton per m^2. Standard atmospheric pressure is 760 mmHg = 1.033 kg/cm^2 = 14.7 lb/in^2 = 101.325 kPa = 1.01325 bar. 1 torr = 1/760 of a standard atmosphere pressure = 1 mmHg. (Evangelista Torricelli, 1608–1647, Italian physicist and mathematician).

The metric system was adopted in France in January 1840.

Prefixes

Factor	Prefix	Symbol
10^{18}	exa	E
10^{15}	peta	P
10^{12}	tera	T
10^9	giga	G
10^6	mega	M
10^3	kilo	K
10^{-1}	deci	d
10^{-2}	centi	c
10^{-3}	milli	m
10^{-6}	micro	μ
10^{-9}	nano	n
10^{-10}	Angstrom	Å
10^{-12}	pico	p
10^{-15}	femto	f
10^{-18}	atto	a

Strengths of solutions

$$0.1\% = 1 \text{ mg/ml}$$
$$0.5\% = 5 \text{ mg/ml}$$
$$1\% = 10 \text{ mg/ml}$$
$$20\% = 200 \text{ mg/ml}$$

PHARMACOKINETICS

Zero-order kinetics: rate of elimination of a drug is independent of its concentration (e.g. alcohol).

First-order kinetics: elimination is exponential, i.e. the rate of change is proportional to the absolute value, so that concentration (C) decreases with time (t) thus:

$$-dC/dt = kC \quad \text{or} \quad C = C_o \cdot e^{-kt} \quad (C_o \text{ is initial concentration})$$

Elimination rate constant is k.
Time constant is the time taken for the concentration to decline to $1/e$ of its initial value, and equals $1/k$.
Half-life $(T_{1/2})$ is the time taken for the concentration to be halved, and equals $(\log_e 2)/k$ or $0.693/k$.
Volume of distribution (Vd) is the apparent volume of water into which a drug disperses after administration. Calculated from the initial dilution by extrapolating the concentration–time curve back to time zero.
Clearance is the volume of plasma from which a drug is completely removed in unit time. It equals: $k \times Vd$ or $(0.693 \times Vd)/T_{1/2}$. It is also the total dose administered divided by the area under the concentration–time curve. Drug half-life therefore depends on the two independent variables, clearance and volume of distribution.
Extraction ratio of a drug by a particular organ is the fraction cleared at each pass, or its arteriovenous concentration difference divided by the arterial concentration.
Organ clearance is organ blood flow $\times$ the extraction ratio.

PHARMACODYNAMICS

Drugs often act on specific receptors. The fraction of the receptors occupied (and therefore the response) is $[D]/(Kd + [D])$ where $[D]$ is drug concentration and Kd is the dissociation constant of the drug–receptor complex. The dose–response curve is thus hyperbolic, but the sigmoid log(dose)–response curve is often used as it displays a wide range of doses.

Agonists combine with receptors to initiate a response.
Competitive antagonists combine with, and block, receptors but produce no response.
Non-competitive antagonists have exceptionally strong receptor affinity.
Partial agonists can produce a response, but always less than that caused by a full agonist.
Intrinsic activity (of a partial agonist) is the ratio of its greatest response to that of a full agonist.
Efficacy is the maximum effect of an agonist.
Potency is the dose required to produce a given effect.
Hysteresis is when the effect of a given plasma concentration is less when it is rising than when it is falling (due to slow kinetics of the drug with the receptor).
Therapeutic index or ratio is the mean lethal dose divided by the mean effective dose, i.e. LD_{50}/ED_{50}, or kill/cure doses.
Tolerance is a decreasing response to a drug, despite a constant plasma level.
Down-regulation may be a cause of this – a decrease in receptor numbers.
Tachyphylaxis is another cause – exhaustion of a transmitter.

BEHAVIOUR OF GASES

Boyle's Law (1662; Robert Boyle, 1627–1691, English chemist). Volume (V) is inversely proportional to pressure (P) of a given mass of gas, at a constant temperature (T).

Charles' Law (1787; Jacques Alexandre Cesar Charles, 1746–1823, French physicist). Volume of a given mass of gas is proportional to its absolute temperature, if its pressure remains constant. (T = Centigrade temperature $+273°$).

Boyle's and Charles' laws can be expressed as $PV = nRT$ for ideal gases, where n is the number of moles of gas present and R is the molar gas constant.

Dalton's Law of Partial Pressures (1801; John Dalton, 1766–1844, Manchester chemist). The (partial) pressure of a component gas in a mixture of gases equals the pressure which that quantity of gas would produce were it alone. Thus, the total pressure of a mixture of gases equals the sum of the individual partial pressures.

Avogadro's Law (1811; Amadeo Avogadro, 1776–1856, Italian physicist). Equal volumes of gas at the same temperature and pressure contain the same numbers of molecules. One gram-molecular weight (mole) of gas occupies 22.4 litres STP (760 mmHg and 0°C), and contains 6.02×10^{23} molecules (the Avogadro constant). Thus, the volume of vapour produced by evaporation of 1 ml of a volatile agent (molecular weight MW and liquid density d) is $22400 \times d/MW$. For halothane this volume of vapour at 20°C is 227 ml, and for isoflurane 195 ml. Thus, 1 ml of liquid isoflurane will yield 19.5 litres of a 1% vapour.

Graham's Law of Diffusion (1831; Thomas Graham, 1805–1869, Scottish physician and chemist). The rate of diffusion of a gas varies inversely as the square root of its density or molecular weight.

Henry's Law (1803; William Henry, 1774–1836, English chemist).[1] At equilibrium between a gas and a liquid exposed to it, the partial pressure of the gas in the liquid equals its partial pressure in the gas phase. Henry's Law states that the amount of gas dissolved at any temperature is proportional to its partial pressure. The lower the temperature, the more can dissolve.

Solubility of Gas in Liquid (1894; Wilhelm Ostwald, 1853–1932, Russian–German physical chemist. Nobel prize-winner, 1909). The *Ostwald coefficient* (λ) is the amount of gas which dissolves in unit volume of solvent, measured under the conditions of temperature and pressure at which solution takes place. The *Bunsen coefficient* (α) is the amount of gas at STP which dissolves in unit volume of solvent at a partial pressure of 760 mmHg. The two coefficents are related:

$$\lambda = \alpha \times \text{absolute temperature of solvent}/273$$

and are identical at 0°C. The partition coefficient of a gas between two phases or solvents is the ratio of the amounts dissolved in equal volumes of each. If one phase is gas it is the same as the Ostwald coefficient.

Vapours: an 'ideal' gas in which the only interactions between molecules are collisions cannot be liquefied. This is not true for a real gas provided the temperature is low enough and the pressure high enough. Above its *critical temperature* a gas cannot be liquefied, however high the pressure. The *critical pressure* is that needed to liquefy a gas at its critical temperature. A *vapour* is a gas below its critical temperature. At room temperature both CO_2 and N_2O are vapours. A vapour in equilibrium with its liquid is said to be *saturated*, and its pressure is the *saturated vapour pressure* (SVP). The SVP increases non-linearly with temperature, and can be calculated from the Antoine equation.[2] The *boiling point* of a liquid is the temperature at which the saturated vapour pressure equals the ambient atmospheric pressure. *Relative humidity* is actual water vapour pressure as a percentage of the SVP at a given temperature.

FLUID FLOW

Laminar flow through tubes is described by Poiseuille's (1799–1868) law.[3] This states that flow rate (Q) is:

$$\Delta P \cdot \pi r^4 / 8 \eta l$$

where: ΔP is the pressure difference; r and l are the tube's radius and length; η is the viscosity of the fluid.

Turbulent flow occurs when flow exceeds a critical value. Turbulence is facilitated by irregularities and corners in the tube. Conversion from laminar to turbulent flow increases resistance, which itself becomes roughly proportional to flow. The dimensionless Reynolds number[4] (Re) must exceed 2000 for turbulence to occur. Re = diameter × density × average velocity/viscosity.

RESPIRATORY CALCULATIONS

Inspired partial pressure of oxygen: $PIO_2 = FIO_2 \times$ (barometric pressure – SVP of water at body temperature).
Respiratory quotient: CO_2 production/O_2 consumption.
Alveolar gas equation: alveolar PO_2 = inspired PO_2 – (alveolar or arterial PCO_2)/respiratory quotient.
Shunt equation: shunt flow/total pulmonary blood flow = (end-capillary CO_2 – arterial CO_2)/(end-capillary CO_2 – mixed venous CO_2).
Oxygen content of blood: O_2 saturation × [Hb] × 1.34/100.
Bohr equation for physiological dead space: ratio of physiological dead space to tidal volume = (arterial PCO_2 – mixed expired PCO_2)/(arterial PCO_2 – inspired PCO_2).
Compliance: volume change per unit change in pressure gradient.
Resistance: pressure difference/gas flow.

STATISTICS

Descriptive terms

Mean: sum of the observations divided by their number.
Median: the observation which, on a distribution curve, has half the number of observations lying above and below it.
Mode: the most frequent observation, the highest point on the curve.
Range: distance between the smallest and largest observation.
Normal (or Gaussian) distribution has a symmetrical, bell-shaped curve, and parametric tests may be used to draw conclusions.

Variance: measure of the scatter of observations around their mean. The sum of the squares of the differences between the individual observation and their mean, divided by their number.

Standard deviation: square root of the variance. For a normal distribution, 68% of data lies within 1 SD of the mean, 95% within 2 SD, and 99.7% within 3 SD.

Standard error of the mean: SD divided by the square root of n.

Coefficient of variation: SD as a percentage of the mean.

Inferential tests

Test the data to calculate (for example) a *probability*, *P*, of the differences between two groups being due to chance. $P < 0.05$ means that the probability of an event occurring by chance is less than 5% (1 in 20), and is a commonly chosen level of statistical significance.

Type I error: the null hypothesis is wrongly rejected (no difference really existed).

Type II error: when it is wrongly accepted (a real difference does exist).

Student's t test:[5] applied when the observations are 30 or less. A calculation of 't' is made, the observed difference between the sample means divided by the calculated standard error of the difference between the means. A table of t values is then used to read the P value. The distributions must be normal with similar variances.

Chi-squared test (χ^2): tests for an association between different characteristics by comparing occurrences of data. The data is not normally distributed, but belongs to several discrete categories, e.g. numbers of patients who vomit after different drugs. It should not be used for small numbers (5 or less). χ^2 is the sum of the squares of the difference between the observed number and the expected number, divided by the expected number.

Correlation and regression: regression analysis places a line of best fit through a group of points plotted with the independent variable on the x-axis (abscissa) and the dependent variable on the y-axis (ordinate). The regression or correlation coefficient (r) measures how scattered the data points are about this line. Values of 1 and −1 indicates a perfect fit to lines with a positive and negative slope respectively. Zero indicates no correlation.

Confidence intervals: 95% confidence limits of data are often preferred, rather than calculating P values, both for parametric and non-parametric tests.

SOME USEFUL ADDRESSES

The Royal College of Anaesthetists
48/49 Russell Square, London WC1B 4JY
Tel: 0171 813 1900

College of Anaesthetists of the Royal College of Surgeons in Ireland
123 St Stephen's Green, Dublin 2
Tel: +353 01 402 2234

The Association of Anaesthetists of Great Britain and Ireland
9 Bedford Square, London WC1B 3RA
Tel: 0171 631 1650

Royal Society of Medicine
1 Wimpole Street, London W1M 8AE
Tel: 0171 290 2900

Committee on Safety of Medicines
Market Towers, 1 Nine Elms Lane, London SW8 5NQ
Tel: 0171 720 2188

General Medical Council
44 Hallam Street, London W1N 6AE
Tel: 0171 580 7642

Medical Protection Society
33 Cavendish Square, London W1M 0PS
Tel: 0171 399 1300

Medical Defence Union
3 Devonshire Place, London W1N 2EA
Tel: 0171 486 6181

Medical and Dental Defence Union of Scotland
Mackintosh House, 120 Blyths Wood Street, Glasgow G2 4EH
Tel: 0141 221 5858

European Academy of Anaesthesiology
PO Box 33, 3001 Heverlee 1, Belgium
Tel: +32 16 405151

World Federation of Societies of Anesthesiologists
(Hon. Sec. Dr A. E. E. Meursing)
Department of Anaesthetics, SKZ/AZR, Sh 3.601,
Rotterdam 2015 GJ, The Netherlands
Tel: +31 10 464 6020

American Society of Anesthesiologists
520 N. Northwest Highway, Park Ridge, IL 60068–2573, USA

Australian and New Zealand College of Anaesthetists
'Ulimaroa', 630 St Kilda Road, Melbourne, Victoria 3004, Australia
Tel: +61 03 510 6299

Canadian Anaesthetists Society
1 Eglinton Avenue East, Suite 208, Toronto, Ontario M4P 4A1, Canada
Tel: +1 416 480 0602

The Faculty of Anaesthetists, The College of Medicine of South Africa
17 Milner Road, Rondebosch 7700, Republic of South Africa

International Anesthesia Research Society
2 Summit Park Drive, No. 140, Cleveland, OH 44131, USA
Tel: +1 216 642 1124

REFERENCES

1 Henry W. *Phil. Trans. R. Soc.* 1803, **93,** 29.
2 Rodgers R. C. and Hill G. E. *Br. J. Anaesth.* 1978, **50,** 415.
3 Poiseuille J. L. M. *C. R. Acad. Sci. Paris* 1840, **11,** 1041; Hagen A. *Ann. Phys. Leipzig* 1839, **46,** 423.
4 Reynolds O. *Phil. Trans.* 1883, **174,** 935.
5 Gosset W. S. *Biometrica* 1908, **6,** 1.

Index